Chinese Herbal Medicine: Formulas and Strategies

Chinese Herbal Medicine: Formulas and Strategies

Edited by Lydia Stephens

☐ SYRAWOOD
PUBLISHING HOUSE

New York

Published by Syrawood Publishing House,
750 Third Avenue, 9th Floor,
New York, NY 10017, USA
www.syrawoodpublishinghouse.com

Chinese Herbal Medicine: Formulas and Strategies
Edited by Lydia Stephens

International Standard Book Number: 978-1-64740-103-0 (Hardback)

Cataloging-in-Publication Data

Chinese herbal medicine : formulas and strategies / edited by Lydia Stephens.
    p. cm.
Includes bibliographical references and index.
ISBN 978-1-64740-103-0
1. Medicine, Chinese. 2. Herbs--Therapeutic use--China. 3. Medicinal plants--China.
4. Botany, Medical--China. 5. Materia medica, Vegetable--China. I. Stephens, Lydia.
RS131.64 .C45 2022
610.951--dc23

TABLE OF CONTENTS

PREFACE

Over the recent decade, advancements and applications have progressed exponentially. This has led to the increased interest in this field and projects are being conducted to enhance knowledge. The main objective of this book is to present some of the critical challenges and provide insights into possible solutions. This book will answer the varied questions that arise in the field and also provide an increased scope for furthering studies.

Chinese herbal medicine is a branch of traditional medicine that is based on the ancient Chinese medical practices. It primarily focuses on the utilization of the elements and extracts derived from plants. It also uses human, animal and mineral products that are sometimes poisonous. Various methods are used for the classification of Chinese herbal medicine. They include the four natures, the five flavors, the meridians and the specific function. The most common herbs used in Chinese herbal medicine are ginseng, ginkgo, mushrooms, wolfberry, astragalus, salvia, cinnamon, licorice, bupleurum and atractylodes. Chinese herbal medicines are usually prepared by decoction in which the herbal materials such as stems, roots, rhizomes and bark are boiled to dissolve their chemicals. This book discusses the fundamentals as well as modern approaches of Chinese herbal medicine. It will also provide interesting topics for research which interested readers can take up. It is appropriate for students seeking detailed information in this area as well as for experts.

I hope that this book, with its visionary approach, will be a valuable addition and will promote interest among readers. Each of the authors has provided their extraordinary competence in their specific fields by providing different perspectives as they come from diverse nations and regions. I thank them for their contributions.

Editor

An investigation of fungal contamination on the surface of medicinal herbs in China

Run-sheng Zheng[1,2†], Wen-li Wang[1,2†], Jing Tan[1,2], Hui Xu[1,2*]●, Ruo-ting Zhan[1,2] and Wei-wen Chen[1,2]

Abstract

Background: The dried parts of medicinal herbs are susceptible to the infection of fungi during pre- or post-harvest procedure. This study aimed to investigate the presence of fungi and their metabolites mycotoxins on the surface of medicinal herbs collected from China.

Methods: Forty-five retail samples of 15 different medicinal herbs were collected from 3 different regions in China. Then the potential fungi were immediately washed off from the surface of each sample with 0.1% Tween-20 followed by incubation of the rinse on petri-dish with potato dextrose agar containing chloramphenicol at 28 °C. The obtained fungi were isolated as single colonies and then characterized by morphology and molecular identification using internal transcribed spacer (ITS) sequencing with extracted DNA. Meanwhile, the mycotoxin-producing potential of the isolates was studied by liquid chromatography-tandem mass spectrometry (LC-MS/MS).

Results: A total of 126 fungi were identified from the surface of samples by morphology and ITS sequencing, with *Aspergillus* and *Penicillium* genera as the predominant contaminants. The mycotoxin-producing potential analysis showed that 6 of 8 *A. versicolor* isolates could produce sterigmatocystin. All 3 *A. aculeatus* isolates produced ochratoxin A, but only 1 of 3 *A. flavus* strains produced aflatoxins B_1 and B_2 without G_1 and G_2. Although the sample contamination ratios were high ($\geq$95.6%), there was no significant difference ($\chi^2 = 1.05$, $P = 1.0$) among the samples from 3 regions, which demonstrates the prevalent fungal contamination in the herbal medicines.

Conclusion: The prevalent contamination phenomenon of fungi and high potential risk of sterigmatocystin and ochratoxin A were observed in 45 medicinal herbs collected from China.

Background

With the popular and extensive use of medicinal herbs all over the world, safety issues related to the contamination with microbial organisms has become a major concern [1–4]. Most of fungi are toxigenic in nature, and some other non-toxigenic species may impart a mouldy odour and taste [5]. In the pre-harvest stage, medicinal herbs are susceptible to indigenous fungi in the soil where they were grown. The dried part of medicinal herbs may be exposed to fungal contamination during post-harvest.

Different taxonomic groups of fungi were detected in medicinal plant samples collected from different regions, suggesting *Aspergillus* and *Penicillium* groups as the most predominant genera [6–8]. Many species of *Aspergillus* and *Penicillium* genera are known mycotoxin-producers, which may pose a great threat to public health [5].

Mycotoxigenic fungi could produce a wide variety of mycotoxins. Aflatoxins (B_1, B_2, G_1, and G_2) are a family of structurally related toxic secondary metabolites which mainly produced by certain strains of *Aspergillus flavus* (*A. flavus*) and *Aspergillus Parasiticus* (*A. parasiticus*) [9, 10]. Aflatoxin B_1 (AFB_1) was classified as a Group I carcinogen by the World Health Organization for Research on Cancer in 1993 [11]. Sterigmatocystin (ST), the stable intermediate in the final steps of aflatoxin biosynthesis

*Correspondence: zyfxsherry@gzucm.edu.cn

†Run-sheng Zheng and Wen-li Wang contributed equally to this work

[1] Research Centre of Chinese Herbal Resource Science and Engineering, Guangzhou University of Chinese Medicine, Guangzhou, China

Full list of author information is available at the end of the article

in the aflatoxin-producing fungi *A. flavus* and *A. parasiticus*, was proven to be another carcinogenic mycotoxin [12]. Some certain stains, e.g., *A. versicolor*, *A. sydowi*, *A. nidulans*, *Bipolaris*, *Chaetomium* and *Emericella* spp. could also produce ST [13–16]. Produced by *P. verrucosum*, *P. nordicum* and *A. carbonarius* [17–19], another mycotoxin ochratoxin A (OTA) could cause a series of adverse effects in animals and humans, including teratogenicity, immunotoxicity, genotoxicity and mutagenicity [20–22].

This study aimed to investigate the presence of fungi on the surface of 45 medicinal herbs samples of fifteen herbs collected from Hunan, Hubei and Guangxi Province, China, by the characterization of morphology and ITS sequencing, followed by analysis of mycotoxigenic potential of isolated fungi using LC-MS/MS for the measurement of AFB_1, AFB_2, AFG_1, AFG_2, ST and OTA.

Methods
Chemicals and reagents
Standard solutions of AFB_1, AFB_2, AFG_1 and AFG_2, and OTA and ST powder standards were purchased from Supelco Sigma-Aldrich (St Louis, MO, USA). Potato dextrose agar (PDA) with chloramphenicol (0.1 g/L) was obtained from Huan-Kai (Guangzhou, China). LC-grade acetonitrile and methanol were bought from Merck (Darmstadt, Germany). Ultra-pure water was obtained from a Millipore Q system (Millipore, France). The other reagents were of analytical grade and bought from local producers.

Samples collection
Fifteen kinds of most commonly-used medicinal herbs (Table 1) were chosen for analysis. During July and August of 2010, about 30 g of each kind of medicinal herb were purchased from a random herbal medicine store in Hunan, Hubei and Guangxi province (China), respectively. The herbs were authenticated by an experienced pharmacist for traditional Chinese medicine according to Chinese Pharmacopeia [23]. Each sample was instantly put into a sterile polythene bag, sealed properly, shipped to the laboratory and stored at 4 °C prior to use. The detail information of each sample was given as Additional file 1: Table S1. The samples were processed as soon as possible to avoid second contamination.

Isolation of the fungi
Five grams of each sample (2.5 g was used for flower samples) was mixed with 30 mL 0.1% Tween-20 and vortexed (Vortex-5, Qilinbeier, China) for 3 min. Then the mixture was filtrated through a disposable syringe with sterile cotton and the filtrate was centrifuged (3-18 K, Satorius, Germany) at 2600×*g* for 10 min. After dissolving the pellet in 300 μL sterile 40% glycerol, serial decimal dilutions were performed. For incubation, 100 μL aliquots of each dilution were plated in duplicate onto PDA containing chloramphenicol (0.1 g/L), which were cultured at 28 °C for 7–10 days. Meanwhile, a sample without medicinal herbs was prepared in parallel and used as the negative control. The fungal colonies were then transferred to fresh PDA plates to obtain pure cultures, with 0.1% Tween-20 as negative control.

Morphological observation
The purified isolates were cultured with 1 or 3 point inoculations for 7 days on PDA at 28 °C. When the colony characteristics and pigment production were noted, the conidia and conidial head were observed microscopically (Smart, Optec, China) for morphological identification by lactophenol cotton blue stain. Taxonomic identification results were classified based on Manual of fungal Identification into Aspergillus, Penicillium and Fuscicladium *etc* [24–27].

Molecular identification by ITS primers
After the pure isolates were grown on PDA at 28 °C for 7 days, the mycelia were harvested. DNA extraction was performed using the Lysis Buffer for Microorganism to Direct PCR kit (Takara, Dalian, China) according to the manufacturer's instructions. Fungal mycelium was added to 50 μL lysis buffer and incubated at 80 °C for 15 min. After centrifugation, the supernatant was collected and used as the polymerase chain reaction (PCR) template. Positive control was performed with the standard strain *Aspergillus flavus* NRRL3357.

PCR amplification was performed in a 50 μL reaction prepared by mixing 25 μL 2× Power *Pfu* PCR Mixture (Bioteke, Beijing, China), 2.5 μL oligonucleotide primers (10 μmol/L) and 5 μL DNA template. Two pairs of primers (Table 2) were used to amplify ITS1, 5.8S and ITS2 in rDNA regions. The novel primers of Wen1-F and Wen1-R were designed according to the ITS sequences of *Penicillium expansu* (AJ005676.1) and *P. janthinellum* (GU565108.1). The amplification program was as follows: pre-denaturation at 95 °C for 5 min; 35 cycles of 30 s at 95 °C, 30 s at 55 °C and 1 min at 72 °C; and final extension at 72 °C for 10 min. The sequence analysis was performed at Huada Co. Ltd. (Guangzhou, China) and the sequencing results were analysed with the BLAST program of the National Centre for Biotechnology Information (NCBI) by searching NCBI nucleotide database (RRID:SCR_004860) for identification of the genus and species of the isolates.

Table 1 Number of different fungal species isolated from different medicinal herbs

Name of Samples	No. of samples	Fungal species[a]									
		A. flavus	A. versicolor	A. aculeatus	Other Aspergillus spp.	Euro-tium spp.	Penic-illium spp.	Clados-porium spp.	Fusa-rium spp.	Others	Total
Bulbus Fritillariae cirrhosae	3	–[b]	–	–	–	1	2	–	–	1	4
Cortex Eucommiae	3	–	–	–	–	–	2	–	–	1	3
Cortex Magnoliae officinalis	3	–	–	–	0	1	–	–	–	1	2
Flos Carthami	3	2	–	–	2	1	2	–	–	6	13
Flos Lonicerae japonicae	3	–	–	–	–	1	2	–	–	0	3
Fructus Lycii	3	1	1	–	1	–	–	–	–	4	7
Herba Andrographis	3	–	1	–	3	4	5	2	–	3	18
Radix Angelicae sinensis	3	–	–	1	1	1	3	–	1	–	7
Radix Astragali	3	–	–	–	3	–	2	3	–	4	12
Radix Codcnopsitis Pilosulas	3	–	–	1	–	–	5	–	1	1	8
Radix et Rhizoma Glycyrrhizae	3	–	2	1	2	–	2	1	1	6	15
Radix Notoginseng	3	–	1	–	1	–	2	–	–	2	6
Radix Panacis quinque-folii	3	–	–	–	–	–	3	2	–	6	11
Radix Pseudostellariae	3	–	1	–	–	–	3	1	–	–	5
Semen Armeniacae amarae	3	–	2	–	2	5	2	1	–	–	12
Total	45	3	8	3	14	14	35	10	3	36	126

[a] The strains were deposited in Research Centre of Chinese Herbal Resource Science and Engineering, Guangzhou University of Chinese Medicine, Guangzhou, China
[b] Not found

Table 2 Oligonucleotide primers used for molecular identification

Primer name	Primer sequence	Amplification product (bp)	Annotation	Gene targeted
Wen1-F	5′–TCCAACCTCCCACCCGTGTTTA–3′	400	This study	ITS1-5.8S-ITS2
Wen1-R	5′–AAGCCCCTACGCTCGAGGA–3′			
ITS1	5′–TCCGTAGGTGAACCTGCG–3′	500 ~ 700	[32]	
ITS4	5′–TCCTCCGCTTATTGATATGC–3′			

Mycotoxin-producing potential analysis

The assay was to aim to determine AFB_1, AFB_2, AFG_1, AFG_2, OTA and ST. Therefore, only the potential producer,according to literatures, were screened and the other 16 strains were excluded. Among the total isolates obtained from the samples, 110 strains potentially producing 6 mycotoxins were grown in Sabouraud dextrose medium (SD) at 28 °C for 10 days. Then 5 mL the culture broth was extracted with ethyl acetate followed by dichloromethane [28] and the organic layers were combined and then evaporated to dryness. After that, the residues were dissolved in 1.5 mL ethanol and injected into liquid chromatography-tandem mass spectrometry (LC–MS/MS) for determination of AFB_1, AFB_2, AFG_1, AFG_2, OTA and ST. Meanwhile, the standard strain *Aspergillus flavus* NRRL3357 were used as positive control.

Liquid chromatography separation of 10 μL sample was performed on a Hypersil GOLD C_{18} (100 × 2.1 mm, 3 μm) column. The mobile phase consisted of (A) water containing 4 m mol/L NH_4Ac–0.1% HCOOH and (B) methanol and the flow rate was 300 μL/min. A gradient elution program was applied: 0–10 min, 20–85% B; 10–15 min, 85–100% B; 15–20 min, 100% B. The mass spectrometer was operated in the ESI^+ mode using selective reaction monitoring (SRM). High-purity nitrogen was used as the drying and ionisation gas. Argon was used as the collision gas for collision-induced dissociation. The capillary voltage was set at 3.50 kV and the capillary temperature was 350 °C. The SRM transitions used to detect mycotoxins were listed in Table 3 and chromatograms of 6 mycotoxins in standard solution and representative samples were showed in the Fig. 1.

Statistical analysis

Software RStudio (R version 3.2.2) [29] was used for the data analysis, where the comparison of fungal contamination ratios was performed by Pearson's Chi squared test with simulated P value (based on 2000 replicates).

Results and discussion
Fungal contamination

The association between fungal species and herbal medicines is not fully understood due to the complicated contamination causes including extrinsic (environmental and geographical) and intrinsic (constituents of each herbal species) factors [30, 31]. Forty-five samples of 15 common medicinal herbs were investigated in this study to reveal the main contaminating fungi and provide some relevant references for quality control on medicinal herbs in China.

In this study, morphological analysis as well as molecular identification using ITS sequencing were applied to analyse fungal diversity. As not all the strains could be amplified by the primer pair ITS1/ITS4 [32], a novel primer pairs Wen1F/Wen1R were designed for the ITS regions of the fungi by Primer-BLAST of NCBI (Table 2). A total of 126 isolated strains were successfully amplified. It is notable that the primers of Wen1F/Wen1R tended to be biased towards the amplification of *Aspergillus* and *Penicillium*, which agreed with the view on the potential primers bias during PCR in fungal diversity exploring [33].

As a result, 126 strains were isolated (Table 1) illustrating the two main genera identified were *Aspergillus* (28 isolates) and *Penicillium* (35 isolates). Among

Table 3 The ESI-MS/MS parameters, retention time, SRM transitions and LOD for 6 mycotoxins

Mycotoxin	RT (min)	Precursor ion (m/z)	Product ions (m/z)	Collision energy (eV)	LOD (ng/L)
Aflatoxin B_1	10.20	313 $[M + H]^+$	285/241	23/37	5.20
Aflatoxin B_2	9.82	315 $[M + H]^+$	287/259	27/31	6.30
Aflatoxin G_1	9.41	329 $[M + H]^+$	243/200	27/45	10.60
Aflatoxin G_2	8.96	331 $[M + H]^+$	313/245	26/30	5.80
Ochratoxin A	13.22	404 $[M + H]^+$	239/358	25/15	25.00
Sterigmatocystin	13.44	325 $[M + H]^+$	281/310	36/25	1.56

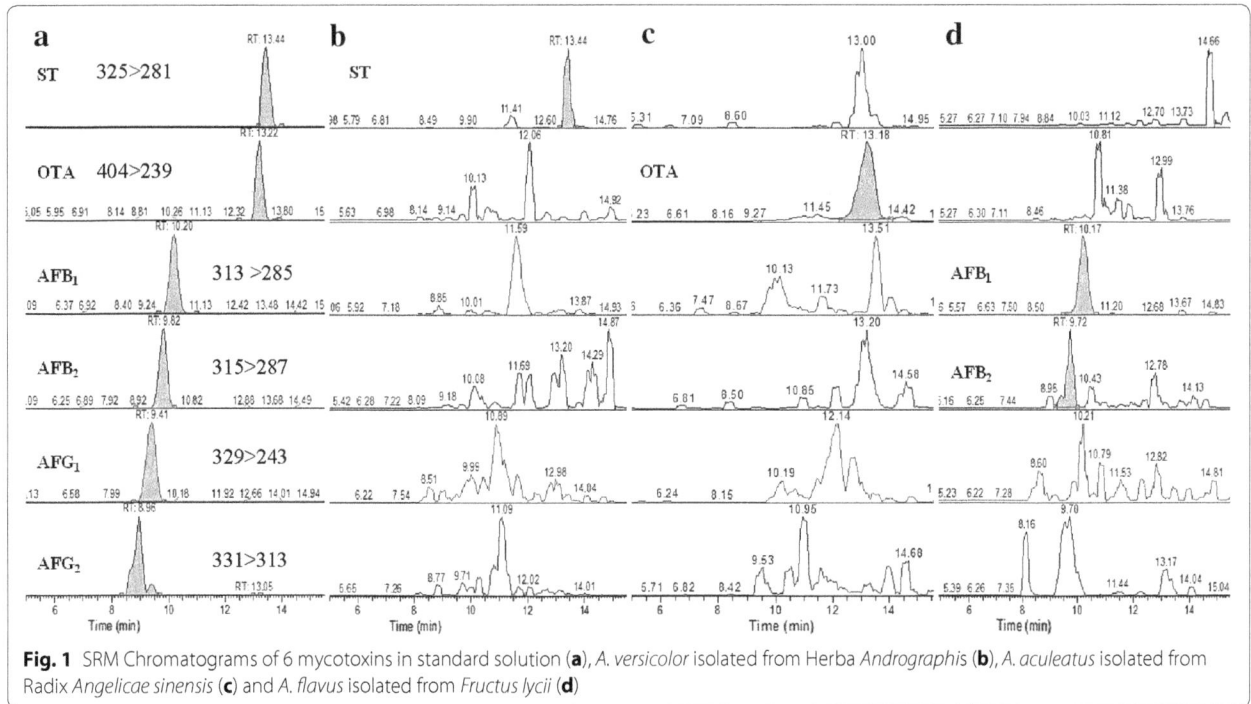

Fig. 1 SRM Chromatograms of 6 mycotoxins in standard solution (**a**), *A. versicolor* isolated from Herba *Andrographis* (**b**), *A. aculeatus* isolated from Radix *Angelicae sinensis* (**c**) and *A. flavus* isolated from *Fructus lycii* (**d**)

of 28 *Aspergillus* recovered, *A. versicolor* (8 strains) was the dominant species, followed by the *A. fumigatus* (4 strains), *A. aculeatus* (3 strains) and *A. flavus* (3 strains). Other members of the *Aspergillus* group were detected at lower level. The colonies and microscopic morphologies of *A. flavus*, *A. aculeatus* and *A. versicolor* isolated from Fructus *Lycii*, Radix *Angelicae Sinensis* and Radix *et* Rhizoma *Glycyrrhizae*, respectively, were shown in Fig. 2.

Although the average of fungal contamination ratio (95.6%) are extremely high in 45 samples collected from 3 places (93.3, 93.3, 100% for samples from Hubei, Hunan and Guangxi, respectively), Pearson's Chi squared test indicated there is no significant difference among 3 groups by $P = 1.0$. This further proved the prevalent fungal contamination phenomenon across the collected herbal medicine and should rise our attention.

Overall, the observation of *Aspergillus* and *Penicillium* spp. as the most frequently contaminant was consistent with previous reports. Efuntoye [30] found that *A. niger*, *A. flavus*, *F. moniliforme*, *Trichoderma viride*, *P. expansum* and *Mucor fragilis* were the dominant species in sundried herbs. Roy et al. [34] reported that 52% of 152 samples were contaminated with species from the *Aspergillus* genus, while Halt [35] found that the most predominant fungi detected in 62 samples of medicinal plant material and 11 herbal tea samples were *Aspergillus* and *Penicillium*.

In comparison, fungi from other genera including *Eurotium*, *Cladosporium* was detected at a low incidence in this study, which was also consistent with the study from Song et al. [3]. *Cladosporium* spp. is the common and widespread fungi on land and in air [36, 37]. Although there are no publications regarding its ability of producing toxin, they do produce odours likely relating to some volatile organic compounds.

Mycotoxigenic potentials of the fungal isolates

As documented in Table 3, the LC-MS/MS method showed an outstanding sensitive, with the limit of detection (LOD) from 1.56 to 25.00 ng/L determined in 3 times of the ratio of signal to noise (S/N). The data on the mycotoxin-producing potentials of the fungal isolates were presented in Table 4. Of the 3 *A. flavus* isolates, only 1 strain from Fructus *Lycii* produced AFB_1 and AFB_2 but not AFG_1 and AFG_2. The inability of the other 2 strains to produce aflatoxins might be a result of some mutation in the biosynthetic gene cluster of aflatoxins [38].

Another mycotoxin ST, which was overlooked in many reports except a study of mycotoxins screening in medicinal herbs [39], presented in 6 of the 8 *A. versicolor* isolates by the analysis of LC-MS/MS. To evaluate human exposure to this mycotoxin and more importantly, monitor medicinal herbs for existing or future legal compliance, suitable and simple analytical procedures are necessary

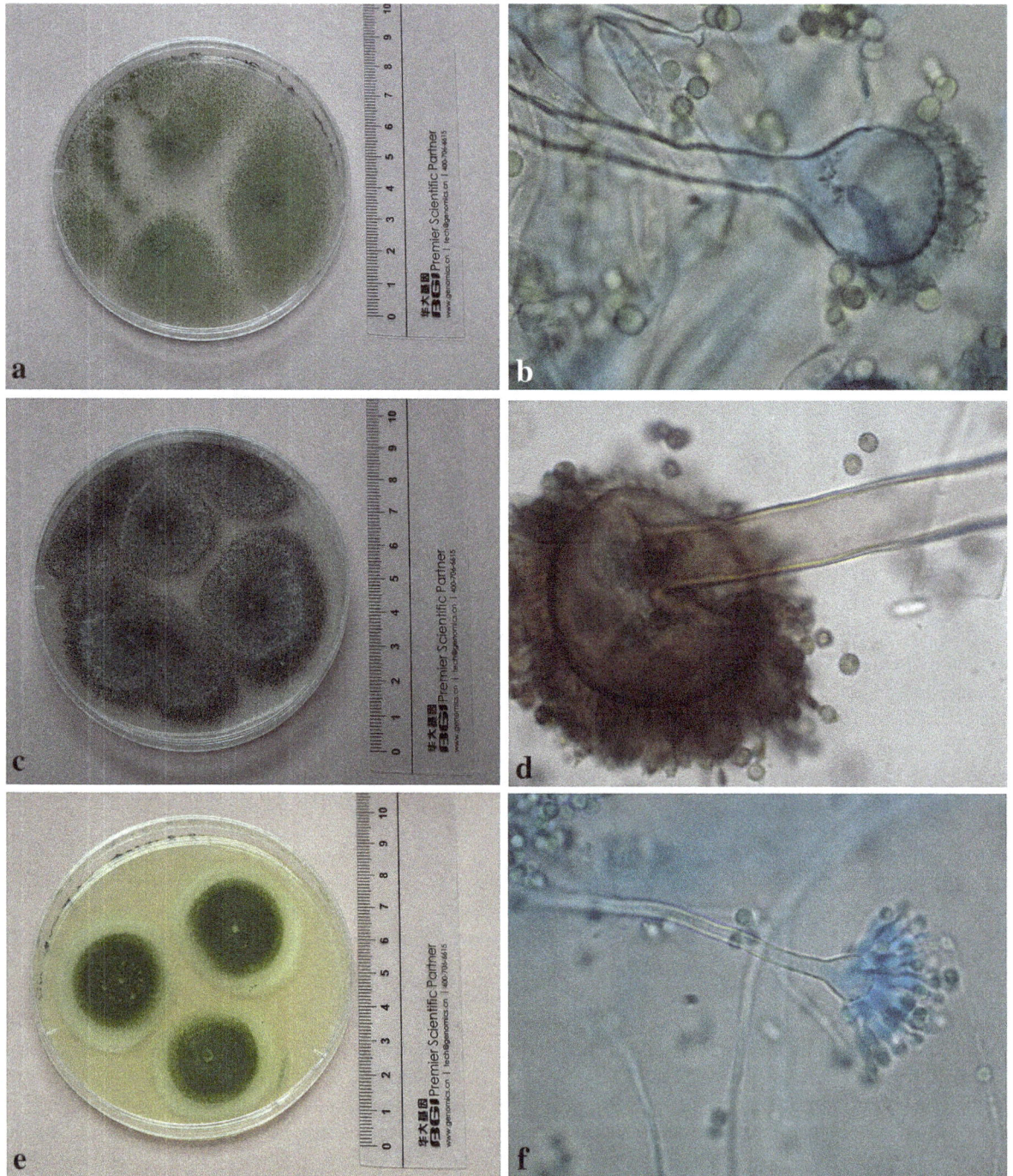

Fig. 2 Colony morphologies and microscopic characteristic of some fungal isolates. **a**, **b** *A. flavus*; **c**, **d** *A. aculeatus*; **e**, **f** *A. versicolor*. **a**, **c** and **e** Colonies after incubation for 7 days at 25 °C on PDA. **b**, **d** and **f** conidial heads and conidiophores. Magnification 10 × 100

to precisely analyse it and its contamination phenomenon in these samples even all the medicinal herbs.

Consistent to Blank et al. [40], all the *A. aculeatus* strains isolated in this study produced OTA. Although it has been reported that a number of *Penicillium* strains are OTA producers [17, 19, 41], none of 35 *Penicillium*

strains in this study produced OTA, which has to be further confirmed. Moreover, the contaminant *A. fumigatus* still should not be neglected, even though neither the *A. fumigatus*, *Cladosporium* spp. strains nor the *Penicillium* spp. produced detectable mycotoxins. Because *A. fumigatus* is thermos-tolerant and has the ability to excrete

Table 4 Toxigenic potentials of the isolates from 45 samples of medicinal herbs

Fungi	Source	No. of strains isolated	No. of positive strains	Toxin production[a]
A. flavus	Flos Carthami	2	0	_[b]
A. flavus	Fructus Lycii	1	1	AFB_1, AFB_2
A. versicolor	Radix et Rhizoma Glycyrrhizae	2	2	ST
A. versicolor	Semen Armeniacae amarae	2	1	ST
A. versicolor	Herba Andrographis	1	1	ST
A. versicolor	Radix Pseudostellariae	1	1	ST
A. versicolor	Fructus Lycii	1	1	ST
A. versicolor	Radix Notoginseng	1	0	–
A. aculeatus	Radix et Rhizoma Glycyrrhizae	1	1	OTA
A. aculeatus	Radix Codcnopsitis pilosulas	1	1	OTA
A. aculeatus	Radix Angelicae sinensis	1	1	OTA

[a] Mycotoxins determined including AFB_1, AFB_2, AFG_1, AFG_2, OTA and ST

[b] Below the detection limits

hydrolytic extracellular enzymes that consequently allow opportunistic colonisation in lung tissue [42].

Conclusion

The prevalent contamination phenomenon of fungi observed in 45 medicinal herbs collected from China and the mycotoxigenic potential of some fungal isolates suggested appropriate procedures should be engaged to protect medicinal herbs from being contaminated.

Abbreviations

AFB$_1$: aflatoxin B$_1$; AFB$_2$: aflatoxin B$_2$; AFG$_1$: aflatoxin G$_1$; AFG$_2$: aflatoxin G$_2$; ITS: internal transcribed spacer; LC-MS/MS: liquid chromatography-tandem mass spectrometry; LOD: limit of detection; NCBI: National Centre for Biotechnology Information; OTA: ochratoxin A; PCR: polymerase chain reaction; PDA: potato dextrose agar; SD: sabouraud dextrose medium; SRM: selective reaction monitoring; ST: sterigmatocystin.

Authors' contributions

HX conceived and designed the study and performed the data analysis. RSZ, WLW and JT performed the experiments, analyzed data and wrote the manuscript. RTZ and WWC collected, authenticated medicinal herb samples and revised the manuscript. All authors have read and approved the final manuscript.

Author details

[1] Research Centre of Chinese Herbal Resource Science and Engineering, Guangzhou University of Chinese Medicine, Guangzhou, China. [2] Key Laboratory of Chinese Medicinal Resource from Lingnan, Ministry of Education, Guangzhou University of Chinese Medicine, Guangzhou, China.

Acknowledgements

This work was financially supported by the Project Based Personnel Exchange Program between the China Scholarship Council and the German Academic Exchange Service, and the Science and Technology Project of Guangdong Province (Grant No. 2015A030401083). The authors thank Mr. Li Dingmiao and Mr. Chen Jiamin for their technical assistance and Miss Chen Huizhi for her comments on the manuscript.

Competing interests

The authors declare that they have no competing interests.

References

1. Limyati DA, Juniar BL. Jamu Gendong, a kind of traditional medicine in Indonesia: the microbial contamination of its raw material and endproduct. J Ethnopharmacol. 1998;63:201–8.
2. Rizzo I, Vedoya G, Maurutto S, Haidukowski M, Varsavsky E. Assessment of toxigenic fungi on Argentinean medicinal herbs. Microbiol Res. 2004;159:113–20.
3. Song MF, Chen J, Li XL, Tang DY, Sun BD, Gao WW. Primary investigation of contaminating fungi on Panax notoginseng and Amomum tsaoko in Yunnan. Zhong Guo Zhong Yao Za Zhi. 2012;37:1734–6.
4. Song MF, Chen J, Li XL, Tang DY, Sun BD, Gao WW. Primary investigation of contaminating fungi on Gynostemma pentaphyllum in Yunnan. Shi Zhen Guo Yi Guo Yao. 2012;23:2016–7.
5. Sekar P, Yamnam N, Ponmurugan K. Screening and characterization of mycotoxin producing fungi from dried fruits and grains. Adv Biotech. 2008;7:12–5.
6. Aziz NH, Youssef YA, El-Fouly MZ, Moussa LA. Contamination of some common medicinal plant samples and spices by fungi and their mycotoxins. Bot Bull Acad Sinica. 1998;39:279–85.
7. Bugno A, Almodovar AAB, Pereira TC, Pinto TJA, Sabino M. Occurrence of toxigenic fungi in herbal drugs. Braz J Microbiol. 2006;37:47–51.
8. Moorthy K, Prasanna I, Thajuddin N, Arjunan S, Gnanendra TS, Zahir Hussain MI. Occurrence of mycopopulation in spices and herbal drugs. Int J Biol Technol. 2010;1:6–14.
9. Kim DM, Chung SH, Chun HS. Multiplex PCR assay for the detection of aflatoxigenic and non-aflatoxigenic fungi in meju, a Korean fermented soybean food starter. Food Microbiol. 2011;28:1402–8.
10. Mateo EM, Gil-Serna J, Patino B, Jiménez M. Aflatoxins and ochratoxin A in stored barley grain in Spain and impact of PCR-based strategies to assess the occurrence of aflatoxigenic and ochratoxigenic Aspergillus spp. Int J Food Microbiol. 2011;149:118–26.
11. International Agency for Research on Cancer (IARC). IARC monographs on the evaluation of carcinogenic risks to humans. Some naturally occurring substances: food items and constituents, heterocyclic aromatic amines and mycotoxins. Iyon: IARC Press; 1993. p. 362.

12. Yu J, Chang PK, Cary JW, Wright M, Bhatnagar D, Cleveland TE, Payne GA, Linz JE. Comparative mapping of aflatoxin pathway gene clusters in *Aspergillus parasiticus* and *Aspergillus flavus*. Appl Environ Microbiol. 1995;61:2365–71.

13. Lepom P, Kloss H. Production of sterigmatocystin by *Aspergillus versicolor* isolated from roughage. Mycopathologia. 1988;101:25–9.

14. Rabie CJ, Lübben A, Marais GJ, van Vuuren HJ. Enumeration of fungi in barley. Int J Food Microbiol. 1997;35:117–27.

15. Atalla MM, Hassanein NM, El-Beih AA, Youssef YA. Mycotoxin production in wheat grains by different Aspergilli in relation to different relative humidities and storage periods. Nahrung. 2003;47:6–10.

16. Versilovskis A, De Saeger S. Sterigmatocystin: occurrence in food-stuffs and analytical methods—an overview. Mol Nutr Food Res. 2010;54:136–47.

17. Pitt JI. Penicillium viridicatum, Penicillium verrucosum, and production of ochratoxin A. Appl Environ Microbiol. 1987;53:266–9.

18. Horie Y. Productivity of ochratoxin A of Aspergillus carbonarius in Aspergillus section Nigri. Nippon Kingakukai Kaiho. 1995;36:73–6.

19. Lund F, Frisvad JC. *Penicillium verrucosum* in wheat and barley indicates presence of ochratoxin A. J Appl Microbial. 2003;95:1117–23.

20. Kuiper-Goodman T, Scott PM. Risk assessment of the mycotoxin ochratoxin A. Biomed Environ Sci. 1989;2:179–248.

21. O'Brien E, Dietrich DR. Ochratoxin A: the continuing enigma. Crit Rev Toxicol. 2005;35:33–60.

22. Pfohl-Leszkowicz A, Manderville RA. Ochratoxin A: an overview on toxicity and carcinogenicity in animals and humans. Mol Nutr Food Res. 2007;51:61–99.

23. Chinese Pharmacopeia Commission. The 2015 Edition of Pharmacopoeia of the People's Republic of China, vol. 1. Beijing: China Medical Science and Technology Press; 2015.

24. Wei J. Manual of fungal identification. Shanghai: Shanghai Scientific & Technical Publisher; 1979.

25. Qi Z. Fungi of China: Aspergillus and Related Teleomorphs, vol. 5. Beijing: Science Publisher; 1997.

26. Kong H. Fungi of China (Vol. 35): Penicillium and Related Teleomorphs. Beijing: Science Publisher; 2007.

27. Zhang Z. Fungi of China (Vol. 14): Gladxporism, Fusicladium, Pyricularia. Beijing: Science Publisher; 2003.

28. Delmulle B, De Saeger S, Adams A, De Kimpe N, Van Peteghem C. Development of a liquid chromatography/tandem mass spectrometry method for the simultaneous determination of 16 mycotoxins on cellulose filters and in fungal cultures. Rapid Commun Mass Spectrom. 2006;20:771–6.

29. R Core Team. R: a language and environment for statistical computing. Vienna: R Foundation for Statistical Computing; 2015.

30. Efuntoye MO. Fungi associated with herbal drug plants during storage. Mycopathologia. 1996;136:115–8.

31. Mandeel QA. Fungal contamination of some imported spices. Mycopathologia. 2005;159:291–8.

32. Sampietro DA, Marín P, Iglesias J, Presello DA, Vattuone MA, Catalan CAN, Gonzalez Jaen MT. A molecular based strategy for rapid diagnosis of toxigenic Fusarium species associated to cereal grains from Argentina. Fungal Biol. 2010;114:74–81.

33. Bellemain E, Carlsen T, Brochmann C, Coissac E, Taberlet P, Kauserud H. ITS as an environmental DNA barcode for fungi: an in silico approach reveals potential PCR biases. BMC Microbiol. 2010;10:189.

34. Roy AK, Sinha KK, Chourasia HK. Aflatoxin contamination of some common drug plants. Appl Environ Microbiol. 1988;54:842–3.

35. Halt M. Moulds and mycotoxins in herb tea and medicinal plants. Eur J Epidemio. 1998;14:269–74.

36. Crous PW, Braun U, Schubert K, Groenewald JZ. Delimiting Cladosporium from morphologically similar genera. Stud Mycol. 2007;58:33–56.

37. Chiba S, Okada S, Suzuki Y, Watanuki Z, Mitsuishi Y, Igusa R, Sekii T, Uchiyama B. Cladosporium species related Hypersensitivity Pneumonitis in household environments. Intern Med. 2009;48:363–7.

38. Wilkinson JR, Kale SP, Bhatnagar D, Yu J, Ehrlich KC. Expression profiling of non-aflatoxigenic *Aspergillus parasiticus* mutants obtained by 5-azacytosine treatment or serial mycelial transfer. Toxins. 2011;3:932–48.

39. Zheng RS, Wang WL, Xu H, Zhan RT, Chen WW. Simultaneous determination of aflatoxin B_1, B_2, G_1, G_2, ochratoxin A and sterigmatocystin in traditional Chinese medicines by LC-MS-MS. Anal Bioanal Chem. 2014;406:3031–9.

40. Blank G, Nwoko U, Frohlich A, Marquardt R. Ochratoxin A production in relation to the growth morphology of Aspergillus alutaceus. Food Sci Technol. 1998;31:210–4.

41. Geisen R, Mayer Z, Karolewiez A, Färber P. Development of a real time PCR system for detection of *Penicillium nordicum* and for monitoring ochratoxin A production in foods by targeting the ochratoxin polyketide synthase gene. Syst Appl Microbiol. 2004;27:501–7.

42. St Leger RJ, Screen SE. In vitro utilization of mucin, lung polymers, plant cell walls and insect cuticle by *Aspergillus fumigatus*, *Metarhizium anisopliae* and *Haematonectria haematococca*. Mycol Res. 2000;104:463–71.

2

Effects of pretreatment with methanol extract of Peucedani Radix on transient ischemic brain injury in mice

So-Youn Jung[1†], Kyoung-Min Kim[1†], Suin Cho[2†], Sehyun Lim[3], Chiyeon Lim[4] and Young Kyun Kim[1*]

Abstract

Background: Stroke is the second most common cause of death and may result in various disabilities; thus, identification of neuroprotective therapeutic agents is important. Peucedani Radix (PR), the root of *Angelica decursiva*, is a well-known remedy for damp and phlegm in Korean medicine and has also been shown to exert antioxidant and anti-inflammatory activities. This study was performed to investigate the mechanism underlying the anti-inflammatory effect of methanol extract of PR (PRex) on cerebral ischemic injury.

Methods: C57BL/6 male mice were orally administered PRex (20, 60, or 200 mg/kg) at 2 days, 1 day, and 1 h prior to middle cerebral artery occlusion (MCAO). Twenty-four hours after MCAO, the infarct volume was measured and the neurological deficit score was assessed. The inflammatory-related substances in the ipsilateral hemisphere were determined by western blotting, DCFH-DA assay, TBARS assay, and ELISA.

Results: PRex pretreatment significantly decreased the infarct volume at 24 h after MCAO. Moreover, PRex effectively suppressed the expression of iNOS, ROS, MDA, and pro-inflammatory cytokines, such as IL-1β and TNF-α, in brain tissue of mice with MCAO-induced brain injury.

Conclusions: PRex protected neurons from ischemic brain injury in mice through its antioxidant and anti-inflammatory activities. Our results suggested that PR could be a promising candidate in the therapy of ischemia-induced brain damage.

Keywords: Peucedani Radix, *Angelica decursiva*, Stroke, Anti-inflammation

Background

The clinical signs of stroke, which arise from a focal disorder of cerebral function that results from the occlusion of blood vessels or hemorrhage, include diverse speech and motor disorders or death [1, 2]. As the quality of life for patients and their families may be irreversibly diminished, the prevention and treatment of stroke are very important, and results from stroke are highly correlated with the extent of brain tissue damage from oxidative damage and neuroinflammation [3, 4]; thus, research

into anti-inflammatory and neuroprotective therapeutic interventions is warranted.

To investigate the efficacy of therapeutic agents against ischemia-induced brain damage, which accounts for approximately 80% of the types of stroke [5], an animal model with similar pathological changes as those in the human body is necessary. The rodent model of middle cerebral artery occlusion (MCAO), which is reproducible and minimally invasive, is commonly used in stroke research [6, 7]. The intraluminal filament method devised by Koizumi et al. [8], and later modified by Longa et al. [9], has been widely used because it allows reperfusion post occlusion [10]. Gupta et al. studied the neuroprotective effect of a combination of *Zizyphus jujuba* and silymarin [11], Gim et al. researched the antioxidant activities of curcumin treatment in rats with

*Correspondence: lab3402201@gmail.com
†So-Youn Jung, Kyoung-Min Kim, and Suin Cho contributed equally to this work
1 College of Korean Medicine, Dong-Eui University, Yangjeong-ro, Busanjin-gu, Busan 47227, Republic of Korea
Full list of author information is available at the end of the article

MCAO-induced cerebral ischemia [12], and Na et al. reported the antioxidant and anti-inflammatory activities of 6-shogaol pretreatment in MCAO-injured mice [13].

Peucedani Radix (PR), the root of *Angelica decursiva* Franchet et Savatier, has been used traditionally as a remedy in Korean medicine for thick phlegm, cough, asthma, and upper respiratory tract infections [14]. Many studies of the pharmacological activities of PR have been recently undertaken. Lim et al. found that the methanol extract of PR had significant inhibitory activity against lung inflammation [15] and Zhao et al. reported that the constituents of PR, predominantly umbelliferone 6-carboxylic acid, could be used for the treatment of oxidative stress-related inflammatory diseases [16]. Coumarins from *A. decursiva* were demonstrated to be effective in the treatment of type 2 diabetes and inflammation-associated disorders [17, 18]. These studies demonstrated the antioxidant and anti-inflammatory activities of PR, which may offer a potential treatment for cerebral damage as oxidative stress and inflammation are responsible for ischemic injury and can eventually result in neuronal death [19]. Although the various cytoprotective actions of PR have been extensively investigated, its effects against ischemia-induced brain damage have not been determined. Hence, to determine whether PR inhibits ischemic brain damage, we observed infarct volumes, neurological deficits, and inflammatory mediators in mice with MCAO-induced brain injury after PRex pretreatment.

Methods
PR treatment
PR was purchased from Naemomedah (Kwangmyoung-dang Medicinal Herbs, Ulsan, Korea) and authenticated by Dr. Cho (Pusan National University School of Korean Medicine, Yangsan, Korea). Due to difficulties of maintaining consistent qualities of herbal extracts, fingerprinting data of the PRex were obtained for future study using high performance thin layer chromatography (HPTLC) method (Additional file 1: Figure S1). A voucher specimen (No. PD16-0322) was deposited in the low temperature room of the laboratory. For solvent extraction, PR (200 g) was immersed in methanol (1000 mL), left at room temperature for 5 days, and the supernatant fluid was collected. This process was repeated for the PR residue. The first and second supernatant fluid were filtered with filter paper and concentrated to dryness; finally, a total of 64 g PR extract (PRex) was obtained (32% yield). PRex was dissolved in dimethyl sulfoxide (DMSO), diluted with 0.9% normal saline, filtered through a 0.45-µm pore sized syringe filter, and adjusted to the concentrations of 20, 60, and 200 mg/kg.

Animal model
The experimental protocol involving animals was approved by the ethics committee of PNU (Pusan National University; Approval Number PNU-2016-1087). The Minimum Standards of Reporting Checklist (Additional file 2) contain details of the experimental design, and statistics, and resources used in this study. Male SPF C57BL/6 mice (Daehan Biolink, Chungbuk, Korea) (22–25 g) were housed in a temperature- and humidity-controlled environment under a 12-h light/dark cycle and given food and water ad libitum for at least 7 days prior to the experiment. Three mice were housed in each cage. The mice were randomly divided into five groups with a minimum of eight mice in each group: the sham control group, in which the animals underwent surgery, but were not subjected to MCAO; the MCAO control group, in which the animals did not receive PRex pretreatment, but were subjected to MCAO; and the 20, 60, and 200 mg/kg PRex pretreated MCAO groups, in which the animals received PRex treatment at 20, 60, or 200 mg/kg, respectively, and were subjected to MCAO. The animals were orally administered 20, 60, or 200 mg/kg of body weight at 2 days, 1 day, and 2 h prior to the MCAO procedure (Fig. 1); in the other groups, mice received an equivalent amount of normal saline instead of PRex. Mice in the MCAO control group and the PRex groups were subjected to MCAO. Isofluorane gas (2%) was added to a mixture of 70% N_2O and 30% O_2 to produce the inhalation anesthetic. During the operation, rectal temperature was maintained at 36.5 ± 0.5 °C via a heating pad and relative cerebral blood flow (rCBF) was monitored using a Laser-Doppler blood flow system (moorVMS-LDF, Moor Instruments, Devon, UK). The general procedure of Koizumi et al. [8] was employed, with some modifications. The hair on the chest and neck of the animal was cleanly removed using a clipper and the skin was cut. After the branches of the left common carotid artery (LCCA) were confirmed, the left external carotid artery (LECA), left internal carotid artery (LICA), and surrounding connective tissues were carefully arranged under a stereo microscope (Nikon 745, Tokyo, Japan) to secure a clear view.

The LECA and the LCCA were bound with 4/0 silk sutures (Ethicon Inc., NJ, USA) to temporarily obstruct the flow of the LICA. A filament (11-mm length of 8/0 nylon suture with a silicon-coated tip, Ethicon, Scotland) was inserted slowly through the LICA to the origin of the LMCA to occlude the LMCA. The inserted filament was fixed with blood vessels and left for 2 h to ensure an ischemic period. Subsequently, the filament was removed to allow reperfusion. During the 2-h period, rCBF was reduced to < 20%, but sharply increased to > 90% of

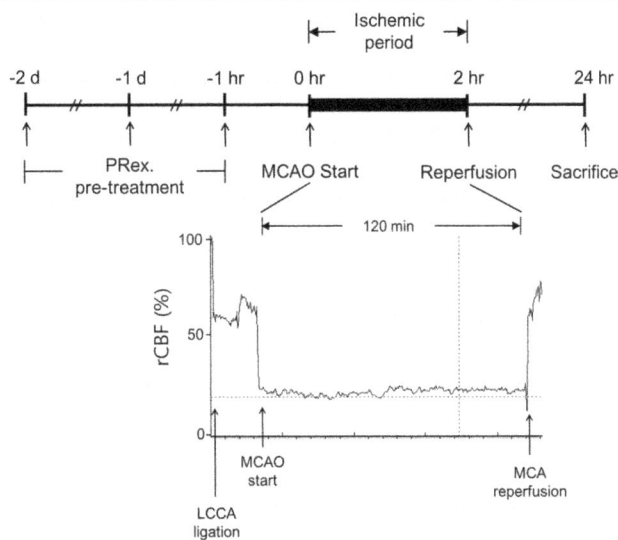

Fig. 1 Design of the MCAO model. The mice were pretreated with methanol extract of Peucedani Radix (PRex) for three consecutive days before MCAO and the mice were killed 24 h after MCAO. During the ischemic conditioning, the relative cerebral blood flow (rCBF) was monitored by using Laser-Doppler flowmetry. *LCCA* left common carotid artery, *MCA* middle cerebral artery

baseline during reperfusion, which indicated that the MCAO procedure was successful. The skin was immediately sutured and the animal was awakened from anesthesia. In the sham control group, the sham operation consisted of binding of the LECA and ligation of the LCCA, but the LMCA was not occluded; finally, the incised muscle and skin were sutured. The mice were euthanized by CO_2 inhalation at 24 h after MCAO.

Measurement of infarct volume

The brains harvested at 24 h after the MCAO procedure were immediately sliced into 1-mm coronal sections from the olfactory bulb to just before the cerebellum and 10 sections were cut per brain. The sections were incubated with 2% 2,3,5-triphenyltetrazolium chloride (TTC) solution for 17 min at 25 °C and then soaked in 10% neutral buffered formalin for more than 2 h. Relative edema and infarct volumes were computed by Image J software (NIH, Maryland, USA) from digital images obtained by a digital camera.

Neurological deficit scores

Twenty hours after MCAO, neurological deficit scores were assessed by using the following five-point scale: 0, no neurological deficit; 1, an incomplete extension of right forepaw and a reduced grip when tail pulled; 2, voluntary movement in all directions and turning to the right when tail pulled; 3, walking or circling to the right and sensitive to nociception when stimulated; 4, no response to stimulation or stroke-related death.

Western blot analysis

The mice brains of ischemic hemisphere were dissected and homogenized in modified phosphate buffered saline (PBS) containing 150 mM NaCl, 1 mM EDTA, 50 mM Tris, and 1:100 (v/v) of proteinase inhibitor. The expression level of inducible nitric oxide synthase (iNOS) in the mouse brains was then assessed by western blotting.

Total proteins were isolated using a protein extraction solution (pro-prep, iNtRON, Gyeonggi-do, Korea). The cell lysates were obtained by centrifugation at $13,250 \times g$ for 10 min at 4 °C. Equal amounts of proteins were separated in sodium-dodecyl sulfate polyacrylamide gels and transferred to PVDF membranes (Millipore, Darmstadt, Germany), which were blocked using 5% skim milk in TBST buffer for 1 h at room temperature and then incubated overnight at 4 °C with specific antibodies for iNOS (1:500) and β-actin (1:1000). Subsequently, the membranes were incubated with horse radish peroxidase (HRP)-conjugated goat anti-rabbit IgG pAb (1:5000) and HRP-conjugated goat anti-mouse IgG pAb (1:3000) for 2 h. The membranes were then treated with ECL solution (GenDEPOT, Houston, TX, USA) and the protein bands were detected by a photosensitive luminescent analyzer system (Amersham™ Imager 600, UK). The band intensities were analyzed using Image J (NIH, Maryland, USA) to determine the relative protein quantities in comparison with β-actin. iNOS antibody were obtained from Cell Signaling (Danvers, MA, USA), and secondary antibodies goat anti-rabbit IgG pAb was obtained from Enzo Life Sciences (Farmingdale, NY, USA).

Inflammatory cytokine analysis

The brain tissue of ischemic hemisphere was homogenized in PBS (pH 7.4) (5% w/v) and the resultant homogenates were clarified at $10,000 \times g$ for 5 min at 4 °C. The post-mitochondrial supernatants were obtained by a second centrifugation step at $10,000 \times g$ for 20 min at 4 °C and used for enzyme-linked immunosorbent assays (ELISAs) (Abcam, Cambridge, MA, USA). The levels of IL-1β and TNF-α in the brain tissue were measured by ELISA using a commercially available kit in accordance with the manufacturer's instructions. The detection limit of the assay was 0.1 ng/mL. The absorbance of the reaction products at 450 nm was measured by using a microplate reader.

Determination of ROS

To measure the production of reactive oxygen species (ROS) and malondialdehyde (MDA), ROS generation in the brain was determined in tissue homogenates by using dichlorofluorescein diacetate (DCFH-DA) [20]. The tissue homogenate was incubated with 1 mM 2′,7′-dichlorodihydrofluorescein diacetate for 30 min at 37 °C. The absorbance was measured by using a fluorescence microplate reader at an excitation wavelength of 485 nm and an emission wavelength of 535 nm.

Estimation of oxidative stress markers

To measure oxidative stress in the injured brain tissue, level of malondialdehyde (MDA), a biomarker of lipid peroxidation, was estimated. The level of MDA in the injured hemispheres was examined using the TBARS (thiobarbituric acid-reactive substances) Assay Kit (Cayman Chemical, Ann Arbor, MI) [21]. The optical density (OD) was read at 540 nm by a spectrophotometer and the results were defined as μM/μg wet tissue.

Histological staining

The harvested brain tissue was fixed in 10% formalin, dehydrated by alcohol, and embedded in paraffin. The sections of the tissue were cut into 3-μm thick slices on the glass slides, deparaffinized by xylene, and stained with hematoxylin and eosin (H&E) or cresyl violet (CV) to observe the histological changes in brain tissue after MCAO-injury by using a microscope (ZEISS AXIO, Carl Zeiss, Oberkochen, Germany).

Statistical analysis

One-way ANOVA was used to determine the statistical significance of differences. The data were expressed as the mean ± standard deviations (STDEVs). SPSS 23.0 version was used to perform the statistical analyses and p values of ≤ 0.05 were considered statistically significant.

Results

Effects of PRex on infarct volumes and behavioral deficits

The regions of infarction were represented by TTC staining. The sham operation induced no damage, but MCAO caused a relatively wide range of damage in the ipsilateral hemispheres (mean ± SD; 121.167 ± 12.671 mm^3). However, significantly smaller infarct lesions were found in the 60 or 200 mg/kg PRex pretreated MCAO groups than in the MCAO control group (60 mg/kg, 101.0 ± 7.874 mm^3; 200 mg/kg, 97.167 ± 9.867 mm^3) (Figs. 2, 3a). The neuronal deficit scores were significantly higher in mice with MCAO. PRex pretreatment did not significantly reduce motor behavioral scores compared with the MCAO control (Fig. 3b).

Effects of PRex on iNOS expression

As determined by the western blot analysis to identify protein changes in harvested brain sections at 24 h after MCAO, the inducible NOS (iNOS) level was significantly higher than that of the sham controls. However, mice in the 200 mg/kg group had significantly lower iNOS levels than did the mice in the MCAO control group (Fig. 4a).

Effects of PRex on pro-inflammatory cytokine levels

The effects of PRex on brain inflammation after MCAO injury were evaluated by the measurement of the levels of pro-inflammatory cytokines. The brains of MCAO-injured mice exhibited higher concentrations of IL-1β (mean ± SD: 642 ± 89 pg/mL) and TNF-α (487 ± 87 pg/mL) compared with levels in the sham-operated mice (IL-1β, 186 ± 13 pg/mL; TNF-α, 123 ± 45 pg/mL). However, PRex pretreatment significantly suppressed the expression of IL-1β (200 mg/kg, 428 ± 29 pg/mL) and TNF-α (60 mg/kg, 342 ± 62 pg/mL; 200 mg/kg, 339 ± 53 pg/mL) (Fig. 4b, c).

Effects of PRex on ROS production and lipid peroxidation

To examine the antioxidant effect of PRex, the contents of ROS and MDA in the brain were measured. The ROS and MDA levels were significantly elevated in the MCAO group (mean ± SD: ROS, 221 ± 17%; MDA, 1.60 ± 0.19 nmol/mg) compared with that in the sham operated group (ROS, 105 ± 6%; MDA, 0.70 ± 0.03 nmol/mg). However, the ROS (200 mg/kg, 132 ± 16%) and MDA levels (60 mg/kg, 1.20 ± 0.12 nmol/mg; 200 mg/kg, 0.90 ± 0.21 nmol/mg) were significantly lower in the PRex-administered groups (Fig. 5a, b).

Effects of PRex on histological changes in brain tissue

To confirm the histological changes in brain tissue 24 h after MCAO, the tissue was stained by H&E or CV. The brain tissue was more strongly stained red by H&E in

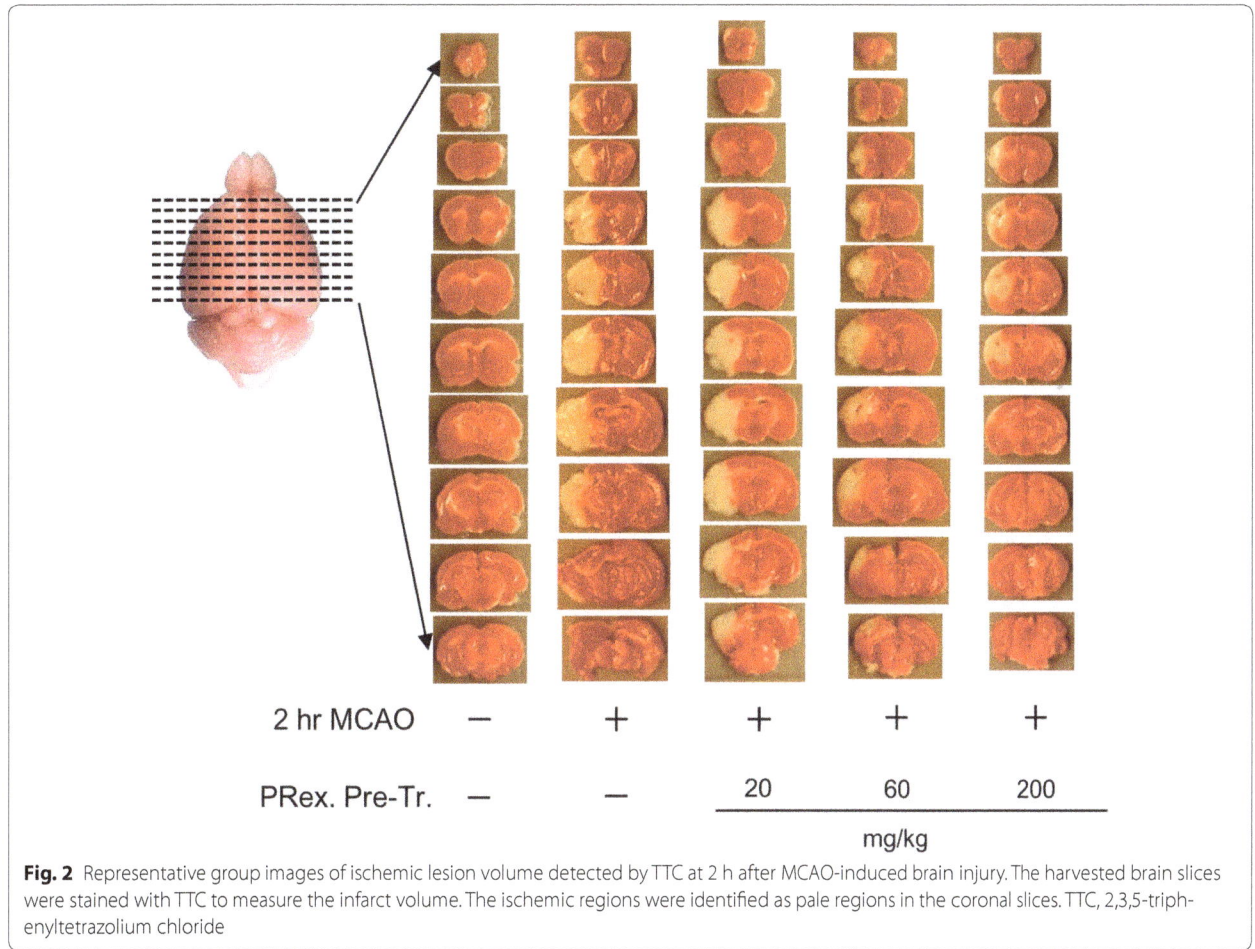

Fig. 2 Representative group images of ischemic lesion volume detected by TTC at 2 h after MCAO-induced brain injury. The harvested brain slices were stained with TTC to measure the infarct volume. The ischemic regions were identified as pale regions in the coronal slices. TTC, 2,3,5-triphenyltetrazolium chloride

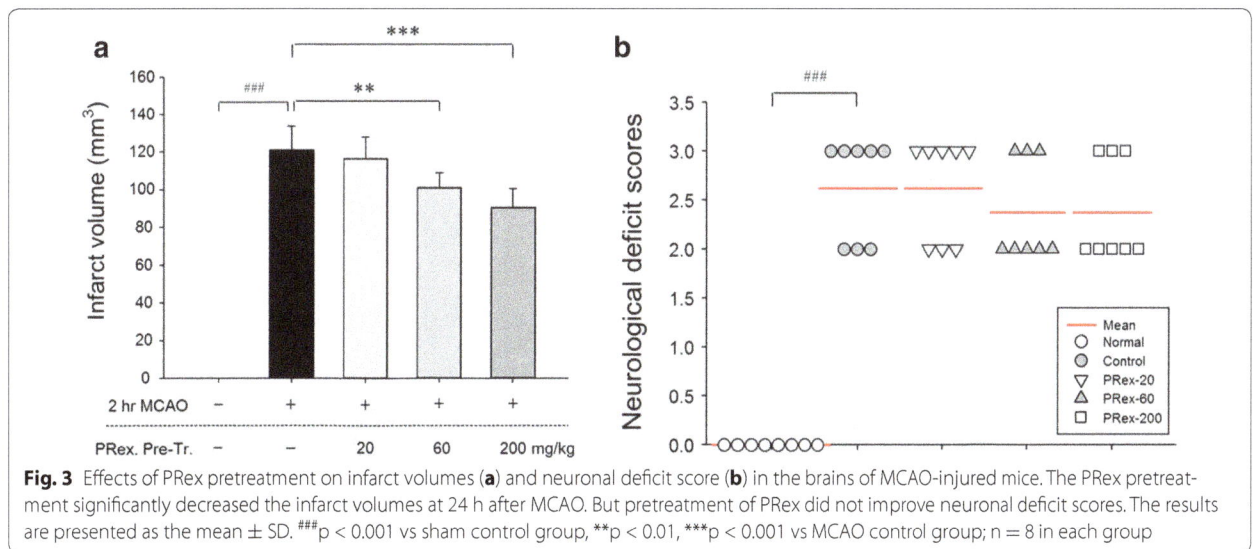

Fig. 3 Effects of PRex pretreatment on infarct volumes (**a**) and neuronal deficit score (**b**) in the brains of MCAO-injured mice. The PRex pretreatment significantly decreased the infarct volumes at 24 h after MCAO. But pretreatment of PRex did not improve neuronal deficit scores. The results are presented as the mean ± SD. ###p < 0.001 vs sham control group, **p < 0.01, ***p < 0.001 vs MCAO control group; n = 8 in each group

the MCAO control group than in the sham controls. At the highest concentration of PRex, the brain tissue was more strongly stained blue than that observed for the MCAO control group (Fig. 6a). In the MCAO control group, fewer purple-stained neurons were observed than in the sham controls; however, in the PRex pretreatment

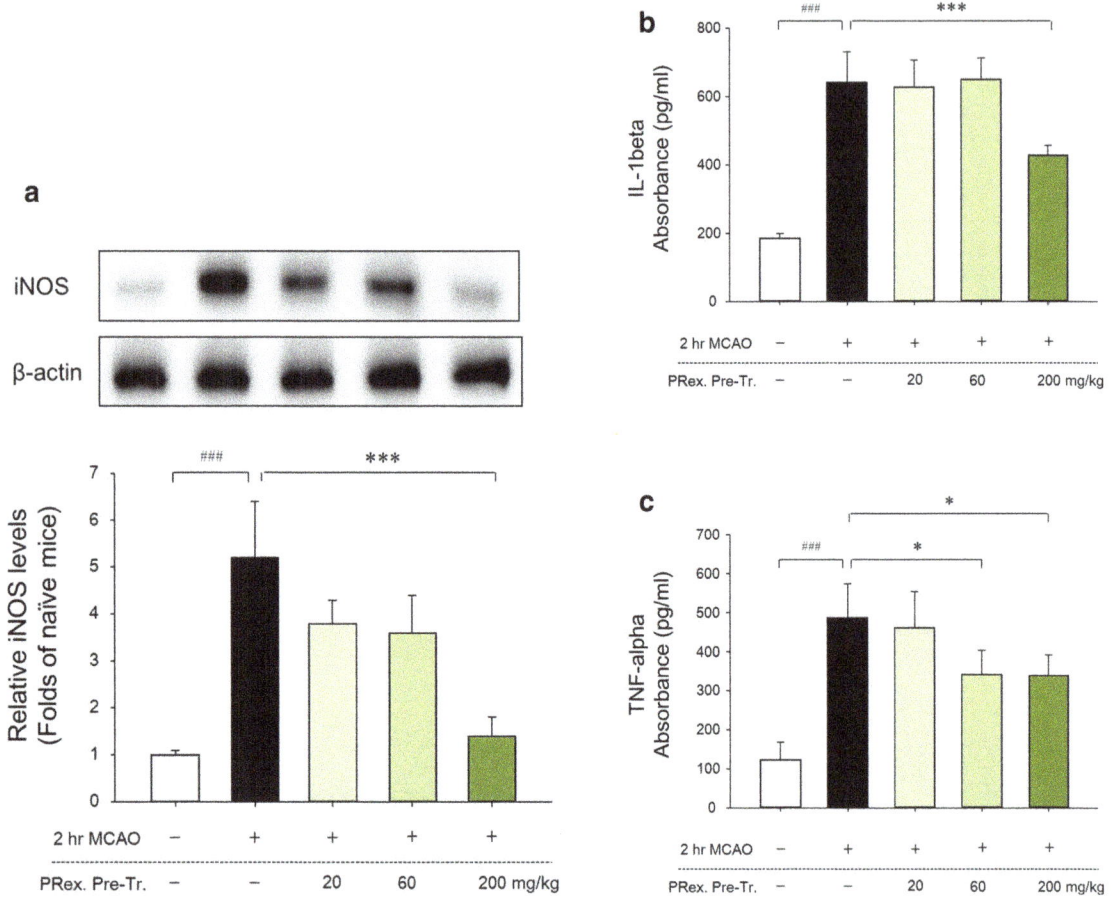

Fig. 4 Effects of PRex pretreatment on iNOS (**a**), IL-1β (**b**), and TNF-α (**c**) in the brains of MCAO-injured mice. PRex pretreatment significantly decreased iNOS level in the mouse model of ischemic brain stroke (**a**). Representative western blots and quantitative analysis of iNOS expression show the effect of PRex on iNOS expression in brain tissue. The IL-1β and TNF-α levels were measured by using a commercially available ELISA kit. The results are presented as the mean ± SD. $^{###}p < 0.001$ vs sham control group, $^*p < 0.05$, $^{***}p < 0.001$ vs MCAO control group; n = 8 in each group

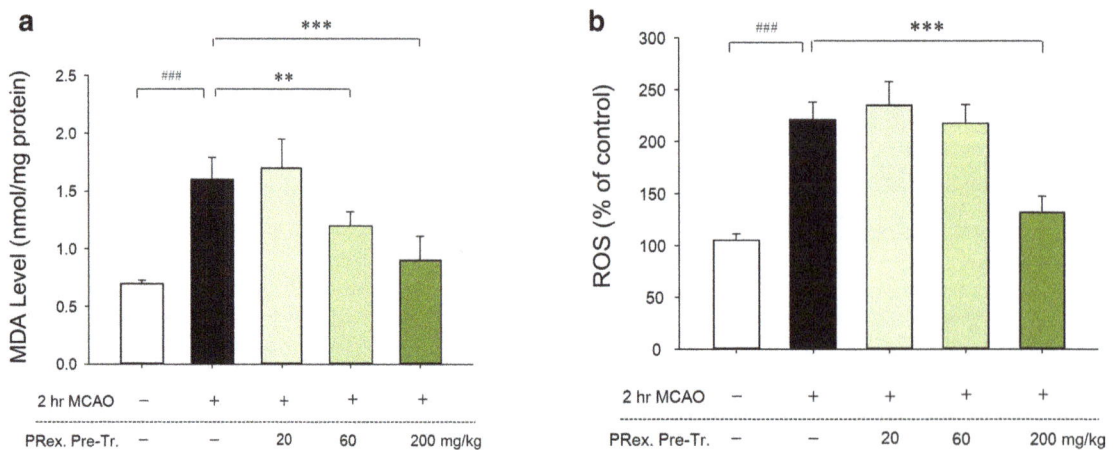

Fig. 5 Effects of PRex on ROS (**a**) and MDA levels (**b**) in the brains of MCAO-induced mice. The results are presented as the mean ± SD. $^{###}p < 0.001$ vs sham control group, $^{**}p < 0.01$, $^{***}p < 0.001$ vs MCAO control group; n = 8 in each group

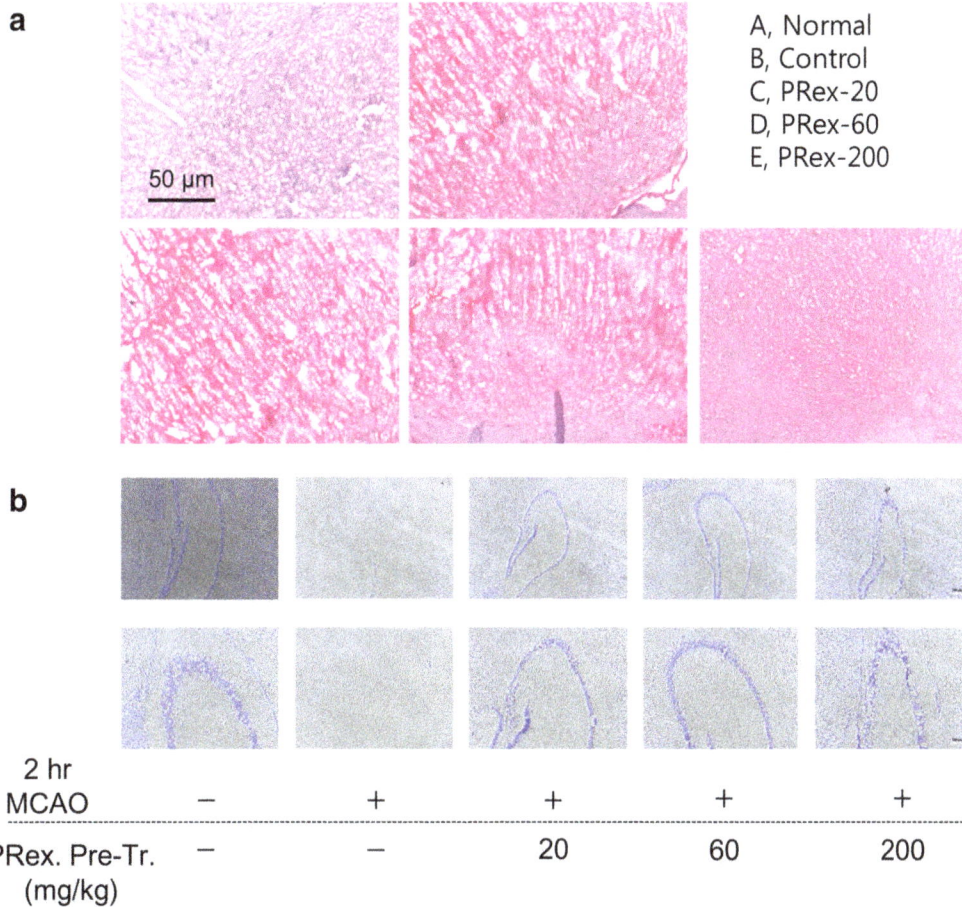

Fig. 6 Effects of PRex pretreatment on histological change in the brains of MCAO-injured mice stained by hematoxylin and eosin (**a**), and by cresyl violet (**b**). Red staining indicates nuclear damage. Neurons dyed by cresyl violet are stained purple

groups, they appeared more often than in the MCAO control group (Fig. 6b).

Discussion

Globally, stroke has been the second most common cause of death for 15 years; more than six million deaths were attributed to stroke in 2015 [22]. Ischemia-induced brain damage accounts for approximately 80% of the types of stroke[5] and may result in permanent disability, which severely impairs dependence and precipitates a large social expense. Furthermore, the incidence of stroke in young adults is experiencing an upward trend [23]. Therefore, the prevention and recovery of stroke are important issues.

In Korean medicine, ischemic brain damage is one of the diseases included in sudden hit by the wind (卒中風) and classified as fire-heat pattern (火熱證), Yin deficiency pattern (陰虛證), Qi deficiency pattern (氣虛證), and the dampness-phlegm pattern (濕痰證) [24]. The dampness-phlegm pattern of stroke has a significant relationship with metabolic syndrome and obesity [25], which are prominent causes of stroke.

PR is a representative herb that expels damp and phlegm, and it has long been used as a therapeutic agent for thick phlegm, upper respiratory tract infections, and asthma [14]. PR was not mentioned as a major therapeutic agent, but it has been reported to exert antioxidant and anti-inflammatory activities [15–18, 26], which are potentially related to the treatment of ischemia-induced brain damage.

When stroke occurs, the cell death that results from the deprivation of oxygen and glucose consequently results in cerebral damage [27, 28]. Although various mechanisms participate in the pathological process of stroke, considerable evidence has indicated that inflammation plays an important role in its progression [29–31]. The inflammatory responses caused by excitotoxicity and oxidative stress owing to hypoperfusion in ischemic areas lead to blood–brain barrier dysfunction and cell death [32].

Although several pharmacological agents were found to be effective in animal models, they did not work in humans [33, 34]. Laboratory experimental conditions did not reflect the factors that influenced stroke in the human population, nevertheless, the most applicable and frequently chosen animal models for research stroke are rodents [33, 35]. The MCAO injury to rodents, the most commonly used surgical procedure to produce stroke, damages the subcortical and cortical structures that mimic human cerebral infarcts in terms of the size and the affected structures [36]. Inflammation has been reported to play an important role in the pathogenesis of ischemic stroke; the brain responds to ischemic injury with an acute and prolonged inflammatory process that can be characterized by the rapid activation of resident cells, the production of pro-inflammatory mediators, and the infiltration of various types of inflammatory cells [37]. Over 1000 drugs have been tested in animal models; of these, 114 underwent clinical evaluation, but a larger proportion of the agents studied previously have failed. Despite the many clinical trials conducted, rt-PA remains the only agent shown to improve stroke outcome and therefore the optimum treatment of cerebral focal ischemia has remained as one of the major challenges of clinical medicine [33–38].

In this study, we evaluated the anti-inflammatory effect of PRex on ischemia-induced brain damage in a mice model. PRex pretreatment was found to reduce the infarct volumes in mice brains 24 h after MCAO (Figs. 2, 3a), but did not significantly improve the neurological behavioral deficits (Fig. 3b). In addition, histological staining indicated that PRex pretreatment protected the nucleus and neuronal cells. Hematoxylin stains the nucleus blue and eosin stains the cytoplasm red; hence, tissues with damaged nuclei appear red. CV stains neurons; in this study, the lighter purple staining indicates greater damage to the neurons of the brain tissues around the hippocampus. In the present study, the tissue stained red by H&E after MCAO injury became more blue as the concentration of PRex pretreatment increased (Fig. 6a) and the reduction in the area stained purple by CV after MCAO-induced brain injury was increased in the PRex pretreatment groups (Fig. 6b).

Nitric oxide synthase (NOS) enzymes, including endothelial NOS (eNOS), neuronal NOS (nNOS), and inducible NOS (iNOS), are important in the maintenance of homeostasis through the production of NO from L-arginine. eNOS and nNOS produce low physiological levels of NO; iNOS consistently produces large amounts of NO through inflammatory cytokines and bacterial products. NO can exert cytotoxicity through the formation of strong oxidant peroxynitrite with superoxide, especially in inflammatory responses. iNOS promotes

inflammation and acts synergistically with other inflammatory mediators. In the brain, the increase in iNOS mRNA and protein after ischemia led to NO production and DNA damage. Therefore, the inhibition of iNOS activity could be critical for the suppression of inflammation in the ischemic brain [39–44]. In the current study, PRex pretreatment was shown to reduce the effects on increased iNOS expression in MCAO-induced brain damage (Fig. 4a).

Among the cytokines known to be associated with inflammation in stroke [45], interleukin-1 (IL-1) and TNF-α were reported to aggravate cerebral injury; in contrast, interleukin-6 (IL-6), interleukin-10 (IL-10), and transforming growth factor-β (TGF-β) were shown to be neuroprotective [46]. In the early stage of focal cerebral ischemia, pro-inflammatory cytokines, such as IL-1β and TNF-α, promote the expression of adhesion-like glycoprotein P and E-selectin and the stimulation of leukocytes attached to the activated vascular endothelium [47]. In the present study, PRex was found to significantly ameliorate the MCAO-induced upregulation of IL-1β and TNF-α expression (Fig. 4b, c).

After ischemia has started, energy depletion causes mitochondrial dysfunction and early generation of ROS and reactive nitrogen species (RNS) [19], the accumulation of which triggers inflammation through the initiation of a chain of harmful cell responses [48]. ROS are molecules derived from small oxygen species, including the superoxide anion radical ($O_2 \cdot -$), hydroxyl radical (OH·), and certain non-radicals, such as hydrogen peroxide (H_2O_2) and the oxygen singlet ($^1O_2$) [27]. Among these oxidants, the superoxide anion is the most destructive because it can cause cytotoxicity in combination with NO [49]. In this study, PRex pretreatment effectively inhibited the increase in the ROS and MDA levels caused by MCAO-induced brain injury (Fig. 5a, b). MDA is a lipoperoxidation product that is used as an indicator of oxidative stress [50].

Consequently, PRex pretreatment suppressed infarction in mice brains after MCAO through decreased oxidative stress, owing to reduced iNOS and ROS, and the regulation of the expression of pro-inflammatory factors, such as IL-1β and TNF-α. These results indicate that neuro-protective effects of PRex could be mediated by anti-oxidative and anti-inflammatory mechanisms in MCAO mice model ((Additional file 1: Figure S2).

Based on above results, PR could be regarded as promising agent for the prevention or initial treatment of stroke through the inhibition of inflammatory responses in cerebral infarction. However, further pharmacological studies on the effects of the pretreatment of other extracts of PR on stroke, the components of PR that affect each pathway of ischemia-induced brain damage, and the effects of PR treatment after cerebral damage are required to establish to clinical applications.

Conclusions

To demonstrate the effects of PRex pretreatment on ischemia-induced brain damage, the infarct volumes in the brain, the neurological deficit scores, and the expression of oxidative stress factors and inflammatory cytokines were observed at 24 h after MCAO-induced brain injury in mice. The results indicated that PRex pretreatment significantly decreased the infarct volume in mice brains after MCAO, but resulted in no significant reduction in the neurological behavioral deficit. PRex pretreatment significantly inhibited the expression of iNOS and the levels of ROS and MDA in mice brains after MCAO. PRex pretreatment significantly suppressed the expression of IL-1β and TNF-α in mice brains after MCAO. In conclusion, PRex pretreatment reduced the infarct volumes in the brains of mice with MCAO-induced brain injury through interference in the inflammatory responses of ischemic brain injury. Our results indicated that PR could be a potential candidate for the prevention or treatment of cerebral stroke.

Abbreviations

PR: Peucedani Radix; PRex: methanol extract of Peucedani Radix; MCAO: middle cerebral artery occlusion; DCFH-DA: dichlorofluorescein diacetate; TBARS: thiobarbituric acid-reactive substances; ELISA: enzyme-linked immunosorbent assay; iNOS: inducible nitric oxide synthase; ROS: reactive oxygen species; MDA: malondialdehyde; IL: interleukin; TNF-α: tumor necrosis factor alpha.

Authors' contributions

SYJ, KMK and YKK designed the study. SYJ, KMK and SC performed the experiments. SL and CY conducted statistical analysis. SC and YKK wrote the manuscript. All authors read and approved the final manuscript.

Author details

[1] College of Korean Medicine, Dong-Eui University, Yangjeong-ro, Busanjin-gu, Busan 47227, Republic of Korea. [2] School of Korean Medicine, Pusan National University, Yangsan, Gyeongnam 50612, Republic of Korea. [3] School of Public Health, Far East University, Chungbuk 27601, Republic of Korea. [4] College of Medicine, Dongguk University, Ilsandong-gu, Gyeonggi-do 10326, Republic of Korea.

Acknowledgements
Not applicable.

Competing interests
The authors declare that they have no competing interests.

Consent for publication
Not applicable.

Funding
Not applicable.

References

1. WHO Monica Project Principal Investigators. The World Health Organization MONICA Project (monitoring trends and determinants in cardiovascular disease): a major international collaboration. J Clin Epidemiol. 1988;41(2):105–14.
2. Roth S, Liesz A. Stroke research at the crossroads—where are we heading? Swiss Med Wkly. 2016;146:w14329.
3. Chamorro A, Dirnagl U, Urra X, Plana AM. Neuroprotection in acute stroke: targeting excitotoxicity, oxidative and nitrosative stress, and inflammation. Lancet Neurol. 2016;15(8):869–81.
4. Barlow SJ. Identifying the brain regions associated with acute spasticity in patients diagnosed with an ischemic stroke. Somatosens Mots Res. 2016;33(2):104–11.
5. Poisson SN, Glidden D, Johnston SC, Fullerton HJ. Deaths from stroke in US young adults, 1989–2009. Neurology. 2014;83(23):2110–5.
6. Durakan A, Tatlisumak T. Handbook of clinical neurology stroke, part 1 basic and epidemiological aspects. New York: Elsevier; 2009. p. 1–464.
7. Kim D. Animal models of stroke. Brain Neurorehabilit. 2011;4(1):1–11.
8. Koizumi JYY, Nakazawa T, Ooneda G. Experimental studies of ischemic brain edema. I. A new experimental model of cerebral embolism in rats in which recirculation can be introduced in the ischemic area. Jpn J Stroke. 1986;8:1–8.
9. Longa EZ, Weinstein PR, Carlson S, Cummins R. Reversible middle cerebral artery occlusion without craniectomy in rats. Stroke. 1989;20:84–91.
10. Macrae IM. Preclinical stroke research-advantages and disadvantages of the most common rodent models of focal ischaemia. Br J Pharmacol. 2011;164:1062–78.
11. Gupta S, Gupta YK. Combination of Zizyphus jujuba and silymarin showed better neuroprotective effect as compared to single agent in MCAo-induced focal cerebral ischemia in rats. J Ethnopharmacol. 2017;197:118–27.
12. Gim SA, Koh PO. Change of Peroxiredoxin-5 expression by curcumin treatment in cerebral ischemia. J Agric Life Sci. 2016;50(3):129–39.
13. Na JY, Song K, Lee JW, Kim S, Kwon J. Pretreatment of 6-shogaol attenuates oxidative stress and inflammation in middle cerebral artery occlusion-induced mice. Eur J Ethnopharmacol. 2016;788:241–7.
14. Cooperative Textbook Compilation Committee of National Korean Medical College: Herbal medicine. Seoul: Young-Lim Pub; 2007. p. 495–6.
15. Lim HJ, Lee JH, Choi JS, Lee SK, Kim YS, Kim HP. Inhibition of airway inflammation by the roots of Angelica decursiva and its constituent. columbianadin. J Ethnopharmacol. 2014;155(2):1353–61.
16. Zhao D, Islam MN, Ahn BR, Jung HA, Kim BW, Choi JS. In vitro antioxidant and anti-inflammatory activities of Angelica decursiva. Arch Pharm Res. 2012;35(1):179–92.
17. Ishita IJ, Nurul Islam M, Kim YS, Choi RJ, Sohn HS, Jung HA, Choi JS. Coumarins form Angelica decursiva inhibit lipopolysaccharide-induced nitrite oxide production in RAW 264.7 cells. Arch Pharm Res. 2016;39(1):115–26.
18. Ali MY, Jannat S, Jung HA, Jeong HO, Chung HY, Choi JS. Coumarins from Angelica decursiva inhibit α-glucosidase activity and protein tyrosine phosphatase 1B. Chem Biol Interact. 2016;252:93–101.
19. Lo EH, Dalkara T, Moskowitz MA. Mechanisms, challenges and opportunities in stroke. Nat Rev Neurosci. 2003;4:399–414.
20. Ruan Q, Liu F, Gao Z, Kong D, Hu X, Shi D, Bao Z, Yu Z. The anti-inflammaging and hepatoprotective effects of huperzine A in D-galactose-treated rats. Mech Ageing Dev. 2013;134(3–4):89–97.
21. Dawn-Linsley M, Ekinci FJ, Ortiz D, Rogers E, Shea TB. Monitoring thiobarbituric acid-reactive substances (TBARs) as an assay for oxidative damage in neuronal cultures and central nervous system. J Neurosci Methods. 2005;141(2):219–22.

22. WHO: The top ten causes of death. Fact sheet no. 310. Geneva: World Health Organization; 2014;http://www.who.int/mediacentre/factsheets/fs310/en/. Accessed 24 Apr 2017.

23. Bejot Y, Delpont B, Giroud M. Rising stroke incidence in young adults: more epidemiological evidence, more questions to be answered. J Am Heart Assoc. 2016. doi:10.1161/JAHA.116.003661.

24. Lee JA, Lee JS, Kang BK, Ko MM, Mun TU, Cho KH, Bang OS. Report on the Korean standard pattern identification for stroke-III. Korean J Orient Int Med. 2011;32(2):232–42.

25. Min IK, Kim CH, Hwang JW, Park JY, Lee SY, Choi WW, Na BJ, Park SW, Jung WS, Moon SK, Park JM, Ko CN, Cho KH, Kim YS, Bae HS. The relation of dampness-phlegm and metabolic syndrome in acute stroke patients. J Korean Orient Med. 2009;30(1):109–19.

26. Kim KH: The analysis of the prescriptions used for stroke in Pung (風) chapter in Donguibogam. Doctoral Dissertation. Dongguk University. 2011.

27. Rodríguez JCG. Acute Ischemic stroke. Rijeka: InTech; 2012. p. 29–58.

28. Moskowitz MA, Lo EH, Iadecola C. The science of stroke: mechanisms in search of treatments. Neuron. 2010;67(2):181–98.

29. Barone FC, Feuerstein GZ. Inflammatory mediators and stroke: new opportunities for novel therapeutics. J Cereb Blood Flow Metab. 1999;19:819–34.

30. Samson Y, Lapergue B, Hosseini H. Inflammation and ischaemic stroke: current status and future perspectives. Rev Neurol (Paris). 2005;161:1177–82.

31. Muir KW, Tyrrell P, Sattar N, Warburton E. Inflammation and ischaemic stroke. Curr Opin Neurol. 2007;20:334–42.

32. Lakhan SE, Kirchgessner A, Hofer M. Inflammatory mechanisms in ischemic stroke: therapeutic approaches. J Transl Med. 2009;7:97.

33. Casals JB, Pieri NC, Feitosa ML, Ercolin AC, Roballo KC, Barreto RS, Bressan FF, Martins DS, Miglino MA, Ambrósio CE. The use of animal models for stroke research: a review. Comp Med. 2011;61(4):305–13.

34. Freitas GR, Noujaim JK, Haussen SR, Yamamoto FI, Novak EM, Gagliardi RJ. Neuroprotective agents in stroke: national opinion. Arq Neuropsiquiatr. 2005;63:889–91.

35. Wessmann A, Chandler K, Garosi L. Ischaemic and haemorrhagic stroke in the dog. Vet J. 2009;180:290–303.

36. Rossmeisl JH Jr, Rohleder JJ, Pickett JP, Duncan R, Herring IP. Presumed and confirmed striatocapsular brain infarctions in 6 dogs. Vet Ophthalmol. 2007;10:23–36.

37. Jin R, Yang G, Li G. Inflammatory mechanisms in ischemic stroke: role of inflammatory cells. J Leukoc Biol. 2010;87(5):779–89.

38. De la Ossa NP, Davalos A. Neuroprotection in cerebral infarction: the opportunity of new studies. Cerebrovasc Dis. 2007;24:153–6.

39. Nathan C. Nitric Oxide as a secretary product of mammalian cells. FASEB J. 1992;6:3051–64.

40. Alderton WK, Cooper CE, Knowles RG. Nitric oxide synthases: structure, function and inhibition. Biochem J. 2001;357(3):593–615.

41. Beckman JS, Beckman TW, Chen J, Marshall PA, Freeman BA. Apparent hydroxyl radical production by peroxynitirite: implications for endothelial injury from nitric oxide and superoxide. Proc Natl Acad Sci. 1990;87:1620–4.

42. Moncada S, Higgs EA. Endogenous nitric oxide: physiology, pathology and clinical relevance. Eur J Clin Invest. 1991;21(4):361–74.

43. Iadecola C, Zhang F, Xu S, Casey R, Ross ME. Inducible nitric oxide synthase gene expression in brain following cerebral ischemia. J Cereb Blood Flow Metab. 1995;15:378–84.

44. Iadecola C, Zhang F, Xu X. Inhibition of inducible nitric oxide synthase ameliorates cerebral ischemic damage. Am J Physiol. 1995;268:R286–92.

45. Han HS, Yenari MA. Cellular targets of brain inflammation in stroke. Curr Opin Investig Drugs. 2003;4:522–9.

46. Allan SM, Rothwell NJ. Cytokines and acute neurodegeneration. Nat Rev Neurosci. 2001;2:734–44.

47. Zhang R, Chopp M, Zhang Z, Jiang N, Powers C. The expression of P- and E-selectins in three models of middle cerebral artery occlusion. Brain Res. 1998;785:207–14.

48. Mukhopadhyay P, Horváth B, Zsengellér Z, Bátkai S, Cao Z, Kechrid M, Holovac E, Erdélyi K, Tanchian G, Liaudet L, Stillman IE, Joseph J, Kalyanaraman B, Pacher P. Mitochondrial reactive oxygen species generation triggers inflammatory response and tissue injury associated with hepatic ischemia-reperfusion: therapeutic potential of mitochondrially-targeted antioxidants. Free Radic Biol Med. 2012;53(5):1123–38.

49. Chan PH. Reactive oxygen radicals in signaling and damage in the ischemic brain. J Cereb Blood Flow Metab. 2001;21:2–4.

50. Dotan Y, Lichtenberg D, Pinchuk I. Lipid peroxidation cannot be used as a universal criterion of oxidative stress. Prog Lipid Res. 2004;43(3):200–27.

3

Rapid identification of growth years and profiling of bioactive ingredients in *Astragalus membranaceus* var. mongholicus (*Huangqi*) roots from Hunyuan, Shanxi

Hua-Sheng Peng[1,2†], Jun Wang[1,3†], He-Ting Zhang[1], Hai-Yan Duan[1], Xiao-Mei Xie[1*], Ling Zhang[1], Ming-En Cheng[1,4] and Dai-yin Peng[1,4*]

Abstract

Background: The content of medicinal bioactive constituents in *huangqi* is affected by plant age. In this study, we devised a quick and convenient method for determining the age of *huangqi*, which was cultivated in Hunyuan County (Shanxi Province).

Methods: 1, 2, 3, 4, 5, 8, 10 growth years *huangqi* had 38 samples, all samples were collected separately. The growth rings in these samples were observed after making paraffin section and freehand-section. The relationship between growth rings and its growth years was analyzed by SPSS 19.0 software. Histochemical localization of total flavones and saponins in *huangqi* was determined by color reactions. The concentration of four flavonoids and two saponins in the roots of *huangqi* of different ages and different organizational structure (normal roots and rotten heart roots) were determined by HPLC-DAD and HPLC-ELSD. The results were analyzed by SPSS 19.0 software.

Results: All *huangqi* samples had clear growth rings, and the statistical result about growth rings (X) and growth years (Y) showed significant correlation ($r = 1$, $P = 0.000$). The calibration curves of these six ingredients showed good linearity respectively, with significant correlation. All relative standard deviations (RSDs) of precision, recovery, repeatability, and stability experiments were less than 2%. Roots of 5-year-old plants contained the highest concentrations of total flavonoids and saponins. Saponin concentrations increased toward the center of the roots, whereas the four flavonoids showed an opposite trend in tissue distribution.

Conclusion: The growth year of *huangqi* (Hunyuan County, Shanxi Province) could be determined soon and conveniently by naked eyes after staining phloroglucinol-HCl solution on freehand section. The content of saponins and flavonoids in rotten heart root and the surrounding normal tissues were affected by the formation and the extent of rotten heart.

Keywords: Growth rings, Freehand section, Rotten heart, Histochemical localization, Concentration

Background

Astragali Radix, also known as *huangqi*, is a well-known Chinese herbal medicine. It is derived from the herbs *Astragalus membranaceus* var. *mongholicus* and *A. membranaceus* [1]. The main active compounds in *huangqi* are polysaccharides, saponins, flavonoids, and various trace elements [2–5]. *Huangqi* has immunoregulation properties, cardiovascular and cerebrovascular protection, and anticancer, antiviral, antiaging, and antidiabetic effects [6–12].

Geo-authentic medicinal materials (*Dao-di*) are produced in the natural conditions and ecological

*Correspondence: xiexiaomei9401@sina.com; pengdy@ahtcm.edu.cn
†Hua-Sheng Peng and Jun Wang contributed equally to this work
[1] School of Pharmacy, Anhui University of Chinese Medicine, Hefei 230031, China
Full list of author information is available at the end of the article

environment, e.g., the cultivation, harvesting, and processing techniques, leading to enhanced quality and clinical effects, compared with the original plant [13]. In the Qing dynasty, Shanxi Province became the *Dao-di* production area of *huangqi* [14], and Hunyuan County in Shanxi Province is currently one of the *Dao-di* production areas [15]. The accumulation of certain secondary metabolites in *huangqi* is related to the number of years of growth [16]. Consequently, the accurate and rapid determination of age is beneficial for evaluating the quality of *huangqi*. Growth rings have been discovered in the roots of many perennial herbs and have been used to identify plant age [17–22]. Growth rings have been found in *huangqi* and could be used to determine the age of samples [23].

The bioactive constituents of medicinal plants are often concentrated in particular tissues of the root [24, 25]. The quality evaluation standard of *huangqi* in Chinese pharmacopoeia is the contents of astragaloside A and calycosin-7-glucoside [1]. Flavonoid and saponin concentrations vary in the different tissue layers of *huangqi* [25, 26]. To date, however, there have been no studies that have investigated the influence of rotten heart on the distribution and concentration of bioactive constituents in *huangqi*.

In this study, we aimed to identify the age of *huangqi* cultivated in Hunyuan County (Shanxi Province) using a convenient method and to profile the main bioactive constituents. *Huangqi* of different ages were collected for anatomical examination and analysis of biochemical composition. This multidisciplinary approach enabled us to determine the affects of age, rotten heart, and tissue on the concentrations of the main active compounds.

Methods
Plant materials
Semi-wild *huangqi* of 1, 2, 3, 4, 5, 8, and 10 years of age was collected separately from Hunyuan County (Table 1) in September 2012. 1-year-old *huangqi* had 5 samples; 2-year-old *huangqi* had 8 samples; 3-year-old *huangqi* had 8 samples; 4-year-old *huangqi* had 8 samples; 5-year-old *huangqi* had 5 samples; 8-year-old *huangqi* had 3 samples and 10-year-old *huangqi* had 1 sample. The above-ground parts were retained as plant specimens. The roots were dried in the sun for experimental analysis. The roots of 8-year-old *huangqi* were categorized into normal roots and rotten heart roots. All samples were authenticated by Professor Huasheng Peng (School of Pharmacy, Anhui University of Chinese Medicine) with reference to the Flora of China [27].

Chemicals and reagents
The internal standards calycosin-7-glucoside and astragaloside A were purchased from the National Institutes for

Table 1 Sample information and number of growth rings observed using two different methods

Age (years of growth)	Number of specimen	TRR	TRM
1	5	0	1
2	8	1	2
3	8	2	3
4	8	3	4
5	5	4	5
8	3	a	8
10	1	a	10

TRR the number of growth rings observed with the naked eye after staining of transverse sections with phloroglucinol–HCl reagent, *TRM* the number of growth rings observed using light microscopy

a The number of growth rings was not clearly observed after staining of transverse sections with phloroglucinol–HCl reagent

Food and Drug Control (Beijing, China). Calycosin, formononetin, and astragaloside II were purchased from the Traditional Chinese Medicine Standardization Research Center (Shanghai, China). Ononin was purchased from Vic Biological Technology (Sichuan, China). Acetonitrile (TEDIA, USA) was chromatographically pure and the water was ultrapure from Milli-Q (Merck Millipore, USA). All other reagents were of analytical grade.

Transverse section analysis
Segments of the roots of 10-year-old *huangqi* (length 80 cm, diameter 2.9 cm) were cut transversely (5 mm thick) at 5-cm intervals from the root-head to the root-tail. These segments were used to prepare paraffin sections. The paraffin sections were prepared as follows: initially, the segments were placed in FAA solution (70% ethanol:formaldehyde:acetic acid, 90:5:5) for over 24 h. The segments were then dehydrated using a gradient series of alcohol, and thereafter embedded in paraffin. Subsequently, the embedded roots were serially sectioned at 10–15-μm thickness using a Leica RM2265 rotary microtome. The serially sectioned samples were placed on clear slides in a consecutive order and then baked for more than 24 h. Each section was then deparaffinized and stained with safranin-fast green and safranin reagent. The parenchyma stained green and the vascular tissue stained red. The microscopic structure of different parts of the root and the development of normal tissues and rotten tissues were observed by light microscopy (Leica DM6000B; Leica Microsystems, IL, Germany).

Huangqi samples of 1, 2, 3, 4, and 5 years of age were used for microscopic examination of growth rings. Root segments were cut at approximately 2 cm from the root-head, excluding any rotten tissue. Parts of the segments were cut (5 mm thick), and from these, paraffin sections were prepared (as described previously) for light microscopic observation. Other parts of the segments were sectioned at 1-mm thickness by hand and stained with phloroglucinol-HCl. The growth rings in these sections were counted with the naked eye and also under a light microscope.

Histochemical analysis

Huangqi samples were sectioned using a freezing microtome (Leica CM1850 UV, 30–40 μm) at 20–40-μm thickness, and the sections were stained with 5% sodium hydroxide solution. After few minutes, the sections were observed using fluorescence microscopy (Leica DM6000B; Leica Microsystems, Fluo, Germany) with a green filter (Leica Microsystems, Germany) and an emission wavelength of 420 nm. *Huangqi* samples were also sectioned using a freezing microtome (Leica CM1850 UV, 30–40 μm) at 20–40-μm thickness, and the sections were stained with 5% vanillin-sulfuric acid solution. After few minutes, saponins may become red or purple. Sections for a negative control experiment were treated with 70% alcohol for 1 month to remove flavonoids and saponins. These sections were then stained with 5% sodium hydroxide solution or 5% vanillin-sulfuric acid solution, as described previously.

HPLC analysis

Preparation of different Huangqi tissues

Huangqi samples were classified into three categories based on the extent of rotten tissue: (A) "normal," (B) "small rotten heart" (rotten tissue <1/3 of the total diameter), and (C) "large rotten heart" (rotten tissue ≥1/3 of the total diameter). Each category comprised three root samples. The normal and "small rotten heart" root samples were sliced (3 mm thick). The normal root slices were then divided into seven parts: periderm (Pd), secondary phloem (SPh) (outside to inside: SPh1 and SPh2), and secondary xylem (SX) (outside to inside: SX1, SX2, SX3, and SX4). The "small rotten heart" samples were partitioned using the same steps, but rotten heart (Ho) included the secondary xylem. The "large rotten heart" root samples were cut into six parts: Pd, SP (outside to inside: SPh1, SPh2), and SX (outside to inside: SX1, SX2) and Ho. All samples were crushed, dried at 60 °C, and sieved through a No. 4 mesh(diameter 250 ± 9.9 μm; Yu Ding Standard Screen Factory, Shaoxing, Zhejiang Province).

Preparation of test sample solutions

Flavonoids   In this study, we used the sample solution preparation method for *Huangqi* described in the Pharmacopoeia [1]. One gram of sample powder was reflux heated in 50 mL methanol for 4 h. The reduced weight was then complemented with methanol and the extract was well hand shaken and filtered. Twenty-five milliliters of the filtered fluid was recovered and dried. The residue was dissolved in methanol in a 5-mL volumetric flask and methanol was added to the scale line.

Saponins   Four grams of sample powder was soaked in 40 mL methanol in a Soxhlet extractor overnight, and then reflux heated for 4 h. The filtered fluid was recovered and dried. The residue was dissolved in 10 mL water. The samples were then extracted four times with 40 mL of water-saturated n-butyl alcohol. The n-butyl alcohol–water extracts were then pooled and washed four times with ammonia solution. The ammonia solution was discarded after each wash. The n-butyl alcohol fraction was dried. The residue was dissolved with methanol in a 5-mL volumetric flask and methanol was added to the scale line. Each sample preparation was performed in triplicate.

HPLC conditions

The samples were analyzed using an Agilent 1260 HPLC system (Agilent, USA), equipped with DAD and ELSD (Agilent) detectors. Flavonoids and saponins were separated on a Kromasil C18 column (250 × 4.6 mm, 5 μm; Sweden). For flavonoids, the mobile phase consisted of acetonitrile (A) and 0.2% formic acid (B) 0–12 min, 20–37% A; 12–16 min, 37–40% A; 16–22 min, 40–50% A; 22–28 min, 50%–95 A; 28–32 min, 95–20% A; 32–42 min, 20% A. The sample injection volume was 20 μL, the flow rate was 1 mL/min, and the column temperature was 30 °C. The UV detection was set at 254 nm. For saponins, the mobile phase was acetonitrile:water (36:64), and the flow rate was 1 mL/min. For ELSD detection, the tube temperature was 100 °C, and the spray chamber temperature was 30 °C. The carrier gas was N_2, the flow rate was 1.5 mL/min, and sample injection volume was 20 μL. The column temperature was 30 °C.

Statistical analysis

The standard curves of the HPLC method, the correlation between growth rings and age, and correlations between the concentrations of the six examined bioactive constituents (calycosin, calycosin-7-glucoside, formononetin, ononin, astragaloside A, and astragaloside II) and age were analyzed using SPSS 19.0 software. The T test we used was two-sided. P value <0.05 indicated that there was significant difference, whereas P ≥ 0.05 indicated that there was no significant difference. Data of the concentration of six compounds are expressed as the mean ± standard deviations.

Information of experimental design and resources

The information of experimental design, statistics, and resources used in this study are attached in Minimum standards of reporting checklist as Additional file 1.

Results

Anatomy of *huangqi*

The typical secondary structure of *huangqi* from Shanxi Province consists primarily of a periderm and secondary vascular tissue (Fig. 1a). The periderm consisted of a cork layer, cork cambium, and phelloderm. The secondary vascular tissue was developed and included secondary xylem, vascular cambium, and secondary phloem. The secondary phloem consisted of many fiber bundles. The phloem rays were curved, with fissures close to the periderm. The vascular cambium consisted of five to seven layers of cells forming a circular line. The xylem rays consisted of two to three rows of cells and several bundle-like wood fibers were observed. The vessels were individually dispersed or gathered into small clusters of two to six vessels.

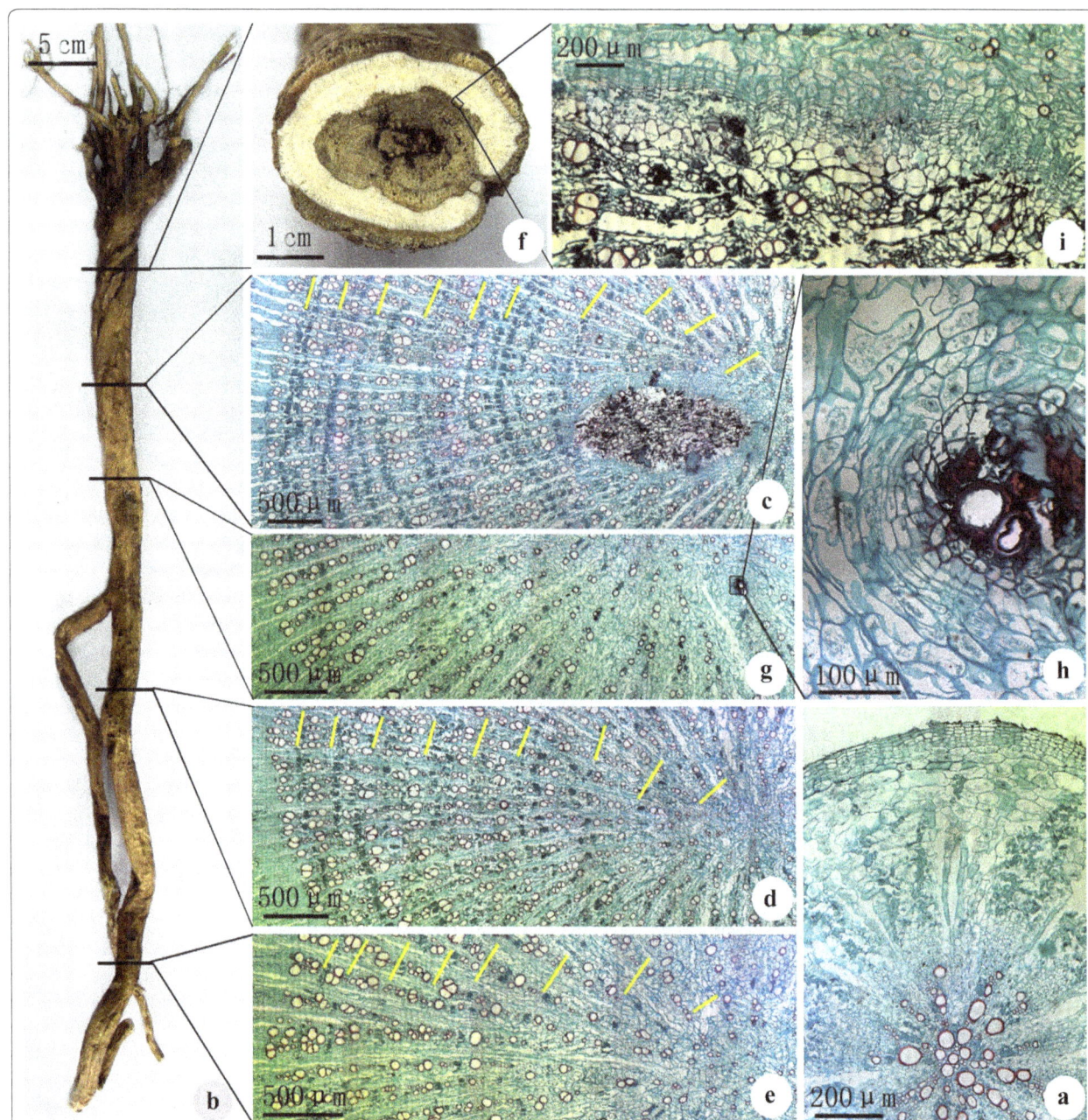

Fig. 1 Pictures of the root anatomy of *Huangqi* from Hunyuan County, Shanxi Province. **a** Secondary structure of the root. **b** Macroscopic examination. **c** Rotting microstructure in the *upper portion* of the root. **d** *Middle portion* of the root. **e** *Lower portion* of the root. **f** Cross-section of rotten heart root. **g**, **h** Early development of the rotten heart at low and high magnifications. **i** Microscopic cross-sectional examination at the junction of healthy and rotten tissue. The *yellow arrows* represent growth rings

In the xylem, clusters of wide and narrow vessels were arranged alternatively as radial arrays. The clusters of wide vessels consisted of two to six large-diameter vessels, whereas numerous fiber bundles accompanied the clusters of narrow vessels. This alternating radial arrangement of wide and narrow vessels, together with the connection of vessels arranged in a tangential direction, forms very distinct growth rings. There were ten growth rings in the zone 20–40 cm from the root-head (Fig. 1b, c), nine in the zone 40–55 cm from the root-head, (Fig. 1b, d), and eight in the zone 55–70 cm from the root-head (Fig. 1b, e). Growth rings were evident from the root-head to the root-tail of *huangqi*, with the number decreasing toward the root-tail.

Rotten heart is primarily composed of decaying root tissue, which is similar to the structure of the periderm. In thick *huangqi*, a rotten heart is typically found in the area <30 cm from the root-head (Fig. 1b, f). The circle of parenchyma cells surrounding the clusters of vessels in the secondary xylem was transformed into cork cambium (Fig. 1g, h). The cork layer extended inward, causing necrosis in the secondary xylem. The growth rings were, however, still clearly visible. The cork cambium in the secondary xylem may became inactive. However, the peripheral parenchyma cell layer was converted to new cork cambium, producing inner cork layers. As this abnormal cambium production continued, the abnormal cork layer gradually increased in thickness. This portion of the secondary xylem gradually progressed from necrosis to decay (Fig. 1f, i).

Relationship between growth rings and actual age in *Huangqi*

After staining of the transverse sections with phloroglucinol-HCl, the growth rings became clearly visible red rings. The paraffin sections showed that the growth rings were composed of large-caliber vessels. These vessels were bound by clear layers of late wood (Fig. 2), More growth rings were identified by light microscopy than by unaided observation because the innermost growth ring was barely visible with the naked eye after phloroglucinol-HCl staining (Table 1). In *huangqi* roots of less than 5 years of age, the number of growth rings observed with the naked eye after staining with phloroglucinol-HCl plus 1 was equal to the actual number of growth rings. SPSS 19.0 software was used to analyze the correlation between growth rings (X) and age (Y). The result showed a significant correlation ($Y = X$, $r = 1.000$, $P = 0.000$).

Validation of the HPLC method

Flavonoids and saponins were quantified by single-point calculation and two-point calculation (Additional file 2). The calibration curves of calycosin, calycosin-7-glucoside,

formononetin, ononin, astragaloside A, and astragaloside II all showed good linearity, with significant correlation coefficient (Table 2). The limits of detection (LODs; $S/N = 0.1$) and limits of quantification (LOQs; $S/N = 44$) for flavonoids and saponins were <6 ng and 16 ng, respectively. The performance parameters evaluated were as follows: precision, recovery, repeatability, and stability at 0, 5, 10, 15, 20, 25, and 30 h. All relative standard deviations (RSDs) were <2%.

Affect of age on the bioactive constituents in *Huangqi*

Huangqi samples of different ages were analyzed by HPLC for the concentrations of four flavonoids and two saponins (Additional file 3). The correlations between years of growth and the four flavonoids were as follows: calycosin-7-glucoside ($P = 0.88$, $r = 0.08$), ononin ($P = 0.848$, $r = -0.102$), calycosin ($P = 0.859$, $r = -0.095$), and formononetin ($P = 0.657$, $r = -0.233$). There were thus no significant correlations between these four flavonoids and years of growth. Among these four flavonoids, formononetin was the most abundant and ononin the least for the sample ages examined (Fig. 3). Concentrations of the other two intermediate flavonoids were largely equivalent during this period. However, the amount of all flavonoids, with the exception of ononin, was two-fold higher during the 2nd to 5th year of growth than during the 1st and 8th years of growth. In contrast, the roots had similar saponins concentration during the first 5 years of growth, followed by proportional decreases in astragaloside A and astragaloside II concentrations in the 8th year of growth (Fig. 3). Astragaloside A was consistently the main saponin, with concentrations >threefold higher than astragaloside II. The SPSS analysis results for the relationship between years of growth and astragaloside A revealed a high correlation ($P = 0.029$, $r = -0.909$). The relationship between years of growth and astragaloside II also showed high correlation ($P = 0.012$, $r = -0.858$).

Histochemical localization of flavonoids and saponins in *Huangqi*

Flavonoids were concentrated in the secondary xylem to a greater extent than in the secondary phloem (Fig. 4A1) compared with the negative control segments (Fig. 4A2). In contrast, saponins were concentrated to a greater extent in the periderm and secondary phloem than in the secondary xylem of *huangqi* (Fig. 4A3). Negative control segments showed no staining of the periderm, secondary xylem, or secondary phloem (Fig. 4A4).

HPLC analysis of flavonoids and saponins in the different tissues of *Huangqi*

The different tissue layers in *Huangqi* roots exhibited different compositions of flavonoids and saponins. In

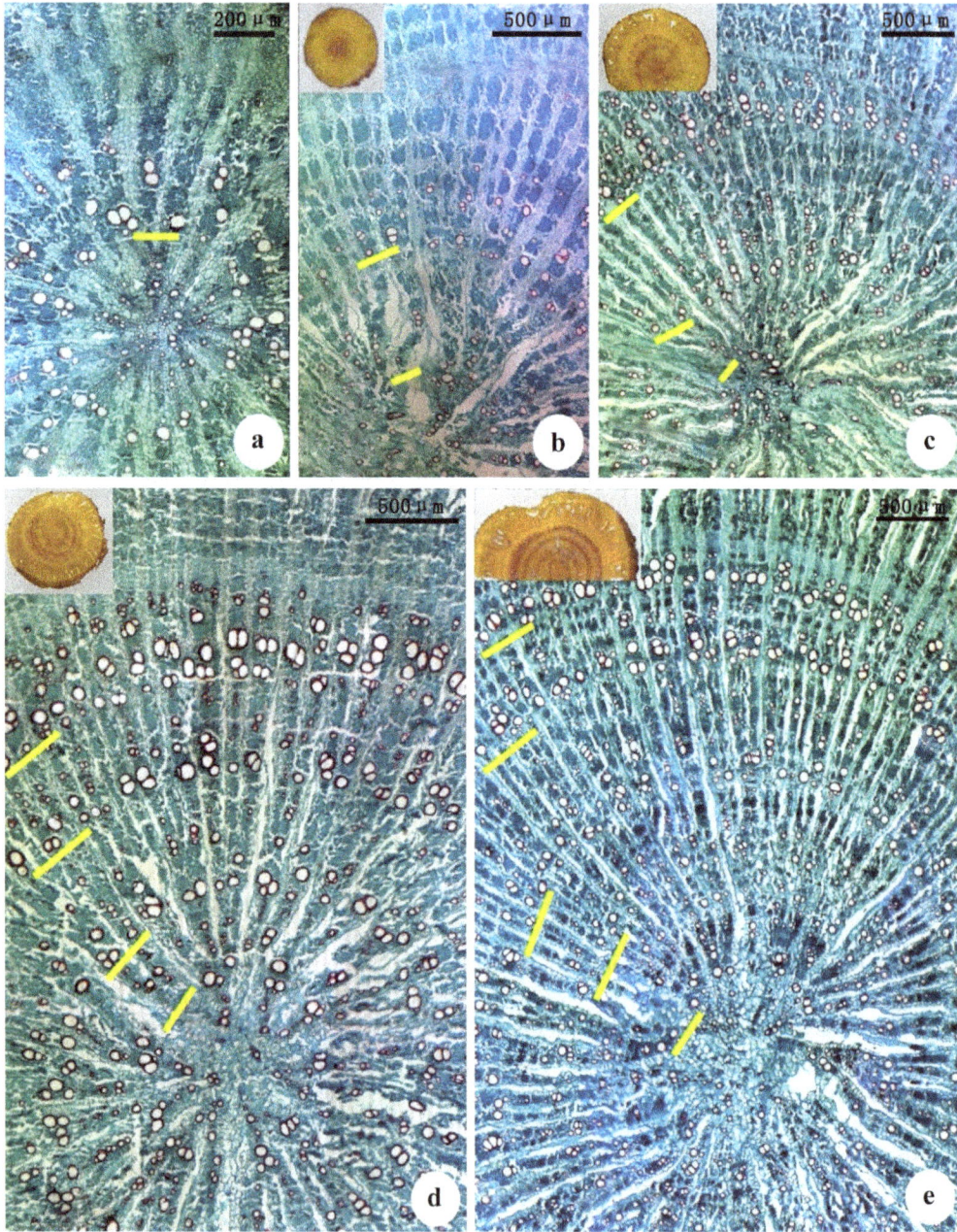

Fig. 2 The growth rings in *huangqi* from Hunyuan County, Shanxi Province. **a** Growth rings in 1-year-old roots; **b** growth rings in 2-year-old roots; **c** growth rings in 3-year-old roots; **d** growth rings in 4-year-old roots; **e** growth rings in 5-year-old roots

normal roots, the total concentration of the four flavonoids (ononin, calycosin, calycosin-7-glucoside, and formononetin) decreased toward the periderm (secondary xylem > secondary phloem > periderm) and increased toward the cambium (Fig. 4b). Ononin, calycosin, and calycosin-7-glucoside showed the same distribution pattern, with concentration decreasing toward the periderm (secondary xylem > secondary phloem > periderm).

In contrast, formononetin concentration gradually increased from the periderm to the cambium, with the highest concentration in the secondary xylem adjacent to the cambium. In the secondary xylem, however, formononetin concentration gradually decreased toward the center of the root.

In the rotten heart roots, the distribution and total concentration of the four flavonoids were similar to

Rapid identification of growth years and profiling of bioactive ingredients in Astragalus membranaceus...

25

Table 2 The standard curves of four flavonoids and two saponins

Compound	Linear regression equation[a]	Correlation coefficient (r)	Linear range (µg)	P value
Calycosin	$Y = 5273.7X - 0.7002$	0.9999	0.0795–1.4310	0.0000
Calycosin-7-glucoside	$Y = 3214.5X + 110.92$	0.9996	0.1236–5.3560	0.0000
Formononetin	$Y = 745.58X + 13.24$	0.9999	0.0924–6.1600	0.0000
Ononin	$Y = 4175.4X + 11.209$	0.9999	0.0350–0.7000	0.0000
Astragaloside A	$Y = 1.4106X + 2.3673$	0.9995	0.3054–30.540	0.0000
AstragalosideII	$Y = 1.5954X + 1.8899$	0.9996	0.4240–16.9600	0.0000

[a] For flavonoids, Y is the peak area score of analyte, X is the concentration of analyte (µg/mL); For saponins, Y is the logarithm of peak area score, X is the logarithm of concentration

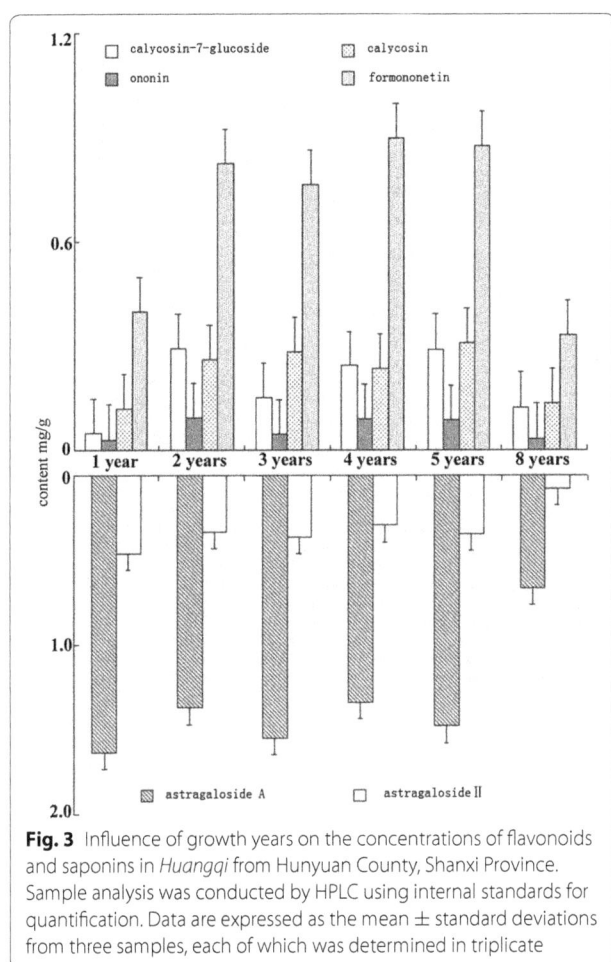

Fig. 3 Influence of growth years on the concentrations of flavonoids and saponins in *Huangqi* from Hunyuan County, Shanxi Province. Sample analysis was conducted by HPLC using internal standards for quantification. Data are expressed as the mean ± standard deviations from three samples, each of which was determined in triplicate

those in the normal roots. However, in the rotten heart structure, the concentrations of the four flavonoids were proportionally lower than those in the surrounding normal tissue. In the periderm, flavonoid concentrations were not affected by the size of the rotten heart. In normal secondary xylem and secondary phloem, the total concentration of the four flavonoids in rotten heart root was significantly higher than that in normal roots.

Calycosin-7-glucoside and ononin were not affected in the rotten heart structure; however, in normal secondary xylem and secondary phloem, calycosin and calycosin-7-glucoside concentrations increased with an increase in the extent of rotten heart.

In normal roots, the concentrations of astragaloside A and astragaloside II in the periderm were significantly higher than those in secondary xylem and secondary phloem. The total concentration of the two saponins was higher in rotten roots than in normal roots and their concentration distribution in different tissues was dependent on the size of the rotten heart. The rotten structures accumulated the two saponins (Additional file 3).

Affect of rotten heart on flavonoids and saponins in 8-year-old *Huangqi*

Total concentrations of the four flavonoids (ononin, calycosin, calycosin-7-glucoside, and formononetin) and two saponins (astragaloside A and astragaloside II) were determined by HPLC (Additional file 3). The flavonoids were not significantly affected by the development of a rotten heart (Fig. 5). In contrast, the concentration of astragaloside A in normal roots was approximately three times higher than that in rotten roots, whereas astragaloside II was not detected in rotten roots. The saponin concentrations of *huangqi* are thus selectively decreased if a rotten heart develops.

Discussion
Identification of the age of *Huangqi*

The number of years of growth and the growth region both affect the quality of *huangqi*. Hunyuan County (Shanxi Province) is the main production region of *Daodi huangqi*, which has a long lifespan. One growth ring includes one ring of larger vessels and one ring of narrower vessels. The larger vessels develop in the growing seasons (spring and summer), whereas the narrower vessels develop later (autumn). The growth rings in *huangqi* roots are located in the xylem [22, 23]. *Huangqi* from Hunyuan County has clearly visible growth rings, and

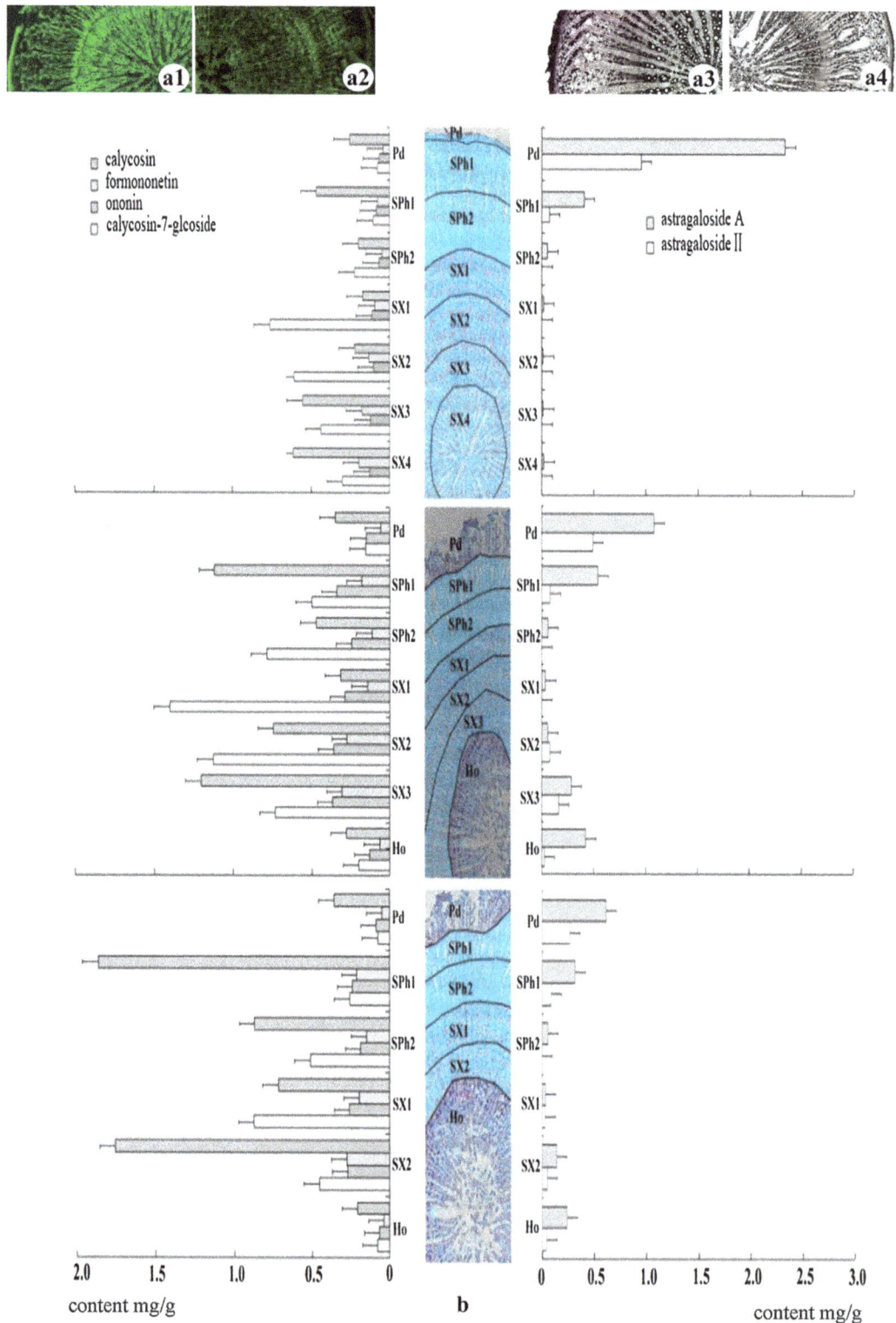

Fig. 4 Quantitative localization of the main flavonoids and saponins in *huangqi*. (**a1**) Segment stained with 5% sodium hydroxide solution compared with the negative control segment (**a2**). (**a3**) Segment stained with 5% vanillin-sulfuric acid solution or unstained compared with the negative control segment (**a4**). **b** The concentration of four flavonoids and two saponins in different tissues. Data are expressed as the mean ± standard deviations from three samples, each of which was determined in triplicate. The slices were divided into seven areas, from the outside to inside, as follows: Pd, periderm; SPh1 and SPh2, secondary phloem zones 1–2; SX1, SX2, SX3, and SX4, secondary xylem zones 1–4; Ho, rotten heart

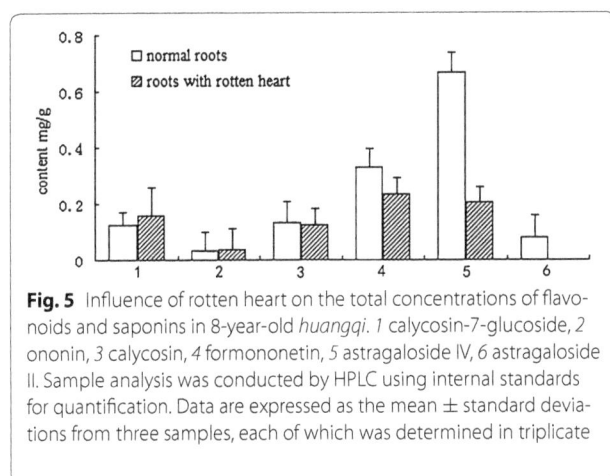

Fig. 5 Influence of rotten heart on the total concentrations of flavonoids and saponins in 8-year-old *huangqi*. *1* calycosin-7-glucoside, *2* ononin, *3* calycosin, *4* formononetin, *5* astragaloside IV, *6* astragaloside II. Sample analysis was conducted by HPLC using internal standards for quantification. Data are expressed as the mean ± standard deviations from three samples, each of which was determined in triplicate

the number of growth rings correspond to the plants' real age. For *huangqi* that has been cultivated for less than 5 years, a very simple and convenient method for determining the number of years of growth is staining of hand-sliced sections with phloroglucinol-HCl, and observing with the naked eye.

Tissue-specific flavonoid and saponin profiles in *Huangqi*

The concentration of two saponins (astragaloside A and astragaloside II) decreases toward the center in normal *huangqi*, whereas the concentration of four flavonoids (ononin, calycosin, calycosin-7-glucoside, and formononetin) showed the opposite trend. These results are consistent with the findings of a previous study [16]. This contrasting trend in concentration distribution between flavonoids and saponins in different tissues could be a general characteristic of *huangqi*, regardless of the growth region or year of growth.

Rotten heart disrupts flavonoids and saponins in *Huangqi*

In old huangqi plants, there is a high likelihood that the root-head will be hollow. The development of a rotten heart does not affect the distribution and accumulation of the four main flavonoids and two main saponins in normal tissue. However, in rotten heart, the concentrations of flavonoids and saponins were distinct from those in the surrounding normal secondary xylem. The concentrations of the four flavonoids in the rotten heart were similar to those in the periderm, but significantly lower than those in the secondary xylem and secondary phloem. As the rotten heart becomes larger, the distribution of flavonoids and saponins changed.

The rotten heart in *huangqi* is typically removed before the medicinal compounds are extracted, which increases the concentration of flavonoids but decreases the concentration of saponins. Thus, the pharmacological activities of *huangqi* may vary depending on the extent of rotten

heart, as a consequence of changes in the concentrations of flavonoids and saponins.

Conclusion

The growth year of *huangqi* (Hunyuan County, Shanxi Province) could be determined very simply and conveniently by naked eye. The content of total flavonoids and saponins in *huangqi* reached the maximum at 5-year-old. The rotten heart in *huangqi* influenced the distribution and concentration of bioactive constituents.

Abbreviations
Pd: periderm; SPh: secondary phloem; SX: secondary xylem; Ho: hollow structure.

Authors' contributions
DYP and XMX substantial contributions to the conception or design of the work. JW, HSP and MEC analysis and interpretation of data for the work. JW and HSP drafting the work and revising it critically for important intellectual content. JW, ZL, ZHT and HYD final approval of the version to be published; All authors read and approved the final manuscript.

Author details
[1] School of Pharmacy, Anhui University of Chinese Medicine, Hefei 230031, China. [2] State Key Laboratory Breeding Base of Dao-di Herbs, China Academy of Chinese Medical Sciences, Beijing 100700, China. [3] School of Pharmacy, Bozhou Vocational and Technical College, Bozhou 236800, China. [4] Institute of TCM Resources Protection and Development, Anhui Academy of Chinese Medicine, Hefei 230031, People's Republic of China.

Acknowledgements
The authors wish to acknowledge Liang-Ping Zha, Anhui University of Chinese Medicines.

Competing interests
The authors declare that they have no competing interests.

Consent for publication
All of authors consent to publication of this study in Journal of Chinese Medicine.

Funding
This research was supported by the National Natural Science Foundation of China (81573543) and the central project significant increase or decrease at the corresponding level "Rare traditional Chinese medicine resources sustainable utilization of capacity building" (2060302).

References
1. Pharmacopoeia Commission of the People's Republic of China. Chinese pharmacopoeia, vol. 1. Beijing: China Medical Science Press; 2015. p. 302.
2. Niu YG, Wang HY, Xie ZH, Whent M, Gao XD, Zhang X, Zhou S, Yao WB. Structural analysis and bioactivity of a polysaccharide from the roots of

Astragalus membranaceus (Fisch) Bge. var. *mongolicus* (Bge.) Hsiao. Food Chem. 2011;128:620–6.

3. Yan Q, Zhu L, Kumar N, Jiang Z, Huang L. Characterisation of a novel monomeric lectin (AML) from *Astragalus membranaceus* with anti-proliferative activity. Food Chem. 2010;122:589–95.

4. Yang ZG, Sun HX, Fang WH. Haemolytic activities and adjuvant effect of *Astragalus membranaceus* saponins (AMS) on the immune responses to ovalbumin in mice. Vaccine. 2005;23:5196–203.

5. Yu DH, Bao YM, Wei CL, An LJ. Studies of chemical constituents and their antioxidant activities from *Astragalus mongholicus* Bunge. Biomed Environ Sci. 2005;18:297–301.

6. Chu SS, Jiang GH, Liu ZL. Insecticidal compounds from the essential oil of Chinese medicinal herb *Atractylodes chinensis*. Pest Manag Sci. 2011;67:1253–7.

7. Luo YM, Qin Z, Hong Z, Zhang XM, Ding D, Fu JH, Zhang WD, Chen J. Astragaloside IV protects against ischemic brain injury in a murine model of transient focal ischemia. Neurosci Lett. 2004;363:218–23.

8. Shao BM, Xu W, Dai H, Tu PF, Li ZJ, Gao XM. A study on the immune receptors for polysaccharides from the roots of *Astragalus membranaceus*, a Chinese medicinal herb. Biochem Biophy Res Commun. 2004;320:1103–11.

9. Tan BK, Vanitha J. Immunomodulatory and antimicrobial effects of some traditional Chinese medicinal herbs: a review. Xian Dai Yao Wu Hua Xue. 2004;11:1423–30.

10. Wang PC, Zhang ZY, Ma XF, Huang Y, Liu XW, Tu PF, Tong TJ. HDTIC-1 and HDTIC-2, two compounds extracted from Astragali Radix, delay replicative senescence of human diploid fibroblasts. Mech Ageing Dev. 2003;124:1025–34.

11. Zhao YZ, Wang WT, Wang F, Zhao KR, Han YM, Xu WR, Tang LD. Effects of Astragaloside IV on heart failure in rats. Chin Med. 2009;4(1):6.

12. Jin M, Zhao K, Huang Q, Shang P. Structural features and biological activities of the polysaccharides from *Astragalus membranaceus*. Inter J Biol Macromol. 2014;64:257–66.

13. Zhao Z, Guo P, Brand E. The formation of Dao-di medicinal materials. J Ethnopharmacol. 2012;140:476–81.

14. Qin XM, Li ZY, Sun HF, Zhang LZ, Zhou R, Feng QI, Li AP. Status and analysis of Astragali radix resource in China. China J Chin Mater Med. 2013;38:3234–8.

15. Duan QM. Study on the biological characters of *astragalus membranaceus* (Fisch.) bge. Yangling: North West Agriculture and Forestry University; 2005.

16. Zhang YL, Liu N, Liu S, Yang SQ, Zhang SY. Comparative study on flavone chemical constituents extracted from different annual *Astragalus membranaceus*. J Med Sci Yanbian Univ. 2011;34:34–7.

17. Dietz H, Schweingruber FH. Annual rings in native and introduced forbs of lower Michigan, USA. Can J Bot. 2002;80:642–9.

18. Dietz H, Ullmann I. Age-determination of dicotyledonous herbaceous perennials by means of annual rings: exception or rule? Ann Bot. 1997;80:377–9.

19. Liu YB, Zhang QB. Growth Rings of Roots in Perennial Forbs in Duolun Grassland, Inner Mongolia, China. J Integr Plant Biol. 2007;49:144–9.

20. Yang DY, Cai SQ, Wang X, Yang WL, Tani T, Yamaji S, Namba T. Study on identification of wild and cultirated Radix Scutellariae in different growing years. Zhong Guo Zhong Yao Za Zhi. 2005;30:1728–35.

21. Zha LP, Cheng ME, Peng HS. Identification of ages and determination of paeoniflorin in roots of *Paeonia lactiflora* Pall. From four producing areas based on growth rings. Microsc Res Tech. 2012;75:1191–6.

22. Liu J, Yang H, Zhu X, Zhao Z, Chen H. Comparative study of wild and cultivated Astragali Radix in Daqingshan district in Wuchuan of Neimenggu. Zhong Guo Zhong Yao Za Zhi. 2011;36:1577–81.

23. Yu KZ, Liu J, Guo BL, Zhao ZZ, Hong H, Chen HB, Cai SQ. Microscopic research on a multi-source traditional Chinese medicine, Astragali Radix. J Nat Med. 2014;68:340–50.

24. Su WH, Zhang GF, Li XH, Ou XK. Relationship between accumulation of secondary metabolism in medicinal plant and environmental condition. Zhong Cao Yao. 2005;36:1415.

25. Kwon H, Hwang J, Lee SK, Park YD. Astragaloside content in the periderm, cortex, and xylem of *Astragalus membranaceus* root. Chin J Nat Med. 2013;67:850–5.

26. Song JZ, Yiu HH, Qiao CF, Han QB, Xu HX. Chemical comparison and classification of Radix Astragali by determination of isoflavonoids and astragalosides. J Pharm Biomed Anal. 2008;47:399–406.

27. Chinese Academy of Sciences, China flora editorial Committee. Flora of China, vol. 42. Beijing: Science Press; 1993. p. 133.

4

A network pharmacology-based strategy deciphers the underlying molecular mechanisms of Qixuehe Capsule in the treatment of menstrual disorders

Yanqiong Zhang[1], Xia Mao[1], Jing Su[1], Ya Geng[2], Rui Guo[3], Shihuan Tang[1], Junfang Li[3], Xuefeng Xiao[3], Haiyu Xu[1*] and Hongjun Yang[1]

Abstract

Background: QiXueHe Capsule (QXHC) is a Chinese patent drug that is extensively used for the treatment of menstrual disorders. However, its underlying pharmacological mechanisms have not been fully elucidated.

Methods: A list of QXHC putative targets were predicted using MetaDrug. An interaction network using links between QXHC putative targets and the known therapeutic targets of menstrual disorders was constructed. QXHC candidate targets were also identified via calculating the topological feature values of nodes in the network. Additionally, molecular docking simulation was performed to determine the binding efficiency of QXHC compound-putative target pairs.

Results: A total of 1022 putative targets were predicted for 311 chemical components containing in QXHC. Following the calculation of topological features of QXHC putative target-known therapeutic target of menstrual disorder network, 66 QXHC candidate targets for the treatment of menstrual disorders were identified. Functionally, QXHC candidate targets were significantly associated with several biological pathways, such as VEGF and Chemokine signaling pathways, Alanine/aspartate/glutamate metabolism, Long-term depression and T/B cell receptor signaling pathway. Moreover, molecular docking simulation demonstrated that there were 20 pairs of QXHC chemical component-candidate target had the strong binding free energy.

Conclusions: This novel and scientific network pharmacology-based study holistically deciphers that the pharmacological mechanisms of QXHC in the treatment of menstrual disorders may be associated with its involvement into hemopoiesis, analgesia, nutrients absorption and metabolism, mood regulation, as well as immune modulation.

Keywords: Traditional Chinese Medicine, Chinese herbal formula, Menstrual disorders, Network pharmacology, Molecular docking simulation

Background

Menstrual disorders, including painful cramps during bleeding, abnormally heavy bleeding, or not having any bleeding, are problems which may affect the normal menstrual cycle of females [1]. Recent epidemiologic studies have declared its high prevalent rates, such as secondary amenorrhea (2.6–8.5%), irregular menstruations (11.3–26.7%) and dysmenorrheal (50%) in adult females [2–5]. Clinically, abnormal uterine bleeding accounts for nearly 20% of outpatient visits and 25% of gynecology-related operations, which may seriously influence the quality of life, mental state and even future fertility of females [6, 7]. Regular menstruation is the periodic shedding of endometrium and blood from the uterus after monthly ovulation, which is regulated by the

*Correspondence: hy_xu627@163.com
[1] Institute of Chinese Materia Medica, China Academy of Chinese Medical Sciences, No. 16, Nanxiaojie, Dongzhimennei, Beijing 100700, China
Full list of author information is available at the end of the article

neuroendocrine hypothalamic-pituitary-ovary axis [8]. Any apparent changes in menstruation patterns are considered as menstrual disorders [9]. Some lifestyle factors could exert a continued influence on the abnormal bleeding of uterus, such as body weight, food habits, physical activities and delivery types (normal vaginal delivery and caesarian section) [9, 10]. Organic pathological changes including polycystic ovary, endometriosis, hypogonadism and even tumors also lead to menstrual disorders [11]. In the current clinics, there exist several medical treatment or surgical options in treating various patterns of menstrual disorders, aiming to adjust the neuroendocrine hypothalamic-pituitary-ovary axis. First-line medical treatment for menstrual disorders include luteal-phase progestins, danazol, tranexamic acid and hormone-releasing intrauterine system [12]. If medications fail or are not well received by patients, the conservative surgery (endometrial ablation and laparoscopic surgery), hysterectomy and developing molecular-targeted therapy may be performed [13]. Although significant improvements in patients' outcome have been achieved in recent years, there have been a number of potential side effects of the conventional therapeutic strategies which are used in the treatment of menstrual disorders. For example, some patients may experience syndromes including breast tenderness, weight gain, nausea, tiredness and irregular vagina bleeding after receiving the conventional treatment. Moreover, there also exist high risks of disease recurrence or exacerbation [14]. Therefore, more effective and safer therapeutic approaches are urgently demanded for the patients with menstrual disorders.

Traditional Chinese medicine (TCM), as an important part of complementary and alternative medical systems, is characterized by comprehensive medical effects and has been extensively used in clinical practice for thousands of years in Asian countries, especially in China, Japan, North and South Korea [15]. A classic literature titled "*The Inner Canon of Huangdi*" has described the origin and formation of menstrual disorders in ancient China. In TCM theory, the generation and regulation of menstruation are closely related to the functions of liver (blood storage and *"qi"* regulation), spleen (source of blood and *"qi"*; digestion and absorption of nutrients) and kidney (essence storage and the root of congenital constitution) systems. The dysfunctions of the three systems accompanying with the deficiency of blood and *"qi"*, and meridian congestion may result in the occurrence of menstrual disorders [16]. Several Chinese herbal formulae and patent drugs are extensively used for the treatment of abnormal bleeding of uterus in clinics. Among them, QiXueHe Capsule (QXHC) is a commonly used multi-herb Chinese patent drug with a satisfactory efficacy, and is prepared under the principle of promoting

blood circulation and regulating *"qi"* circulation. It consists of fifteen Chinese herbs including the principle herbs *Angelica sinensis* (Danggui, DG) and *Radix Paeoniae Rubra* (Chishao, CS); the ministerial herbs *Ligusticum wallichii* (Chuanxiong, CX), seed of *Prunus persica*(L.)*Batsch* (Taoren, TR), *Carthamus tinctorius* (Honghua, HH), *Radix Bupleuri* (Chaihu, CH), *Cyperus rotundus* (Xiangfu, XF), *Salvia miltiorrhiza* (Danshen, DS), *Rhizoma Corydalis* (Yanhusuo, YHS) and *Platycodon grandiflorum* (Jigen, JG); the adjunctive herbs *Fructus Aurantii* (Zhiqiao, ZQ), *Lindera aggregate* (Wuyao, WY) and *Achyranthes bidentata* (Niuxi, NX); the messenger herbs *Rhizoma Cimicifugae* (Shenma, SM) and *Glycyrrhiza uralensis* (Gancao, GC). Among them, DG, CS and CX excel in nourishing blood and promoting its circulation, accompanied by TR and HH to remove blood stasis [17–19]. DS, YHS and JG can activate the circulation of blood and *"qi"* to alleviate pain, on the basis of a TCM theory "when there is stagnation, there is pain, and vice versa" [20, 21]. Moreover, the herbal pair CH and XF act on liver for alleviating *"qi"* stagnation, as well as, ZQ and WY/NX combination, respectively, exert effects on spleen and kidney to reinforce their functions [22–24]. The messenger herbs SM and GC play a role in guiding the actions of all herbs to a certain area of the human body, and harmonizing and integrating the effects of all herbs in this formula [25, 26]. Growing evidence shows the pharmacological and biochemical actions of the chemical components containing in QXHC. For example, Z-ligustilide in DG, total glycosides in CS, tanshinone IIA and phenolic acids in DS, and licoricidin in GC, may exert obvious anti-inflammatory, anti-tumor and anti-hepatotoxic effects [27–30]. However, the underlying pharmacological mechanisms of QXHC acting on menstrual disorders have not been fully elucidated due to a lack of appropriate research approaches to Chinese herbal formulae.

Network pharmacology, firstly proposed by Hopkins AL, has become a powerful tool in elucidating complex and holistic mechanisms of TCM with the rapid progress of systems biology, bioinformatics and polypharmacology [31–34]. It illustrates the intricate interactions among genes, proteins and metabolites related to diseases and drugs from a network perspective, which is consistent with the multi-component and multi-target nature of TCM. The integration of network pharmacology and TCM are shifting the conventional "one target, one drug" paradigm to "multi-target, multi-component drug" strategy [35]. In recent years, our research groups have identified the candidate drug target of various TCM herbal formulae acting on the corresponding diseases using a series network pharmacology-based strategies. To investigate the underlying pharmacological mechanisms of

QXHC, we here performed a three-step analysis: (1) Predicting QXHC putative targets; (2) Illustrating a drug target-disease gene network using the interactions between QXHC putative targets and the known therapeutic targets of menstrual disorders-related diseases, and identifying the QXHC candidate targets for the treatment of menstrual disorders; (3) Validating the binding efficiency of chemical components containing in QXHC to the corresponding candidate targets using molecular docking simulation. Figure 1 depicts a flowchart of the technical strategy used in this study.

Methods
The Minimum Standards of Reporting Checklist contains details of the experimental design, and statistics, and resources used in this study (Additional file 1).

Data preparation
Chemical components of each herb containing in QXHC
Chemical components of each herb containing in QXHC were obtained from a chemistry database [36] (http://www.organchem.csdb.cn/scdb/main/slogin.asp, updated on 2014-05-05), which is specialized in storing chemical related information, including chemical and crystal structures, spectra, reactions, syntheses, as well as thermophysical data. In total, we collected the structural information of 54 components for CH, 8 components for CS, 28 components for CX, 29 components for DS, 61 components for DG, 50 components for GC, 28 components for HH, 15 components for JG, 20 components for NX, 8 components for SM, 17 components for TR, 6 components for WY, 11 components for XF, 13 components for YHS and 28 components for ZQ. The molecular files of all the chemical components were downloaded from ChemSpider (http://www.chemspider.com/, updated on 2011-12-23) and saved in *.sdf format.

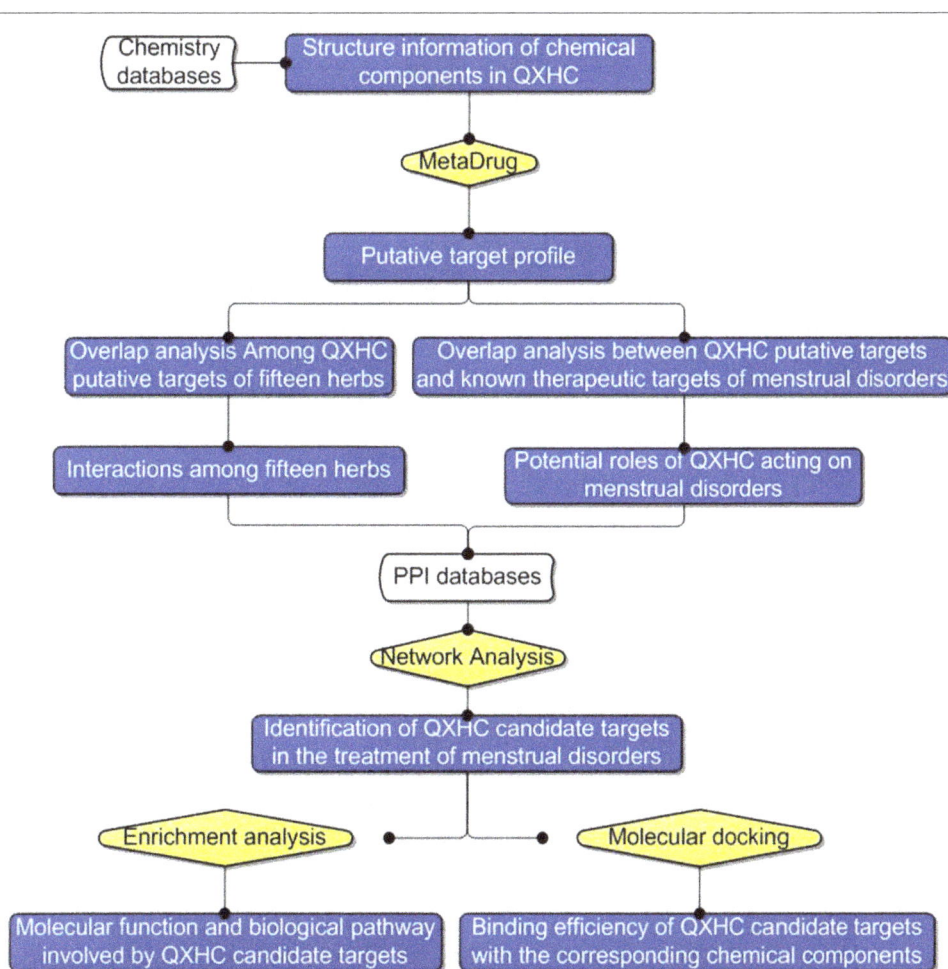

Fig. 1 A schematic diagram of the network pharmacology-based strategies for unraveling the pharmacological mechanisms of QXHC acting on menstrual disorders

Known therapeutic targets for the treatment of menstrual disorders

Known therapeutic targets for the treatment of menstrual disorders were obtained from the DrugBank database [37] (http://www.drugbank.ca/, version, 4.3). We only selected the drug-target interactions whose drugs are approved by the Food and Drug Administration, USA (FDA) for treating menstrual disorders. All target gene/protein identifiers (IDs) were converted into the corresponding gene symbol/UniProtKB-Swiss-Prot ID to facilitate further data analyses. After removing redundant entries, 37 known therapeutic targets for the treatment of menstrual disorders were collected. Detailed information about these known therapeutic targets is provided in Additional file 2: Table S1.

Protein-protein interaction (PPI) data

PPI data were imported from the following PPI databases, including Human Annotated and Predicted Protein Interaction Database (HAPPI, http://bio.informatics.iupui.edu/HAPPI/, Version 31.2) [38], Reactome (http://www.reactome.org/, Version 37) [39], Online Predicted Human Interaction Database (OPHID, http://ophid.utoronto.ca, Version 1.71) [40], InAct (http://www.ebi.ac.uk/intact/, Version 2.0) [41], Human Protein Reference Database (HPRD, http://www.hprd.org/, Release 8) [42], Molecular interaction Database (MINT, http://mint.bio.uniroma2.it/mint/download.do, Aug-2011) [43], Database of Interacting Proteins (DIP, http://dip.doe-mbi.ucla.edu/dip/, Jan-2010) [44] and PDZBase (http://icb.med.cornell.edu/services/pdz/start, 2004) [45].

Prediction of QXHC putative targets

The putative targets of chemical components containing in QXHC were predicted by MetaDrug from GeneGo, Inc. which combines chemical structural analysis tools, a structure-activity database, and a systems biology database of molecular interactions, canonical signaling and metabolic pathways, and gene-biological property associations [46, 47]. Putative targets of certain chemical components were predicted by comparing the structure of the certain chemical components to that of known drugs. The targets of known drugs with high structural similarity (the structural similarity score is higher than 0.8) were identified as the putative targets of the certain chemical components.

Gene Ontology (GO) and pathway enrichment analyses

GO and pathway enrichment analyses were performed using the application of database for Annotation, Visualization and Integrated Discovery [48] (DAVID, http://david.abcc.ncifcrf.gov/home.jsp, version 6.7), on the basis of the information obtained from GO (http://www.geneontology.org) [49] and KEGG pathway database [50] (Kyoto Encyclopedia of Genes and Genomes, http://www.genome.jp/kegg/, Last updated, Oct 16, 2012), respectively.

QXHC putative targets-known therapeutic targets for menstrual disorders interaction network construction and analysis

QiXueHe Capsule putative targets-known therapeutic targets for menstrual disorders interaction network (drug target-known disease therapeutic targets network) was constructed using the links among QXHC putative targets and known therapeutic targets for menstrual disorders. The PPI data were collected from eight existing PPI databases as listed above [38–45]. The network was visualized by Navigator software (version 2.2.1).

Then, the nodes, the degree of which are higher than the median value of the degree of all nodes in the network, were identified as hubs. After that, the hub network was constructed using the direct interactions among hubs. To identify the major hubs, 4 topological features of nodes, including 'Degree', 'Node-betweenness', 'Closeness', and 'K-value', were calculated. The definitions of the above topological features have been described in our previous studies [51–53]. Hubs, the four topological feature values of which are all higher than the corresponding median values, were identified as major hubs in the hub network.

Molecular docking simulation

Molecular docking simulation was carried out to evaluate the binding efficiency of QXHC candidate targets with the corresponding chemical components containing in QXHC using the program LibDock implemented in Discovery Studio (Accelrys, San Diego, CA). We collected all the crystal structures of QXHC candidate targets from the RCSB protein data bank (PDB, http://www.pdb.org/, updated on 2014-3-11) and selected the relatively higher resolution crystal structures with the ligands. The virtual screening protocol LibDock was used to calculate the docking scores for binding efficiency assessment. Compounds to be docked were prepared via the Prepare Ligand protocol to give 3D coordinates and confirmation. Number of Hotspots generated by LibDock was set as 100 for each case while the remaining parameters were unchanged. After docking, binding poses of compounds were assessed by LibDock Score and visual inspection to identify the correct poses. The pairs of target-component which had higher docking than 100 (the median value of all docking scores) were indicated that these QXHC candidate targets had strong binding efficiency with the corresponding chemical components.

Results

Putative target profile of QXHC

A total of 1022 putative targets were predicted for 311 chemical components of 15 herbs containing in QXHC, including 261 putative targets for CH, 78 for CS, 352 for CX, 664 for DG, 211 for DS, 286 for GC, 263 for HH, 65 for JG, 384 for NX, 64 for SM, 258 for TR, 106 for WY, 96 for XF, 84 for YHS and 188 for ZQ (Additional file 2: Table S2). Among them, 31 putative targets of QXHC have been identified as the known therapeutic targets for the treatment of menstrual disorders according to the data obtained from the DrugBank database. Among 15 herbs containing in QXHC, CS (functions as a principle herb in QXHC and plays a role in promotion of blood circulation to remove blood stasis), XF (functions as a ministerial herb, and can relieve "*qi*" stagnation in liver), YHS (functions as a ministerial herb, and plays a role in the regulation of "*qi*"), JG (functions as an adjunctive herb, and can tonify "*qi*") and SM (functions as a messenger herb, and invigorates "*qi*") shared the most common potential targets (more than 50% of their putative targets) with the other herbs, suggesting that CS, XF, YHS, JG and SM may link with other herbs more closely.

Pathways involved by QXHC putative targets consistent with the therapeutic effects of the corresponding herbs

To get an initial sense of the biological processes and pathways enriched by QXHC putative targets, we performed the functional enrichment analysis based on GO and KEGG Pathway database. As shown in Fig. 2, the biological processes and pathways involved by QXHC putative targets are often associated with the main therapeutic effects of the corresponding herbs. Especially, the herbs DG and CS have been indicated to play a role in activating blood circulation and enriching blood during the progression of menstrual disorders [17]; Accordingly, the putative targets of the two herbs were significantly associated with amyotrophic lateral sclerosis pathway, cardiac muscle contraction and various nutrient metabolic pathways, such as alanine, aspartate and glutamate metabolism, arginine and proline metabolism, as well as Glycine, serine and threonine metabolism; Herbs DS, TR, HH and CX function as ministerial drugs in QXHC, and has been found to exert synergistic effects with herbs DG and CS mainly in removing blood stasis and regulating blood circulation [18–20], in line with which, our enrichment analysis revealed that the putative targets of these herbs were involved into several hemopoiesis-related pathways, including amyotrophic lateral sclerosis, vascular smooth muscle contraction and VEGF signaling pathways; In the TCM theory, the main biological functions of the liver in human body is to regulate the circulation of "*qi*", and the stagnation of "*qi*" often leads to the occurrence of diseases and depression [54]; Interestingly, our pathway enrichment analysis revealed that the putative targets of herbs CH, XF, YHS and JG were significantly

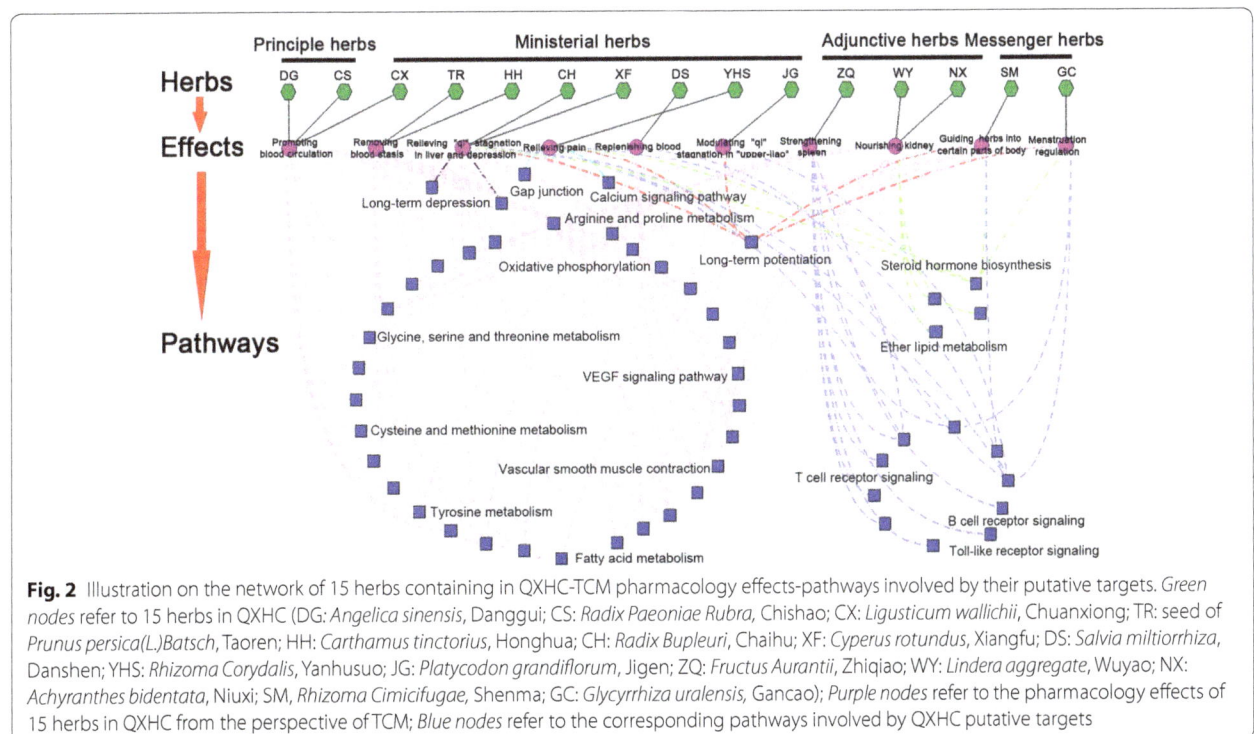

Fig. 2 Illustration on the network of 15 herbs containing in QXHC-TCM pharmacology effects-pathways involved by their putative targets. *Green nodes* refer to 15 herbs in QXHC (DG: *Angelica sinensis*, Danggui; CS: *Radix Paeoniae Rubra*, Chishao; CX: *Ligusticum wallichii*, Chuanxiong; TR: seed of *Prunus persica(L.)Batsch*, Taoren; HH: *Carthamus tinctorius*, Honghua; CH: *Radix Bupleuri*, Chaihu; XF: *Cyperus rotundus*, Xiangfu; DS: *Salvia miltiorrhiza*, Danshen; YHS: *Rhizoma Corydalis*, Yanhusuo; JG: *Platycodon grandiflorum*, Jigen; ZQ: *Fructus Aurantii*, Zhiqiao; WY: *Lindera aggregate*, Wuyao; NX: *Achyranthes bidentata*, Niuxi; SM, *Rhizoma Cimicifugae*, Shenma; GC: *Glycyrrhiza uralensis*, Gancao); *Purple nodes* refer to the pharmacology effects of 15 herbs in QXHC from the perspective of TCM; *Blue nodes* refer to the corresponding pathways involved by QXHC putative targets

associated with various emotion regulation-related pathways, such as long-term potentiation, long-term depression and neuroactive ligand-receptor interaction; It has been indicated that the adjunctive drugs WY and NX, and the messenger drug GC assist with DG and CS in nourishing the kidney and strengthening spleen for the treatment of menstrual disorders [24–26]. Here, we found that the putative targets of herbs DG, WY, NX, ZQ and GC were significantly associated with the pathways involved in the absorption and metabolism of various nutrients, including alanine, aspartate and glutamate metabolism, arginine and proline metabolism and phenylalanine metabolism; Moreover, the putative targets of ZQ may frequently play a role in immune modulation-related pathways, such as T/B cell receptor signaling pathways.

Pharmacological mechanisms of QXHC acting on menstrual disorders

From the above functional enrichment analysis, we were able to infer that QXHC could alleviate the pathological changes of menstrual disorders. Then, we asked which putative targets played crucial roles in the therapeutic effects of QXHC and how they interacted with each other. To address this problem, the interaction network using the links among QXHC putative targets and the known therapeutic targets of menstrual disorders (drug target-disease gene network, Additional file 2: Table S3) was constructed. This network consisted of 695 nodes and 4455 edges. A total of 362 hubs were identified since they had many connections with other nodes in the network. After that, the hub network was constructing using the direct interactions among hubs, and then, four topological features, including degree, betweenness, closeness and k-value, were calculated for each hub to screen the major hubs with topological importance. As a result, 89 major hubs were identified. Among them, 66 major hubs, which were QXHC putative targets, were considered as QXHC candidate targets in the treatment of menstrual disorders (Additional file 2: Table S4).

Moreover, further pathway enrichment analysis demonstrated that QXHC candidate targets were significantly associated with hemopoiesis-related pathways, such as VEGF signaling pathway and Vascular smooth muscle contraction; Analgesia-related pathways, such as MAPK signaling pathway, Wnt signaling pathway and Chemokine signaling pathway; Nutrient absorption and metabolism-related pathways, such as aminoacyl-tRNA biosynthesis, alanine, aspartate and glutamate metabolism, and insulin signaling pathway; Emotion regulation-related pathways, such as long-term potentiation, neurotrophin signaling pathway, long-term depression and gap junction; As well as immune modulation-related

pathways, such as T/B cell receptor signaling pathway and Toll-like receptor signaling pathway. Figure 3 illustrated the relationship among herbs, chemical components, QXHC candidate targets and the associated pathways.

Among QXHC candidate targets, PRKCA (for DG, DS and CH), PTGS2 (for CS, CX, HH and TR), NOS3 (for DG and NX), SRC (for DG and NX) and PRKCB (for DS, CH, CX and ZQ) were involved into VEGF signaling pathway, which plays a crucial role in the formation of new blood vessels from existing vessels [55]. In addition, PRKCA (for DG, DS and CH), PRKACA (for CH, CX and HH), PPP1CC (for DS, DG and HH), CALM1 (for CH, CX, HH, TR and WY) and PRKCB (for DS, CH, CX and ZQ), all function as components in the pathway of vascular smooth muscle contraction. The smooth muscle cells directly affect the contraction of the vascular wall and thus modulate the alterations of blood vessel lumen. The changes in vascular smooth muscle contraction seriously influences blood pressure. On this basis, accumulating therapeutic strategies have been developed to be involved into the regulation of vascular smooth muscle cells during various pathological processes [56]. Generally, the normal menstrual cycle is featured by changes in radial artery distensibility in the ovulatory phase, which may be caused by the reduced estrogen in vascular smooth muscle tone. It has also been reported that vascular smooth muscle contraction may influence the arterial stiffening in the luteal phase due to a complex hormonal environment [57]. Therefore, QXHC may activate blood circulation and enrich blood by targeting its candidate targets that were components of VEGF signaling pathway and vascular smooth muscle contraction.

Moreover, dysmenorrhea is one of the most common menstrual disorders experienced by females, and is characterized by painful uterine cramps during the menses. It adversely affects the daily life and social performance of females [1]. Among QXHC candidate targets, PRKACA (for DG, DS and CH), TP53 (for GC), RAC2 (for YHS), JUN (for ZQ), RAC1 (for YHS) and PRKACA (for CH, CX, HH and TR) are involved into both MAPK and Wnt signaling pathways. MAPK signaling pathway plays important roles in the formation and transduction of neuropathic pain and numerous drugs in clinics produce analgesic effect through this signaling pathway [58]. It is also implicated in endometriosis pathogenesis. RAC1 is essential for the integrin-induced MAPK activation and its up-regulation contributes to the activation of MAPK pathway in patients with endometriosis [59]. The tumor suppressor TP53 is down-regulated throughout the menstrual cycle and might act as molecular targets for the diagnosis of endometriosis [60]. Wnt signaling pathway is involved into the development of nervous systems,

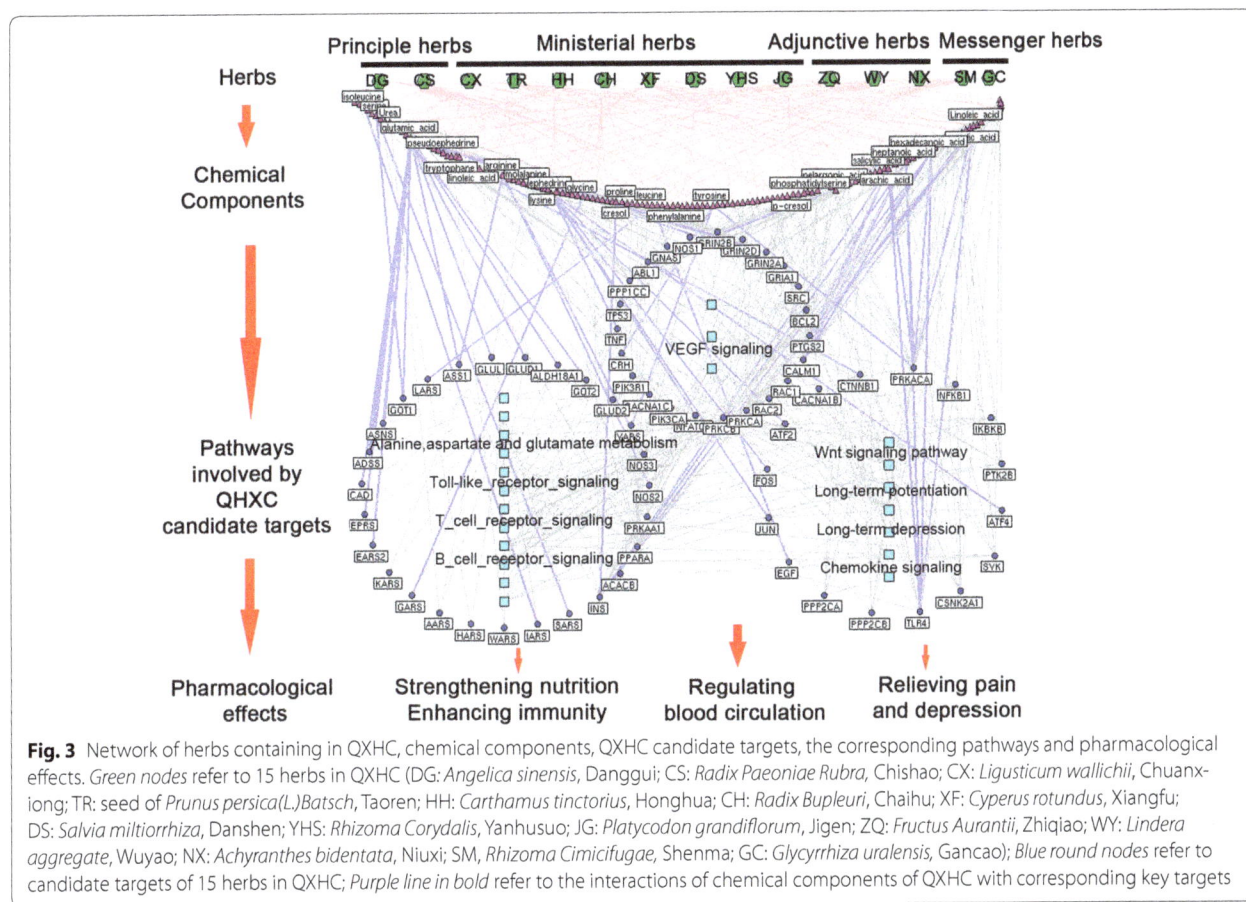

Fig. 3 Network of herbs containing in QXHC, chemical components, QXHC candidate targets, the corresponding pathways and pharmacological effects. *Green nodes* refer to 15 herbs in QXHC (DG: *Angelica sinensis*, Danggui; CS: *Radix Paeoniae Rubra*, Chishao; CX: *Ligusticum wallichii*, Chuanxiong; TR: seed of *Prunus persica(L.)Batsch*, Taoren; HH: *Carthamus tinctorius*, Honghua; CH: *Radix Bupleuri*, Chaihu; XF: *Cyperus rotundus*, Xiangfu; DS: *Salvia miltiorrhiza*, Danshen; YHS: *Rhizoma Corydalis*, Yanhusuo; JG: *Platycodon grandiflorum*, Jigen; ZQ: *Fructus Aurantii*, Zhiqiao; WY: *Lindera aggregate*, Wuyao; NX: *Achyranthes bidentata*, Niuxi; SM, *Rhizoma Cimicifugae*, Shenma; GC: *Glycyrrhiza uralensis*, Gancao); *Blue round nodes* refer to candidate targets of 15 herbs in QXHC; *Purple line in bold* refer to the interactions of chemical components of QXHC with corresponding key targets

and participants in the development of neuropathic pain after nerve injury and cancers [61]. Notably, Wnt signaling pathway has been proved to regulate the proliferation of menstrual blood derived stem cells by the trans-localization of activated-β-catenin protein [62]. It could also balance the estrogen-induced proliferation and progesterone-induced differentiation in the duration of menses [63]. These findings suggest that analgesic effect may be one of the main pharmacological actions of QXHC.

Accumulating studies have indicated that vegan diets may be a cause of menstrual disorders and thus, the absorption and metabolism of nutrients is indispensible in maintaining normal menstrual cycles [64]. According to our data, several QXHC candidate targets, such as INS (for CH, CX, DG and HH), PRKACA (for CH, CX and HH), PPP1CC (for JG, GC, NX and SM) and CALM1 (for CH, CX, HH, TR and WY), were all significantly associated with Insulin signaling pathway, which may be implicated into many biological processes, including lipid synthesis and storage, protein and glycogen synthesis, as well as cell growth and survival [65]. The defects in insulin signaling pathway often lead to insulin resistance, which is an important risk factor for metabolic

dysfunctions and other diseases [66]. Hence, our data here indicated that QXHC candidate targets were significantly associated with nutrients-related pathways for the normal absorption and metabolism of nutrients.

From the perspective of TCM, the function of the liver system is closely related to emotion regulation. Chinese herbs that can act on the liver to regulate *"qi"* circulation may efficiently improve the patients' emotional states in clinics [67]. The spleen belongs to a primary hematopoietic and peripheral lymphoid organ that is implicated in breakdown of aged erythrocytes, and T/B-like cells for antigen capturing, antigen presentation, as well as initiation of the adaptive immune response [68]. Nourishing spleen can improve patients' immune indexes and enhance their immune function [69]. QXHC candidate targets, such as PRKCA (for DG, DS, CH, CH and ZQ), GRIN2B (for HH, TR, CS, DG and NX), ATF4 (for ZQ), GRIN2D (shared by 15 herbs), GRIN2A (for CH, HH, TR, CS and DG), GRIA1 (for DG and NX), PPP1CC (for DG, GC, NX and CX) and CALM1 (for CH, CX, HH, TR and WY) were enriched in emotional regulation pathways. Long-term depression and long-term potentiation are persistent modifications of the synaptic strength that were induced by different rises of intracellular calcium ion concentration respectively [70]. In the neostriatum, long-term depression may exert synaptic efficiency by storing motor skills within the basal ganglia, and this synaptic plasticity is regarded to be correlated with some cognitive and emotional activities, which is modulated by cortical-striatal-pallidal-thalamic loops. Striatal long-term potentiation has been considered as a potential therapeutic target for various mood disorders [71, 72]. ATF4 is one member of ATF/cAMP response element binding protein family that can negatively regulate synaptic plastic and memory. Its knockdown causes profound impairment in the induction of two forms of synaptic plasticity long-term depression and long-term potentiation [73]. The mRNA expression of GRIA1 related to these two pathways were significantly decreased at the cerebellar postsynaptic density of mouse cerebellum exposed to arsenic, which is a neurotoxin that induces dysfunction of learning and memory [74].

Binding efficiency of QXHC candidate targets with the corresponding chemical components containing in QXHC

Molecular docking is one of the most frequently used structure-based drug design method and has wide range of applications in molecular recognition event analysis, such as binding energies and molecular interactions [75]. LibDock is a powerful high-throughput docking program that is on the strength of the algorithm developed by Diller and Merz to guide the molecular docking using protein binding site features. LibDock scoring could execute predictions of binding energy on the basis of the binding efficiency of ligand-receptor complexes with a high speed and a substantial degree of accuracy [76]. In the current study, a docking score is an indication of the binding efficiency between the chemical components containing in QXHC and the corresponding candidate targets for the treatment of menstrual disorders molecular targets. As listed in Additional file 2: Table S5, a total of 41 pairs of QXHC candidate targets (n=24) and the corresponding chemical components (n=21) were delivered into docking. As shown in Table 1, 20 pairs of chemical component-QXHC candidate target interactions had strong binding free energy, since their docking scores were higher than the median value of all pairs.

Discussion

Menstrual disorders are a group of female diseases with a high prevalence [1]. Short- or long-term uncomfortable feelings on females seriously impair their life quality. Increasing evidence suggests that multi-component therapeutics, which is characterized by the simultaneous actions of two or more agents on multiple targets, may be efficient in controlling complex diseases. Of note,

Table 1 Docking scores of QXHC candidate targets with the corresponding chemical components containing in QXHC

Herbs	Chemical_components	Major_targets	Libdockscores
CH	hexadecanoic_acid	ABL1	109.602
CH	hexadecanoic_acid	PRKACA	104.17
CH	hexadecanoic_acid	TLR4	100.788
CX	Linoleic_acid	PTGS2	117.673
CX	arachic_acid	ABL1	119.662
CX	arachic_acid	PRKACA	119.296
CX	arachic_acid	TLR4	112.936
DG	arginine	ASS1	107.341
DG	arginine	NOS2	106.253
DG	phosphatidylserine	PRKACA	119.477
DG	tryptophane	WARS	112.00
HH	arachic_acid	ABL1	119.662
HH	arachic_acid	PRKACA	119.296
HH	arachic_acid	TLR4	112.936
HH	linoleic_acid	PTGS2	117.673
NX	arginine	ASS1	107.341
NX	arginine	NOS2	106.253
NX	tryptophane	WARS	112
TR	linoleic_acid	PTGS2	117.673
TR	tryptophane	WARS	112.00

Chinese herbal formulae are considered to be an empirical system of multi-components and multi-targets, and specialize in treating diseases in an integrative manner. The rapid development of network pharmacology-based methods provide new possibilities to identify active multi-components and their interactions with the corresponding targets and diseases. In the current study, we combined drug target prediction, network analysis and target validation to reveal the associations among the chemical components of each herb containing in QXHC, their candidate targets and menstrual disorders-related pathways. Our main findings are summarized as follows:

1. A total of 1022 putative targets of 15 herbs in QXHC were predicted, and gave us a first glance at the investigation of the pharmacological mechanisms of QXHC acting on menstrual disorders;
2. QXHC candidate targets in the treatment of menstrual disorders are significantly associated with several biological pathways, such as VEGF and Chemokine signaling pathways, Alanine, aspartate and glutamate metabolism, Long-term depression and T/B cell receptor signaling pathway, which are involved into the major pathological processes of menstrual disorders, including abnormal menstrual bleeding, dysmenorrhea, malnutrition, emo-

tional disturbances, as well as immune dysregulation, respectively.

3. Further molecular docking simulation confirmed that 20 pairs of QXHC candidate targets and the corresponding chemical components had the strong binding free energy.

In conclusion, the current study provides a novel and scientific approach to holistically decipher that the pharmacological mechanisms of QXHC in the treatment of menstrual disorders may be associated with its involvement into hemopoiesis, analgesia, nutrients absorption and metabolism, mood regulation, as well as immune modulation. However, this pilot study was performed on the basis of data analysis, and further experimental experiments were demanded to validate these hypotheses.

Abbreviations
QXHC: QiXueHe Capsule; TCM: Traditional Chinese medicine; DG: *Angelica sinensis*; CS: *Radix Paeoniae Rubra*; CX: *Ligusticum wallichii*; TR: seed of *Prunus persica*(L.)*Batsch*; HH: *Carthamus tinctorius*; CH: *Radix Bupleuri*; XF: *Cyperus rotundus*; DS: *Salvia miltiorrhiza*; YHS: *Rhizoma Corydalis*; JG: *Platycodon grandiflorum*; ZQ: *Fructus Aurantii*; WY: *Lindera aggregate*; NX: *Achyranthes bidentata*; SM: *Rhizoma Cimicifugae*; GC: *Glycyrrhiza uralensis*; FDA: Food and Drug Administration, USA; PPI data: protein–protein interaction data; HAPPI: human annotated and predicted protein interaction database; OPHID: online predicted human interaction database; HPRD: human protein reference database; MINT: molecular interaction database; DIP: database of interacting proteins; GO: gene ontology; DAVID: database for annotation, visualization and integrated discovery; KEGG: kyoto encyclopedia of genes and genomes; ALS: amyotrophic lateral sclerosis.

Authors' contributions
XH & ZY & YH conceived and designed the experiments; ZY & MX analyzed the data; MX and ZY wrote the paper. The other authors contributed materials and analysis tools. All authors read and approved the final manuscript.

Author details
[1] Institute of Chinese Materia Medica, China Academy of Chinese Medical Sciences, No. 16, Nanxiaojie, Dongzhimennei, Beijing 100700, China. [2] School of Basic Medicine, Shandong University of Traditional Chinese Medicine, Jinan 250300, China. [3] College of Pharmacy, Tianjin University of Traditional Chinese Medicine, Tianjin 300193, China.

Acknowledgements
Not applicable.

Funding
This study was supported by the National Basic Research Program of China (973 Program, No. 2015CB554406), the National Key Technology R & D Program of China (2011BAI07B08), the National Natural Science Foundation of China (81202793) and Beijing Nova Program (No. Z1511000003150126).

Competing interests
The authors declare that they have no competing interests.

Consent for publication
Not applicable.

References
1. Kazama M, Maruyama K, Nakamura K. Prevalence of dysmenorrhea and its correlating lifestyle factors in Japanese female junior high school students. Tohoku J Exp Med. 2015;236(2):107–13.
2. Slap GB. Menstrual disorders in adolescence. Best Pract Res Clin Obstet Gynaecol. 2003;17(1):75–92.
3. Pettersson F, Fries H, Nillius SJ. Epidemiology of secondary amenorrhea. I. Incidence and prevalence rates. Am J Obstet Gynecol. 1973;117(1):80–6.
4. Bachmann GA, Kemmann E. Prevalence of oligomenorrhea and amenorrhea in a college population. Am J Obstet Gynecol. 1982;144(1):98–102.
5. Woodman J, Pitkin J. Menstrual disturbances. J Obstet Gynecol Rep Med. 2010;20(11):329–34.
6. Abenhaim HA, Harlow BL. Live births, cesarean section and the development of menstrual abnormalities. IJGO. 2006;92(2):111–6.
7. Goldstein SR. Menorrhagia and abnormal bleeding before the menopause. J BEST Pract Res Clin Obstet Gynaecol. 2004;18(1):59–69.
8. Su Y, Kong GL, Su YL, Zhou Y, Lv LF, Wang Q, Huang BP, Zheng RZ, Li QZ, Yuan HJ, Zhao ZG. Correlation analysis of the PNPLA7 gene polymorphism and susceptibility to menstrual disorder. Genet Mol Res. 2015;14(1):1733–40.
9. Nahidi F, Bagheri L, Jannesari S, Alavi Majd H. Relationship between delivery type and menstrual disorders: a case-control study. J Res Health Sci. 2011;11(2):83–90.
10. Wiksten-Almström M, Hirschberg AL, Hagenfeldt K. Prospective followup of menstrual disorders in adolescence and prognostic factors. Acta Obstet Gynecol Scand. 2008;87(11):1162–8.
11. Rigon F, De Sanctis V, Bernasconi S, Bianchin L, Bona G, Bozzola M, Buzi F, Radetti G, Tatò L, Tonini G, De Sanctis C, Perissinotto E. Menstrual pattern and menstrual disorders among adolescents: an update of the Italian data. Ital J Pediatr. 2012;14(38):38.
12. Marjoribanks J, Lethaby A, Farquhar C. Surgery versus medical therapy for heavy menstrual bleeding. Cochrane Database Syst Rev. 2016;2:CD003855.
13. Eizenberg DH. Update on treatment of menstrual disorders. Med J Aust. 2003;179(8):454–5.
14. Ghezzi F, Beretta P, Franchi M, Parissis M, Bolis P. Recurrence of ovarian endometriosis and anatomical location of the primary lesion. Fertil Steril. 2001;75(1):136–40.
15. Yao Y, Zhang X, Wang Z, Zheng C, Li P, Huang C, Tao W, Xiao W, Wang Y, Huang L, Yang L. Deciphering the combination principles of Traditional Chinese Medicine from a systems pharmacology perspective based on Ma-huang Decoction. J Ethnopharmacol. 2013;150(2):619–38.
16. Sun W, Feng XJ, Feng X. Research progress of traditional Chinese medicine in the treatment of female menstrual disorder. WORLD CLINICAL DRUGS. 2012; 12(33): 722–725. WORLD CLINICAL.
17. Wang Y, Li G, Zhou Y, Yin D, Tao C, Han L, Yue X, Pan Y, Yao Y, Peng D, Xu F. The difference between blood-associated and water-associated herbs of Danggui-Shaoyao San in theory of TCM, based on serum pharmacochemistry. Biomed Chromatogr. 2016;30(4):579–87.
18. Zhang D, Duan X, Deng S, Nie L, Zang H. Fingerprint analysis, multi-component quantitation, and antioxidant activity for the quality evaluation of Salvia miltiorrhiza var. alba by high-performance liquid chromatography and chemometrics. J Sep Sci. 2015;38(19):3337–44.
19. Lu Y, Ning H, Jiang X, Yang R, Song D, Yuan H. Metabolomics reveals hippocampal metabolic fluctuations of postoperative fatigue syndrome and anti-fatigue effect of Carthamus tinctorius L extract in rat model. Biomed Chromatogr. 2015 Nov 17. doi: 10.1002/bmc.3649.
20. Yin ZY, Li L, Chu SS, Sun Q, Ma ZL, Gu XP. Antinociceptive effects of dehydrocorydaline in mouse models of inflammatory pain involve the opioid receptor and inflammatory cytokines. Sci Rep. 2016;6:27129.

21. Zhang L, Wang Y, Yang D, Zhang C, Zhang N, Li M, Liu Y. Platycodon grandiflorus—an ethnopharmacological, phytochemical and pharmacological review. J Ethnopharmacol. 2015;164:147–61.
22. Jiang Y, Zhang Y, Chen W, Liu C, Li X, Sun D, Liu Z, Xu Y, Mao X, Guo Q, Lin N. Achyranthes bidentata extract exerts osteoprotective effects on steroid-induced osteonecrosis of the femoral head in rats by regulating RANKL/RANK/OPG signaling. J Transl Med. 2014;12:334.
23. Wang F, Gao Y, Zhang L, Bai B, Hu YN, Dong ZJ, Zhai QW, Zhu HJ, Liu JK. A pair of windmill-shaped enantiomers from Lindera aggregata with activity toward improvement of insulin sensitivity. Org Lett. 2010;12(14):3196–9.
24. Xiong X, Peng W, Chen L, Liu H, Huang W, Yang B, Wang Y, Xing Z, Gan P, Nie K. Traditional Chinese medicine Zhiqiao-Houpu herb-pair induce bidirectional effects on gastric motility in rats. J Ethnopharmacol. 2015;175:444–50.
25. Kim SH, Lee SE, Oh H, Kim SR, Yee ST, Yu YB, Byun MW, Jo SK. The radioprotective effects of bu-zhong-yi-qi-tang: a prescription of traditional Chinese medicine. Am J Chin Med. 2002;30(1):127–37.
26. Wang X, Zhang H, Chen L, Shan L, Fan G, Gao X. Liquorice, a unique "guide drug" of traditional Chinese medicine: a review of its role in drug interactions. J Ethnopharmacol. 2013;150(3):781–90.
27. Chao WW, Lin BF. Bioactivities of major constituents isolated from Angelica sinensis (Danggui). Chin Med. 2011;6:29. doi:10.1186/1749-8546-6-29.
28. Lin MY, Chiang SY, Li YZ, Chen MF, Chen YS, Wu JY, Liu YW. Anti-tumor effect of Radix Paeoniae Rubra extract on mice bladder tumors using intravesical therapy. Oncol Lett. 2016;12(2):904–10.
29. Ma XH, Ma Y, Tang JF, He YL, Liu YC, Ma XJ, Shen Y, Cui GH, Lin HX, Rong QX, Guo J, Huang LQ. The Biosynthetic pathways of tanshinones and phenolic acids in salvia miltiorrhiza. Molecules. 2015;20(9):16235–54.
30. Park SY, Kwon SJ, Lim SS, Kim JK, Lee KW, Park JH. Licoricidin, an active in the hexane/ethanol extract of glycyrrhiza uralensis, inhibits lung metastasis of 4t1 murine mammary carcinoma cells. Int J Mol Sci. 2016;17(6):E934.
31. Hopkins AL. Network pharmacology. Nat Biotechnol. 2007;25(10):1110–1.
32. Lee S. Systems biology—a pivotal research methodology for understanding the mechanisms of traditional medicine. J Pharmacopuncture. 2015;18(3):11–8.
33. Zhang GB, Li QY, Chen QL, Su SB. Network pharmacology: a new approach for chinese herbal medicine research. Evid Based Complement Alternat Med. 2013;2013:621423.
34. da Hao C, Xiao PG. Network pharmacology: a Rosetta Stone for traditional Chinese medicine. Drug Dev Res. 2014;75(5):299–312.
35. Li S. Exploring traditional chinese medicine by a novel therapeutic concept of network target. Chin J Integr Med. 2016;22(9):647–52.
36. Tao W, Xu X, Wang X, Li B, Wang Y, Li Y, Yang L. Network pharmacologybased prediction of the active ingredients and potential targets of Chinese herbal Radix Curcumae formula for application to cardiovascular disease. J Ethnopharmacol. 2013;145:1–10.
37. Wishart DS, Knox C, Guo AC, Cheng D, Shrivastava S, Tzur D, Gautam B, Hassanali M. DrugBank: a knowledgebase for drugs, drug actions and drug targets. Nucleic Acids Res. 2008;36:D901–6.
38. Chen JY, Mamidipalli S, Huan T. HAPPI: an online database of comprehensive human annotated and predicted protein interactions. BMC Genomics. 2009;10(Suppl 1):S16.
39. Matthews L, Gopinath G, Gillespie M, Caudy M, Croft D, de Bono B, Garapati P, Hemish J, Hermjakob H, Jassal B, Kanapin A, Lewis S, Mahajan S, May B, Schmidt E, Vastrik I, Wu G, Birney E, Stein L, D'Eustachio P. Reactome knowledgebase of human biological pathways and processes. Nucleic Acids Res. 2009;37:D619–22.
40. Brown KR, Jurisica I. Online predicted human interaction database. Bioinformatics. 2005;21:2076–82.
41. Aranda B, Achuthan P, Alam-Faruque Y, Armean I, Bridge A, Derow C, Feuermann M, Ghanbarian AT, Kerrien S, Khadake J, Kerssemakers J, Leroy C, Menden M, Michaut M, Montecchi-Palazzi L, Neuhauser SN, Orchard S, Perreau V, Roechert B, van Eijk K, Hermjakob H. The IntAct molecular interaction database in 2010. NucleicAcids Res. 2010;38:D525–31.
42. Keshava Prasad TS, Goel R, Kandasamy K, Keerthikumar S, Kumar S, Mathivanan S, Telikicherla D, Raju R, Shafreen B, Venugopal A, Balakrishnan L, Marimuthu A, Banerjee S, Somanathan DS, Sebastian A, Rani S, Ray S, Harrys Kishore CJ, Kanth S, Ahmed M, Kashyap MK, Mohmood R, Ramachandra YL, Krishna V, Rahiman BA, Mohan S, Ranganathan P, Ramabadran

S, Chaerkady R, Pandey A. Human protein reference database—2009 update. Nucleic Acids Res. 2009;37:D767–72.
43. Ceol A, Chatr Aryamontri A, Licata L, Peluso D, Briganti L, Perfetto L, Castagnoli L, Cesareni G. MINT, the molecular interaction database: 2009 update. Nucleic Acids Res. 2010;38:D532–9.
44. Lehne B, Schlitt T. Protein-protein interaction databases: keeping up with growing interactomes. Hum Genomics. 2009;3:291–7.
45. Beuming T, Skrabanek L, Niv MY, Mukherjee P, Weinstein H. PDZBase: a protein–protein interaction database for PDZ-domains. Bioinformatics. 2005;21:827–8.
46. GeneGo. Personal communication. MetaDrug Analysis Report. Prepared for NTP by GeneGo Inc. Tricolsan. Last updated on August 14, 2009.
47. Zhang YQ, Wang SS, Zhu WL, Ma Y, Zhang FB, Liang RX, Xu HY, Yang HJ. Deciphering the pharmacological mechanism of the Chinese formula Huanglian-Jie-Du decoction in the treatment of ischemic stroke using a systems biology-based strategy. Acta Pharmacol Sin 2015;36(6):724–33.
48. Dennis G Jr, Sherman BT, Hosack DA, Yang J, Gao W, Lane HC, Lempicki RA. DAVID: database for Annotation, Visualization, and Integrated Discovery. Genome Biol. 2003;4(5):P3.
49. Gene Ontology Consortium. Creating the gene ontology resource: design and implementation. Genome Res. 2001;11(8):1425–33.
50. Wixon J, Kell D. The Kyoto encyclopedia of genes and genomes–KEGG. Yeast. 2000;17(1):48–55.
51. Guo Q, Zhong M, Xu H, Mao X, Zhang Y, Lin N. A systems biology perspective on the molecular mechanisms underlying the therapeutic effects of Buyang Huanwu Decoction on ischemic stroke. Rejuvenation Res. 2015;18(4):313–25.
52. Xu H, Zhang Y, Lei Y, Gao X, Zhai H, Lin N, Tang S, Liang R, Ma Y, Li D, Zhang Y, Zhu G, Yang H, Huang L. A Systems biology-based approach to uncovering the molecular mechanisms underlying the effects of Dragon's blood tablet in colitis, involving the integration of chemical analysis, ADME prediction, and network pharmacology. PLoS ONE. 2014;9(7):e101432.
53. Zhang Y, Mao X, Guo Q, Bai M, Zhang B, Liu C, Sun Y, Li S, Lin N. Pathway of PPAR-gamma coactivators in thermogenesis: a pivotal traditional Chinese medicine-associated target for individualized treatment of rheumatoid arthritis. Oncotarget. 2016;7(13):15885–900.
54. Li HM, Ye ZH, Zhang J, Gao X, Chen YM, Yao X, Gu JX, Zhan L, Ji Y, Xu JL, Zeng YH, Yang F, Xiao L, Sheng GG, Xin W, Long Q, Zhu QJ, Shi ZH, Ruan LG, Yang JY, Li CC, Wu HB, Chen SD, Luo XL. Clinical trial with traditional Chinese medicine intervention "tonifying the kidney to promote liver regeneration and repair by affecting stem cells and their microenvironment" for chronic hepatitis B-associated liver failure. World J Gastroenterol. 2014;20(48):18458–65.
55. Lee HT, Chang YC, Tu YF, Huang CC. VEGF-A/VEGFR-2 signaling leading to cAMP response element-binding protein phosphorylation is a shared pathway underlying the protective effect of preconditioning on neurons and endothelial cells. J Neurosci. 2009;29(14):4356–68.
56. Brozovich FV, Nicholson CJ, Degen CV, Gao YZ, Aggarwal M, Morgan KG. Mechanisms of vascular smooth muscle contraction and the basis for pharmacologic treatment of smooth muscle disorders. Pharmacol Rev. 2016;68(2):476–532.
57. Giannattasio C, Failla M, Grappiolo A, Stella ML, Del Bo A, Colombo M, Mancia G. Fluctuations of radial artery distensibility throughout the menstrual cycle. Arterioscler Thromb Vasc Biol. 1999;19(8):1925–9.
58. Anand P, Shenoy R, Palmer JE, Baines AJ, Lai RY, Robertson J, Bird N, Ostenfeld T, Chizh BA. Clinical trial of the p38 MAP kinase inhibitor dilmapimod in neuropathic pain following nerve injury. Eur J Pain. 2011;15(10):1040–8.
59. Ping S, Ma C, Liu P, Yang L, Yang X, Wu Q, Zhao X, Gong B. Molecular mechanisms underlying endometriosis pathogenesis revealed by bioinformatics analysis of microarray data. Arch Gynecol Obstet. 2016;293(4):797–804.
60. Arimoto T, Katagiri T, Oda K, Tsunoda T, Yasugi T, Osuga Y, Yoshikawa H, Nishii O, Yano T, Taketani Y, Nakamura Y. Genome-wide cDNA microarray analysis of gene-expression profiles involved in ovarian endometriosis. Int J Oncol. 2003;22(3):551–60.
61. Xu Z, Chen Y, Yu J, Yin D, Liu C, Chen X, Zhang D. TCF4 Mediates the Maintenance of Neuropathic Pain Through Wnt/β-Catenin Signaling Following Peripheral Nerve Injury in Rats. J Mol Neurosci. 2015;56(2):397–408.

62. Kazemnejad S, Khanmohammadi M, Zarnani A, Nikokar I, Saghari S. Role of Wnt signaling on proliferation of menstrual blood derived stem cells. J Stem Cells Regen Med. 2013;9(1):14–8.

63. Wang Y, Hanifi-Moghaddam P, Hanekamp EE, Kloosterboer HJ, Franken P, Veldscholte J, van Doorn HC, Ewing PC, Kim JJ, Grootegoed JA, Burger CW, Fodde R, Blok LJ. Progesterone Inhibition of Wnt/β-Catenin Signaling in Normal Endometrium and Endometrial Cancer. Clin Cancer Res. 2009;15(18):5784–93.

64. Griffith J, Omar H. Association between vegetarian diet and menstrual problems in young women: a case presentation and brief review. J Pediatr Adolesc Gynecol. 2003;16(5):319–23.

65. Zhang J, Liu F. Tissue-specific Insulin Signaling in the Regulation of Metabolism and Aging. IUBMB Life. 2014;66(7):485–95.

66. Scazzocchio B, Varì R, Filesi C, Del Gaudio I, D'Archivio M, Santangelo C, Iacovelli A, Galvano F, Pluchinotta FR, Giovannini C, Masella R. Protocatechuic acid activates key components of insulin signaling pathway mimicking insulin activity. Mol Nutr Food Res. 2015;59(8):1472–81.

67. Yang DJ, Pan HR, Zou MF, Yang H. The influence of Chinese herbs that can smooth "qi" stagnation in liver for relieving depression and strengthening spleen on the emotion states of patients suffering from irritable bowel syndrome and its relations with cortisol. Clin J Trad Chin Med. 2011;23(10):882–3.

68. Ali A, Rexroad CE, Thorgaard GH, Yao J, Salem M. Characterization of the rainbow trout spleen transcriptome and identification of immune-related genes. Front Genet. 2014;5:348.

69. Yang B, Su YH. Relationship between Spleen in Traditional Chinese Medicine and Its Corresponding Viscera in Modern Medicine. J Anhui Trad Chin Med coll. 2008;27(1):8–11.

70. Atwood BK, Lovinger DM, Mathur BN. Presynaptic long-term depression mediated by Gi/o-coupled receptors. Trends Neurosci. 2014;37(11):663–73.

71. Calabresi P, Pisani A, Mercuri NB, Bernardi G. Lithium treatment blocks long-term synaptic depression in the striatum. Neuron. 1993;10(5):955–62.

72. Calabresi P, De Murtas M, Bernardi G. The neostriatum beyond the motor function: experimental and clinical evidence. Neuroscience. 1997;78(1):39–60.

73. Pasini S, Corona C, Liu J, Greene LA, Shelanski ML. Specific down-regulation of hippocampal ATF4 reveals a necessary role in synaptic plasticity and memory. Cell Rep. 2015;11(2):183–91.

74. Zhang C, Li S, Sun Y, Dong W, Piao F, Piao Y, Liu S, Guan H, Yu S. Arsenic downregulates gene expression at the postsynaptic density in mouse cerebellum, including genes responsible for long-term potentiation and depression. Toxicol Lett. 2014;228(3):260–9.

75. Diller DJ, Merz KM Jr. High throughput docking for library design and library prioritization. Proteins. 2001;43(2):113–24.

76. Rao SN, Head MS, Kulkarni A, LaLonde JM. Validation studies of the site-directed docking program libdock. J Chem Inf Model. 2007;47(6):2159–71.

5

Revealing topics and their evolution in biomedical literature using Bio-DTM

Qian Chen[1], Ni Ai[2], Jie Liao[2], Xin Shao[2], Yufeng Liu[2] and Xiaohui Fan[2*] ⓘ

Abstract

Background: Valuable scientific results on biomedicine are very rich, but they are widely scattered in the literature. Topic modeling enables researchers to discover themes from an unstructured collection of documents without any prior annotations or labels. In this paper, taking ginseng as an example, biological dynamic topic model (Bio-DTM) was proposed to conduct a retrospective study and interpret the temporal evolution of the research of ginseng.

Methods: The system of Bio-DTM mainly includes four components, documents pre-processing, bio-dictionary construction, dynamic topic models, topics analysis and visualization. Scientific articles pertaining to ginseng were retrieved through text mining from PubMed. The bio-dictionary integrates MedTerms medical dictionary, the second edition of side effect resource, a dictionary of biology and HGNC database of human gene names (HGNC). A dynamic topic model, a text mining technique, was used to emphasize on capturing the development trends of topics in a sequentially collected documents. Besides the contents of topics taken on, the evolution of topics was visualized over time using ThemeRiver.

Results: From the topic 9, ginseng was used in dietary supplements and complementary and integrative health practices, and became very popular since the early twentieth century. Topic 6 reminded that the planting of ginseng is a major area of research and symbiosis and allelopathy of ginseng became a research hotspot in 2007. In addition, the Bio-DTM model gave an insight into the main pharmacologic effects of ginseng, such as anti-metabolic disorder effect, cardioprotective effect, anti-cancer effect, hepatoprotective effect, anti-thrombotic effect and neuroprotective effect.

Conclusion: The Bio-DTM model not only discovers what ginseng's research involving in but also displays how these topics evolving over time. This approach can be applied to the biomedical field to conduct a retrospective study and guide future studies.

Background

The scientific study of biomedicine is very active but all of the profound results are widely scattered in the literature. The information (Additional file 1: Figure S1), the number of journals and indexed citations in MED-LINE, has been increasing at a considerable rate, so that it becomes a challenging task for researchers to keep up-to-date with relevant scientific information [1, 2]. In response, continuous improvement of PubMed Web service is made by the National Center for Biotechnology Information (NCBI) and many Web tools are developed to fulfill quick and efficient systematic search and retrieve as well as comparable literature search service [3, 4]. Furthermore, great progress has been made in text mining, a technique in conjunction with machine learning and computational statistics [5]. Except several approaches specifically for small and homogenous document collections [6], text mining approaches are designed for rapidly analyzing large quantities of literature to extract meaningful information and yield valuable insights [7,

*Correspondence: fanxh@zju.edu.cn; xiaohui.fan@outlook.com
[2] Pharmaceutical Informatics Institute, College of Pharmaceutical Sciences, Zhejiang University, Hangzhou 310058, China
Full list of author information is available at the end of the article

8]. Some text mining approaches, like CRAB [9], Spark-Text [8], SWIFT-Review [10] and other topic models [11, 12], have been successfully applied to knowledge discovery in the growing body of literature [1]. Topic modeling, a statistical solution to summarizing large archives of documents, has gained increasing attention in recent years [12]. It enables researchers to discover the themes from an unstructured collection of documents without any prior annotations or labels. latent Dirichlet allocation (LDA), proposed by David M. Blei in 2003, is the most basic topic model [13]. The primary assumptions of LDA are that words in a document are exchangeable and documents exhibit multiple topics. Along with the rapid development of topic modeling in machine learning, there have emerged plenty of exciting extensions of LDA. With the increasing interest on authorship attribution, Michal et al. presented an author-topic model (ATM) which simultaneously focused on the content of documents and the interests of authors [14]. David et al. developed a correlated topic model (CTM) remedying the limitation of LDA without the ability to model topic correlation [15]. When applied to the articles from Science published from 1990 to 1999, the CTM obtained a better fit of the large document collections than LDA [16]. Daniel et al. introduced labeled LDA (L-LDA), a supervised topic model, for addressing the problem of multi-labeled document classification. L-LDA significantly outperformed SVMs on some document collections [17]. Furthermore, many implementations for topic modeling are available. The MATLAB topic modeling toolbox brings topic modeling tools to scientists for free scientific use. Topic models and lda are two R packages for fitting topic models, but they employ different estimation techniques [18, 19].

Latent Dirichlet allocation models and other extensions are successfully used for organization of massive documents, find patterns in a large collections of information and classifying multi-label text. These models assume that the order of documents is of no great importance. The assumption is obviously unrealistic when analyzing long-running collections, such as news, scientific journals or search query commercial textual information. For someone, especially business professionals, scholars and politicians, it is important to keep abreast of tracing the evolution of their related fields, so that they can make correct judgments on some critical problems and take further actions in time. To resolve the problem, several topic models have been developed for fitting how topics evolving over time. Levent et al. proposed a generative model, called segmented author-topic model (S-ATM), for discovering scientific topics and the evolution of topics over time effectively [20]. Online topic model (OLDA) captures not only the thematic patterns but also their

changes over time even when a new set of related documents appears [21]. Another LDA-style topic model, topics over time (TOT), can summary a mass of collections and how the structure changes over time with the assumption that topic discovery is determined by both word co-occurrences and temporal information [22]. However, there is another probabilistic time series model, dynamic topic model (DTM), developed for capturing the topic evolution by grouping corpus of documents sequentially. Compared with TOT, DTM fits the models on a series of discretized time slices, for instance by date. The strong assumption of DTM is that topics at current time slice have smoothly evolved from the corresponding topics at previous time slice. It means that the kth topic in one epoch only depends on the kth topic in its previous epoch. In the field of machine learning, some promising extensions of DTM have been proposed in order to meet different needs [23–25]. These changes improve or extend the methodology. In addition, the presentation of results from topic models has become another promising direction [26]. Some tools have been designed to visualize trend analysis of dynamic topic models [27, 28].

Ginseng, one of famous and precious medicinal materials, has a history of more than 2000 years for human health and medicine in China and Asia. The traditional belief holds that various properties of ginseng, such as tonic effect, can modulate the unbalanced situation of human body. With the addition of significant effects on many situations, ginseng is widely used in traditional Chinese medicine (TCM). According to statistics, at least 3500 TCM formulae contain ginseng, which is the main form of TCM [29]. For example, in *Shanghan Lun*, a classical set of TCM formula which was compiled by a famous doctor Zhang Zhongjing in han dynasty, ginseng is not only one of the well-known herbs, it is used in nearly a fifth of the formulae to benefit many situations. To complement diets or maintain health, ginseng has gained popularity in the West over the last two decades. According to two recent national health interview surveys in the United States, ginseng is widely used as a dietary supplement and is one of the ten most used natural products among both adults and children [30, 31]. Based on the results from PlantLIBRA plant food supplements (PFS) consumer survey, ginseng is the fourth most frequently used botanicals in Germany, Italy, the United Kingdom and six other European countries [32]. Due to the popularity of ginseng and its high efficacy, many new technologies and strategies were applied to studying ginseng and more and more ginseng-related scientific articles are published every year [33–35]. Additional file 1: Figure S2 showed that the number of ginseng-related articles published every year has always been on the rise. As always, there has been a keen interest in ginseng's research using advanced techniques. Furthermore, retrospective summaries of previous studies has always contribute to great achievements in science. As we mentioned before, topic modeling has been used in medical and biological sciences [36, 37]. To our knowledge, scientific literature is the predominant resource, but has not yet been applied to interpreting the temporal evolution of research domains, like ginseng-related research. The inherent hypothesis of DTM closely matches the formation of scientific research ideas, which proceed gradually in an orderly way. In this paper, taking ginseng as an example, DTM was employed to do a retrospective study and capture the temporal evolution of the research domain of ginseng.

Methods

System overview

In this paper, a Bio-DTM was established by combining DTM and a bio-dictionary to help researchers mine the related topics how developing over time in a large amount of biomedical documents. Figure 1 illustrates an overview of our Bio-DTM, mainly including four components, documents pre-processing, bio-dictionary construction, dynamic topic models and topics analysis and visualization. Matlab (R2013a) and R (3.1.1) were used to process data in this study. The Additional file 2: Minimum standards of reporting checklist contains details of the experimental design, and statistics, and resources used in this study.

Documents pre-processing

Documents pre-processing is mainly divided into three steps. The first is to collect the target documents. Then useful information is extracted from the collection of text documents. Lastly, it needs to reduce the noise of the

extracted raw data. In the example of this paper, scientific articles pertaining to ginseng were retrieved through text mining with keyword 'ginseng [Title/Abstract]' up to the publication date at 2017/7/31 from PubMed. The title, abstract and year of publication were extracted from each scientific article. Then the document-words matrix was generated and then subjected to filtered process. In a raw article, it contains any sort of punctuation and hyphenation. So a bag of words was extracted from the original articles by removing punctuation and stop words. Then stemming process was employed to convert inflected words to their roots so that mapping related words to the same stem as far as possible. It naturally simplifies the feature space through reducing the number of words of each article.

Bio-dictionary construction

The Bio-DTM in the paper is a dynamic sequential probabilistic model for a text corpus considered as a bag of words. Thus a dictionary of biomedical domain becomes a necessity. The bio-dictionary used in this paper integrates MedTerms medical dictionary, SIDER2, a dictionary of biology and HGNC four resources. MedTerms medical dictionary written by physicians contains a considerable number of classical and contemporary medical terms. SIDER2, the second edition of side effect resource, is used to obtain names of side effects that are extracted from public documents and package inserts. The sixth edition of a dictionary of biology edited by Elizabeth Martin and Robert S. Hine covers primary terms of biology, biophysics and biochemistry. HGNC provides a unique and meaningful names for known human genes. Approved symbol, previous symbols and synonyms of human genes were all included. Considering that the Bio-DTM is based on single word, all collected terms were split apart into individual word. Just like with documents pre-processing, stop words and hyphenations were removed and stemming process was performed to optimize the established Bio-dictionary.

Dynamic topic models

Latent Dirichlet allocation, introduced by David Blei et al. in 2003, is a generative probabilistic model for text corpora and collections of discrete data. The basic purpose is to facilitate organizing and summarizing information about a large number of electronic files which users are interested in. It's the most important theoretical concept that each document belongs to a multinomial distribution over topics, and each topic is associated with a multinomial distribution over a set of words which are simply assumed to be exchangeable. At present, it has becoming more and more popular to analyze how topics evolving over time, especially in the fields of academia

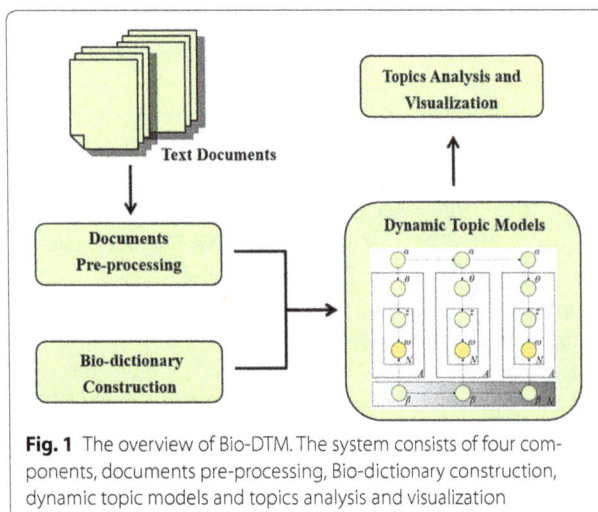

Fig. 1 The overview of Bio-DTM. The system consists of four components, documents pre-processing, Bio-dictionary construction, dynamic topic models and topics analysis and visualization

and business. A dynamic topic model, an extension of the LDA model, emphasizes on capturing the development trends of topics in a sequentially collected documents. In a dynamic topic model, all documents are grouped by time slice and the primary assumption is that topics of this time slice evolve from topics of the previous time slice.

Topics analysis and visualization

After the topics were obtained via Bio-DTM, the topmost frequent words of each topic were listed. The main research contents of topics were analyzed according to the words with the highest frequency. The evolution of topics was detected based on the probabilities of topics at every time slice. ThemeRiver [28], a prototype system, was employed to visualize the evolution of topics over time within a large collection of documents related to ginseng in this paper.

Results

Text documents for DTM

A MEDLINE format result with 5857 ginseng-related articles was downloaded from PubMed by setting the keyword 'ginseng [Title/Abstract]' and the publication date from 1975/01/01 to 2017/7/31. But only 5394 articles with available abstract were used for the study. The title, abstract and year of publication of each article were extracted from the MEDLINE result. The main content of per-article is represented by its title and abstract. The number of time-slices depends on the information of publication year. All articles fall into 16 time-slices and the first four time-slices cover all documents published from 1975 to 2005, about 400 articles per slice.

Bio-dictionary construction

The bio-dictionary used in this paper mainly includes four sources, MedTerms medical dictionary, SIDER2, a dictionary of biology and HGNC. MedTerms medical dictionary contains 16,392 medical terms. SIDER2

records 5373 side effects. A dictionary of biology provides 5492 biological terms. HGNC has 19,094 known human genes. Because of the bag-of-words assumption, all of these sources were concatenated together and were separated into single word. The bio-dictionary ultimately contains 67,696 words by two operations, stemming and removing duplicate.

Documents pre-processing

The corpus of ginseng in the paper possesses 5394 documents. Every document holds explicit timestamp and textual information consisting of title and abstract. All documents were spilt into 16 groups according to their timestamps, because DTM is an discrete-time model and there is clearly a large discrepancy in the number of ginseng-related literature published per year. Textual information was transformed into a word-frequency matrix. After documents pre-processing, there were only 5384 paper left for analysis. For every document, the DTM format includes the number of unique words qualified in the bio-dictionary, the serial number of words and the number of occurrences of these words. Table 1 shows the number of documents in each time slice.

Dynamic topic models

A subset of 5384 articles about ginseng from PubMed has been analyzed on a 20-topic dynamic topic model, spilt into 16 time slices between 1975 and 2017. Every topic has changed smoothly across time. For every topic, its topmost frequent words were extracted based on its probability of occurrence in 16 time slices. Table 2 listed 20 discovered topics and its most representative words.

Topics visualization

Figure 2 illustrates the evolution of 20 topics from 1975 to 2017 discovered from a large collection of ginseng-related articles. The river, horizontally flowing from left to right, represents the whole collection time shaft and colored currents represent topics. The changing width of

Table 1 The number of documents in each time slice

The serial number of slice	The publication date of paper	The number of paper	The serial number of slice	The publication date of paper	The number of paper
1	1975–1995	389	9	2010	248
2	1996–2000	402	10	2011	343
3	2001–2003	411	11	2012	382
4	2004–2005	340	12	2013	410
5	2006	212	13	2014	426
6	2007	206	14	2015	439
7	2008	210	15	2016	432
8	2009	239	16	2017	295

Table 2 The topmost frequent words for 20 topics after fitting to the ginseng-related articles by Bio-DTM

Topic ID	Topmost frequent words of topic
1	Renal, genom, amino, biosynthesi, clone, cultivar, yeast, cdna, athlet, polymorph
2	Stem, skin, leaf, bone, dri, phenol, marrow, stage, fibroblast, wound
3	Infect, radic, scaveng, heat, virus, substrat, cyp3a4, influenza, hydroxyl, pgp
4	Diet, muscl, cholesterol, fat, glycosid, adipocyt, ppargamma, antibodi, ampk, insulin
5	Fraction, polysaccharid, ferment, pesticid, residu, column, frg, transit, neutral, pectin
6	Strain, soil, genus, nov, warfarin, polar, bacterium, minor, dsm, genom
7	Cam, tcm, irradi, hair, radiat, sperm, exhaust, alkalin, train, contamin
8	Channel, ca2, cardiac, relax, oocyt, contract, muscl, eno, lpa, ion
9	Injuri, women, fatigu, myocardi, estrogen, ischemia, menopaus, syndrom, cerebr, ischem
10	Pharmacokinet, ion, formula, prescript, ppd, rhizom, ppt, urin, raw, excret
11	Cultiv, temperatur, wild, seed, white, embryo, genet, flower, somat, pathogen
12	Cancer, lung, colon, intak, metastasi, colorect, ventricular, pulmonari, failur, mmp9
13	Diabet, intestin, insulin, toler, digoxin, absorpt, pancreat, beta, grg1, morphin
14	Apoptosi, macrophag, nfkappab, ros, cox2, cancer, mitochondri, angiogenesi, arrest, p38
15	Transform, medium, hairi, transgen, cold, degrad, spectroscopi, biomass, ml1, callus
16	Breast, vaccin, adjuv, discrimin, prostat, skin, fingerprint, antibodi, metabolom, antigen
17	Pressur, hepat, oil, ethanol, metal, aqueous, allerg, hepatotox, fibrosi, asthma
18	Platelet, lymphocyt, spleen, aggreg, pain, cisplatin, nrf2, antiplatelet, milk, camp
19	Berri, behavior, alcohol, depress, memori, swim, ach, learn, avoid, erectil
20	Neuron, cognit, memori, hippocampus, drink, behavior, glutam, energi, astrocyt, task

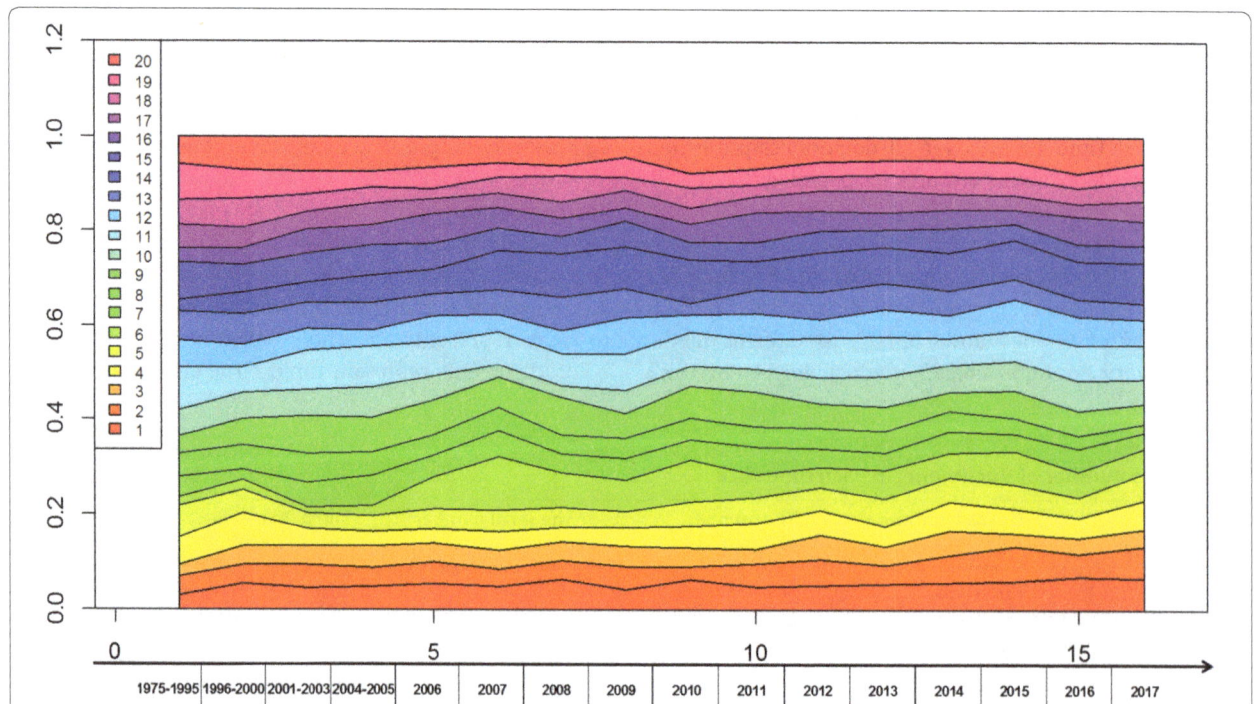

Fig. 2 Visualization of ginseng-related topics discovered by Bio-DTM. The river stands for the 20 topics and their evolution over 16 time slices. The river, horizontally flowing from left to right, represents the whole collection time shaft from 1975 to 2017 and different colored currents represent the 20 topics, respectively. The width variation of every river visually depicts changes in strength or popularity of the corresponding topic over time slice

a river visually depicts transient changes in strength or popularity of the corresponding topic.

Discussion

In this paper, we developed a Bio-DTM model by extending the DTM model to reveal topics and their evolution in biomedical literature. PubMed, accessing primarily the MEDLINE database, provides abundant biomedical literature for free. MEDLINE contains over 5600 biomedical journals from all around the world and the abstract coverage dates back to 1946. The Bio-DTM model in this paper emphasizes on bio-terms occurred in biomedical literature. A restricted bio-vocabulary was used as input parameter to measure their distribution on topics. The bio-vocabulary integrates MedTerms medical dictionary, SIDER2, a dictionary of biology and HGNC four databases, including genes, side effects, diseases and so on. Finally, 5384 articles with available abstract and a bio-dictionary covering 67,696 words are available for Bio-DTM model. All documents were spilt into 16 groups according to their timestamps and textual information was transformed into a word-frequency matrix. Textual information, consisting of title and abstract, was optimized by two restricted restrictions. One is the total frequency of words more than once. The second is that only words with a term frequency-inverse document frequency (tf-idf) a bit more than the first quartile were included. Tf-idf reflects how important a word is to a document in a corpus by a method of numerical statistic. So the second restriction allows to elide words which have low frequency as well as those occurring in many documents.

Twenty topics have been discovered from the large collection of ginseng-related articles and the most representative words of every topic were list in Table 2. Topic 1 focuses on the landscape, such as ginsenoside biosynthesis, physiological traits, polymorphism, of ginseng or the differences among ginseng cultivars by genomic and transcriptomic studies. Topic 6 reminded that the cultivation of ginseng is one of the major research fields of ginseng. The research contents of topic 9 mainly involved in the application of ginseng in dietary supplements, complementary and integrative health practices. Based on the content of topic 10, it is primarily on pharmacokinetics of ginseng and Chinese herbal formulae containing ginseng. Besides, the Bio-DTM model gave us insight into the main pharmacologic effects of ginseng, like anti-aging effect (topic 2), immunomodulatory activity (topic 3), anti-metabolic disorder effect (topic 4), cardioprotective effect (topic 8), anti-cancer effect (topic 12), anti-diabetic activity (topic 13), anti-inflammatory and anti-apoptosis activities (topic 14), hepatoprotective effect (topic 17), anti-thrombotic effect (topic 18), anti-depressive effect (topic 19) and neuroprotective effect (Topic 20).

To better display how topics change over time, ThemeRiver, a prototype system, was employed to visualize topic variations over time. Figure 2 illustrates the evolution of 20 topics from 1975 to 2017 discovered from a large collection of ginseng-related articles. The river horizontally flows from left to right, which represents the whole collection time shaft. Each colored current represents one topic. The changing width of a river visually depicts changes in strength or popularity of the corresponding topic.

The width variation of each current reflects the matching topic strength at each time slice. For example, in Fig. 2 the topic 9 increases the relative popularity in the early twentieth century as indicated by broadening the spring green current. As shown in Fig. 3a, c, topic 9 showed that ginseng was used for dietary supplements, complementary and integrative health practices. Under the condition of legislative favors, in 1999, the National Center for Complementary and Alternative Medicine (NCCAM), a division of the National Institutes of Health (NIH), had been established to explore complementary and alternative healing practices in the context of rigorous science. According to NIH state-of-the-science conference statement on management of menopause-related symptoms in 2005, ginseng may be favorable for some menopausal symptoms, such as daily mood symptoms and sleep disturbances, and with one's overall sense of well-being [38]. According to the 2002 National Health Interview Survey, 19% of adults took natural products and ginseng was the second most commonly used natural products [39]. While in 2007, 17.7% of American adults took natural products and ginseng came in fifth follow after fish oil/omega 3/DHA, glucosamine, echinacea and flaxseed oil or pills [40]. Moreover, in the light of nutraceutical guidelines for endocrine practice in 2003, ginseng is one of dietary supplements and nutraceuticals used in functional medicine for stress and menopause conditions [41]. These all contribute to the popularity of topic 9 in the beginning of the twentieth century.

From Fig. 3b, d, it is obvious that topic 6 mainly has with respect to the planting of ginseng, especially symbiosis and allelopathy. The width variation of this topic in the Fig. 2 reflect that it has become stronger since the mid-twentieth century. In the past for a long time, people had to cut forest to cultivate ginseng because of the unable successively cultivation. Aiming at improving ecological conditions, the Chinese government initiated the Natural Forest Protection Program and the Slope Land Conversion Program in the twentieth century [42]. The ecological rehabilitation projects not only protect existing natural forests from excessive cutting but also plan to restore natural forests in particular in ecologically sensitive areas [43]. Therefore, research of growing

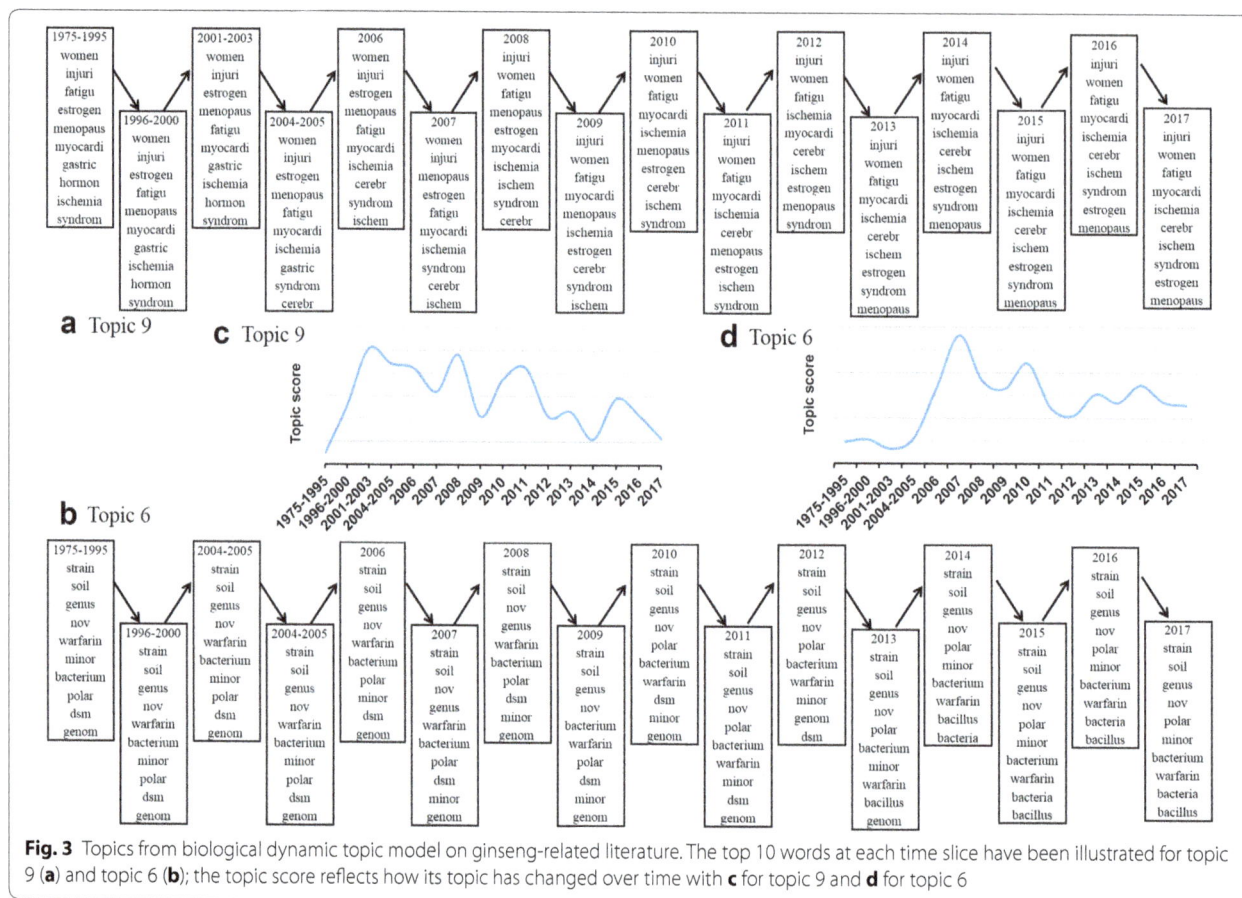

Fig. 3 Topics from biological dynamic topic model on ginseng-related literature. The top 10 words at each time slice have been illustrated for topic 9 (**a**) and topic 6 (**b**); the topic score reflects how its topic has changed over time with **c** for topic 9 and **d** for topic 6

and cultivation on ginseng should be enhanced and it needs to make the fullest use of each part of the plant, such as leaf, flower and stem [44, 45]. To obtain high-quality ginseng and improve the productivity of ginseng, the research highlights have been turned to endophytic microorganisms and allelopathy [46, 47]. There are many reports on endophytes in ginseng and their roles, such as plant growth promotion and antifungal activity [48, 49]. As shown in Fig. 3d, the content of topic 6 became a research hotspot in 2007.

Conclusion

In this paper, we have employed the Bio-DTM to model the evolution of ginseng-related topics. The main advantage is that the inherent hypothesis of DTM, that topics supposed to evolve smoothly from their previous state, closely matches the formation of scientific research ideas. The DTM model not only discovers what ginseng's research is involving in but also displays how these top-ics have evolved over time. This approach is well-suited for conducting a retrospective study as well as has a wide application in biomedical field.

Abbreviations
DTM: dynamic topic model; LDA: latent Dirichlet allocation; TOT: topics over time; tf–idf: term frequency–inverse document frequency; L-LDA: labeled latent Dirichlet allocation; CTM: correlated topic model.

Authors' contributions
XF and QC conceived and designed the study. QC, XS and JL collected and checked the data. QC and NA performed the study and analyzed the data. JL and YL realized visualization. QC and NA wrote the manuscript text. All authors read and approved the final manuscript.

Author details
[1] School of Pharmaceutical Sciences, Wenzhou Medical University, Wenzhou 325035, China. [2] Pharmaceutical Informatics Institute, College of Pharmaceutical Sciences, Zhejiang University, Hangzhou 310058, China.

Acknowledgements
Not applicable.

Competing interests
The authors declare that they have no competing interests.

Consent for publication
Not applicable.

Funding
This work was financially supported by the National Project for TCM Standardi-
zation (No. ZYBZH-C-ZJ-60), the National Natural Science Foundation of China
(No. 81373893) and the National youth top-notch talent support program.

References
1. Rebholz-Schuhmann D, Oellrich A, Hoehndorf R. Text-mining solutions for biomedical research: enabling integrative biology. Nat Rev Genet. 2012;13:829–39.
2. Fleuren WW, Alkema W. Application of text mining in the biomedical domain. Methods. 2015;74:97–106.
3. Lu Z. PubMed and beyond: a survey of web tools for searching biomedi-cal literature. Database. 2011;2011:baq036.
4. Wildgaard LE, Wildgaard LE, Lund H, Lund H. Advancing PubMed? A comparison of third-party PubMed/Medline tools. Libr Hi Tech. 2016;34:669–84.
5. Allahyari M, Pouriyeh S, Assefi M, Safaei S, Trippe ED, Gutierrez JB, et al. A brief survey of text mining: classification, clustering and extraction techniques. arXiv preprint arXiv:1707.02919. 2017.
6. Yeganova L, Kim W, Kim S, Wilbur WJ. Retro: concept-based clustering of biomedical topical sets. Bioinformatics. 2014;30:3240–8.
7. Holzinger A, Schantl J, Schroettner M, Seifert C, Verspoor K. Biomedical text mining: state-of-the-art, open problems and future challenges. In: Interactive knowledge discovery and data mining in biomedical infor-matics. Berlin: Springer; 2014. p. 271–300.
8. Ye Z, Tafti AP, He KY, Wang K, He MM. Sparktext: biomedical text mining on big data framework. PLoS ONE. 2016;11:e0162721.
9. Guo Y, Séaghdha DO, Silins I, Sun L, Högberg J, Stenius U, et al. CRAB 2.0: a text mining tool for supporting literature review in chemical cancer risk assessment. In: COLING (Demos); 2014. p. 76–80.
10. Howard BE, Phillips J, Miller K, Tandon A, Mav D, Shah MR, et al. SWIFT-Review: a text-mining workbench for systematic review. Syst Rev. 2016;5:87.
11. Altena AJ, Moerland PD, Zwinderman AH, Olabarriaga SD. Understand-ing big data themes from scientific biomedical literature through topic modeling. J Big Data. 2016;3:23.
12. Liu L, Tang L, Dong W, Yao S, Zhou W. An overview of topic modeling and its current applications in bioinformatics. SpringerPlus. 2016;5:1608.
13. Blei DM, Ng AY, Jordan MI. Latent dirichlet allocation. J Mach Learn Res. 2003;3:993–1022.
14. Rosen-Zvi M, Griffiths T, Steyvers M, Smyth P. The author-topic model for authors and documents. In: Proceedings of the 20th conference on uncertainty in artificial intelligence. Banff, Canada: AUAI Press; 2004. p. 487–94.
15. Blei DM, Lafferty JD. Correlated topic models. In: Advances in neural information processing systems; 2005. p. 113–20.
16. Blei DM, Lafferty JD. A correlated topic model of science. Ann Appl Stat. 2007;1:17–35.
17. Ramage D, Hall D, Nallapati R, Manning CD. Labeled LDA. A supervised topic model for credit attribution in multi-labeled corpora. In: Proceed-ings of the 2009 conference on empirical methods in natural language processing: Volume 1-Volume 1. Singapore: Association for Computa-tional Linguistics; 2009. p. 248–56.
18. Grün B, Hornik K. topicmodels: an R package for fitting topic models. J Stat Softw. 2011;40:1–30.
19. Chang J. lda: collapsed Gibbs sampling methods for topic models. R Package 'lda'; 2015. https://cran.r-project.org/web/packages/lda/lda.pdf.
20. Bolelli L, Ertekin Ş, Giles CL. Topic and trend detection in text collections using latent dirichlet allocation. In: Boughanem M, Berrut C, Mothe J, Soule-Dupuy C, editors. Advances in information retrieval. Heidelberg: Springer; 2009. p. 776–80.
21. AlSumait L, Barbará D, Domeniconi C. On-line lda: adaptive topic models for mining text streams with applications to topic detection and tracking. In: Data mining, 2008 ICDM '08 eighth IEEE international conference on: IEEE; 2008. p. 3–12.
22. Wang X, McCallum A. Topics over time: a non-Markov continuous-time model of topical trends. In: Proceedings of the 12th ACM SIGKDD interna-tional conference on knowledge discovery and data mining. Philadel-phia, PA, USA: ACM; 2006. p. 424–33.
23. Takahashi Y, Utsuro T, Yoshioka M, Kando N, Fukuhara T, Nakagawa H, et al. Applying a burst model to detect bursty topics in a topic model. In: Isahara H, Kanzaki K, editors. Advances in natural language processing. Heidelberg: Springer; 2012. p. 239–49.
24. Zhang X, Wang T. Topic tracking with dynamic topic model and topic-based weighting method. J Softw. 2010;5:482–9.
25. Tang S, Zhang Y, Wang H, Chen M, Wu F, Zhuang Y. The discovery of burst topic and its intermittent evolution in our real world. China Commun. 2013;10:1–12.
26. Liu S, Zhou MX, Pan S, Song Y, Qian W, Cai W, et al. Tiara: interactive, topic-based visual text summarization and analysis. ACM Trans Intell Syst Technol. 2012;3:25.
27. Günnemann N, Derntl M, Klamma R, Jarke M. An interactive system for visual analytics of dynamic topic models. Datenbank-Spektrum. 2013;13:213–23.
28. Havre S, Hetzler B, Nowell L. ThemeRiver: visualizing theme changes over time. In: IEEE symposium on information visualization 2000 INFOVIS 2000 Proceedings. Salt Lake City, UT: IEEE; 2000. p. 115–23.
29. Song C, editor. A set of Chinese formulae with ginseng. Beijing: China Medical Science Press; 2006.
30. Clarke TC, Black LI, Stussman BJ, Barnes PM, Nahin RL. Trends in the use of complementary health approaches among adults: United States, 2002–2012. Natl Health Stat Rep. 2015;79:1–16.
31. Black LI, Clarke TC, Barnes PM, Stussman BJ, Nahin RL. Use of complemen-tary health approaches among children aged 4–17 years in the United States: National Health Interview Survey, 2007–2012. Natl Health Stat Rep. 2015;78:1–19.
32. Garcia-Alvarez A, Egan B, de Klein S, Dima L, Maggi FM, Isoniemi M, et al. Usage of plant food supplements across six European countries: findings from the PlantLIBRA consumer survey. PLoS ONE. 2014;9:e92265.
33. Lo Y-T, Li M, Shaw P-C. Identification of constituent herbs in ginseng decoctions by DNA markers. Chin Med. 2015;10:1.
34. Lee YS, Park H-S, Lee D-K, Jayakodi M, Kim N-H, Koo HJ, et al. Integrated transcriptomic and metabolomic analysis of five *Panax ginseng* cultivars reveals the dynamics of ginsenoside biosynthesis. Front Plant Sci. 2017;8:1048.
35. Lee M-H, Rhee Y-K, Choi S-Y, Cho C-W, Hong H-D, Kim K-T. Quality and characteristics of fermented ginseng seed oil based on bacterial strain and extraction method. J Ginseng Res. 2017;41:428–33.
36. Rider AK, Chawla NV. An ensemble topic model for sharing healthcare data and predicting disease risk. In: Proceedings of the international conference on bioinformatics, computational biology and biomedical informatics. Washington DC, USA: ACM; 2013. p. 333–40.
37. Bisgin H, Liu Z, Kelly R, Fang H, Xu X, Tong W. Investigating drug reposi-tioning opportunities in FDA drug labels through topic modeling. BMC Bioinform. 2012;13:S6.
38. Anonymous. NIH State-of-the-Science Conference Statement on man-agement of menopause-related symptoms. NIH consensus and state-of-the-science statements; 2005. p. 1–38.
39. Barnes PM, Powell-Griner E, McFann K, Nahin RL. Complementary and alternative medicine use among adults: United States, 2002. In: Seminars in integrative medicine. Amsterdam: Elsevier; 2004. p. 54–71.
40. Barnes P, Bloom B, Nahin R. Complementary and alternative medicine use among adults and children: united States. Natl Health Stat Rep. 2007;2008:1–23.
41. Mechanick JI, Brett EM, Chausmer AB, Dickey RA, Wallach S. American Association of Clinical Endocrinologists medical guidelines for the clinical use of dietary supplements and nutraceuticals. Endocr Pract.

2003;9:417–70.

42. Junfei M, Changhe L, Bohua Y. Impacts of sloping land conversion program on the vegetation in loess hilly and gully area of northern Shaanxi. Ecol Econ. 2009;5:160–7.

43. Yin R, Xu J, Li Z, Liu C. China's ecological rehabilitation: the unprecedented efforts and dramatic impacts of reforestation and slope protection in western China. China Environ Ser. 2005;6:17–32.

44. Wu J, Basila D. Antihyperglycemic effects of total ginsenosides from leaves and stem of *Panax ginseng*. Acta Pharmacol Sin. 2005;26:1104–10.

45. Shi W, Wang Y, Li J, Zhang H, Ding L. Investigation of ginsenosides in different parts and ages of *Panax ginseng*. Food Chem. 2007;102:664–8.

46. CHEN C-B, LIU J-Y, WANG Y-Y, YAN S, XU S-Q. Allelopathy of Ginseng Rhizosphere and its effect on germination of seed. J Jilin Agric Univ. 2006;5:014.

47. Bernards MA, Yousef LF, Nicol RW. The allelopathic potential of ginsenosides. Allelochemicals: biological control of plant pathogens and diseases. Berlin: Springer; 2006. p. 157–75.

48. Vendan RT, Yu YJ, Lee SH, Rhee YH. Diversity of endophytic bacteria in ginseng and their potential for plant growth promotion. J Microbiol. 2010;48:559–65.

49. Cho KM, Hong SY, Lee SM, Kim YH, Kahng GG, Lim YP, et al. Endophytic bacterial communities in ginseng and their antifungal activity against pathogens. Microb Ecol. 2007;54:341–51.

6

Glossogyne tenuifolia (Hsiang-ju) extract suppresses T cell activation by inhibiting activation of c-Jun N-terminal kinase

Jer-Yiing Houng[1†], Tzong-Shyuan Tai[2,3†], Shu-Ching Hsu[4,5], Hsia-Fen Hsu[1], Tzann-Shun Hwang[6], Chih-Jiun Lin[7] and Li-Wen Fang[1*]

Abstract

Background: *Glossogyne tenuifolia* (GT) (*Hsiang-ju*) is a Chinese herbal medicine previously exhibited an anti-inflammatory activity. This study aimed to investigate the effect of GT ethanol extract (GTE) on T cell-mediated adaptive immunity.

Methods: Human peripheral blood mononuclear cells (PBMCs) and Jurkat T cells were activated by phytohemagglutinin in the presence of various doses (3.13–50 μg/mL) of GTE. The effect of GTE on T cell activation was examined by a proliferation assay of activated PBMCs and the level of the activation marker CD69 on the surface of activated Jurkat T cells. Apoptosis was determined by propidium iodide staining in hypotonic solution. Signaling pathway molecules were assessed by western blotting.

Results: *Glossogyne tenuifolia* ethanol extract was demonstrated to inhibit T cell activation, not only in the proliferation of human PBMCs at the concentrations of 12.5, 25 and 50 μg/mL ($P = 0.0118, 0.0030$ and 0.0021) but also in the CD69 expression in Jurkat cells, which was not due to the cytotoxicity of GTE. The presence of GTE did not change the activity of nuclear factor kappa-light-chain-enhancer of activated B cells or extracellular signal-regulated kinase upon T cell activation. In addition, GTE significantly reduced activation of c-Jun N-terminal kinase (JNK) ($P = 0.0167$) and p38 ($P = 0.0278$). Furthermore, decreased JNK activation mediated the preventive effect of GTE on T cell activation-induced cell death (AICD).

Conclusion: *Glossogyne tenuifolia* ethanol extract inhibited T cell activation of Jurkat cells and freshly prepared human PBMCs due to suppression of JNK activity. Furthermore, GTE inhibited AICD by blocking prolonged JNK phosphorylation in activated T cells. Taken together, the anti-inflammatory effects exerted by GTE were mediated via suppression of JNK phosphorylation in T cell activation.

Background

Inflammation is a normal host defense mechanism against infection, involving not only innate but also adaptive immunity. However, uncontrolled inflammation may lead to tissue damage and cause autoimmune or autoinflammatory diseases. In autoinflammatory diseases, such as type 2 diabetes and obesity, macrophages in innate immunity become dysfunctional [1]. In contrast, autoimmune diseases, such as rheumatoid arthritis, inflammatory bowel disease, type 1 diabetes, psoriasis, lupus, and multiple sclerosis, are often mediated by lymphocytes of adaptive immunity rather than macrophages [1]. T cells are the dominant dysfunctional cells or initiators during the development of autoimmune diseases [1].

Anti-inflammatory drugs have several adverse side effects. *Glossogyne tenuifolia* (GT) (*Hsiang-ju*) is a perennial herb of *Asteraceae* that is distributed from south Asia to Australia. GT is a Chinese medicine used in antipyretic, hepatoprotective, and anti-inflammatory remedies

*Correspondence: fanglw@isu.edu.tw
†Jer-Yiing Houng and Tzong-Shyuan Tai contributed equally to this work
[1] Department of Nutrition, I-Shou University, No.8, Yida Rd., Yanchao District, Kaohsiung City 82445, Taiwan
Full list of author information is available at the end of the article

[2, 3]. Previous studies have shown that GT extract possesses pharmacological activities of antioxidation [4–6], cytotoxicity against several cancer cell lines [4, 7], protection against endothelial cell injury [8], and prevention of osteoclast-related diseases such as osteoporosis [9]. In addition, GT exhibited activity in immunomodulation [10–12]. GT extract downregulated the gene expression of inducible nitric oxide synthase and cyclooxygenase-2, as well as the production of proinflammatory cytokines upon stimulation by lipopolysaccharide (LPS) in Raw 264.7 cells [10] and human peripheral blood mononuclear cells (PBMCs) [11]. However, the effect of GT on adaptive immune cells, such as T cells, remains unclear.

Currently, the discovery of safe natural products for the treatment of inflammatory disorders focuses on inhibition of macrophage activity [13]. However, cells of the adaptive immune system, such as T and B cells, mediate inflammatory processes of some inflammatory diseases such as rheumatoid arthritis and inflammatory bowel disease. Molecules of the activation pathway of T cells might be a good target for modulation of these inflammatory diseases [1]. Resting T cells are in the G0 phase of the cell cycle. In response to T cell receptor (TCR) ligation, mitogenic stimulation, or a combination of a phorbol ester and calcium ionophore, T cells activate and transduce activation signals, leading to their proliferation. TCRs initiate signaling cascades that lead to activation of downstream mitogen-activated protein kinases (MAPKs) and nuclear factor kappa-light-chain-enhancer of activated B cells (NF-κB) [14]. Extracellular signal-regulated kinase (ERK), c-Jun N-terminal kinase (JNK) and p38 MAPK are important MAPKs involved in T cell activation. Cell proliferation and differentiation into effector cells as well as the production of interleukin (IL)-2 reflect the degree of T cell activation, and a lack of either MAPK or NF-κB impairs T cell activation-induced proliferation and IL-2 production [15].

Activated T cells undergo apoptosis upon re-stimulation, which is called activation-induced cell death (AICD). AICD is a critical mechanism to eliminate autoreactive lymphocytes in the immune system and maintain immune tolerance and homeostasis [16]. During cancer progression, the immune system acts as a significant barrier. Immune cells, such as CD8+ cytotoxic T lymphocytes (CTLs), CD4+ helper T cells, and natural killer cells, contribute to immunosurveillance and tumor elimination [17]. In antitumor immunotherapy, AICD of T cells is believed to be the key event leading to the failure of anti-tumor effects [18, 19]. Several studies of cancer immunotherapy using different approaches have highlighted inhibition of AICD to rescue activated T cells, thereby enhancing anti-tumor immune responses [18–21]. In adoptive cancer immunotherapy [22], tumor antigen-specific T cells are susceptible to AICD upon encountering the tumor antigen, causing the low success rate of cancer immunotherapy. Phosphorylation of JNK is critical for AICD of melanoma antigen-specific primary CTLs, and blocking JNK activation prevents AICD of CTLs [20, 23, 24]. This study aimed to investigate the effect of GT ethanol extract (GTE) on T cell-mediated adaptive immunity.

Methods

Preparation of GTE

GT plant materials were purchased from an herb store in Penghu Island, Taiwan, and deposited as the number of ISU-JYH-001 in the Herbarium of I-Shou University (Kaohsiung City, Taiwan). The nucleotide sequences of internal transcribed spacer (ITS) 1, ITS2, and 5.8S rDNA were isolated from this plant, and the species was confirmed by the NCBI DNA database [4]. Dry whole plant materials were ground into powder. GT (5.3 kg) was extracted with 20 L of 95% ethanol at room temperature for 1 day and repeated for three times. The extracted solutions were filtered through medicinal gauze. The GTE was obtained by removing the solvent with a rotary evaporator (VP-60DJ, Panchum Co., Kaohsuing City, Taiwan) and drying in a freeze drier (FD8530, Panchum Co.). The total dry weight of this extract was 777 g, and the extraction yield was 14.7%. The quality of the herb extract was monitored by high performance liquid chromatography (L-7100, Hitachi, Tokyo, Japan) analysis using luteolin and luteolin-7-glucoside (Sigma Chemicals Co., St Louis, MO, USA) as the principle control standards [4, 9]. The dry GTE was dissolved in dimethyl sulfoxide (DMSO) at the concentration 50 mg/mL as the GTE stock. The final GTE concentrations (3.13, 6.3, 12.5, 25 and 50 μg/mL) were made by culture medium dilution. The DMSO was added no more than 0.1% (v/v) and used as a mock control in this study.

Cell culture and human PBMC preparation

Human PBMCs were prepared from the whole blood and human leukemia cell line Jurkat was obtained from American Type Cell Collection (ATCC, Manassas, VA, USA). Human PBMCs and leukemic Jurkat cells were grown in RPMI-1640 medium (GE Healthcare, Piscataway, NJ, USA) with 10% fetal bovine serum (FBS; Thermo Fisher Scientific Inc., Waltham, MA, USA), 1% penicillin/streptomycin (Sigma-Aldrich, St. Louis, MO, USA), and 2 mM L-glutamine (Sigma-Aldrich) at 37 °C in a humidified atmosphere with 5% CO_2. Human PBMCs were isolated from whole blood using a Ficoll-Paque plus density gradient [25]. Whole bloods from healthy volunteers were mixed with the same volume of Hank's balanced salt solution (HBSS; Thermo Fisher, St. Louis, MO, USA).

The blood-HBSS mixture was layered over Ficoll-Paque PLUS (GE Healthcare) 1:1 (v/v) and centrifuged (5810R, Eppendorf, Hamburg, Germany) (400×g) for 20 min at 25 °C with the break off. The PBMC layer at the interface was collected and washed with HBSS three times by centrifugation (300×g) for 5 min at 4 °C. The PBMCs were suspended in RPMI-1640 medium. The study protocols were approved by the Institutional Review Board of the Research Ethics Committee of National Health Research Institutes (EC1001101) (Additional file 1).

Western blotting

For each sample, 1×10^6 cells were washed with phosphate buffered saline (PBS; pH 7.2) and lysed in freshly prepared cell lysis buffer (20 mM Tris–HCl, pH 7.5, 150 mM NaCl, 1 mM Na₂EDTA, 1 mM EGTA, 1% Triton X-100, 2.5 mM sodium pyrophosphate, 1 mM β-glycerophosphate, 1 mM Na₃VO₄, 1 μg/mL leupeptin, and 1 mM phenylmethanesulfonyl fluoride). The cell lysate was separated from debris by centrifugation at 13,200×g for 10 min at 4 °C. The protein concentration was measured by Bio-Rad Protein Assay Dye Reagent (Bio-Rad Laboratories, Hercules, CA, USA). An aliquot of 20 μg protein was separated on a 10% polyacrylamide gel and transferred onto a polyvinylidene fluoride membrane (EMD Millipore, Billerica, MA, USA). The membranes were subsequently blocked with 5% dry skim milk in Tris-buffered saline (TBS; pH 7.5). The membranes were hybridized with the indicated primary antibody at 4 °C overnight, washed three times with 0.05% TBST solution (50 mM Tris–Cl, pH 7.5, 150 mM NaCl, and 0.05% Tween-20) for 10 min, and then hybridized with a horseradish peroxidase (HRP)-conjugated secondary antibody at room temperature for 1 h. After washing three times with 0.05% TBST for 10 min each, the membrane was incubated with Luminata™ Western HRP Substrates (EMD Millipore). The signals were detected using Image Lab software Version 2.0 (Bio-Rad Laboratories).

T cell proliferation and activation assay

PBMCs (1×10^5) were pretreated with GTE (3.13, 6.3, 12.5, 25 and 50 μg/mL) for 30 min and then activated by 2.5 μg/mL phytohemagglutinin (PHA) in each well of a 96-well plate for 48 h. An aliquot of 0.5 μCi ^{3}H-thymidine was added to each well. After 20 h of incubation, the cells were harvested with a FilterMate 96-well harvester (PerkinElmer Inc, Waltham, MA, USA) for a proliferation assay. The radioactivity (counts per minute, CPM) was measured to quantify cell proliferation with a microplate scintillation and luminescence counter (TopCount NXT, Packard Instrument Co, Meriden, CT, USA). Jurkat cells (1×10^5) were pretreated with GTE (25 μg/mL) for 30 min and then stimulated by 10/80 ng/

mL 12-O-tetradodecanoyl-phorbol-13-acetate (PMA)/ionomycin (P/I) in each well of a 96-well plate for 24 h. Cells were then harvested for surface marker staining. To detect NF-κB activation, phosphorylation of nuclear factor of kappa light polypeptide gene enhancer in B-cells inhibitor (IκB) and p65 proteins were determined by western blotting. Jurkat cells (1×10^6) were pretreated with GTE (25 μg/mL) for 30 min and then stimulated by PHA (2.5 μg/mL) for 0, 1, and 3 h. Cell lysates were then prepared for western blot analysis. To detect MAPK activation (p-ERK, p-p38, and p-JNK), 1×10^6 Jurkat cells were pretreated with GTE (25 μg/mL) for 30 min and then stimulated with 2.5 μg/mL PHA for 0, 10 and 20 min. Cell lysates were then prepared for western blotting. Primary antibodies against p-IκB (#2859, 1:500), p-p65 (#3033, 1:2000), p-ERK (#9101, 1:3000), p-p38 (#4511, 1:1000), and p-JNK (#4671, 1:500) were purchased from Cell Signaling Technology (Beverly, MA, USA). Primary antibodies against α-tubulin (#2871, 1:3000) was purchased from Epitomics Inc. (Burlingame, CA, USA). Primary antibodies against ERK2 (sc-154, 1:5000), p38 (sc-535, 1:3000), and JNK1 (sc-1648, 1:1000), and an HRP-conjugated secondary antibody were purchased from Santa Cruz Biotechnology (Dallas, TX, USA).

Cell surface staining

Jurkat cells (1×10^5) were stimulated with P/I (10/80 ng/mL) for 24 h. The cells were then stained with CD69-PE (12-0699, 1:50, eBioscience, San Diego, CA, USA) in staining buffer (PBS with 1% FBS) on ice for 20 min and then washed three times with staining buffer. The CD69-positive population was evaluated by a flow cytometer (FACSCalibur; BD Biosciences). Data were analyzed with FlowJo software (BD Biosciences). The signal obtained for the cells treated without or with GTE alone and stained with mouse IgG1 isotype control-PE (12-4714, 1:50, eBioscience) was used as a control respectively.

Apoptosis assay

Apoptosis was determined by propidium iodide (PI) (Sigma-Aldrich) staining [26]. PBMCs or Jurkat cells (1×10^5) were treated with various concentrations of GTE (3.13, 6.3, 12.5, 25 and 50 μg/mL) in each well of a 96-well plate for 24 h. Harvested cells were suspended in a hypotonic solution (0.1% sodium citrate, 0.1% Triton X-100, and 20 μg/mL PI). The extent of the sub-G0/G1 peak representing apoptotic cells was measured by gating on cells stained in the region below the G0/G1 peak. The apoptotic sub-G0/G1 population was examined by flow cytometry and analyzed with FlowJo software (BD Biosciences).

AICD assay

Healthy female Balb/c mice were obtained from National Laboratory Animal Center (NLAC, Taipei, Taiwan) at 4 weeks of age. The animals were maintained in cages (5 mice/cage) under standard conditions. The mice were euthanized by use of CO_2 exposure. $CD4^+$ T cells isolated from the splenocytes of C57BL/6 mice were activated by antibodies against CD3 (16-0031, eBioscience) and CD28 (16-0281, eBioscience) (1 and 2 μg/mL, respectively) in the presence of 100 U/mL IL-2 for 5 days. The activated T cells were washed three times and reactivated by the anti-CD3 (16-0031, eBioscience) antibody (0.5 μg/mL) for 8 h. The cells were then harvested for an apoptosis assay. All animal experiments were performed in accordance with protocols approved by the Institutional Animal Care and Use Committee of I-Shou University (IACUC-ISU-96002) (Additional file 2). The combination of P/I and sodium orthovanadate (Na_3VO_4) induces significant AICD in Jurkat T cells [27]. Jurkat cells (1×10^5) were pretreated with GTE (25 μg/mL) for 30 min and then activated by P/I (10/80 ng/mL) and 1.5 mM Na_3VO_4 in each well of a 96-well plate for 24 h. The cells were then harvested for an apoptosis assay.

Statistical analyses

Each experiment was performed at least three times and measured in triplicates. The data were presented as mean ± standard deviation (SD). Each GTE-treated group was compared to the respective mock-treated (DMSO) control group. Statistical differences were analyzed by Student's t-test ($*P < 0.05$, $**P < 0.01$ and $***P < 0.001$). Data were analyzed using GraphPad Prism software (GraphPad Software, La Jolla, CA, USA).

Information of experimental design and resources

Details of our experimental design and statistics and all resources used in this study were included in Additional file 3.

Results

Inhibitory effects of GTE on the activation of T cells and PBMCs

Mitogen stimulation hydrolyzes membrane polyphosphoinositides to inositol trisphosphate (IP3) and diacylglycerol (DAG). Then, IP3 releases Ca^{2+} into the cytosol, and DAG activates protein kinase C (PKC). These synergistic effects lead to progression of the cell cycle and proliferation of T cells [28, 29]. A combination of phorbol esters, which activates PKC, and a calcium ionophore, which increases the intracellular Ca^{2+} concentration, mimic the signals triggered by the TCR or mitogen stimulation and can be used as agents for T cell activation. In addition, CD69 is an early activated surface molecule on T cells, and expression of CD69 has been frequently used as an indicator for T cell activation [30].

GTE has been reported to exert an inhibitory effect on LPS-treated macrophage and human PBMC activation [10, 11]. To further explore the influence of GTE on adaptive immunity, we examined the effect of GTE on the activation of T cells. PHA (a mitogen) or a combination of PMA (a phorbol ester) and ionomycin (a calcium ionophore) were used to activate T cells. First, Jurkat cells were pretreated with 25 μg/mL GTE for 30 min and then P/I were added to induce T cell activation for 24 h. The expression of CD69 was used as the T cell activation marker [31]. Figure 1a

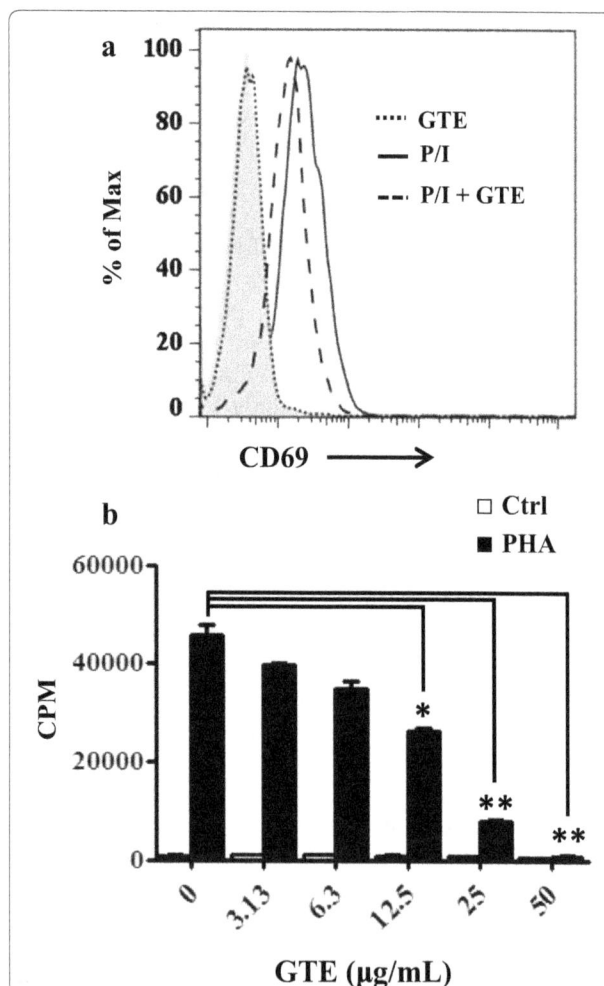

Fig. 1 GTE blocks T cell activation. **a** CD69 induction decreased in GTE-treated Jurkat T cells. Jurkat T cells were activated by PMA/ionomycin alone (P/I; *solid line*) or with 25 μg/mL GTE (*long dashed line*). GTE treatment alone (*short dashed line*) was used as a control. The cells were stained with an anti-CD69-PE antibody. The CD69-positive cells were then analyzed by flow cytometry. Data were assessed with FlowJo software. **b** Decreased proliferation of GTE-treated PBMCs. Freshly purified PBMCs were pretreated with various doses of GTE for 30 min and then stimulated by 2.5 μg/mL PHA. Cell proliferation was examined by ^{3}H-thymidine incorporation after a 20 h pulse with 0.5 μCi/well ^{3}H-thymidine. Data are expressed as counts per minute (CPM) of ^{3}H-thymidine uptake. A significant difference from the vehicle is indicated as $*P < 0.05$ or $**P < 0.01$

shows that GTE treatment reduced the fluorescence intensity of CD69-PE on P/I-activated Jurkat cells. The mean fluorescence intensity (MFI) was determined after analyzing 10,000 cells. The MFI changes of GTE and mock control were expressed as the fold changes relative to the individual group without P/I stimulation. The relative MFI fold changes of GTE-treated and mock control were 2.69 ± 0.01

and 4.14 ± 0.12 respectively. These data demonstrated that GTE administration decreased P/I-induced CD69 expression on P/I-activated Jurkat cells ($P = 0.0044$). In addition, the proliferation of primary T cells, representing successful activation of T cells, was used to evaluate T cell activation of PHA-stimulated PBMCs. Proliferation of PBMCs triggered with PHA (2.5 µg/mL) was suppressed by GTE/PHA

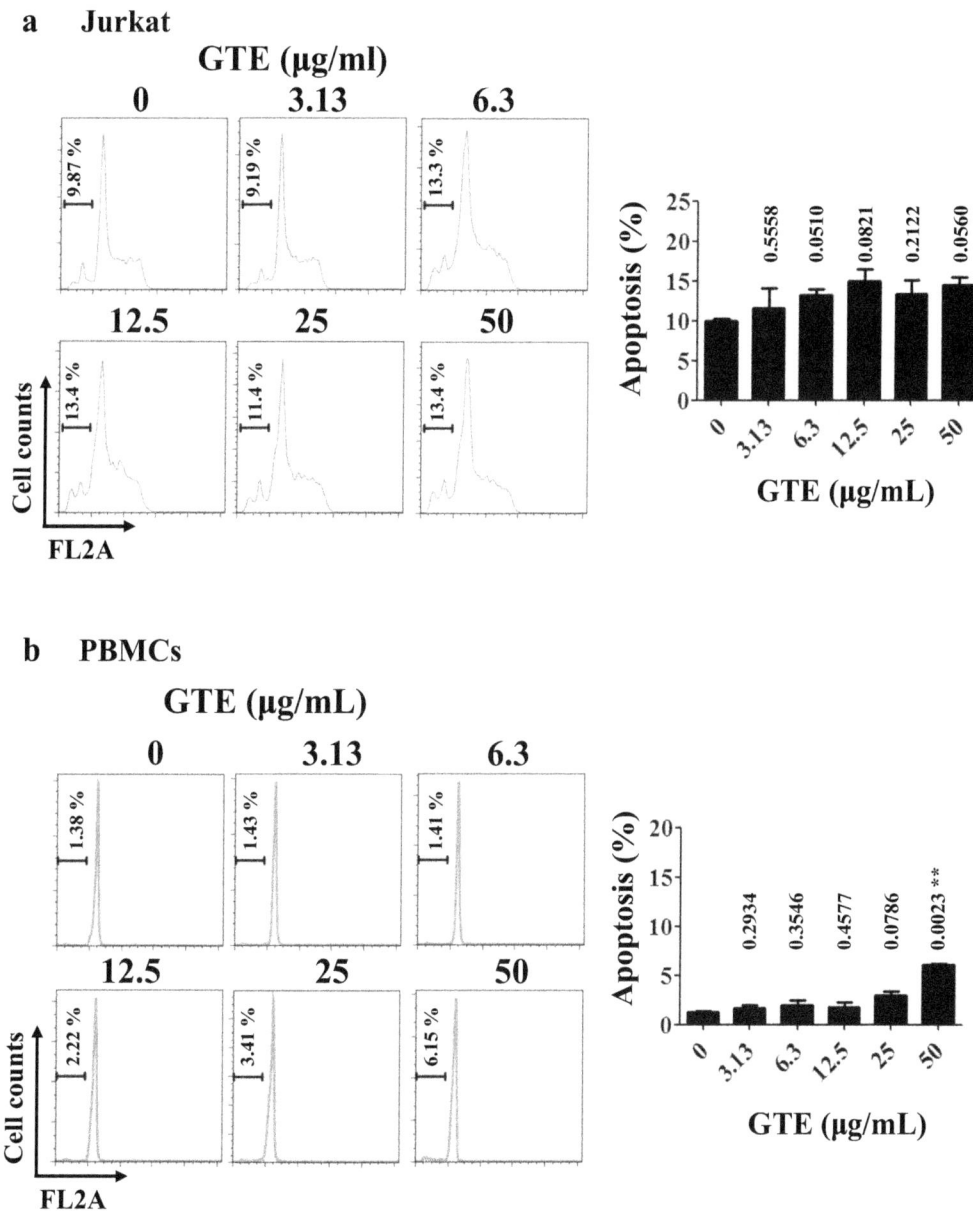

Fig. 2 GTE does not induce apoptosis of Jurkat cells or PBMCs. Jurkat cells (**a**) and PBMCs (**b**) were treated with GTE at the concentrations indicated for 24 h. The cells were stained with 20 µg/mL propidium iodide (PI) in a hypotonic solution (0.1% sodium citrate and 0.1% Triton X-100). The apoptotic cells were then analyzed by flow cytometry. Data were analyzed with FlowJo software. The *left panel* is the original apoptosis data. The *right panel* is quantitative data. The extent of the sub-G0/G1 peak representing apoptotic cells was measured by gating on cells in the region below the G0/G1 peak. Numbers above the *bar* in the *right panel* of Jurkat cells (**a**) and PBMCs (**b**) are P-values relative to the control group. A significant difference from the control is indicated as **P < 0.01

cotreatment compared with PHA treatment alone at the GTE concentrations of 12.5, 25 and 50 μg/mL ($P = 0.0118$, 0.0030 and 0.0021) (Fig. 1b). The results of ^{3}H-thymidine incorporation of PHA-activated PBMCs from four individual donors showed the suppressive trend of GTE in a dose-dependent manner (Additional file 4). The inhibitory effect of GTE on CD69 expression of activated Jurkat T cells (Fig. 1a) correlated well with the proliferation of PHA-stimulated human PBMCs in which GTE inhibited PHA-induced proliferation by up to 80% at 25 μg/mL (Fig. 1b). These results indicated that the GTE inhibited activation of both Jurkat T cells and human PBMCs.

Cytotoxic effect of GTE on Jurkat T cells and PBMCs

Cytotoxic activity of GTE has been reported in certain cancer cell lines such as HepG2, Hep3B, MDA-MB-231, and MCF-7 [4, 7, 32]. This study showed that the death of cancer cells was mediated through the apoptotic pathway. The downregulating effect of GTE on T cell activation could be due to a cytotoxic effect on T cells. Thus, to determine whether GTE has a cytotoxic effect on T cells, Jurkat cells were cultured in the presence of various doses of GTE for 24 h, and then the degree of apoptosis was examined. Figure 2a shows minimal apoptosis in Jurkat cells (<20%) treated with GTE at up to 50 μg/mL. In addition, almost no apoptosis was observed in PBMCs treated with GTE at less than 25 μg/mL (Fig. 2b). Because GTE did not induce apoptosis of human PBMCs at 25 μg/mL, this dosage was used for the following activation assay. These results suggested that the inhibitory effect of GTE on T cell activation was not due to a cytotoxic effect.

GTE down-regulated JNK phosphorylation, but not NF-κB activities, in activated human T cells

The T cell activation signal activates multiple downstream molecules including phosphorylation of MAPKs and NF-κB. It has been shown that inhibition of the DNA-binding activity of NF-κB upon PHA stimulation is significant at a high dosage of GTE (up to 150 μg/mL) but insignificant at a low GTE dose (less than 100 μg/mL) [12]. In this study, we further examined GTE effects on NF-κB activity in T cell activation signaling. In the NF-κB activation pathway, IκB is phosphorylated and undergoes degradation upon PHA stimulation. We therefore evaluated IκB phosphorylation upon T cell activation. Figure 3 shows that GTE-treated Jurkat cells displayed similar levels of IκB phosphorylation upon PHA stimulation. The phosphorylation of RelA/p65, one of the NF-κB members, regulates NF-κB transcriptional activity [33]. We found that RelA/p65 phosphorylation was normal after co-treatment with GTE (Fig. 3). These data suggest that the deficiency of T cell activation in the presence of GTE is independent of the NF-κB pathway.

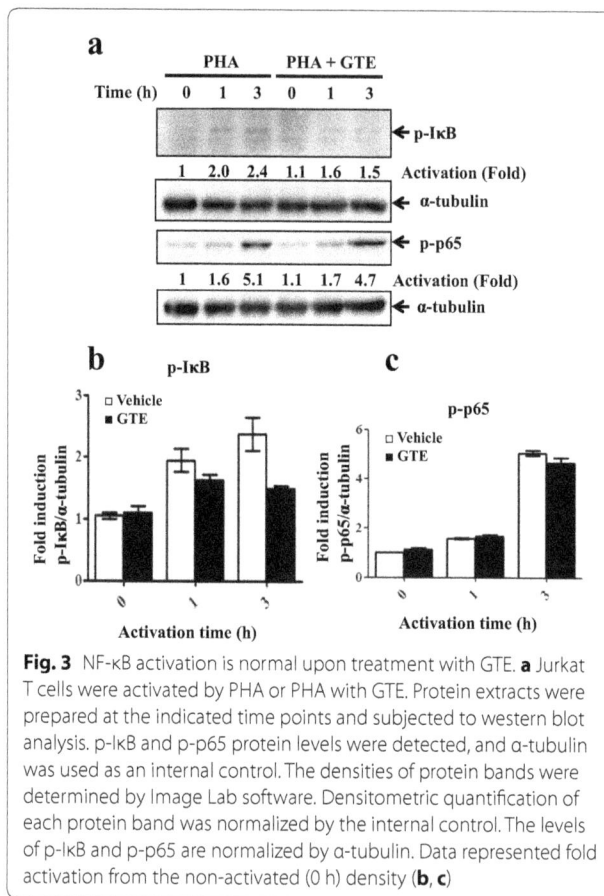

Fig. 3 NF-κB activation is normal upon treatment with GTE. **a** Jurkat T cells were activated by PHA or PHA with GTE. Protein extracts were prepared at the indicated time points and subjected to western blot analysis. p-IκB and p-p65 protein levels were detected, and α-tubulin was used as an internal control. The densities of protein bands were determined by Image Lab software. Densitometric quantification of each protein band was normalized by the internal control. The levels of p-IκB and p-p65 are normalized by α-tubulin. Data represented fold activation from the non-activated (0 h) density (**b**, **c**)

Because NF-κB signaling was normal in GTE-treated Jurkat cells, we mapped the signal defect in these cells. In addition to NF-κB signaling, the activities of MAPKs are important for T cell activation. Thus, we further examined the activity of three major MAPKs, ERK, p38 MAPK, and JNK, after stimulation. T cell activation increased ERK phosphorylation, and GTE administration did not alter the phosphorylation status of ERK (Fig. 4a, b). GTE slightly inhibited p38 MAPK phosphorylation after stimulation with PHA for 20 min ($P = 0.0278$) (Fig. 4a, c). Notably, JNK phosphorylation was significantly suppressed by GTE in activated Jurkat cells at the activation time 10 and 20 min ($P = 0.0217$ and 0.0167) (Fig. 4a, d). Taken together, the suppression of T cell activation by GTE might be attributed to a slight reduction in p38 activation and profound JNK activation.

GTE attenuated prolonged JNK-induced AICD

JNK is activated by a wide array of stress conditions and mitogenic stimulation. Previous studies have shown that JNK plays an important role in AICD [27]. It is important to examine whether GTE regulates AICD by modulating the activity of JNK. Na_3VO_4, a tyrosine phosphatase

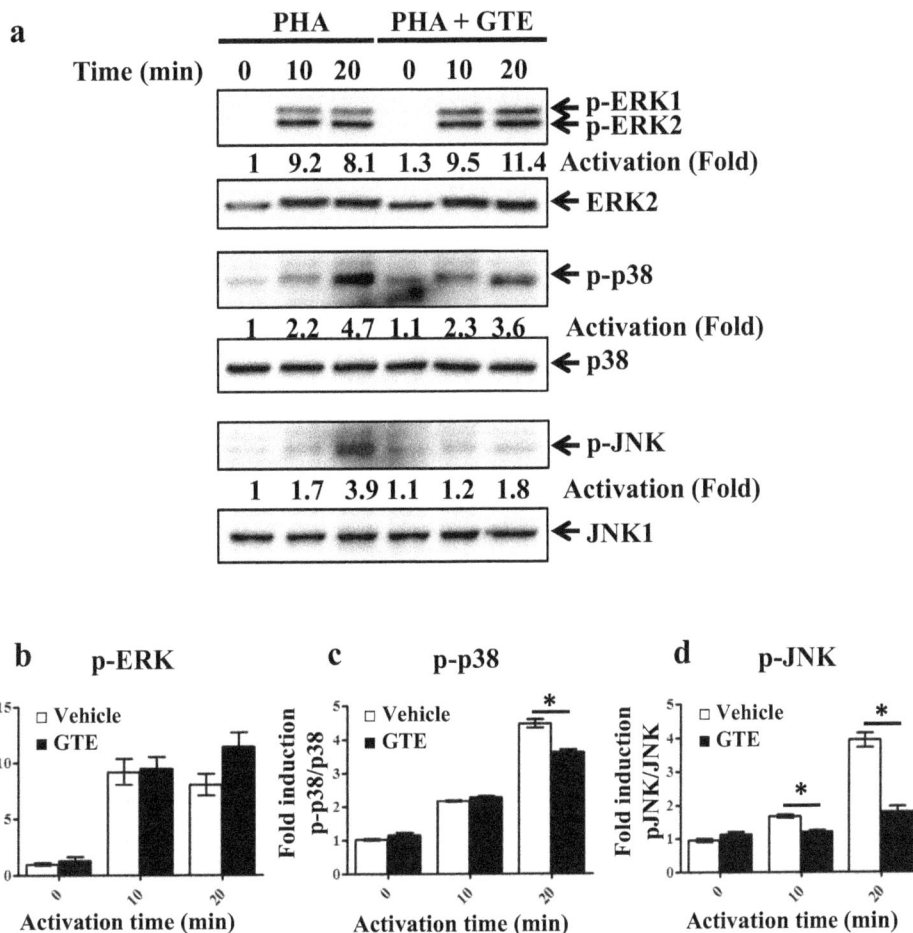

Fig. 4 GTE attenuates JNK and p38 activation. **a** Jurkat T cells were activated by PHA alone or with GTE. Protein extracts were prepared at the indicated time points and subjected to western blot analysis. Activation of ERK, JNK and p38 was measured by phosphorylation of ERK, JNK, and p38. ERK2, JNK1, and p38 served as internal controls. Densitometric quantification of fold inductions of the levels of **b** p-ERK2 relative to ERK2, **c** p-p38 relative to p38, and **d** p-JNK relative to JNK1 protein. The densities of protein bands were determined by Image Lab software. Densitometric quantification of each protein was normalized by the internal control. The level of p-ERK2 was normalized by ERK2. The level of p-p38 was normalized by p38, and the level of p-JNK was normalized by JNK1. Data represented fold activation from the non-activated (0 h) density (**b–d**). A significant difference from the control is indicated as $*P < 0.05$

inhibitor, has been used to prolong JNK activation during T cell activation, whereas the combination of P/I and Na_3VO_4 upon T cell stimulation induces significant AICD in Jurkat T cells [27]. In this study, Na_3VO_4 was also shown to induce apoptosis upon T cell activation by P/I. Furthermore, administration of GTE with Na_3VO_4 or P/I did not induce apoptosis of Jurkat T cells (Fig. 5a). Figure 5a also demonstrates that GTE blocked Na_3VO_4-induced apoptosis in activated Jurkat T cells ($P = 0.0037$). Next, we examined the effect of GTE on AICD in reactivated T cells ex vivo. Naïve CD4 T cells were activated with anti-CD3/CD28 antibodies and maintained in IL2-containing medium for 5 days. The activated CD4 T cells were then re-activated with the anti-CD3 antibody to

trigger AICD. Figure 5b shows that T cells underwent AICD through repeated stimulation of CD3, and GTE inhibited AICD of primary isolated T cells ($P = 0.0016$). These results suggested that GTE might attenuate prolonged JNK-induced AICD.

Discussion

Several studies have investigated the anti-inflammatory mechanism of GTE, but all of them have focused on GTE effects in activated myeloid lineage macrophages [10, 11]. However, the inflammatory effect of GTE on T cells is still unknown. Cells of the adaptive immune system, especially T cells, mediate the tissue damage of some inflammatory diseases such as rheumatoid arthritis and

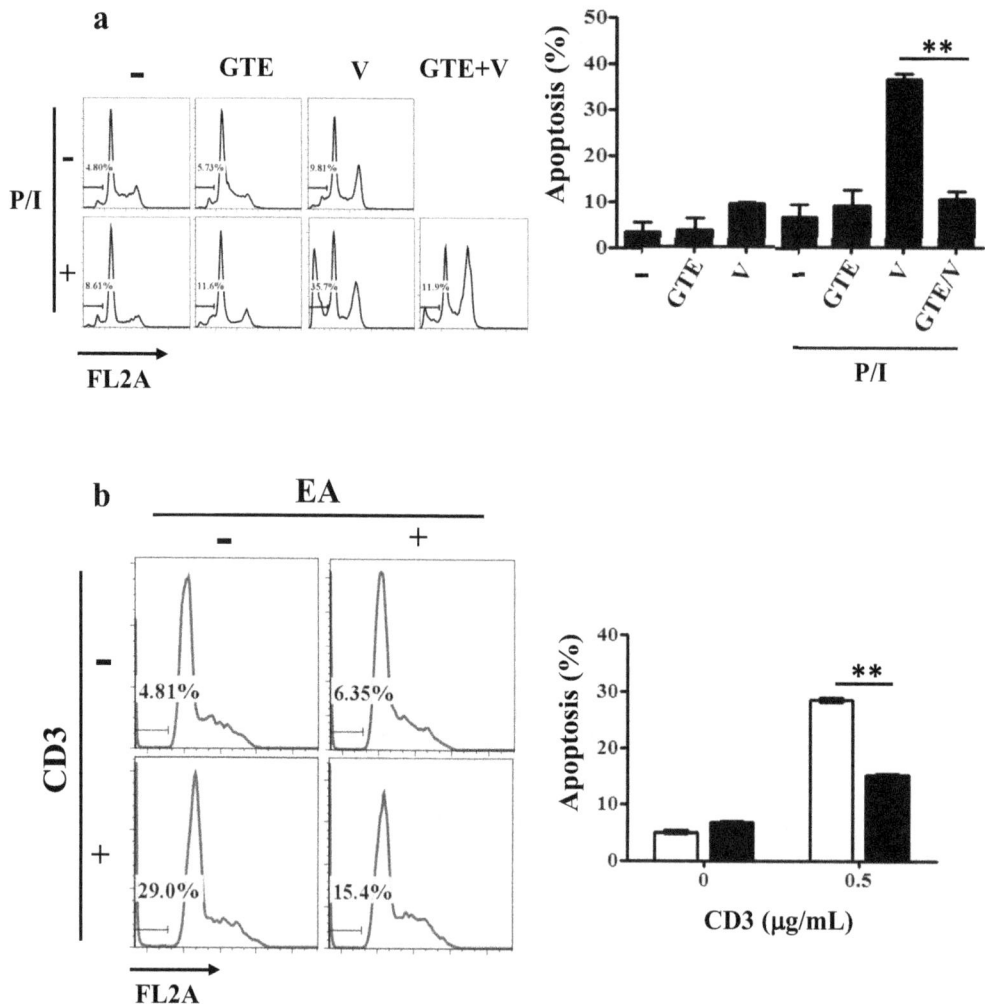

Fig. 5 GTE blocks prolonged JNK-induced AICD. **a** Jurkat cells were treated with GTE, sodium orthovanadate (V; 1.5 mM), and/or PMA/ionomycin (P/I; 50/80 ng/mL) for 24 h. The cells were collected and stained with PI in a hypotonic solution. Apoptotic cells were analyzed by flow cytometry. Data were assessed with FlowJo software. **b** CD4 T cells were isolated from mouse spleen, activated with anti-CD3/CD28 antibodies, and cultured in the presence of IL-2. The activated T cells were re-activated by 0.5 μg/mL anti-CD3 antibody at day 5 and then harvested for an apoptosis assay. The *left panel* is the original apoptosis data. The *right panel* is quantitative data. The extent of the sub-G0/G1 peak representing apoptotic cells was measured by gating on cells in the region below the G0/G1 peak. A significant difference from the control is indicated as **P < 0.01

inflammatory bowel disease [1]. In the present study, we found that GTE suppressed T cell activation in both Jurkat T cells and in human PBMCs (Fig. 1). This suppressive effect was not caused by cytotoxicity of GTE in T cells (Fig. 2).

Previous studies [4, 7] have reported that GTE possessed an anti-cancer activity. GTE showed cytotoxicity in breast cancer cell lines (MDA-MB-231 and MCF-7) and hepatoma cell lines (HepG2 and Hep3B) [4]. The IC_{50} doses of GTE in these susceptible cell lines are 20–30 μg/mL [4]. Our data suggest that PBMCs and Jurkat T cells were resistant to GTE-induced cytotoxicity (Fig. 2).

Ha et al. [12] reported that GTE at a high dose, but not a low dose, inhibited NF-κB activation. In our study, no NF-κB defect in T cell activation was observed with co-treatment at a low concentration of GTE (Fig. 3), although we did find strong inhibition of JNK activity and slight suppression of p38 activity (Fig. 4). LPS treatment induced activation of NF-κB and JNK/p38 [34], it was possible that a low concentration of GTE might also inhibited JNK activity upon LPS treatment in macrophages.

The mechanism by which GTE regulated JNK activity was unclear. One possible mechanism is through the production of reactive oxygen species (ROS) that induce JNK activation to initiate a downstream signal that amplifies ROS production upon stimulation [35]. Previous studies have shown that GTE has an antioxidant activity [4, 5], and the ability of GTE to modulated JNK might be mediated through its activity as a ROS scavenger by blocking the JNK–ROS activation loop.

In adoptive immunotherapy of cancer treatment, AICD of adoptively transferred T cells represents one of the major hurdles to devise an effective immune intervention therapy. Rescuing T cells from AICD might promote anti-tumor immunity [19, 36]. Previous studies have demonstrated that the modulation effect of JNK prevents AICD of adoptively transferred T cells [20, 23]. Our study demonstrated that GTE inhibited JNK activity upon T cell activation and AICD (Figs. 4, 5b). The mechanism of AICD inhibition by GTE might be mediated through modulation of prolonged JNK phosphorylation in activated T cells. In addition to its roles in cell activation and AICD in the immune system, JNK has been shown to be involved in other stress signaling pathways such as those in response to ultraviolet and γ irradiation [37]. Hence, our findings of the effects of GTE on JNK modulation indicate that GTE may have regulatory effects on other cellular responses.

Conclusion
GTE inhibited T cell activation of Jurkat cells and freshly prepared human PBMCs due to suppression of JNK activity. Furthermore, GTE inhibited AICD by blocking prolonged JNK phosphorylation in activated T cells. Taken together, the anti-inflammatory effects exerted by GTE were mediated via suppression of JNK phosphorylation in T cell activation.

Abbreviations
AICD: activation-induced cell death; CPM: counts per minute; CTLs: cytotoxic T lymphocytes; DAG: diacylglycerol; DMSO: dimethyl sulfoxide; ERK: extracellular signal-regulated kinase; FBS: fetal bovine serum; GT: *Glossogyne tenuifolia*; GTE: *Glossogyne tenuifolia* ethanol extract; HBSS: Hank's balanced salt solution; HRP: horseradish peroxidase; IκB: nuclear factor of kappa light polypeptide gene enhancer in B-cells inhibitor; IL-2: interleukin-2; IP3: inositol trisphosphate; ITS: internal transcribed spacer; JNK: c-Jun N-terminal kinases; LPS: lipopolysaccharide; MAPKs: mitogen-activated protein kinases; MFI: mean fluorescence intensity; Na_3VO_4: sodium orthovanadate; NF-κB: nuclear factor kappa-light-chain-enhancer of activated B cells; PBMCs: peripheral blood mononuclear cells; PBS: phosphate buffered saline; PHA: phytohemagglutinin; PI: propidium iodide; P/I: PMA/ionomycin; PKC: protein kinase C; PMA: 12-O-tetradodecanoyl-phorbol-13-acetate; SD: standard deviation; TCR: T cell receptor.

Authors' contributions
LWF, JYH and TST conceived and designed the study. TST performed the flow cytometry experiments. LWF and TST performed the biological experiments. LWF, TST and SCH interpreted the results. TSH, HFH and CJL performed the statistical analysis. LWF, JYH and TST wrote the manuscript. All authors read and approved the final manuscript.

Author details
Department of Nutrition, I-Shou University, No.8, Yida Rd., Yanchao District, Kaohsiung City 82445, Taiwan. [2] Department of Medical Research, E-Da Hospital, Kaohsiung City 82445, Taiwan. [3] School of Medicine for International Students, I-Shou University, Kaohsiung City 82445, Taiwan. [4] National Institute of Infectious Diseases and Vaccinology, NHRI, Miaoli County 35053, Taiwan. [5] Department of Medical Research, Show-Chwan Memorial Hospital, Changhua County 50008, Taiwan. [6] Graduate Institute of Biotechnology, Chinese Culture University, Taipei City 11114, Taiwan. [7] Department of Leisure and Recreation Management, Da-Yeh University, Changhua County 51591, Taiwan.

Acknowledgements
This work was supported by the National Science Council, Taiwan (NSC 97-2313-B-214-001-MY3-002), and I-Shou University, Taiwan (ISU101-04-06 and ISU-103-01-E-01).

Competing interests
The authors declare that they have no competing interests.

Funding
This work was funded by the National Science Council, Taiwan (NSC 97-2313-B-214-001-MY3-002), and I-Shou University, Taiwan (ISU101-04-06 and ISU-103-01-E-01).

References
1. Dinarello CA. Anti-inflammatory agents: present and future. Cell. 2010;140:935–50.
2. Anonymous. Zhong Hua Ben Cao (China Herbal), vol. 7. Shanghai: Shanghai Science and Technology; 1999.
3. Xu HY. Illustrations of Chinese herbs in Taiwan. Taiwan: Committee on Chinese Medicine and Pharmacy, Department of Health, Executive Yuan; 1972.
4. Hsu HF, Houng JY, Chang CL, Wu CC, Chang FR, Wu YC. Antioxidant activity, cytotoxicity, and DNA information of *Glossogyne tenuifolia*. J Agric Food Chem. 2005;53:6117–25.
5. Wu MJ, Huang CL, Lian TW, Kou MC, Wang L. Antioxidant activity of *Glossogyne tenuifolia*. J Agric Food Chem. 2005;53:6305–12.
6. Yang JH, Tsai SY, Han CM, Shih CC, Mau JL. Antioxidant properties of *Glossogyne tenuifolia*. Am J Chin Med. 2006;34:707–20.
7. Hsu HF, Wu YC, Chang CC, Houng JY. Apoptotic effects of bioactive fraction isolated from *Glossogyne tenuifolia* on A549 human lung cancer cells. J Taiwan Inst Chem Eng. 2011;42(4):556–62.
8. Wang CP, Houng JY, Hsu HF, Chen HJ, Huang B, Hung WC, Yu TH, Chiu CA, Lu LF, Hsu CC. *Glossogyne tenuifolia* enhances posttranslational S-nitrosylation of proteins in vascular endothelial cells. Taiwania. 2011;56(2):97–104.
9. Wang SW, Kuo HC, Hsu HF, Tu YK, Cheng TT, Houng JY. Inhibitory activity on RANKL-mediated osteoclastogenesis of *Glossogyne tenuifolia* extract. J Funct Foods. 2014;6:215–23.
10. Wu MJ, Wang L, Ding HY, Weng CY, Yen JH. Glossogyne tenuifolia acts to inhibit inflammatory mediator production in a macrophage cell line by downregulating LPS-induced NF-κB. J Biomed Sci. 2004;11:186–99.
11. Wu MJ, Weng CY, Ding HY, Wu PJ. Anti-inflammatory and antiviral effects of *Glossogyne tenuifolia*. Life Sci. 2005;76:1135–46.

12. Ha CL, Weng CY, Wang L, Lian TW, Wu MJ. Immunomodulatory effect of *Glossogyne tenuifolia* in murine peritoneal macrophages and splenocytes. J Ethnopharmacol. 2006;107:116–25.

13. Gautam R, Jachak SM. Recent developments in anti-inflammatory natural products. Med Res Rev. 2009;29:767–820.

14. Paul S, Schaefer BC. A new look at T cell receptor signaling to nuclear factor-κB. Trends Immunol. 2013;34:269–81.

15. Dong C, Davis RJ, Flavell RA. MAP kinases in the immune response. Annu Rev Immunol. 2002;20:55–72.

16. Zhang J, Xu X, Liu Y. Activation-induced cell death in T cells and autoimmunity. Cell Mol Immunol. 2004;1:186–92.

17. Hanahan D, Weinberg RA. Hallmarks of cancer: the next generation. Cell. 2011;144:646–74.

18. Kunkele A, Johnson AJ, Rolczynski LS, Chang CA, Hoglund V, Kelly-Spratt KS, Jensen MC. Functional tuning of CARs reveals signaling threshold above which CD8+ CTL antitumor potency is attenuated due to cell Fas-FasL-dependent AICD. Cancer Immunol Res. 2015;3:368–79.

19. Cao K, Wang G, Li W, Zhang L, Wang R, Huang Y, Du L, Jiang J, Wu C, He X, Roberts AI, Li F, Rabson AB, Wang Y, Shi Y. Histone deacetylase inhibitors prevent activation-induced cell death and promote anti-tumor immunity. Oncogene. 2015;34:5960–70.

20. Mehrotra S, Chhabra A, Chattopadhyay S, Dorsky DI, Chakraborty NG, Mukherji B. Rescuing melanoma epitope-specific cytolytic T lymphocytes from activation-induced cell death, by SP600125, an inhibitor of JNK: implications in cancer immunotherapy. J Immunol. 2004;173:6017–24.

21. Friedlein G, El Hage F, Vergnon I, Richon C, Saulnier P, Lecluse Y, Caignard A, Boumsell L, Bismuth G, Chouaib S, Mami-Chouaib F. Human CD5 protects circulating tumor antigen-specific CTL from tumor-mediated activation-induced cell death. J Immunol. 2007;178:6821–7.

22. Chhabra A. Mitochondria-centric activation induced cell death of cytolytic T lymphocytes and its implications for cancer immunotherapy. Vaccine. 2010;28:4566–72.

23. Chhabra A, Mehrotra S, Chakraborty NG, Dorsky DI, Mukherji B. Activation-induced cell death of human melanoma specific cytotoxic T lymphocytes is mediated by apoptosis-inducing factor. Eur J Immunol. 2006;36:3167–74.

24. Mehrotra S, Chhabra A, Hegde U, Chakraborty NG, Mukherji B. Inhibition of c-Jun N-terminal kinase rescues influenza epitope-specific human cytolytic T lymphocytes from activation-induced cell death. J Leukoc Biol. 2007;81:539–47.

25. Ferrante A, Thong YH. A rapid one-step procedure for purification of mononuclear and polymorphonuclear leukocytes from human blood using a modification of the Hypaque-Ficoll technique. J Immunol Methods. 1978;24:389–93.

26. Nicoletti I, Migliorati G, Pagliacci MC, Grignani F, Riccardi C. A rapid and simple method for measuring thymocyte apoptosis by propidium iodide staining and flow cytometry. J Immunol Methods. 1991;139:271–9.

27. Chen YR, Wang X, Templeton D, Davis RJ, Tan TH. The role of c-Jun N-terminal kinase (JNK) in apoptosis induced by ultraviolet C and gamma radiation. Duration of JNK activation may determine cell death and proliferation. J Biol Chem. 1996;271:31929–36.

28. Koyasu S, Suzuki G, Asano Y, Osawa H, Diamantstein T, Yahara I. Signals for activation and proliferation of murine T lymphocyte clones. J Biol Chem. 1987;262:4689–95.

29. Planelles D, Hernandez-Godoy J, Gonzalez-Molina A. Differential effects of the calcium ionophore A23187 and the phorbol ester PMA on lymphocyte proliferation. Agents Actions. 1992;35:238–44.

30. Mardiney M 3rd, Brown MR, Fleisher TA. Measurement of T-cell CD69 expression: a rapid and efficient means to assess mitogen- or antigen-induced proliferative capacity in normals. Cytometry. 1996;26:305–10.

31. Ziegler SF, Ramsdell F, Alderson MR. The activation antigen CD69. Stem Cells. 1994;12:456–65.

32. Hsu HF, Houng JY, Kuo CF, Tsao N, Wu YC. Glossogin, a novel phenylpropanoid from *Glossogyne tenuifolia*, induced apoptosis in A549 lung cancer cells. Food Chem Toxicol. 2008;46:3785–91.

33. Neumann M, Naumann M. Beyond IκBs: alternative regulation of NF-κB activity. FASEB J. 2007;21:2642–54.

34. Guha M, Mackman N. LPS induction of gene expression in human monocytes. Cell Signal. 2001;13:85–94.

35. Chambers JW, LoGrasso PV. Mitochondrial c-Jun N-terminal kinase (JNK) signaling initiates physiological changes resulting in amplification of reactive oxygen species generation. J Biol Chem. 2011;286:16052–62.

36. Tabbekh M, Franciszkiewicz K, Haouas H, Lecluse Y, Benihoud K, Raman C, Mami-Chouaib F. Rescue of tumor-infiltrating lymphocytes from activation-induced cell death enhances the antitumor CTL response in CD5-deficient mice. J Immunol. 2011;187:102–9.

37. Johnson GL, Nakamura K. The c-jun kinase/stress-activated pathway: regulation, function and role in human disease. Biochim Biophys Acta. 2007;1773:1341–8.

7

Discrimination of Radix Polygoni Multiflori from different geographical areas by UPLC-QTOF/MS combined with chemometrics

Jin-Fa Tang[1†], Wei-Xia Li[1†], Fan Zhang[1], Yu-Hui Li[1], Ying-Jie Cao[1], Ya Zhao[1], Xue-Lin Li[1*] and Zhi-Jie Ma[2*]

Abstract

Background: Nowadays, Radix Polygoni Multiflori (RPM, Heshouwu in Chinese) from different geographical origins were used in clinic. In order to characterize the chemical profiles of different geographical origins of RPM samples, ultra-high performance liquid chromatography quadrupole time of flight mass spectrometry (UPLC-QTOF/MS) combined with chemometrics (partial least squared discriminant analysis, PLS-DA) method was applied in the present study.

Methods: The chromatography, chemical composition and MS information of RPM samples from 18 geographical origins were acquired and profiled by UPLC-QTOF/MS. The chemical markers contributing the differentiation of RPM samples were observed and characterized by supervised PLS-DA method of chemometrics.

Results: The chemical composition differences of RPM samples derived from 18 different geographical origins were observed. Nine chemical markers were tentatively identified which could be used as specific chemical markers for the differentiation of geographical RPM samples.

Conclusions: UPLC-QTOF/MS method coupled with chemometrics analysis has potential to be used for discriminating different geographical TCMs. Results will help to develop strategies for conservation and utilization of RPM samples.

Keywords: UPLC-QTOF/MS, Radix Polygoni Multiflori, Different geographical origins, Chemical markers, Partial least squared discriminant analysis

Background

Radix Polygoni Multiflori (RPM, Heshouwu in Chinese) is the dried root tuber of *Polygonum multiflorum* Thunb. (Fam. Polygonaceae). As one of the most popular and precious traditional Chinese medicines (TCMs), it is officially documented in the Chinese Pharmacopoeia for calming the nerves, nourishing blood, activating channels and collaterals, tonifying liver and kidneys, and preventing the premature graying of hair. Many 1000 years of clinical practice of TCM has demonstrated the effect of RPM in terms of preventing dementia and improving memory [1]. As a traditional medicine and dietary supplement for health, it has also been considered effective in antiaging and increasing longevity [2, 3]. According to modern researches, RPM has the pharmacological effects of enhancing immunity, anti-atherosclerosis, anti-inflammatory, antibacterial, anti-cancer, anti-mutagenic, antioxidation, increasing DNA repair, and improving adipose metabolism [4–6].

*Correspondence: ydsys507@126.com; lixuelin450000@126.com; 13811647091@163.com
†Jin-Fa Tang and Wei-Xia Li contributed equally to this work
[1] The First Affiliated Hospital of Henan University of Chinese Medicine, No. 19, Renmin Road, Jinshui District, Zhengzhou 450000, People's Republic of China
[2] Beijing Friendship Hospital Affiliated to Capital Medical University, No. 95, Yongan Road, Xuanwu District, Beijing 100050, China

With the extensive application of RPM, its safety has drawn widespread attention. More and more literatures showed that RPM and RPM-containing herbal products had the adverse effects of hepatotoxicity [7]. The RPM dose in the Chinese Pharmacopoeia (2005 edition) is 6–12 g [8]. According to the safety considerations, the recommended dose of RPM was adjusted to 3–6 g in the 2010 edition of the Chinese Pharmacopoeia [9]. In addition, the safety, quality and efficacy of RPM samples may vary greatly because of the different geographical origins. As well known, medicinal herbs in authentic producing areas had the best quality, which can produce the best pharmacological effect. The place where authentic medicinal herbs produced is called the "trueborn area". RPM is widely distributed in China's southwest, central, south, east and other regions, including Sichuan, Yunnan, Guizhou, Chongqing, Guangdong, Guangxi, Jiangsu, Anhui, Hubei, Hunan, Henan, Jiangxi, Shanxi, Gansu and other provinces and cities [10]. Owing to its many origins, the "trueborn area" of RPM is still being studied. It is consensus that the effect of Chinese medicine relies on the role of its multi-component. There are large difference among the chemical composition and content of RPMs because of its different species and origins, which will cause a greater impact on its efficacy. Therefore, the distinction among RPM samples from different origins is essential for determining the trueborn area of RPM and for selecting good quality RPM to treat diseases.

The introduction of new analytical techniques and the application of novel data analysis methods have greatly promoted the quality assurance of TCM. From the literatures summary, we found that fingerprinting quality control of RPM from different geographical origins was determined by thin-layer chromatography (TLC) scanning and high-performance liquid chromatography (HPLC) [11, 12]; the quality of various commercial specifications of RPM and its dregs was evaluated by HPLC [13]; the quality control of RPM from different origins was determined by infrared spectrum (IR), inductively coupled plasma-atomic emission spectrometer (ICP-AES) and LC–mass spectrometry (MS), etc. [14–16]. However, the authentic correlation between geographical distribution regions and chemical variation in RPMs has been rarely reported.

It was reported that RPM mainly contains anthraquinones, stilbene glycosides, phospholipids, phenols, flavonoids, etc. [17]. The present study is aimed to classify and characterize RPM samples from different geographical origins based on the chemical compounds by chemometrics. Chemometrics is an interdisciplinary science involving mathematics and statistics, chemistry and computer science. In recent years, chemometrics have gained more attention along with the development of computer science. Chemometrics combined with liquid chromatography and other spectrometric methods are widely used in many fields concerning TCMs, such as the comparison of different species [18], quality control and modernization of TCM [19]. Herein, eighteen RPM samples from 10 counties of 4 provinces were analyzed using ultra-high performance liquid chromatography quadrupole time of flight mass spectrometry (UPLC-QTOF/MS). And partial least squared discriminant analysis (PLS-DA) of chemometrics approach was applied to classify different RPM samples and find chemical variables that contribute to the differentiation of RPMs. Furthermore, the Progenesis QI software (v2.0, Waters Corporation, Milford, USA) with fast, objective, and reliable characteristics was used for the chemometrics statistical analysis, which had been already used to found the chemical differences among the different extracts of RPM and RPM Praeparata [20], but it only analyzed the differences between the water and ethanol extracts of RPM and RPM Praeparata. Therefore, it would also be feasible to use this method to find different chemical markers among RPMs from different geographical origins. The results can provide more effective strategy guidance for the utilization and domestication of RPM.

Methods
The Minimum Standards of Reporting Checklist (Additional file 1) contains details of the experimental design, and statistics, and resources used in this study.

Chemicals and reagents
Acetonitrile (HPLC grade) and formic acid were purchased from Merck KGaA (Darmstadt, Germany); ultra-pure water was purified by a Milli-Q system (Milford, MA, USA).

Plant materials
Seventeen species of planted or wild RPM samples were collected from 10 counties, 4 provinces of China; and one kind of RPM sample (S13) was purchased from pharmacies (Table 1). All the herbal samples were authenticated by the authors. The corresponding voucher specimens were stored in the laboratory for drug metabolism and pharmacokinetics (DMPK) Research of Herbal Medicines, the First Affiliated Hospital of Henan University of Chinese Medicine.

Sample preparation
The 18 RPM samples were sliced, dried, and powdered. The powdered samples were screened trough no. 4 sieve, respectively; and 0.25 g was extracted with 25 mL 70% ethanol for 30 min by reflux extraction method, cooled at room temperature and weighted. The reduced weight

Table 1 Geographical information of 18 RPM samples

No.	Source	Longitude	Latitude
S1	Cultivated in Xinzhou town, Huangping county, Guizhou province	107.92213	26.98450
S2	Wild, Xinzhou town, Huangping county, Guizhou province	107.92213	26.99918
S3	Wangsi town, Duyun county, Guizhou province	107.51576	26.30596
S4	Huaxi district, Guiyang city, Guizhou province	107.27755	26.73151
S5	Cultivated in Meitan county, Zunyi city, Guizhou province for 2 years	107.45728	28.02350
S6	Cultivated in Meitan county, Zunyi city, Guizhou province for 3 years	107.45728	28.02350
S7	Guizhou Academy of Agricultural Sciences (Huaxi district, Guiyang city, Guizhou province)	107.27755	26.73151
S8	Baiduo village, Shibing county, Guizhou province for 2 years	108.15923	27.14368
S9	Baiduo village, Shibing county, Guizhou province for 3 years	108.15923	27.14368
S10	Niudachang town, Shibing county, Guizhou province for 2 years	107.92594	27.14054
S11	Niudachang town, Shibing county, Guizhou province for 3 years	107.92594	27.14054
S12	Wild, Shibing county, Guizhou province	108.06787	27.12923
S13	Changhao Chinese Medicine Development Co., Ltd. (Shibing county, Guizhou province)	107.94637	26.55361
S14	Zhenjiang town, Gaozhou city, Guangdong province	110.84849	21.94484
S15	Shigu town, Gaozhou city, Guangdong province	110.86943	21.95980
S16	Yangchun city, Guangdong province	111.79154	22.17044
S17	Luanchuan county, Luoyang city, Henan province	111.61577	33.78570
S18	Panzhihua city, Miyi county, Sichuan province	102.11034	26.89069

was complemented by 70% ethanol and mixed well. After standing, the supernatant was filtered through filter paper. During the process, 18 RPM samples were prepared 3 replicates. Before UPLC-QTOF/MS analysis, the filtered supernatant was filtered through a 0.22 μm microporous membrane and 2 μL aliquot was injected.

In addition, quality control (QC) sample was prepared by mixing 100 μL supernatants of 18 geographical RPM samples to validate stability of LC–MS system. It was injected for 3 times before beginning the whole sample list to condition or balance the system. During the analytical run, QC sample was injected every 9 RPM samples to further monitor and investigate the stability and analytical variability of the system. After that, the change degree of the analytical system in the analysis process could be obtained and determined, which was critical for assessing the variation and reliability of the analytical results.

UPLC-QTOF/MS conditions
Samples were analyzed using a Waters ACQUITY UPLC I-Class system (Waters Corporation, Milford, USA). An Acquity UPLC HSS T3 C18 column (2.1 mm i.d. × 100 mm, 1.8 μm) was used for chromatographic separation. All samples were run in a random and non-grouped order. The flow phases consisted of 0.1% formic acid in water (A) and acetonitrile (B). The program of gradient elution was set as follows: 0–16 min, 5–60% B; 16–20 min, 60–100% B. The flow rate was 0.4 mL/min. The temperatures of column oven and auto-sampler were

maintained at 35 and 10 °C during the analysis, respectively. The sample injection volume was 2 μL.

MS spectrometry detection was operated on a Waters Xevo G2-XS QTOF/MS (Waters, Manchester, UK) equipped with the UPLC system through an electrospray ionization (ESI) interface in negative and positive ion modes. The ESI source parameters were maintained as follows: capillary voltage 1.0 kV, cone voltage 40 V, source temperature 110 °C, desolvation temperature 450 °C. Nitrogen was used as cone gas and desolvation gas with flow of 50 and 800 L/h, respectively. Argon was used as collision gases. The acquisition range of MS scanning was from m/z 50 to 1200 Da in MS^E continuum mode. By using a collision energy ramp from 10 to 30 V, the MS/MS fragment information was obtained. The mass accuracy and reproducibility of UPLC-QTOF/MS was validated by the reference lock mass of leucine-enkephalin (ESI$^+$: m/z 556.2771; ESI$^-$: m/z 554.2615) with the concentration of 100 pg/μL and the flow rate of 10 μL/min. Data acquisition was performed using Masslynx™ v 4.1 (Waters, Manchester, UK).

Data processing
All raw data of RPM samples in the LC–MS runs were loaded on Progenesis QI software (v2.0). By using the "assess all runs in the experiment for suitability", QC2 was automatically selected as the alignment reference. Next, the peaks of all other runs were aligned by comparison with QC2. After that, the experiment design (QC group and S1–S18 groups) was set, the peaks of all samples

were picked and convoluted. And then, all data of the peaks were exported into the EZinfo software (v3.0) for PLS-DA analysis. The necessary data were filtered and then were imported into Progenesis QI software (v2.0) to identify the compounds by its powerful Metascope search engine in the software according to the accurate mass, isotope distribution, fragment ions, collision cross-sectional area and many other parameters.

The significant differences of the markers in different RPM species were analyzed by one-way analysis of variance (ANOVA). The results are shown as mean ± SD. The differences were considered statistically significant at $P \leq 0.05$.

Results

Data analysis by Progenesis QI

Multivariate statistical tools was used to observe all differences among the RPM samples from different geographical origins. Firstly, the 3D LC/MS data acquired by Masslynx™ v 4.1 were converted into a 2D ion intensity map as an exact mass retention time (EMRT) pair by using Progenesis QI. During the process, the RPM QC2 sample was automatically selected as the alignment reference by Progenesis QI, and all other RPM samples

were aligned with QC2 as the reference. The representative peak alignment results and chromatograms between QC2 and S14b were shown in Fig. 1. Figure 1a was a vector alignment window, there were 414 vectors; Fig. 1b, c both were 2D ion intensity map. Figure 1c also showed the matching results for peak alignment between QC2 and S9b, the score was 96.1%. The matching score range between QC2 and other RPM sample was from 90.3% (S15c) to 97.9% (S18b). The ordinate of Fig. 1a–c represented the retention time (Rt), and the abscissa of them was m/z. Figure 1d was the total ion chromatograms (TIC), green and purple chromatograms represented QC2 and S9b, representatively.

Then, the experiment was designed, 60 samples were divided into 19 groups, including QC and S1–S18 groups. Next, all peaks of RPM samples were picked and convoluted. The parameters of sensitivity value was set at 3 and the minimum peak width was set at 0.15 min, respectively. Under the condition, the best balance could be obtained with the most true feature ion signals and the least random noise. Total 24,530 peaks were observed in the 2D ion intensity map, which was shown in Additional file 2: Figure S1. The normalization graphs for the RPM samples are shown in Additional file 3: Figure S2.

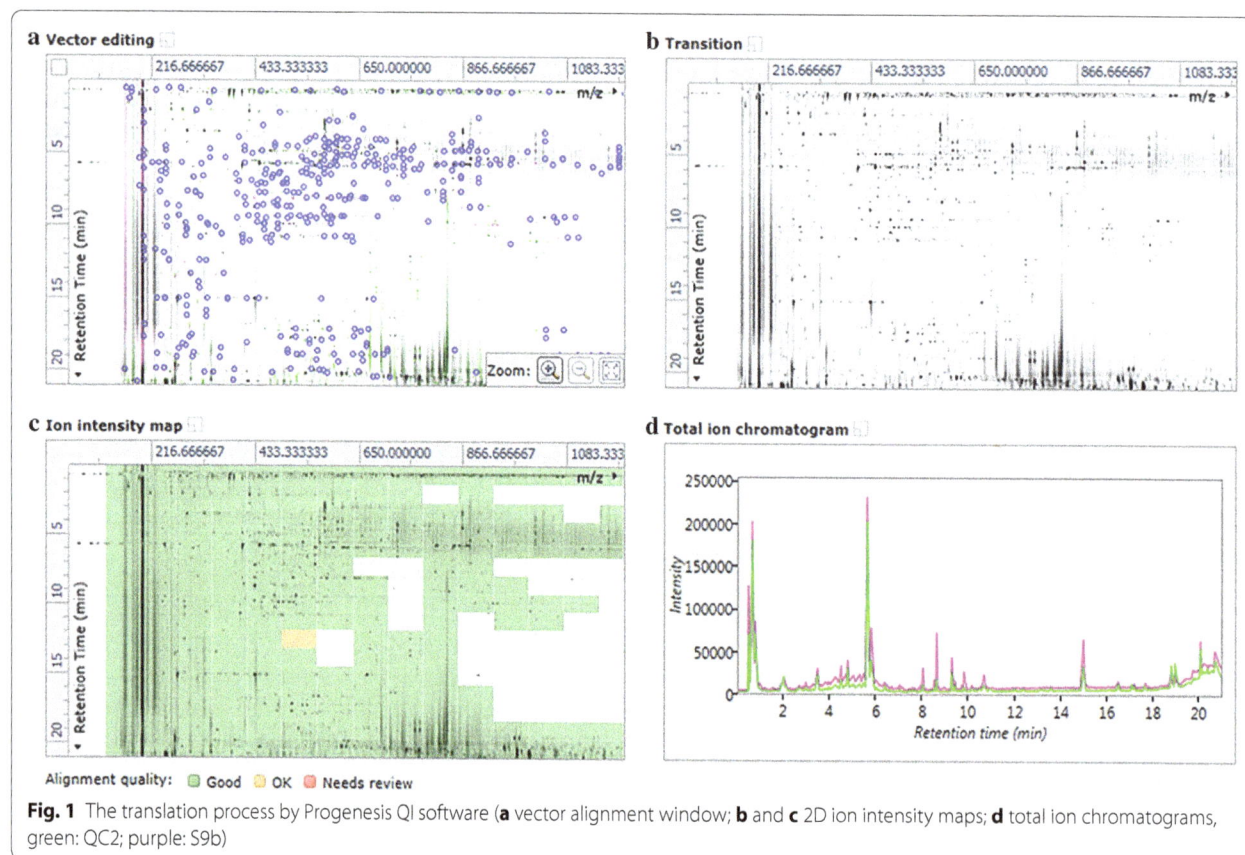

Fig. 1 The translation process by Progenesis QI software (**a** vector alignment window; **b** and **c** 2D ion intensity maps; **d** total ion chromatograms, green: QC2; purple: S9b)

PLS-DA analysis for RPM samples

After that, all data were exported into the EZinfo software (v3.0) for PLS-DA analysis. The outliers and classification trends among the 18 kinds of RPM samples could be observed in PLS-DA results (Fig. 2). In the score plot obtained by PLS-DA, there was a clear differentiation between RPM S1–S12 groups and S13 group, indicating that RPM sample from Changhao Chinese Medicine Development Co., Ltd. was very different from other samples in Guizhou province. RPM samples from Guangdong province (S14–S16 groups) clustered together and separated from Guizhou samples. RPM samples from Henan (S17 group) and Sichuan (S18 group) provinces were closer to Guizhou samples, and located father from Guangdong samples. R^2Y and Q^2 of the PLS-DA model were 0.771 and 0.634, respectively, which suggested that the PLS-DA model had good adaptability and predictability. Among the RPM samples from the same place of Guizhou province, the samples between S1 and S2 clustered together respectively, indicating that cultivated and wild RPM samples in Xinzhou town had significant difference; the separation between S5 and S6, S8 and S9, S10 and S11 indicated that cultivated RPM samples for 2 and 3 years in Meitan county, Baiduo village, and Niudachang town also had significant difference.

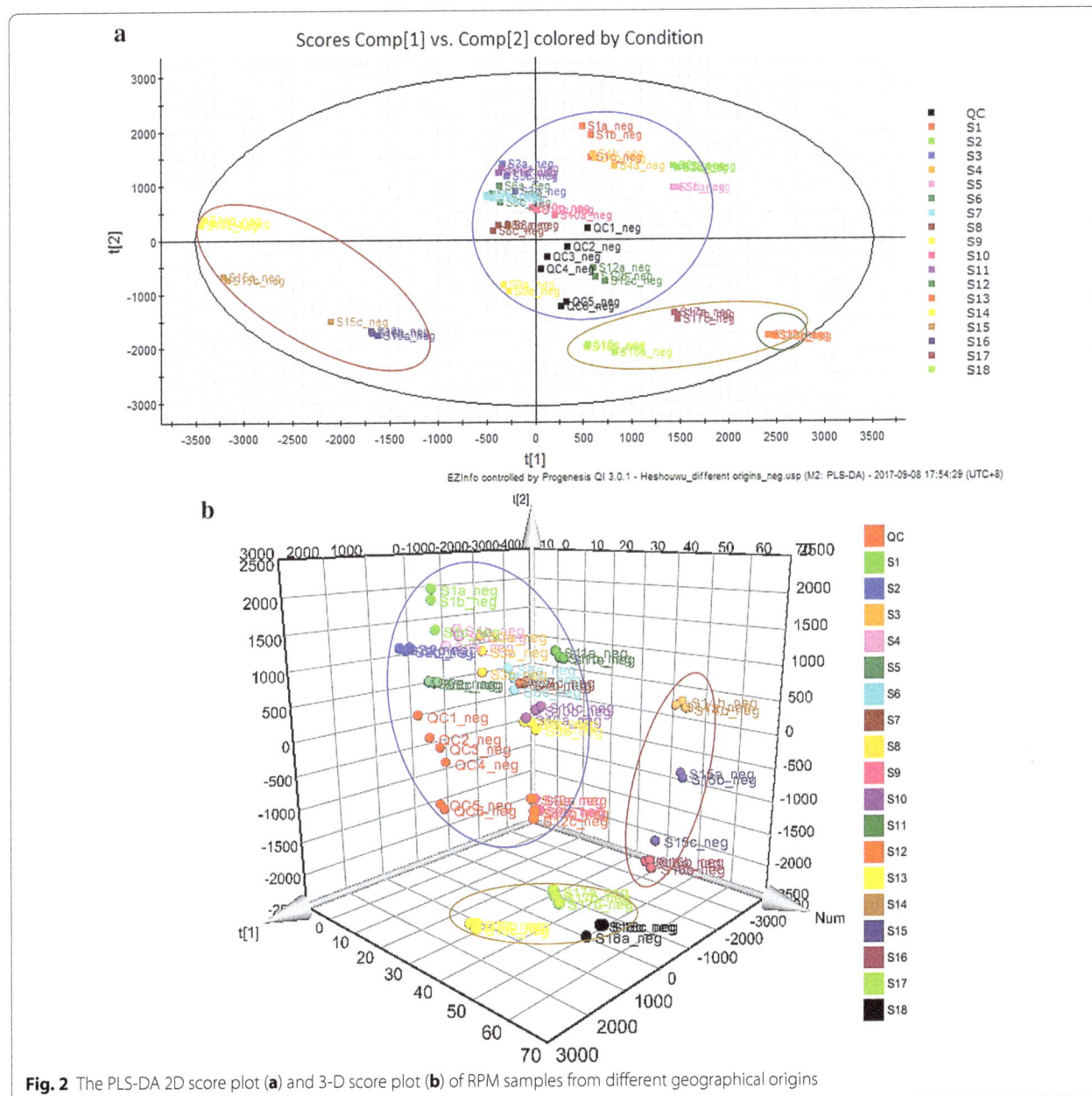

Fig. 2 The PLS-DA 2D score plot (**a**) and 3-D score plot (**b**) of RPM samples from different geographical origins

Identification of chemical markers

Identification of potential chemical markers in RPM samples from different geographical origins was carried out on basis of the retention behavior and mass assignment using Progenesis QI software. First, PLS-DA model was constructed from the EZinfo software. From loading plots (Fig. 3a) and VIP plots (Fig. 3b) of that model, the interested potential biomarkers could be extracted.

Additionally, an ANOVA $P \leq 0.05$, a maximum fold change ≥ 2 and VIP value > 1 were set as the restriction conditions to select the significant changing compounds and reduce the "false discovery rate (FDR)". Next, the Progenesis MetaScope, ChemSpider (http://www.chemspider.com/) and Element composition methods of Progenesis QI software was used for preliminary determination of the chemical markers. The mass tolerance

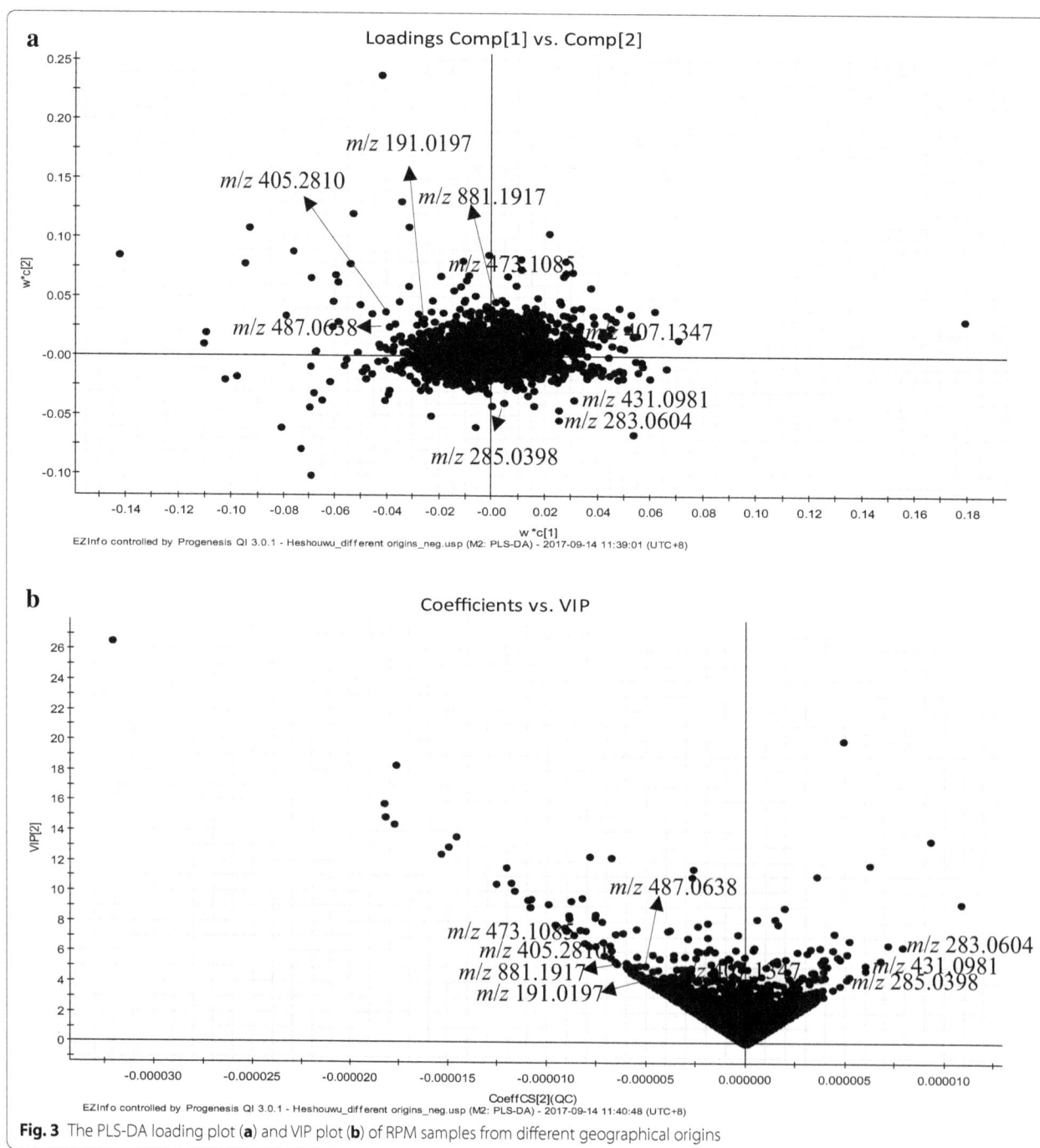

Fig. 3 The PLS-DA loading plot (**a**) and VIP plot (**b**) of RPM samples from different geographical origins

between the measured m/z values and exact mass of the interest compounds, and the relative mass error of the performed theoretical fragmentation both were set to within 5 ppm. Then, under the targeted MS/MS mode, the MS/MS spectrum of chemical markers was obtained. Finally, some chemical markers were identified by comparison with the standard reference; and others were identified by MS/MS spectrum, online database, element composition results, and literatures.

According to the protocol detailed above, 9 chemical markers (**C1–C9**) in RPM samples from different geographical origins were identified (Table 2). Among them, 4 chemical markers including **C1**, **C3**, **C4** and **C9** were identified by comparing with their reference compounds. Other 5 compounds were tentatively identified on basis of their molecular ion information and fragments generated by precursor ions. Herein, the **C5** with Rt-m/z of 8.53–407.1347 in negative ion mode was detailed as an example to illustrate the identification process. Firstly, the accurate mass of the marker

([M−H]$^-$ at m/z 407.1347) was found from the mass spectrum (Fig. 4). Secondly, specific MS/MS information about fragmentation pattern of the marker was acquired from QTOF system. The main fragment ions of the marker in the negative ion spectrum were observed at m/z 245.0819, 230.0948, 202.0635, and 159.0451, which could be the [M−H]$^-$ of lost $-C_6H_{12}O_5$, $-C_6H_{12}O_6$, $-C_8H_{14}O_5$, $-C_{10}H_{19}O_6$, respectively. $C_{20}H_{24}O_9$ was located as the candidate due to its high mass accuracy among the possible compounds. Finally, the chemical compound was identified as torachrysone-8-O-glucoside (**C5**) according to the ChemSpider database and literature [20, 21].

The data of 6 replicates of QC sample were analyzed to evaluate the repeatability of LC–MS method. The relative standard deviations (RSD%) of peak areas, Rt and m/z were 5.73–13.42, 0–0.25 and 0.00012–0.00301%, respectively. QC sample maintained in auto sampler at 4 °C for 4, 8, 12, 24, 28, 32 h were tested to assess the post-preparation stability of samples. The relative errors of peak

Table 2 Chemical markers in RPM samples from different geographical origins by UPLC-QTOF/MS

No.	t (min)	m/z (−)	Fragment information	Compound name	Compound type	Formula	Max fold change	VIP value
C1	0.79	191.0197	191.0197, 173.0091	Citric acid	Organic acids	$C_6H_8O_7$	4.72	4.11
C2	2.86	881.1917	881.1917, 863.1829, 591.1144, 217.0506, 152.0015	3,3′-di-O-Galloyl-procyanidin B2	Polyphenols	$C_{44}H_{34}O_{20}$	8.12	5.12
C3	5.68	405.2810	405.2810, 243.1911, 227.0425, 215.0702, 201.0545, 173.0596	2,3,5,4′-Tetrahydroxystilbene-2-O-glucoside	Stilbene glycosides	$C_{20}H_{22}O_9$	2.01	6.15
C4	8.06	431.0981	431.0981, 269.0455, 265.0506, 263.0350, 253.0506, 241.0506, 227.0350, 224.0478, 210.0322, 182.0373	Emodin-8-O-glucoside	Anthraquinone glycosides	$C_{21}H_{20}O_{10}$	31.99	5.20
C5	8.53	407.1347	407.1347, 245.0819, 230.0948, 202.0635, 159.0451	Torachrysone-8-O-glucoside	Anthraquinone glycosides	$C_{20}H_{24}O_9$	7.78	4.28
C6	8.65	473.1085	473.1085, 456.1062, 431.0983, 269.0455, 265.0506, 253.0506, 240.0428, 227.0350, 224.0478, 210.0322, 182.0373	Emodin-O-(acetyl)-hexoside	Anthraquinone derivatives	$C_{23}H_{22}O_{11}$	4.42	7.54
C7	9.30	487.0638	487.0638, 470.0734, 445.0369, 283.0604, 240.0428, 212.0478, 197.0244, 184.0505, 169.0278	Physcion-O-(acetyl)-hexoside	Anthraquinone derivatives	$C_{23}H_{22}O_{12}$	4.73	3.80
C8	10.18	285.0398	285.0398, 269.0455, 253.0506, 240.0428, 227.0350, 224.0478, 210.0322, 182.0373	Citreorosein	Anthraquinones	$C_{15}H_{10}O_6$	34.91	4.25
C9	12.50	283.0604	283.0604, 240.0428, 212.0478, 197.0244, 184.0505, 169.0278	Physcion	Anthraquinones	$C_{16}H_{12}O_5$	2567.78	6.46

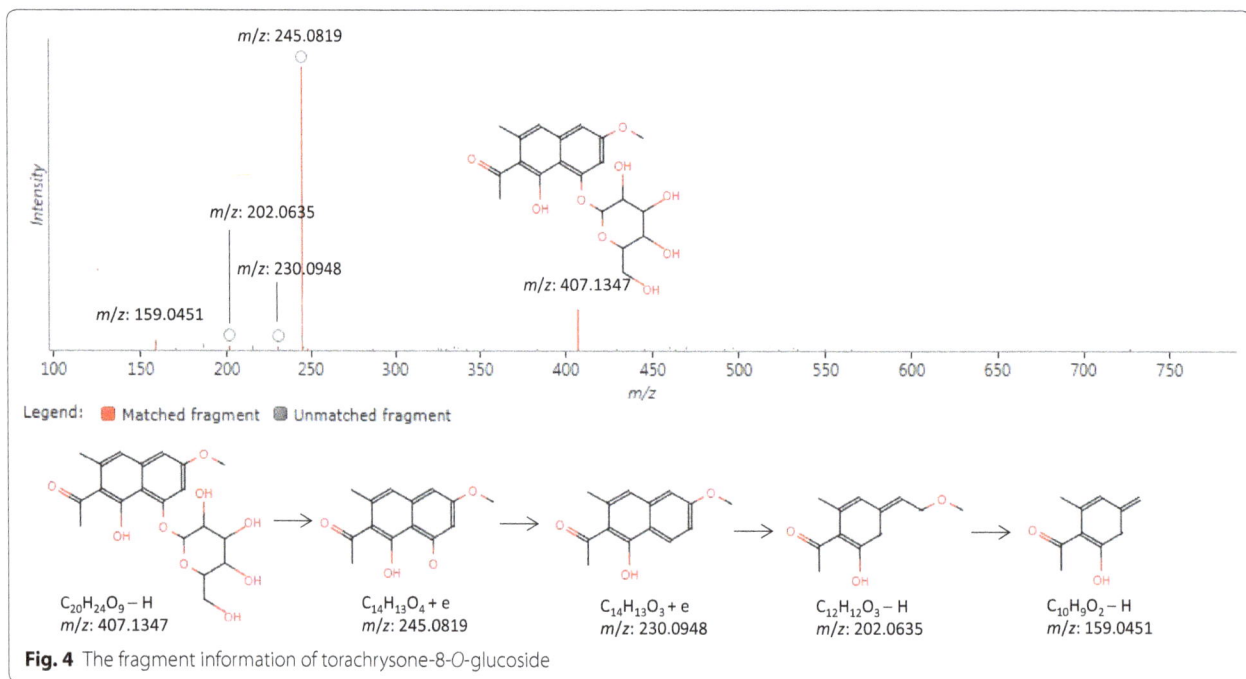

Fig. 4 The fragment information of torachrysone-8-O-glucoside

areas were < 13.42% demonstrating good repeatability and stability of the method.

Furthermore, in order to characterize the differences more clearly, the relative intensity of chemical markers in RPM samples from different geographical origins was shown in Table 3 and Fig. 5. The max fold change of **C1–C9** were 4.72, 8.12, 2.01, 31.99, 7.78, 4.42, 4.73, 34.91 and 2567.78, respectively. And the results of Fig. 5**C9** and Table 3 showed that the content of **C9** in 18 RPM samples had the most different, and the content of **C9** in S18 was the highest, which was about 4 time than S13; the content of **C9** in S2 and S10 were similar, which was lower than S13 and S18, but higher than other 15 RPM samples; the content of **C9** in S1, S3–S9, S11, S12, S14–S17 were similar. The content trend of **C4** (Fig. 5**C4**) in 18 RPM samples was similar with **C9**. The content of **C8** (Fig. 5**C8**) in S9 was the highest; the content of S1, S3, S13, and S16 were lower than S9, but higher than S2, S4–S8, S10–S12, S14, S15, S17 and S18. The content of S4 and S7 was similar, which was higher than other 16 RPM samples. The content of **C5** (Fig. 5**C5**) and **C7** (Fig. 5**C7**) in S5 was the highest, the content of them in S9 was the lowest, but the content of **C7** in S9 was similar with that in S9. The content of **C1** (Fig. 5**C1**) and **C3** (Fig. 5**C3**) in S9 and S14 were the highest, respectively; but the content of them in S13 both were the lowest. The content of **C2** (Fig. 5**C2**) and **C6** (Fig. 5**C6**) in S4 were the highest, but the content of **C2** in S7 was similar with S4; the content of them in S16 both were the lowest, but the content of **C2** (Fig. 5**C2**) in S13 and S15 was almost equal to that of

S16; and the content of **C6** (Fig. 5**C6**) in S14 was almost equal to the content in S16.

Discussion

Because of the clinical benefits, TCM is becoming more and more attractive around the world. Therefore, it is an important issue to carry out the quality control study of TCM for its application and development. To control the quality of Chinese medicine and its products, studying the source of TCMs is a key. In the present study, 18 RPM samples were collected from 10 counties, 4 provinces of China. And 9 representative chemical markers related to the differences among the 18 RPM samples were identified. The content of **C1** and **C8** in S9 were the highest; while the content of **C5** and **C7** in S9 were the lowest. The content of **C1**, **C2** and **C3** in S13 and S18 were the lowest. The content of **C2** and **C6** were the highest. The content of **C3** in S14 was the highest. The content of **C4** and **C9** in S18 were the highest. The content of **C5** and **C7** in S5 were the highest. The results suggested that **C1**, **C5** and **C7** could be used as specific chemical markers for S9 and S5; **C1**, **C2** and **C3** could be used as special chemical markers for S13; **C1**, **C2**, **C3**, **C4** and **C9** could be used as specific chemical markers for S18; **C3** could be used as unique chemical markers for S14. The PLS-DA results of different RPM samples showed that the RPM from Guizhou provinces were different from the RPMs of Guangdong, Henan and Sichuan provinces, indicating that RPM samples from Guizhou province had some similarity. The samples from Guangdong, Henan and

Table 3 The relative intensity of the chemical markers in RPM samples from different geographical origins

Chemical markers	C1	C2	C3	C4	C5	C6	C7	C8	C9
S1	51,705.58 ± 2584.63	11,951.15 ± 645.72	41,725.54 ± 1340.02	6190.75 ± 327.08	38,687.07 ± 1649.29	12,771.68 ± 387.55	93,588.08 ± 1845.63	21,294.27 ± 376.74	200.19 ± 12.50
S2	54,477.74 ± 917.00	8448.42 ± 87.23	38,606.33 ± 469.16	18,825.53 ± 301.36	17,532.28 ± 153.38	11,199.92 ± 238.20	70,742.37 ± 835.72	5498.40 ± 81.59	9020.02 ± 164.72
S3	44,807.13 ± 1130.32	11,820.68 ± 330.10	49,625.66 ± 1886.30	8764.83 ± 106.85	13,463.15 ± 581.06	10,266.89 ± 220.35	32,995.56 ± 377.37	23,010.73 ± 197.83	135.31 ± 6.01
S4	42,325.49 ± 814.97	19,590.50 ± 412.11	35,216.92 ± 2860.68	12,300.10 ± 71.24	39,277.20 ± 327.26	17,174.93 ± 181.83	54,798.00 ± 125.03	6112.91 ± 18.00	32.25 ± 3.28
S5	50,502.99 ± 1160.87	13,260.65 ± 337.26	27,497.91 ± 2333.92	10,675.71 ± 108.05	68,958.14 ± 1118.64	14,959.91 ± 269.53	105,951.47 ± 340.46	5149.43 ± 86.72	142.77 ± 5.33
S6	52,510.17 ± 469.61	13,909.26 ± 26.51	29,965.99 ± 4288.98	5033.78 ± 50.00	38,243.35 ± 601.64	13,510.20 ± 253.37	67,729.01 ± 989.02	2754.53 ± 78.86	112.64 ± 5.46
S7	70,993.90 ± 1120.09	18,915.88 ± 265.25	31,622.93 ± 2802.44	7517.20 ± 59.55	24,700.24 ± 307.49	11,980.72 ± 136.83	57,924.29 ± 528.54	4078.03 ± 49.53	36.85 ± 3.83
S8	53,605.42 ± 785.10	10,332.18 ± 26.08	29,137.10 ± 142.32	7607.70 ± 36.09	26,767.93 ± 389.67	11,810.46 ± 169.16	71,004.30 ± 686.40	9197.88 ± 145.75	419.49 ± 18.62
S9	110,338.57 ± 4435.84	9357.71 ± 360.23	26,242.61 ± 904.28	8703.56 ± 334.27	8860.43 ± 215.65	7481.79 ± 311.97	22,402.21 ± 930.10	85,213.75 ± 2949.23	207.27 ± 6.94
S10	68,329.09 ± 1392.30	10,975.66 ± 244.40	29,228.39 ± 646.70	13,375.96 ± 68.22	32,143.18 ± 499.74	12,191.99 ± 118.92	57,392.75 ± 257.02	3760.47 ± 56.91	4594.62 ± 33.44
S11	83,294.77 ± 1355.53	15,550.55 ± 165.35	34,725.41 ± 338.49	11,433.86 ± 102.78	35,063.82 ± 417.58	13,051.54 ± 162.43	58,825.87 ± 474.70	3568.84 ± 103.00	580.74 ± 14.62
S12	41,004.17 ± 1032.78	6952.98 ± 101.11	26,092.98 ± 252.66	10,560.47 ± 208.07	46,059.83 ± 1052.28	11,851.39 ± 375.25	67,597.12 ± 1589.29	11,122.57 ± 179.55	162.41 ± 4.12
S13	23,363.99 ± 409.93	3334.93 ± 112.08	21,933.99 ± 1748.61	17,956.26 ± 40.22	53,097.08 ± 468.53	10,430.68 ± 150.77	52,453.40 ± 504.74	25,826.56 ± 338.01	23,061.01 ± 317.64
S14	45,590.58 ± 569.55	10,154.77 ± 584.16	56,602.21 ± 661.72	3363.27 ± 49.48	24,145.97 ± 989.02	5032.57 ± 106.25	61,403.82 ± 355.13	2559.13 ± 33.60	319.72 ± 8.80
S15	61,091.53 ± 11,395.42	3528.03 ± 802.85	43,153.78 ± 8584.56	3198.19 ± 365.14	26,207.57 ± 4683.80	5990.59 ± 988.60	59,731.13 ± 9985.09	5800.22 ± 859.43	92.49 ± 7.94
S16	44,684.42 ± 1532.64	3634.70 ± 225.88	29,010.21 ± 859.34	2200.38 ± 79.65	19,619.97 ± 320.79	4492.36 ± 130.95	48,868.69 ± 1139.51	30,643.84 ± 717.00	119.19 ± 4.10
S17	46,299.52 ± 753.18	7457.72 ± 215.09	25,504.16 ± 476.59	12,099.00 ± 86.28	15,555.46 ± 36.35	9026.73 ± 156.75	22,756.80 ± 104.18	11,503.65 ± 83.20	276.60 ± 4.81
S18	27,660.30 ± 536.51	2413.59 ± 48.12	26,851.27 ± 3378.46	70,400.91 ± 2306.84	19,093.18 ± 461.26	9595.14 ± 175.49	27,212.01 ± 692.91	10,298.36 ± 312.60	82,806.08 ± 486.14
QC	50,895.72 ± 5125.28	9259.56 ± 530.38	28,056.00 ± 3725.38	12,474.95 ± 914.73	28,101.47 ± 3305.72	10,350.10 ± 1388.66	52,497.63 ± 4122.08	16,243.25 ± 1997.41	7632.61 ± 928.12

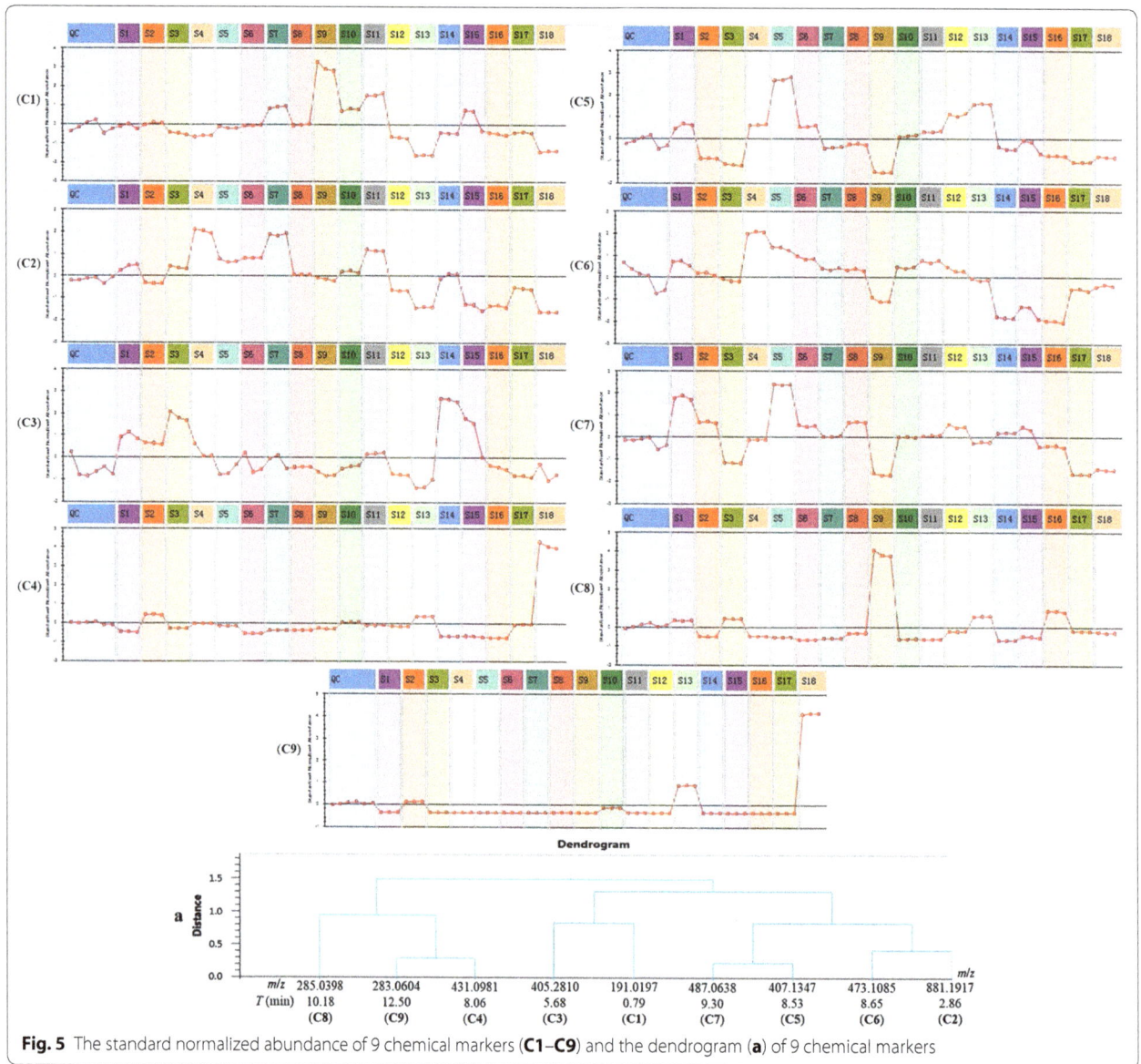

Fig. 5 The standard normalized abundance of 9 chemical markers (**C1–C9**) and the dendrogram (**a**) of 9 chemical markers

Sichuan provinces were also clustered together, respectively. And there were significant difference between the RPM sample for 2 and 3 years.

RPM contains a variety of anthraquinones, stilbene glycosides, phospholipids, phenols, flavonoids and tannins. Stilbene glycosides are a class of natural ingredients with a variety of physiological activities. The most active components including aloe-emodine, emodin, rhein and physcione were identified as the antioxidant anthraquinones [22]. The anthraquinone glycoside from RPM could significantly accelerate T and B lymphocytes proliferation in vitro, improve macrophages phagocytosis, increase TNF secretion activity and activity of NK cells, accelerate mixed lymphocyte reaction, and antagonize restraining effect of lymphocyte proliferation by mitomycin [23].

RPM samples from 18 different geographical origins were discriminated using UPLC-QTOF/MS coupled with chemometrics method in the present study. Those chemical markers with significant pharmacological activities could be used to distinguish the geographical origins of RPM samples. The results will help to develop strategies for protection and utilization of RPM samples. Chemometrics technique has potential to be used for discovering active components and evaluating the therapeutic effect and toxicity of TCMs, related to the complex composition and different growth geographical environment, and help us to find the natural substitute for the geographical origins herb medicine depleting more rapidly.

Conclusion

Classification and distinction of TCMs based on geographical origins are important basis for ensuring their quality and safety. The chemical constitution of RMP samples from different areas were characterized by UPLC-QTOF/MS method. PLS-DA method was applied to classify the samples from different origins. And the marker compounds contributing to the differentiation of RPMs were observed and identified. Nine chemical markers were tentatively identified and semi-quantified in different geographical RPM samples. The individual peak data of those chemical markers with significant content difference in different RPM regions were calculated. Those chemical markers could be applied to distinguish the geographical origins of different geographical RPM samples. The results showed that chemometric technique has potential to be used for discovering active components of TCMs, related to the complex composition and different growth geographical environment, and help us to find the natural substitute for the geographical origins herb medicine depleting more rapidly.

Abbreviations
RPM: Radix Polygoni Multiflori; UPLC-QTOF/MS: ultra-high performance liquid chromatography quadrupole time of flight mass spectrometry; PLS-DA: partial least squared discriminant analysis; TCM: traditional Chinese medicines; TLC: thin-layer chromatography; HPLC: high-performance liquid chromatography; IR: infrared spectrum; ICP-AES: inductively coupled plasma-atomic emission spectrometer; MS: mass spectrometry; DMPK: drug metabolism and pharmacokinetics; QC: quality control; EMRT: exact mass retention time; TIC: total ion chromatograms; ANOVA: analysis of variance; FDR: false discovery rate.

Authors' contributions
JFT and WXL contributed equally to this work. JFT and XLL conceived and designed the study. JFT and YHL collected RPM samples from different geographical areas. WXL and YJC performed the LC–MS analysis experiment and collected the data. FZ and YZ prepared the RPM samples. WXL wrote the manuscript. ZJM involved in the initial experimental design, and provided a great help and careful guide for the twice modification of the manuscript including the data processing analysis and grammar part. All authors read and approved the final manuscript.

Acknowledgements
We are pleased to thank Waters China Ltd. for technical support.

Competing interests
The authors declare that they have no competing interests.

Consent for publication
All of authors consent to publication of this study in journal of Chinese Medicine.

Funding
This work was supported by 2015 Special subject of Chinese medicine research in Henan Province (No. 2015ZY02101).

References
1. Man SC, Chan KW, Lu JH, Durairajan SS, Liu LF, Li M. Systematic review on the efficacy and safety of herbal medicines for vascular dementia. Evid Based Complement Altern Med. 2012. https://doi.org/10.1155/2012/426215.
2. He Y, Wang F, Chen SQ, Liu M, Pan W, Li X. The protective effect of Radix Polygoni Multiflori on diabetic encephalopathy via regulating myosin light chain kinase expression. J Diabetes Res. 2015. https://doi.org/10.1155/2015/484721.
3. Man SC, Chan KW, Lu JH, Durairajan SS, Liu LF, Li M. Systematic review on the efficacy and safety of herbal medicines for vascular dementia. Evid Based Complement Altern Med. 2012. https://doi.org/10.1155/2012/426215.
4. He Y, Wang F, Chen SQ, Liu M, Pan W, Li X. The protective effect of Radix Polygoni Multiflori on diabetic encephalopathy via regulating myosin light chain kinase expression. J Diabetes Res. 2015. https://doi.org/10.1155/2015/484721.
5. He Y, Wang F, Chen SQ, Liu M, Pan W, Li X. The protective effect of Radix Polygoni Multiflori on diabetic encephalopathy via regulating myosin light chain kinase expression. J Diabetes Res. 2015. https://doi.org/10.1155/2015/484721.
6. Hong CY, Lo YC, Tan FC, Wei YH, Chen CF. *Astragalus membranaceus* and *Polygonum multijlorum* protect rat heart mitochondria against lipid peroxidation. Am J Chin Med. 1994;22:63–70.
7. Jung KA, Min HJ, Yoo SS, Kim HJ, Choi SN, Ha CY, Kim HJ, Kim TH, Jung WT, Lee OJ, Lee JS, Shim SG. Drug-induced liver injury: twenty five cases of acute hepatitis following ingestion of *Polygonum multiflorum* Thunb. Gut Liver. 2011;5:493–9.
8. Chinese Pharmacopoeia Commission. Pharmacopoeia of the People's Republic of China. Beijing: China Medical Science Press; 2005. p. 122–3.
9. Chinese Pharmacopoeia Commission. Pharmacopoeia of the People's Republic of China. Beijing: China Medical Science Press; 2010. p. 164–5.
10. Chen Y, Jiang B, Zeng YE. Study on the geographic distribution and ecological environmental characteristics of *Polygonum multiflorum* based on GIS. China Pharm. 2011;22:3726–8.
11. Gao XX, Yan HJ, Liang CQ, Chen XY. Preliminary study on TLC fingerprint of Radix Polygoni Multiflori from different areas. J Chin Med Mater. 2007;30:407–9.
12. Li SF, Zheng CZ, Zhang L, Lan CW, He DX, Yao WF, Shang EX, Ding AW. HPLC fingerprint on roots of *Polygonum multiflorum* from different habitats. Chin Trade Herbal Drugs. 2015;46:2149–54.
13. Liang ZT, Leung NN, Chen HB, Zhao ZZ. Quality evaluation of various commercial specifications of Polygoni Multiflori Radix and its dregs by determination of active compounds. Chem Cent J. 2012;6:53.
14. Yuan YF, Tao ZH, Tian CH, Liu JX, Huang SS. Assessment of *Polygonum multiflorum* based on different origins by infrared spectra and chemometrics. Lishizhen Med Mater Med Res. 2011;22:1835–7.
15. Yan HJ, Fang ZJ. Study on determination and principal component analysis of inorganic elements in *Polygonum multiflorum* from different areas. China J Chin Mater Med. 2008;33:416–9.
16. Zhu ZW, Li J, Gao XM, Amponsem E, Kang LY, Hu LM, Chang YX. Simultaneous determination of stilbenes, phenolic acids, flavonoids and anthraquinones in Radix Polygoni Multiflori by LC–MS/MS. J Pharm Biomed Anal. 2012;62:162–6.
17. Liang ZT, Leung NN, Chen HB, Zhao ZZ. Quality evaluation of various commercial specifications of Polygoni Multiflori Radix and its dregs by determination of active compounds. Chem Cent J. 2012;6:1–7.
18. Chen ML, Chang WQ, Zhou JL, Yin YH, Xia WR, Liu JQ, Liu LF, Xin GZ. Comparison of three officinal species of *Callicarpa* based on a biochemome profiling strategy with UHPLC-IT-MS and chemometrics analysis. J Pharm Biomed Anal. 2017;145:666–74.
19. Liu S, Liang YZ, Liu HT. Chemometrics applied to quality control and metabolomics for traditional Chinese medicines. J Chromatogr B Anal Technol Biomed Life Sci. 2016;1015–1016:82–91.
20. Lin LF, Lin HM, Zhang M, Ni BR, Yin XB, Qu CH, Ni J. A novel method to analyze hepatotoxic components in *Polygonum multiflorum* using ultra-performance liquid chromatography-quadrupole time-of-flight mass spectrometry. J Hazard Mater. 2015;299:249–59.
21. Qiu XH, Zhang J, Huang ZH, Zhu DY, Xu W. Profiling of phenolic constituents in *Polygonum multiflorum* Thunb. by combination of ultra-

high-pressure liquid chromatography with linear ion trap-orbitrap mass spectrometry. J Chromatogr A. 2013;1292:121–31.

22. Zuo Y, Wang C, Lin Y, Guo J. Simultaneous determination of anthraquinones in Radix Polygoni Multiflori by capillary gas chromatography coupled with flame ionization and mass spectrometric detection. J Chromatogr A. 2008;1200:43–8.

23. Sun GB, Guo BJ, Li XE, Huang JN, Xue HB, Sun XB. The effect of anthraquinone glycoside from *Polygonum multiflorum* Thunb. on cellular immunological function in mice. Pharmacol Clin Chin Mater Medica. 2006;22:30–2.

8

Efficacy of Chinese herbal medicine for stroke modifiable risk factors

Wenbo Peng[1], Romy Lauche[1], Caleb Ferguson[2], Jane Frawley[1], Jon Adams[1] and David Sibbritt[1,3*]

Abstract

Background: The vast majority of stroke burden is attributable to its modifiable risk factors. This paper aimed to systematically summarise the evidence of Chinese herbal medicine (CHM) interventions on stroke modifiable risk factors for stroke prevention.

Methods: A literature search was conducted via the MEDLINE, CINAHL/EBSCO, SCOPUS, and Cochrane Database from 1996 to 2016. Randomised controlled trials or cross-over studies were included. Risk of bias was assessed according to the Cochrane Risk of Bias tool.

Results: A total of 46 trials (6895 participants) were identified regarding the use of CHM interventions in the management of stroke risk factors, including 12 trials for hypertension, 10 trials for diabetes, eight trials for hyperlipidemia, seven trials for impaired glucose tolerance, three trials for obesity, and six trials for combined risk factors. Amongst the included trials with diverse study design, an intervention of CHM as a supplement to biomedicine and/or a lifestyle intervention was found to be more effective in lowering blood pressure, decreasing blood glucose level, helping impaired glucose tolerance reverse to normal, and/or reducing body weight compared to CHM monotherapy. While no trial reported deaths amongst the CHM groups, some papers do report moderate adverse effects associated with CHM use. However, the findings of such beneficial effects of CHM should be interpreted with caution due to the heterogeneous set of complex CHM studied, the various control interventions employed, the use of different participants' inclusion criteria, and low methodological quality across the published studies. The risk of bias of trials identified was largely unclear in the domains of selection bias and detection bias across the included studies.

Conclusion: This study showed substantial evidence of varied CHM interventions improving the stroke modifiable risk factors. More rigorous research examining the use of CHM products for sole or multiple major stroke risk factors are warranted.

Keywords: Chinese herbal medicine, Stroke, Risk factor, Prevention

Background

Stroke is the second foremost cause of mortality and a leading cause of serious disability worldwide [1]. The incidence of stroke continues to rise due to societal and lifestyle changes and an aging population [2]. More than 90% of the stroke burden is attributable to its modifiable risk factors such as high blood pressure, high fasting plasma glucose, and high total cholesterol [3]. These stroke risk factors are strongly inter-related and some of them are simultaneous shown as a combined risk factor in people with stroke with higher risk [4, 5]. Previous research has clearly demonstrated the benefits of treating risk factors such as hypertension, diabetes, hyperlipidemia, obesity, atrial fibrillation, or transient ischaemic attack (TIA) for reducing the prevalence of primary stroke [6, 7]. The treatments of major stroke modifiable risk factors are therefore crucial for informing stroke prevention

*Correspondence: David.Sibbritt@uts.edu.au
[3] Australian Research Centre in Complementary and Integrative Medicine (ARCCIM), Faculty of Health, University of Technology Sydney, Level 8, Building 10, 235-253 Jones St, Ultimo, NSW 2007, Australia
Full list of author information is available at the end of the article

strategies and helping achieve improved quality of life of people with those risk factors and lowered associated health care costs [3].

Chinese herbal medicine (CHM)—therapies and products made from any part of medicinal plants (e.g. leaves and roots) and some non-herb based components (e.g. shells and powdered fossil) [8]—has a history of more than 2500 years with a unique theory of diagnosis and treatment, and is considered a modality of complementary medicine in Western countries [9]. CHM has been increasingly used for a wide range of chronic diseases in China and elsewhere in the form of raw plant materials, powers, capsules, tablets and/or liquids [9–11].

Chinese herbal medicine is a field of health care that may offer potential for addressing related risk factors of stroke [12–14]. Many CHM interventions have long been used for the treatments of some stroke risk factors as individual diseases such as Type 2 diabetes [15], hypertension [8] and obesity [16]. However, the research evidence as to whether specific CHM therapies or products may be effective in reducing each individual or mixed major risk factors of stroke remains unclear. The aim of this systematic review is to assess and summarize the efficacy and safety of all relevant CHM interventions for people at greatest risk(s) of stroke.

Methods
Search strategy
Four key bibliographic databases—MEDLINE, CINAHL/EBSCO, SCOPUS, and Cochrane Database of Systematic Reviews—were searched in the systematic review.

This review was designed and conducted in accordance with PRISMA (Preferred Reporting Items for Systematic Reviews and Meta-Analyses) guidelines. The stroke modifiable risk factors identified in this systematic review refer to high blood pressure (hypertension), high cholesterol (hyperlipidemia), irregular pulse (atrial fibrillation), TIA, high blood glucose (diabetes and impaired glucose tolerance (IGT), and overweight (obesity). The literature search employed keyword and MeSH term searches for terms relevant to 'CHM' and terms regarding stroke risk factors (Table 1). The combination of the search results of CHM and stroke risk factors were identified for screening. To obtain all relevant articles, reference lists of published review papers were also reviewed via Google Scholar.

Study selection
The inclusion criteria of literature in the systematic review were: peer-reviewed English-language journal articles focusing upon randomized controlled trials (RCTs) or cross-over studies published in the past 20 years (1996–2016), and articles reporting primary data findings examining the efficacy and safety of any type of CHM interventions (e.g. decoction, capsule, granule, power) on one or more major modifiable risk factors of stroke. Exclusion criteria were (1) published RCT protocols of this research area; (2) quasi- or pseudo-RCTs (3) studies focusing upon the efficacy and safety of CHM for treating stroke or post-stroke symptoms; (4) studies focusing upon the efficacy and safety of CHM for treating the complications of the stroke risk factors;

Table 1 Search terms for the systematic review

Chinese herbal medicine	Chinese herbal medicine [MeSH Term & Keyword] OR Chinese medicine [MeSH Term & Keyword] OR Chinese herb* [Title/Abstract] OR Chinese herbal [Title/Abstract]	
AND		
Stroke risk factors	High blood pressure	Hypertension [MeSH Term & Keyword] OR Blood pressure [MeSH Terms & Keyword] OR Hypertens* [Title/Abstract] OR Prehypertens* [Title/Abstract] OR Systolic [Title/Abstract] OR Diastolic [Title/Abstract] OR
	High cholesterol	Cholesterol [MeSH Term & Keyword] OR Triglycerides [MeSH Term & Keyword] OR Dyslipidemia [MeSH Term & Keyword] OR Epicholesterol [Title/Abstract] OR HDL [Title/Abstract] OR LDL [Title/Abstract] OR Triglyceride* [Title/Abstract] OR Hyperlipidem* [Title/Abstract] OR Lipidem* [Title/Abstract] OR
	Irregular pulse	Cardiac arrhythmias [MeSH Terms & Keyword] OR Atrial fibrillation [MeSH Terms & Keyword] OR Dysrhythmia* [Title/Abstract] OR Cardiac arrhythmia* [Title/Abstract] OR
	Transient ischaemic attack	Transient ischaemic attack [MeSH Terms & Keyword] OR Transient ischaemic attack* [Title/Abstract] OR
	High blood glucose	Diabetes [MeSH Terms & Keyword] OR Mellitus [MeSH Terms & Keyword] OR Impaired glucose tolerance [MeSH Terms & Keyword] OR Diabet* [Title/Abstract] OR NIDDM [Title/Abstract] OR IDDM [Title/Abstract] OR T2DM [Title/Abstract] OR *insulin* [Title/Abstract] OR Glucose [Title/Abstract] OR
	Overweight	Obesity [MeSH Terms & Keyword] OR Overweight [MeSH Terms & Keyword] OR Metabolic syndrome [MeSH Terms & Keyword] OR Obes* [Title/Abstract] OR Adiposity [Title/Abstract] OR Adipos* [Title/Abstract]

* Truncation, referring to all records that have those letters with any ending

(5) conference abstracts; and (6) publications without abstracts.

Data extraction

Titles and abstracts of all citations identified in the initial search were imported to Endnote (Version X7) and duplicates removed. Two of the authors screened all the titles/abstracts to identify articles meeting the inclusion and exclusion criteria independently. When consensus was not reached, the full texts of these unclear papers were retrieved and assessed by these two authors. Disagreements were discussed with a third author.

Data were extracted into a pre-determined table (Table 2) and checked for coverage and accuracy by two of the authors. Any differences in data extraction and interpretation were resolved through discussion amongst all authors. Table 2 includes detailed information on study recruitment, participant characteristics, intervention groups, results of primary outcome measures, study limitations, and CHM safety.

Quality assessment

Two authors independently assessed the methodological quality of the included studies using the Cochrane risk of bias criteria [17]. The characteristics of RCTs that might be related to selection bias (random sequence generation and allocation concealment), performance bias (blinding of participants and personnel), detection bias (blinding of outcome assessment), attrition bias (incomplete outcome data), reporting bias (selective outcome reporting), and other bias were evaluated. Disagreements regarding the risks of bias of some studies were resolved through discussion amongst these two authors (Table 3).

Results

The systematic review reported in this paper has been registered on the PROSPERO (International prospective register of systematic reviews, #CRD42017060107). The PRISMA flowchart of literature search and study/ article selection has been shown in Fig. 1. A total of 2377 papers were identified (2374 via database searches and three additional papers via Google Scholar). After removing duplicates, a total of 2065 papers remained for review. From amongst these, 70 manuscripts were identified for full review following title and abstract screening. Further screening of the full texts identified 46 publications (reporting on 46 RCTs) as eligible for final inclusion in the systematic review. Twelve of the included articles report on the efficacy of CHM for hypertension (1340 participants), 10 for diabetes (2004 participants), eight for hyperlipidaemia (997 participants), seven for IGT (1805 participants), three for obesity (329 participants), and six for the combination of several stroke risk factors (420 participants). No manuscript reported on a trial investigating the efficacy of CHM interventions for the stroke risk factor of transient ischemic attack or atrial fibrillation as a primary outcome. The characteristics of included studies with regards to the CHM interventions for hypertension, diabetes, hyperlipidaemia, IGT, obesity, and combined stroke risk factors are summarized in Table 2.

Hypertension

Eight RCTs were focused upon primary (essential) hypertension [18–25], one with isolated systolic [26], one with elder polarized hypertension [27], and two with hypertension and related cardiovascular diseases [28, 29]. Of the 12 RCTs on CHM for hypertension, 11 RCTs originated from China [18–22, 24–29]. Amongst the hypertension-focused RCTs, one RCT compared 'CHM, biomedicine plus lifestyle' intervention with 'biomedicine plus lifestyle' intervention [27] and showed significant decreased systolic blood pressure (SBP) before and after treatment of both intervention groups and a similar effect on controlling SBP between these two groups after treatment. Another two RCTs compared two different CHM interventions using different inclusion criteria of people with hypertension [19, 21]—these studies both reported a significant decrease of SBP and diastolic blood pressure (DBP) via all the CHM interventions examined with higher effective rate of treatments in the CHM groups than those in the control groups. Another three RCTs compared 'CHM' interventions with 'biomedicine' interventions and employed consistent inclusion criteria regarding SBP (140–179 mmHg) and DBP (90–109 mmHg) of participants, reporting a statistically significant decrease of SBP and DBP before and after treatment of both groups and a similar effect on controlling SBP and DBP between these two groups after treatment [18, 22, 24]. Another six RCTs compared 'CHM plus biomedicine' interventions with 'biomedicine alone' or 'biomedicine plus placebo' interventions [20, 23, 25, 26, 28, 29]. It is noteworthy that two of these six trials [20, 28] examined the efficacy of the same CHM products (Xuezhikang capsule) at different dose levels, demonstrating a significant decrease of SBP and DBP before and after treatment of both intervention groups and a silimar effect on SBP and DBP control between these two groups after treatment. Also amongst these six RCTs, three were three-armed RCTs which compared either 'CHM plus biomedicine' intervention versus 'biomedicine/no intervention,' 'CHM' interventions versus 'CHM plus biomedicine' or 'placebo plus biomedicine' intervention, or two types of preparations of a 'CHM plus biomedicine' intervention versus 'placebo plus biomedicine' intervention [25, 26, 28], showing inconsistent findings

Table 2 Characteristics of the included studies

Author Country Study period	Stroke risk factor	Participants	Intervention groups		Results	Side effects	Limitations
			Treatment group(s)	Control group(s)			
Lin et al. [18] China Sep 2001– Sep 2002	(Primary) Hypertension	*Sample size* n = 102 *CHM group* n = 52; 41 males and 11 females; mean age: 55 years *Control group* n = 50; 41 males and 9 females; mean age: 54 years *Inclusion criteria* SBP: 140–179 mmHg or DBP: 90–109 mmHg; TCM diagnosed for hyperactivity of the liver-yang syndrome	*Tianma gouteng decoction* 150 ml/time, twice daily, 4 weeks *Formulas* Tianma, Niuxi, Sangjisheng, Yimucao, Yejiaoteng, Huangqi, et al.	*Nitrendipine* 10 mg/time, 3 times daily, 4 weeks	*Baseline balance* Yes Significantly decreased SBP and DBP of both CHM and control groups before and after treatment, without significant difference between these two groups after treatment	No side effects	N/A
Li [19] China No information on study period	(Primary) Hypertension	*Sample size* n = 72 *CHM group* n = 46; 18 males and 28 females; mean age: 54 years *Control group:* n = 26; 11 males and 15 females; mean age: 53 years Both groups have cases with coronary heart disease, hyperlipemia, and diabetes *Inclusion criteria* SBP: 140–179 mmHg or DBP: 90–109 mmHg; TCM diagnosed for flaming-up of the liver-fire syndrome	During the intervention, no other drugs *Huanglian fire-purging mixture* 30 ml/time, twice daily, 4 weeks *Formulas* Huanglian, Gouteng, Zexie, Luhui	*Niuhuang Bolus* 1–2 bolus/time, 2–3 times daily, 4 weeks	*Baseline balance* Yes An effective rate (return to the normal range of BP or ≥20 mmHg but not in the normal range) at 60.9% of hypertension in the CHM group and 15.4% in the control group; Significantly decreased cholesterol, TG, blood sugar of the CHM group before and after treatment, without significant difference compared to the control group after treatment	CHM group: Vomiting and distension (n = 1); Slight abdominal pain and diarrhea (n = 3)	N/A
Ye et al. [20] China Feb 2004– Dec 2004	(Primary) Hypertension	*Sample size* n = 55 *CHM group* n = 28 *Control group* n = 27 *Inclusion criteria* SBP: 140–179 mmHg or DBP: 90–109 mmHg; normal LDL-C level; currently no antihypertensive medications or using antihypertensive medications for at least 6 months before screening	*Xuezhikang with Nifedipine* (20 mg/time, twice daily) 1200 mg daily, 72 weeks *Formulas* Red yeast rice	*Placebo with Nifedipine* (20 mg/time, twice daily) 1200 mg daily, 72 weeks	*Baseline balance* Yes No significant differences in BP between the CHM and placebo groups after treatment; 92.8% of the CHM group and 88.9% of the placebo group reached the target BP (<140/90 mmHg)	N/A	N/A

Table 2 continued

Author Country Study period	Stroke risk factor	Participants	Intervention groups		Results	Side effects	Limitations
			Treatment group(s)	Control group(s)			
Zhao et al. [21] China No information on study period	(Primary) Hypertension	*Sample size* n = 79 *CHM group* n = 40; 17 males and 23 females; mean age: 52 years *Control group* n = 39; 18 males and 21 females; mean age: 52 years *Inclusion criteria* SBP: 140–159 mmHg or DBP: 90–99 mmHg; no antihypertensive drugs or stopped taking antihypertensive drugs for 2 weeks; TCM diagnosed for stagnation of phlegm, blood stasis and hyperactivity of the liver-yang syndrome; age: 40–60 years	*Yinian Jiangya Yin* 100 ml/time, twice daily, 15 days *Formulas* Gouteng, Shijueming, Yimucao, Gujia, Banxia, Zhike, et al.	*Tianma Gouteng Yin* 100 ml/time, twice daily, 15 days *Formulas* Tianma, Gouteng, Huangqin, Yejiaoteng, Fushen, Duzhong, et al.	*Baseline balance* Yes Significantly decreased SBP and DBP of both CHM and control groups before and after treatment; Significantly decreased SBP and DBP in the CHM group than those in the control group after treatment; The total effective rate at 95.0% of BP control in the CHM group, while 87.2% in the control group	No side effects	N/A
Zhong et al. [22] China Jan 2006–Dec 2008	(Primary) Hypertension	*Sample size* n = 57 *CHM group* n = 31 *Control group* n = 26 *Inclusion criteria* SBP: 140–179 mmHg or DBP: 90–109 mmHg; daytime BP > 135/85 mmHg or nighttime BP > 120/70 mmHg; age: 18 years and older	During the intervention, no antiplatelet or lipid-lowering drugs and other Chinese patent medicines *Jiangya capsule with Nimodipine simulation* (1 capsule simulation/time, 3 times daily) 4 capsules/time, 3 times daily, 4 weeks *Formulas* Dilong, Nuxi, Haizao, Tianma, Chuanxiong	*Control group 1: Integrative medicine* 4 Jiangya capsule with 1 nimodipine capsule 3 times daily, 4 weeks *Control group 2: Western medicine* 4 Jiangya capsule simulation with 1 nimodipine capsule 3 times daily, 4 weeks	*Baseline balance* Yes Significantly decreased SBP and DBP in both CHM and control groups before and after treatment, without significant difference between these two groups after treatment	N/A	N/A
Yang et al. [23] Taiwan Sept 2008–Aug 2009	(Uncontrolled primary) Hypertension	*Sample size* n = 55 *CHM group* n = 30 *Control group* n = 25 *Inclusion criteria* sitting SBP ≥ 140 mmHg or sitting DBP ≥ 90mHg despite the conventional antihypertensive treatment; TCM diagnosed for hyperactivity of the liver-yang syndrome; age: 18–80 years	*Fufang Danshen capsule* 1000 mg/time, twice daily, 12 weeks *Formulas* Gegen, Juhua, Danshen, Hongjingtian	*Placebo* 12 weeks	*Baseline balance* Yes BP control rate (SBP < 140 mmHg and DBP < 90 mmHg) at 25.5% in the CHM group and 7.3% in the placebo group; More significant decrease of SBP in the CHM group than that of the placebo group after treatment	Mild side effects (e.g. diarrhea, fatigue, common cold) (CHM: n = 13; Control: n = 15)	Small sample size; Short study period

Table 2 continued

Author Country Study period	Stroke risk factor	Participants	Intervention groups		Results	Side effects	Limitations
			Treatment group(s)	Control group(s)			
Tong et al. [24] China Mar 2010–Sep 2010	(Mild to moderate) Hypertension	Sample size n = 219 CHM group n = 106; 61 males and 45 females; mean age: 52 years Control group n = 113; 62 males and 51 females; mean age: 52 years Inclusion criteria SBP: 140–180 mmHg or DBP: 90–110 mmHg; age: 18–65 years; WC ≥ 85 cm (male)/80 cm (female); plus one of the following: (1) TG ≥ 1.7 mmol/l or have received antidyslipidemia treatment; (2) HDL-C < 0.9 mmol/l (male)/1.1 mmol/l (female), or have received the related treatment; (3) FPG ≥ 5.6 mmol/l, diagnosed Type 2 diabetes, or have received glycemic control treatment; (4) TCM diagnosed for liver and stomach damp-heat syndrome	Jiangzhuoqinggan 170 ml/time, twice daily, 4 weeks Formulas Huanglian, Huangbai, Gouteng, Yinyanghuo	Irbesartan 150 mg/time, once daily, 4 weeks	Baseline balance Yes Significantly decreased BP in both CHM and control groups before and after treatment, without significant difference between these two groups after treatment; More significant decrease of daytime and nighttime SBP and DBP in the CHM group than those in the control group after treatment; Significantly decreased WC in the CHM group before and after treatment	N/A	Short study period; No placebo group; Small sample size
Wu et al. [25] China Jan 2010–May 2012	(Primary) Hypertension	Sample size n = 137 CHM group 1 n = 45; 31 males and 14 females; mean age: 50 years CHM group 2 n = 47; 33 males and 14 females; mean age: 48 years Control group n = 45; 29 males and 16 females; mean age: 48 years Inclusion criteria diagnosed primary hypertension for at least 3 months prior to screening; age: 18–75 years; 24 h MBP ≥ 130/80 mmHg, MBP ≥ 135/85 mmHg during waking hours, or MBP ≥ 120/70 mmHg during sleeping hours; or SBP ≥ 140 mmHg and/or DBP ≥ 90 mmHg	CHM group 1: Bushen Qinggan granule with amlodipine (5 mg/time, twice daily) Twice daily, 8 weeks CHM group 2: Bushen Qinggan decoction with amlodipine (5 mg/time, twice daily) Twice daily, 8 weeks Formulas Tianma, Gouteng, Duzhong, Huangqin, Kudingcha	Placebo with amlodipine (5 mg/time, twice daily) Twice daily, 8 weeks	Baseline balance Yes Significantly decreased BP in all three groups before and after treatment; Significant decrease in the daytime SBP in the CHM group 2 than that in the other two groups after treatment; More significant decrease of BP variability in the two CHM groups than those in the placebo group, without significant difference between these two CHM groups after treatment	N/A	N/A

Table 2 continued

Author Country Study period	Stroke risk factor	Intervention groups		Results	Side effects	Limitations
		Treatment group(s)	Control group(s)			
Li et al. [26] China Jun 2007–Jan 2008	(Isolated systolic) Hypertension	*Sample size* n = 241; 98 males and 143 females; mean age: 67 years *CHM group* n = 80 *Control group 1* n = 76 *Control group 2* n = 85 *Inclusion criteria* diagnosed hypertension; after 1-week elution period, sitting SBP: 140–180 mmHg and sitting DBP < 90 mmHg; age: 60–80 years	During the intervention, no other antihypertensive drugs *Jiangya capsule with Nimodipine simulation* (1 capsule simulation/time, 3 times daily) 4 capsules/time, 3 times daily, 4 weeks *Formulas* Dilong, Nuxi, Haizao, Tianma, Chuanxiong	*Control group 1: Integrative medicine 4 Jiangya capsule with 1 nimodipine capsule 3 times daily, 4 weeks Control group 2: Western medicine 4 Jiangya capsule simulation with 1 nimodipine capsule 3 times daily, 4 weeks*	*Baseline balance* Yes Significantly decreased SBP in all three groups before and after treatment; More significant decrease of SBP in the control group 1 than that in the CHM group and control group 2, without significant difference between the CHM group and control group 2 after treatment	Stomach discomfort (CHM: n = 2; Control 2: n = 2); Facial flush and dizziness (Control 2: n = 1)	N/A
Chen et al. [27] China 2006–2010	(Polarized) Hypertension	*Sample size* n = 125 *CHM group* n = 66 *Control group* n = 59 *Inclusion criteria* SBP > 140 mmHg and DBP < 70 mmHg; age: 60 years and older	Diet, exercise, smoking/alcohol advices were provided; no other Western medicine affecting BP *Shiyiwei Shenqi capsule or Dengzhan Shengmai capsule with Amlodipine Besylate tablets and Irbesartan tablets* 3–5 capsules/time, 2–3 times daily, 6 weeks *Formulas Shiyiwei Shenqi capsule*-Danggui, Xixin, Gouqi, Huangqi, Juemingzi, Lurong, et al. *Dengzhan Shengmai capsule*-Wuweizie, Xixin, Ginseng, Maidong	*Amlodipine Besylate tablets and Irbesartan tablets* 5 mg/time, once or twice daily, 6 weeks	*Baseline balance* Yes Significantly decreased SBP and pulse pressure in the CHM group before and after treatment; Significantly decreased SBP in the control group before and after treatment; No significant difference of DBP between the two CHM capsule groups after treatment	Dizziness and weakness (CHM: n = 5; Control: n = 4); Pretibial edema (CHM: n = 4; Control: n = 4); Facial flushing and headache (CHM: n = 4; Control: n = 4); Severe side effects (Control: n = 21)	N/A
Gong et al. [28] China Apr 2007–Apr 2009	Hypertension with cardiac damage	*Sample size* n = 90 *CHM group* n = 32; 19 males and 13 females; mean age: 59 years *Control group 1* n = 30; 18 males and 12 females; mean age: 56 years *Control group 2* n = 28; 15 males and 13 females; mean age: 59 years *Inclusion criteria* SBP ≥ 140 mmHg and/or DBP ≥ 90 mmHg	Co-administered medications: aspirin, β-blockers, calcium antagonists, diuretics *Xuezhikang capsule with Valsartan* (80 mg/time, once daily) 600 mg/time, twice daily, 24 months *Formulas* Red yeast rice	*Control group 1: Valsartan* 80 mg/time, once daily, 24 months *Control group 2: No intervention*	*Baseline balance* Yes Significantly decreased SBP, DBP in all three groups before and after treatment; More significant decrease of SBP, DBP; TO, LVMI in the CHM group and control group 1 than those in the control group 2 after treatment	Nausea and gastric discomfort (CHM: n = 3; Control 1: n = 1; Control 2: n = 2); Skin rash (Control 1: n = 1)	N/A

Table 2 continued

Author Country Study period	Stroke risk factor	Participants	Treatment group(s)	Control group(s)	Results	Side effects	Limitations
Xu et al. [29] China Jan 2006–Apr 2006	Hypertension, hypertension with diabetes, hypertension with coronary heart disease	*Sample size* n = 108 *CHM group* n = 55 *Control group* n = 53 Both groups have cases with diabetes and cases with coronary heart disease *Inclusion criteria* SBP > 140 mmHg or DBP > 90 mmHg; age: 40–80 years	*Qian Yang He Ji with antihypertensive angiotensin II receptor blocker therapy* 35 ml/time, twice daily, 6 months *Formulas* Gouteng, Shengdihuang, Jili, Nvzhenzi	*Antihypertensive angiotensin II receptor blocker* No information of usage	*Baseline balance* Yes Significantly decreased SBP, DBP, pulse pressure, cardioankle vascular index of both CHM and control groups before and after treatment; More significant decrease of SBP, DBP, cardioankle vascular index in the CHM group than those in the control group after treatment	CHM group: serious side effects (n = 5)	N/A
Chao et al. [30] China Sep 2006–Nov 2007	Type 2 diabetes	*Sample size* n = 43; age range: 18–70 *Inclusion criteria* newly diagnosed Type 2 diabetes; FPG ≥ 7 mmol/l and/or OGTT 2hPG ≥ 11.1 mmol/l; BMI: 23–35 kg/m² with poor glucose level after a 1-month diet control (i.e, FPG: 7–10 mmol/l); no antidiabetic drugs before	Diet and exercise advices were provided. During the intervention, no antidiabetic medications *CHM compound* 3 times daily, 3 months *Formulas* Huanglian, Huangqi, Rendongteng	*Placebo* 3 times daily, 3 months	*Baseline balance* Yes Significantly decreased FPG, PPG, HbA1c, BMI in the CHM group before and after treatment, without significant difference between these two groups after treatment	Moderate constipation (CHM: n = 2; Placebo: n = 2)	N/A
Ji et al. [31] China Dec 2007–Oct 2008	Type 2 diabetes	*Sample size* n = 627 (1) Drug naive group; mean age: 54 years *CHM group* n = 153 *Control group* n = 150 (2) Metformin group; mean age: 55 years *CHM group* n = 164 *Control group* n = 160 *Inclusion criteria* diagnosed Type 2 diabetes; age: 21–70 years; BMI: 18–28 or 18–35 kg/m² using metformin at 750 mg/day (or more) for at least 3 months before screening; stable body weight within at least 3 months before screening; FPG: 7.0–13.0 mmol/l and HbA1c >7%	Diet and exercise advices were provided *Drug naive group* Xiaoke pill 5–30 pills daily (according to FPG level), 48 weeks *Formulas* N/A *Metformin group:* Xiaoke pill with Metformin (250 mg/tablet) 5 tablets daily, 48 weeks *Formulas* N/A	*Gilbenclamide* 1.25–7.5 mg daily (according to FPG level), 48 weeks *Gilbenclamide with Metformin* 1.25 mg daily, 48 weeks	*Baseline balance* Yes In drug naive group: Significant 38% lower any hypoglycemia rate and 41% lower mild hypoglycemic episode in the CHM group than those in the control group after treatment; In Metformin group: Significant 24% lower hypoglycemia rate in the CHM group than that in the control group, without significant difference between these two groups in the mild hypoglycemic episode after treatment; In both drug narve group and Metformin groups, no significant difference of the rate of reducing HbA1c <6.5% between the CHM and control groups	Urinary tract infection; Upper respiratory tract infection; Elevated ALT/AST; Dyslipidemia	N/A

Table 2 continued

Author Country Study period	Stroke risk factor	Participants	Intervention groups Treatment group(s)	Control group(s)	Results	Side effects	Limitations
Tong et al. [32] China May 2009– Dec 2009	Type 2 diabetes	*Sample size* n = 480 *CHM group* n = 360 *Control group* n = 120 *Inclusion criteria* early diabetic status; BMI ≥ 24 kg/m²; HbA1c ≥ 7.0%; FPG: 7.0–13.9 mmol/l or 2hPG > 11.1 mmol/l; age: 35–65 years	During the intervention, antihyperlipidemia or antihypertensive drugs remain stable *Tang-Min-Ling-Wan* 6 g/time, 3 times daily, 12 weeks *Formulas* Huangqin, Huanglian, Baishao, Chenpi, Dahuang	*Placebo* 6 g/time, 3 times daily, 12 weeks	*Baseline balance* statistically different in HbA1c and 2hPG between groups Significantly decreased HbAlc, FPG, 2hPG and increased HOMA-β in both CHM and placebo groups before and after treatment; Significant higher proportion of the HbA1c reversed to normal (HbA1c ≤ 6.5%) in the CHM group (47.6%) than that in the placebo group (35.5%) after treatment; More significant decrease of HbAlc, FPG, 2hPG, body weight, BMI, WC and increase of HOMA-β in the CHM group than those in the placebo group after treatment	Mild side effects (CHM: n = 24; Placebo: n = 7); Transient slight ALT elevation (CHM: n = 2); Transient slight AST elevation (CHM: n = 2)	Short study period; No follow-up
Tu et al. [33] China No information on study period	Type 2 diabetes	*Sample size* n = 80 *CHM group* n = 41 *Control group* n = 39 *Inclusion criteria* diagnosed Type 2 diabetes; FPG: 7.0–13.3 mmol/l or 2hPG: 11.1–22.9 mmol/l; age: 18–70 years; normal renal function	Diet and exercise advices were provided *Wumei Wan* 3 packages daily, 12 weeks *Formulas* Huanglian, Huangbai, Ganjiang, Ginseng, Danggui, Huajiao, et al.	*Metformin* 500 mg/time, twice daily, 12 weeks	*Baseline balance* statistically different in gender between groups No significant difference of FPG, PPG, HbA1c between the CHM and control groups after treatment	Side effects (CHM: n = 1)	Short study period; Not double blind trial
Wu and Fan [34] China Oct 2012–Jan 2013	Type 2 diabetes	*Sample size* n = 152 *CHM group* n = 76; 48 males and 28 females; age: 48–66 years *Control group* n = 76; 35 males and 41 females; age: 47–68 years *Inclusion criteria* diabetes symptoms and any plasma glucose ≥ 11.1 mmol/l; FPG ≥ 7.0 mmol/l; 2hPG ≥ 11.1 mmol/l during OGTT	*Self-proposed Chinese herbal medicines with insulin* 1 dose daily, 2 weeks *Formulas* Gujianyu, Zhimu, Gegen, Jineijin, Zexie, Ginseng, et al.	*Insulin injection* Novolin 30R before breakfast and lunch, 2 weeks	*Baseline balance* Yes Significant more 20% decrease of insulin use in the CHM group than that in the control group after treatment; Significant less treatment days and frequency of hypoglycaemia in the CHM group than those in the control group after treatment	N/A	N/A
Cai et al. [35] China No information on study period	Type 2 diabetes	*Sample size* n = 67 *CHM group* n = 37 *Control group* n = 30 *Inclusion criteria* diabetes course < 5 years, fasting serum glucose > 7.0 mmol/l and/or 11.1 mmol/l after meal	Diet and exercise advices were provided *Lycium barbarum Poly-saccharide capsule* 300 mg/day, twice daily, 3 months *Formulas* Gouqi	*Placebo* 300 mg/day body weight, twice daily, 3 months	*Baseline balance* Yes Significantly decreased serum glucose and increased insulinogenic index in the CHM group before and after treatment; Significantly increased HDL in the CHM group than that in the placebo group after treatment	No side effects	Small sample size; Short follow-up

Table 2 continued

Author Country Study period	Stroke risk factor	Participants	Intervention groups Treatment group(s)	Control group(s)	Results	Side effects	Limitations
Lian et al. [36] China Apr 2013–Oct 2013	Type 2 diabetes	*Sample size* n = 186 *CHM group* n = 92 *Control group* n = 94 *Inclusion criteria* diagnosed type 2 diabetes; standard diet control and exercise therapy; taking metformin in a steady dose for over 3 months; HbA1c ≥ 7.0%; FPG: 7.0–13.9 mmol/l or 2hPG ≥ 11.1 mmol/l; BMI: 18–40 kg/m²; age: 18–70 years	Diet and exercise advices were provided *Jinlida with metformin* (1500 mg/kg/day) 1 granule/time, 3 times daily, 12 weeks *Formulas* Shuweicao, Yinyanghuo, Ginseng, Huangjing, Cangzhu, Kushen, et al.	*Placebo with metformin* (1500 mg/kg/day) 1 granule/time, 3 times daily, 12 weeks	*Baseline balance* Yes Significantly decreased HbA1c and increased HOMA-β in the CHM group before and after treatment; More significant decrease of HbA1c, FPG, 2hPG in the CHM group than those in the placebo group after treatment	N/A	Short study period; Small sample size
Zhang et al. [37] China Jan 2011– Dec 2013	Type 2 diabetes	*Sample size* n = 219; 112 males and 107 females; age: 38–74 years *CHM group* n = 109 *Control group* n = 110 *Inclusion criteria* diagnosed type 2 diabetes treated with insulin alone; FPG ≥ 7.0 mmol/l or 2hPG ≥ 11.1 mmol/l; age: 18 years and older; standard food containing100 g of carbohydrate during intervention	*Shen-Qi-Formula with insulin injection* (300 IU), twice daily before breakfast and dinner) 100 ml/time, 3 times daily, 12 weeks *Formulas* Shengdihuang, Huangqi, Zhidahuang, Ginseng, Shanzhuyu, Shuweicao, et al.	*Insulin injection* 300 IU, twice daily before breakfast and dinner, 12 weeks	*Baseline balance:* Yes Significantly decreased FPG, HbA1c in both CHM and control groups before and after treatment; Significantly decreased HOMA-IR and insulin usage level in the CHM group, while significantly increased insulin usage level in the control group, before and after treatment after treatment; More significant decrease of FPG, PPG, HbA1c in the CHM group than those in the control group after treatment	Transient hypoglycemia (Control: N/A n = 1)	
Hu et al. [38] China No information on study period	Type 2 diabetes	*Sample size* n = 112 *CHM group* n = 59 *Control group* n = 53 *Inclusion criteria* newly diagnosed type 2 diabetes (illness course ≤5 years); only taking metformin for treatment; age: 18–75 years; HbA1c: 6.5–9.0% despite taking two 500 mg metformin tablets daily	Diet and exercise advices were provided *Jianyutangkang tablet with Metformin* (1.5 g/time, 3 times daily) 3 tablets/time, 3 times daily, 26 weeks *Formulas* Ciwujia, Zhimu, Guijianyu	*Placebo with Metformin* 1.5 g/time, 3 times daily, 26 weeks	*Baseline balance* Yes Significantly decreased FPG, HbA1c in both CHM and placebo groups before and after treatment; More significant decrease of FPG, HbA1c in the CHM group than those in the placebo group after treatment	No side effects	Small sample size; No group without lifestyle intervention; Almost 25% participants lost from both groups

Table 2 continued

Author Country Study period	Stroke risk factor	Participants	Intervention groups Treatment group(s)	Control group(s)	Results	Side effects	Limitations
Li et al. [39] China Jun 2014– Dec 2014	Type 2 diabetes	Sample size n = 38 CHM group n = 23 Control group n = 15 Inclusion criteria diagnosed Type 2 diabetes; not on a regimen of antidiabetic medical treatment at least 3 months before screening, or on a regimen of anti-diabetic treatment no more than 3 months at any time in the past, or on a stable regimen of metformin monotherapy for at least 8 weeks; age:18–70 years; HbA1c: 7.0–10.0%; FPG ≤ 13 mmol/l; BMI: 19–30 kg/m²	Mulberry twig alkaloid tablet with Acarbose placebo (50 mg/time, 3 times daily) 50 mg–100 mg/time, 3 times daily, 24 weeks Formulas Sangzhi	During the intervention, metformin remains stable Placebo with Acarbose (50–100 mg/time, 3 times daily) 50 mg/time, 3 times daily, 24 weeks	Baseline balance Yes Significantly decreased 1 h and 2 h PPG, HbA1c in the CHM group before and after treatment without significant difference between these two groups after treatment; No significant difference of FPG between the CHM and control groups after treatment	Gastrointestinal side effects (lower in the CHM group than control group) Slightly higher liver and kidney function indices in the CHM group than those in the control group	Short study period; Small sample size; Missing data of BMI in follow-up period
Wang et al. [40] China No information on study period	Hyperlipidemia	Sample size n = 446 CHM group n = 324; 188 males and 136 females; mean age: 56 years Control group n = 122; 73 males and 49 females; mean age: 56 years Inclusion criteria serum TC ≥ 5.95 mmol/l, LDL-C ≥ 3.41 mmol/l, or TG: 2.26-4.52 mmol/l; HDL-C ≤ 1.04 mmol/l (male)/1.16 mmol/l (female); no medication for hyperlipidemia for more than 4 weeks and received dietary advice for 2–4 weeks	During the intervention, no medications affecting serum lipids Monascus purpureus rice preparation 3 tablets (600 mg)/ time, twice daily, 8 weeks Formulas Red yeast rice	Jiaogulan 3 tablets (600 mg)/time, twice daily, 8 weeks Formulas Jiaogulan	Baseline balance Yes Significantly decreased TC, LDL-C, TG in both CHM and control groups before and after treatment; More significant decrease of TC, LDL-C, TG and increase of HDL-C in the CHM group than those in the control group after treatment; Significant higher total effective rate in the CHM group (93.2%) than that in the control group (50.8%)	CHM group: Heartburn; flatulence; Dizziness; Exacerbation of preexisting stomachache	N/A

Table 2 continued

Author Country Study period	Stroke risk factor	Participants	Intervention groups — Treatment group(s)	Intervention groups — Control group(s)	Results	Side effects	Limitations
Yang et al. [41] China Feb 2002– May 2004	Hyperlipidemia	*Sample size* n = 96 *CHM group* n = 56; 31 males and 25 females; mean age: 69 years *Control group* n = 40; 29 males and 11 females; mean age: 68 years Both groups have cases with coronary heart disease, hypertension, and cerebral vascular disease *Inclusion criteria* TC > 5.7 mmol/l and/or TG > 1.7 mmol/l; TCM diagnosed for phlegm-damp and blood stasis syndrome	During the intervention, no other drugs *Danshen Jueming granules* 24 g/time, twice daily *Formulas* Taizishen, Danshen, Juemingzi, Shanzha, Zexie, Chenpi, et al.	*Xuezhikang capsules* 0.8 g/time, 3 times daily	*Baseline balance* Yes Significantly decreased TC, LDL-C in both CHM and control groups before and after treatment; Significantly decreased TG in the CHM group before and after treatment; More significant decrease of TC, LDL-C in the CHM group than those in the control group after treatment	No side effects	N/A
Ai et al. [42] China No information on study period	Hyperlipidemia	*Sample size* n = 60 *CHM group* n = 30 *Control group* n = 30 *Inclusion criteria* BMI < 35 kg/m²; TC ≥ 5.72 mmol/l and TG > 4.52 mmol/l; age: 18 years and older	During the intervention, no other lipid-modulating drugs *Daming capsule* 2 g/time, twice daily, 6 weeks *Formulas* Dahuang, Ginseng, Juemingzi, Danshen	*Pravastatin* 10 mg/time, once daily, 6 weeks	*Baseline balance* statistically different in the serum TG level between groups Significantly decreased in the TC, LDL-C in both CHM and control groups before and after treatment; More significant decrease of TC, LDL-C in the control group than those in the CHM group after treatment	Diarrhea (CHM: n = 8); Myalgia and epigastric discomfort (Control: n = 2)	N/A
Xu et al. [43] China No information on study period	Hyperlipidemia	*Sample size* n = 77 *CHM group* n = 37; 17 males and 20 females; mean age: 59 years *Control group* n = 40; 20 males and 20 females; mean age: 61 years *Inclusion criteria* TC ≥ 5.72 mmol/l or TG ≥ 1.70 mmol/l or HDL-C ≤ 1.04 mmol/l (male)/1.17 mmol/l (female); TCM diagnosed for phlegm-damp and blood stasis syndrome	During the intervention, no drugs affecting the blood lipid metabolism *Antihyperlipidemic decoction* 150 ml/time, twice daily, 8 weeks *Formulas:* Yiyiren, Shengpuhuang, Zexie, Shengshanzha, Huangqi, Juemingzi, et al.	*Zhinbiticose* 1050 mg/time, 3 times daily, 8 weeks	*Baseline balance* Yes Significantly decreased TC, TG, LDL-C, BMI in the CHM group and significantly decreased LDL-C, BMI in the control group, before and after treatment; More significant decrease of TC, TG in the CHM group than those in the control group after treatment; Significantly lower recurrence rate in the CHM group than that in the control group after treatment	No side effects	N/A

Table 2 continued

Author Country Study period	Stroke risk factor	Participants	Intervention groups — Treatment group(s)	Control group(s)	Results	Side effects	Limitations
Hu et al. [44] Hong Kong No information on study period	Hyperlipidemia	*Sample size* n = 40 *CHM group* n = 20; 6 males and 14 females; mean age: 58 years *Control group* n = 20; 10 males and 10 females; mean age: 55 years *Inclusion criteria* diagnosed dyslipidemia with lipid-lowering therapy or fasting LDL-C ≥ 4.1 mmol/l or TG ≥ 1.7 mmol/l; plasma LDL-C ≥ 2.6 mmol/l or ≥ 1.8 mmol/l for those with high cardiovascular risk following lipid-lowering treatment and diet or plasma TG ≥ 1.7 mmol/l following a lipid-lowering diet; age: 18 years and older	*A multiherb formula* 4 capsules in in the morning and 4 capsules in the evening, 12 weeks *Formulas* Shanzha, Zexie, Yumixu, Sangye, Lingzhi, Heshouwu	*Placebo* 4 capsules in the morning and 4 capsules in the evening, 12 weeks	*Baseline balance* statistically different in the LDL-C level between groups More significant decrease of LDL-C in the CHM group than that in the placebo group after treatment; No significant difference of LDL-C in the CHM group before and after treatment	CHM group: n = 11, including one stomach upset; Placebo group: n = 12, including one acid reflux	Not balanced baseline data of the two groups; Small sample size; Lack of consideration of the different types of dyslipidemia
Moriarty et al. [45] USA and China Apr 2011–Aug 2012	Hyperlipidemia	*Sample size* n = 116 *CHM group 1* n = 36; 6 males and 30 females; mean age: 58 years *CHM group 2* n = 42; 13 males and 29 females; mean age: 56 years *Control group* n = 38; 11 males and 27 females; mean age: 56 years *Inclusion criteria* TC ≥ 13.3 mmol/l; LDL-C: 8.9-12.2 mmol/l; TG < 22.2 mmol/l; BMI < 36 kg/m², age: 18 years and older	During the intervention, no lipid-lowering drugs, investigational agent, medications promoting weight loss, agents affecting lipid metabolism *CHM group 1: Xuezhi-kang* 1200 mg 2 capsules (300 mg) and 2 placebo daily, 12 weeks *CHM group 2: Xuezhikang* 2400 mg 4 capsules (300 mg) daily, 12 weeks *Formulas* Red yeast rice	*Placebo* 4 placebo capsules daily, 12 weeks	*Baseline balance* Yes Significantly decreased LDL-C in both two CHM groups before and after treatment, without significant difference between these two groups after treatment; The total effective rates at about 48% of LDL-C by ≥30% in the two CHM groups before and after treatment, without significant difference between these two groups	CHM groups 1, 2: n = 5, not CHM-related side effects (thyroid cancer, pulmonary embolism, fractured leg) Placebo group: n = 3	Not representative data; More females than males; Short treatment period
Heber et al. [46] USA No information on study period	Hyperlipidemia	*Sample size* n = 83; 46 males and 37 females; age: 34–78 years *Inclusion criteria* LDL-C > 4.14 mmol/l and TG < 2.94 mmol/l; no treatment for hypercholesterolemia before; normal liver and renal function	Diet advices were provided *Red yeast rice capsule* 1 capsule (600 mg), 2.4 g daily, 12 weeks *Formulas* Red yeast rice	*Rice powder placebo capsule* 1 capsule (600 mg), 2.4 g daily, 12 weeks	*Baseline balance* Yes Significantly decreased TC, TG, LDL-C in the CHM group before and after treatment; More significant decrease of TC, LDL-C in the CHM group than those in the placebo group after treatment	Placebo group: Rash (n = 1); Headaches (n = 1); Concurrent development of pneumonia (n = 1)	N/A

Table 2 continued

Author Country Study period	Stroke risk factor	Participants	Intervention groups Treatment group(s)	Control group(s)	Results	Side effects	Limitations
Lin et al. [47] Taiwan Dec 2001–Jan 2003	Hyperlipidemia	Sample size n = 79 CHM group n = 39; 23 males and 16 females; mean age: 46 years Control group n = 40; 22 males and 18 females; mean age: 47 years Inclusion criteria TC ≥ 6.22 mmol/l; LDL-C ≥ 4.14 mmol/l; TG ≤ 4.52 mmol/l; age: 18–65 years; BMI < 30 kg/m²; no lipid-lowering drugs 4 weeks before screening	Diet advices were provided Monascus purpureus Went rice 1 capsule (600 mg)/time, twice daily, 8 weeks Formulas Red yeast rice	Rice powder placebo 1 capsule (600 mg)/time, twice daily, 8 weeks	Baseline balance Yes Significantly decreased TC, TG, LDL-C in the CHM group before and after treatment; More significant decrease of TC, TG, LDL-C in the CHM group than those in the placebo group after treatment	CHM group: Drug-related side effects (n = 6)	No record of diets of the participants
Wei et al. [48] China Mar 2006–Sep 2007	Impaired glucose tolerance	Sample size n = 140 CHM group n = 70; 31 males and 39 females; mean age: 51 years Control group n = 70; 32 males and 38 females; mean age: 51 years Inclusion criteria 2hPG: 7.8–11.1 mmol/l; age: 25–70 years; BMI: 18.5–35.0 kg/m²; no IGT treatment before; TCM diagnosed for spleen-stomach dampness-heat syndrome	Tang No.1 granule with IGT knowledge education 2 packets/time, twice daily, 6 months Formulas: Dangshen, Fushen, Huangqi, Shanyao, Huangqin, Huanglian, et al.	IGT knowledge education	Baseline balance Yes Significantly decreased FPG, 2hPG, HbA1c, TG, HOMA-IR in the CHM group before and after treatment;More significant decrease of FPG, 2hPG, HbA1c, TG, HOMA-IR in the CHM group than those in the control group after treatment;More patients with IGT reversed to normal in the CHM group (19.1%) than that in the control group (3.1%)	No side effects	N/A
Gao et al. [49] China No information on study period	Impaired glucose tolerance	Sample size n = 510 CHM group n = 255; 110 males and 145 females; mean age: 49 years Control group n = 255; 112 males and 143 females; mean age: 51 years Inclusion criteria 2hPG: 7.8–11.1 mmol/l after OGTT and FPG > 7.0 mmol/l; age: 25–75 years; BMI: 20–35 kg/m²	Co-administered medications: calcium antagonists, a blockers or ACE antagonists, or β-blockers or thiazide for hypertension control Tangzhiping granule with Standard health care advice 5 g/time, twice daily, 5 days a week Formulas Huanglian, Sangbaipi, Gegen	Standard health care advice	Baseline balance Yes Significantly decreased 2hPG, HbA1c, BMI, FIN, HOMA-IR in the CHM group before and after treatment; More significant decrease of FPG, 2hPG, HbA1c, FIN, HOMA-IR in the CHM group than those in the control group after treatment; More patients with IGT reversed to normal in the CHM group (29.1%) than those in the control group (13.6%) after treatment; Lower risk of IGT patients progressing to Type 2 diabetes in the CHM group (22.2%) than that in the placebo group (43.9%)	Mild abdominal distension (CHM: n = 4; Control: n = 3)	Small sample size; Short follow-up

Table 2 continued

Author Country Study period	Stroke risk factor	Participants	Intervention groups Treatment group(s)	Control group(s)	Results	Side effects	Limitations
Fang et al. [50] China No information on study period	Impaired glucose tolerance	*Sample size* n = 514 *CHM group* n = 257; 136 males and 121 females; mean age: 55 years *Control group* n = 257; 142 males and 115 females; mean age: 55 years *Inclusion criteria* 2hPG: 7.8–11.1 mmol/l and FPG < 7.0 mmol/l; TCM diagnosed for spleen deficiency and dampness syndrome; age: 25–70 years; no IGT treatment before; no participation in clinical trials within the 3 months before screening	*Shenzhu Tiaopi granule with lifestyle intervention* 8.8 g/ time, twice daily, 12 months *Formulas* N/A	*Lifestyle intervention*	*Baseline balance* Yes More patients with IGT reversed to normal in the CHM group (42.2%) than that in the control group (32.9%); Lower risk of IGT patients progressing to Type 2 diabetes in the CHM group (8.5%) than that in the placebo group (15.3%)	CHM group: n = 9 Placebo group: n = 5 Gastrointestinal reactions were the most common side effects	Short follow-up; No consensus about efficacy of the CHM approach
Lian et al. [51] China Aug 2008– Mar 2010	Impaired glucose tolerance	*Sample size* n = 420 *CHM group* n = 210; 98 males and 112 females; mean age: 53 years *Control group* n = 210; 106 males and 104 females; mean age: 52 years *Inclusion criteria* 2hPG: 7.8–11.1 mmol/l after OGTT and FPG > 7.0 mmol/l; age: 25–70 years; no IGT treatment before; no participation in clinical trials within the 3 months before screening	*Tianqi capsule* 5 capsules/time, 3 times daily, 12 months *Formulas* Huangqi, Nvzhenzi, Huanglian, Tianhuafen, Shihu, Jixueteng, et al.	Diet and exercise advices were provided; *Placebo* 5 capsules/time, 3 times daily, 12 months	*Baseline balance* Yes More patients with IGT reversed to normal in the CHM group (63.1%) than that in the control group (46.6%); Lower risk of IGT patients progressing to Type 2 diabetes in the CHM group (18.2%) than that in the placebo group (29.3%)	CHM group: n = 15 Placebo group: n = 11 Gastrointestinal reactions were the most common side effects	Short study period; No data on plasma insulin and HbA1c; Small sample size
Huang et al. [52] China Mar 2013–Jul 2015	Impaired glucose tolerance	*Sample size* n = 120 *CHM group* n = 60; 31 males and 29 females; mean age: 52 years *Control group* n = 60; 35 males and 25 females; mean age: 51 years *Inclusion criteria* 2hPG: 7.8–11.1 mmol/l and FPG < 7.0 mmol/l; age: 30–70 years; no diabetes history; normal blood test, urine, stool, liver and renal function	*Tangyiping granules with lifestyle intervention* 10 g/time, twice daily, 12 weeks *Formulas* Huangqi, Baishao, Huanglian, Danshen, Banxia, Gegen	*Lifestyle intervention*	*Baseline balance* Yes Significantly decreased 2hPG, HbA1c, HOMA-IR, TG in the CHM group before and after treatment; More significant decrease of 2hPG, HbA1c, HOMA-IR, TG in the CHM group than those in the control group after treatment; More patients with IGT reversed to normal in the CHM group (58.3%) than that in the control group (26.7%); Lower risk of IGT patients progressing to Type 2 diabetes in the CHM group (16.7%) than that in the placebo group (31.7%)	No severe side effects	Small sample size; Short follow-up; Insufficient outcome measures

Table 2 continued

Author Country Study period	Stroke risk factor	Participants	Intervention groups — Treatment group(s)	Control group(s)	Results	Side effects	Limitations
Shi et al. [53] China Apr 2014–Oct 2014	Impaired glucose tolerance	*Sample size* n = 61; *CHM group* n = 32; 17 males and 15 females; mean age: 47 years; *Control group* n = 29; 14 males and 15 females; mean age: 50 years; *Inclusion criteria* 2hPG: 7.8–11.1 mmol/l after OGTT and FPG < 7.0 mmol/l; age: 20–80 years; BMI: 18–30 kg/m²	Diet, exercise, smoking/alcohol consumption advices were provided; no other CHM products with similar function; *Jinlida granule* 1 granule (9 g)/time, 3 times daily, 12 weeks; *Formulas* Ginseng, Fuling, Cangzhu, Gegen, Huangjing, Zhimu, et al.	*No drug intervention*	*Baseline balance Yes.* Significantly decreased FPG, 2hPG, HbA1c, HOMA-IR, BMI in the CHM group before and after treatment; More significant decrease of HbA1c, 2hPG, HOMA-IR in the CHM group than those in the control group after treatment; Lower risk of IGT patients progressing to Type 2 diabetes in the CHM group (6.2%) than that in the placebo group (17.2%); More patients with IGT reversed to normal in the CHM group (43.8%) than that in the control group (6.9%)	Gastrointestinal reactions (n = 2)	Short study period; Small sample size
Grant et al. [54] Australia Jun 2007–Dec 2009	Impaired glucose tolerance	*Sample size* n = 71; *CHM group* n = 39; 15 males and 24 females; mean age: 58 years; *Control group* n = 32; 18 males and 14 females; mean age: 60 years; *Inclusion criteria* FPG < 7.0 mmol/l and 2hPG: 7.8–11.0 mmol/l; age: 18 years and older	*Jiangtang Xiaozhi* 3 capsules/time, 3 times daily, 16 weeks; *Formulas* Nvzhenzi, Huangqi, Huanglian, Kunbu, Lizhihe, Jianghuang	*Placebo* 3 capsules/time, 3 times daily, 16 weeks	*Baseline balance Yes.* More significant decrease of fasting insulin, HDL in the CHM group than those in the placebo group after treatment; No information on the efficacy of CHM before and after treatment	CHM group: moderate dizziness (n = 1)	Short study period; Small sample size
Pan et al. [55] China Jul 2003–Aug 2003	Obesity	*Sample size* n = 78; *CHM group* n = 40; 18 males and 22 females; mean age: 41 years; *Control group* n = 38; 17 males and 21 females; mean age: 41 years; *Inclusion criteria* BMI ≥ 25 kg/m²; age: 20–50 years	*Dietary powder* 1 package (9 g)/time, twice daily, 7 weeks; *Formulas* Lotus rhizome, Green tea, Sanqi	*Placebo* 1 package (9 g)/time, twice daily, 7 weeks	*Baseline balance Yes.* Significantly decreased body mass, percentage of body fat, BMI, WC, HC in the CHM group before and after treatment; More significant decrease of body mass, percentage of body fat, BMI, WC, HC in the CHM group than those in the placebo group	Irritability (CHM: n = 1; Placebo: n = 1); Nausea (CHM: n = 2; Placebo: n = 1); Constipation (Placebo: n = 2)	N/A
Zhou et al. [56] China May 2010–Feb 2011	Obesity	*Sample size* n = 134; *CHM group* n = 70; 31 males and 39 females; mean age: 40 years; *Control group* n = 64; 29 males and 35 females; mean age: 40 years; *Inclusion criteria* BMI: 28–40 kg/m²; WC ≥ 85 cm (male)/80 cm (female); age: 18–60 years; TCM diagnosed for qi and phlegm stasis syndrome	*Xin-Ju-Xiao-Gao-Fang (full-dose)* 170 ml decoction/time, twice daily, 24 weeks; *Formulas* Dahuang, Zhishi, Huanglian, Juemingzi	*Xin-Ju-Xiao-Gao-Fang (10% of full-dose)* 170 mL decoction/time, twice daily, 24 weeks	*Baseline balance Yes.* More significant decrease of body weight, WC, HC, FIN in the CHM group than those in the control group after treatment	Minor side effects (e.g. skin rash) (CHM: n = 4; Control: n = 3)	Short study period; No follow-up; No true placebo group

Table 2 continued

Author Country Study period	Stroke risk factor	Participants	Treatment group(s)	Control group(s)	Results	Side effects	Limitations
Lenon et al. [57] Australia No information on study period	Obesity	Sample size n = 117 CHM group n = 59; 10 males and 49 females; mean age: 39 years Control group n = 58; 10 males and 48 females; mean age: 40 years Inclusion criteria BMI ≥ 30 kg/m²; age: 18–60 years	During the intervention, no other medications for obesity management Chinese herbal medicine formula RCM-104 4 capsules/time, 3 times daily, 12 weeks Formulas Green tea, Juemingzi, Huaihua	Placebo 4 capsules/time, 3 times daily, 12 weeks	Baseline balance Yes Significantly decreased body weight, BMI, body fat in the CHM group and increased body weight, BMI, body fat in the placebo group, before and after treatment; More significant decrease of body weight, BMI in the CHM group than those in the placebo group after treatment	Nausea (CHM: n = 4) Headache (CHM: n = 9) Decrease of appetite (Placebo: n = 2)	N/A
Hioki et al. [58] Japan No information on study period	Obesity and impaired glucose tolerance	Sample size n = 81; mean age: 54 years CHM group n = 41 Control group n = 40 Inclusion criteria FPG < 7.0 mmol/l and 2hPG: 7.8–11.1 mmol/l after OGTT	Diet and exercise advices were provided Bofu-tsusho-san 3 times daily, 24 weeks Formulas Jingjie, Bohe, Shigao, Gancao, Lianqiao, Mahuang, et al.	Placebo 3 times daily, 24 weeks	Baseline balance Yes Significantly decreased body weight, WC, HC, TC,TG, LDL-C in both CHM and placebo groups before and after treatment; Significantly decreased fasting insulin, HOMA-IR in the CHM group before and after treatment; More significant decrease of WC in the CHM group than that in the placebo group after treatment	CHM group: Loose bowels (n = 3)	N/A
Gao & Hu [59] China No information on study period	Type 2 diabetes and hyperlipidemia	Sample size n = 80 CHM group n = 40; 22 males and 18 females; mean age: 59 years Control group n = 40; 20 males and 20 females; mean age: 59 years Inclusion criteria FPG > 7.0 mmol/l and blood PG > 6.1 mmol/l	During the intervention, hypoglycemic agents remain stable Taizhi'an capsule with Simvastatin (10 mg daily) 0.9 g/time, 3 times daily, 12 weeks Formulas N/A	Simvastatin 20 mg daily, 12 weeks	Baseline balance Yes Significantly decreased TC, TG, LDL-C and increased HDL-C in the CHM group before and after treatment, without significant difference compared to the control group after treatment	Control group: Slight elevation of ALT (n = 2)	N/A
Poppel et al. [60] Netherlands May 2012–Mar 2013	Hyperlipidemia and hypertension	Sample size n = 20; 14 males and 6 females; mean age: 58 years CHM group n = 9 Control group n = 11 Inclusion criteria fasting LDL-C > 3.5 mmol/l and/or TG > 1.7 mmol/l; age: 40–70 years; SBP > 140 mmHg and/or DBP > 90 mmHg despite taking antihypertensive drugs	Danshen capsules 4 capsules (500 mg)/time, 3 time daily, 4 weeks Formulas Danshen	Placebo 4 capsules (500 mg)/time, 3 time daily, 4 weeks	Baseline balance Yes Significantly increased LDL-C in the CHM group before and after treatment, without significant difference compared to the placebo group; No significant difference of BP between the CHM and placebo groups after treatment	CHM group: Headache (n = 5); Dizziness (n = 3); Change in stool frequency (n = 3); Flatulence (n = 2); Peripheral facial nerve paralysis (n = 1)	Carry-over effect

Table 2 continued

Author Country Study period	Stroke risk factor	Participants	Intervention groups Treatment group(s)	Control group(s)	Results	Side effects	Limitations
Chu et al. [61] China Jan 2008– Dec 2009	Metabolic syndrome	*Sample size* n = 90 *CHM group* n = 60; 28 males and 32 females; mean age: 51 years *Control group* n = 30; 13 males and 17 females; mean age: 50 years *Inclusion criteria* diagnosed central obesity; WC > 90 cm (male)/80 cm (female) and/ or BMI > 25 kg/m²; fasting blood glucose ≥ 6.1 mmol/l and/or 2hPG ≥ 7.8 mmol/l or having diabetes history; TG > 1.7 mmol/l and/ or HDL-C < 0.9 mmol/ l(male)/1.0 mmol/l (female); age: 18–70 years	Diet and exercise advices were provided; During the intervention, no other CHM with hypoglycemic, lipid-lowering and antihypertensive effects *Pǔ'er tea extract capsules* 4 capsules/time, twice daily, 3 months *Formulas* Pǔ'er tea	*Placebo* 4 capsules/time, twice daily, 3 months	*Baseline balance* Yes Significantly decreased BMI, waist-to-hip ratio, TC, TG, LDL-C, 2hPG and increased HDL-C in the CHM group before and after treatment; More significant decrease of BMI, TC, LDL-C, 2hPG and increase of HDL-C in the CHM group than those in the placebo group after treatment	CHM group: Diarrhea (n = 1)	N/A
Chen et al. [62] China Oct 2011–Oct 2012	Hypertension and metabolic syndrome	*Sample size* n = 43 *CHM group* n = 22; 14 males and 8 females; mean age: 49 years *Control group* n = 21; 14 males and 7 females; mean age: 49 years *Inclusion criteria* diagnosed metabolic syndrome; average BP > 135/85 mmHg when awake and > 120/75 mmHg during sleep or SBP ≥ 140 mmHg and/ or DBP ≥ 90 mmHg; age: 18–65 years	Diet and exercise intervention were provided *Yiqi Huajiu formula* 1 bag/time, twice daily, 12 weeks *Formulas* Huangqi, Zexie, Huanglian, Yinchen, Puhuang	*Placebo* 12 weeks	*Baseline balance* Yes Significantly decreased body weight, WC, BMI, FPG, 2hPG, FIN, HOMA-IR, SBP, DBP, daytime SBP, daytime DBP, nighttime SBP in the CHM group before and after treatment; More significant decrease of WC, waist-to-hip ratio, 2hPG, HOMA-IR, FIN, SBP, DBP, daytime SBP and DBP than those in the placebo group after treatment	CHM group: Skin allergy (n = 2)	N/A

Table 2 continued

Author Country Study period	Stroke risk factor	Participants	Intervention groups		Results	Side effects	Limitations
			Treatment group(s)	Control group(s)			
Azushima et al. [63] Japan Jun 2010– Mar 2013	Hypertension and obesity	*Sample size* n = 106 *CHM group* n = 54; 28 males and 26 females; mean age: 59 years *Control group* n = 52; 29 males and 23 females; mean age: 60 years *Inclusion criteria* diagnosed hypertension with a history of antihypertensive treatment more than 4 weeks; BMI > 25 kg/m²; age: 20–79 years	Diet and exercise advices were provided *Bofu-tsusho-san with Antihypertensive therapy* 2.5 g/ time, once daily, 24 weeks *Formulas* Jingjie, Bohe, Shigao, Mahuang, Gancao, Lianqiao, et al.	*Antihypertensive therapy* No further information	*Baseline balance* Yes Significantly decreased daytime SBP, daytime DBP, body weight, BMI in the CHM group before and after treatment; More significant decrease of daytime SBP, body weight, BMI in the CHM group than those in the control group after treatment	CHM group: Gastric irritation (n = 1); Constipation (n = 1); Elevation of serum hepatic enzyme level (n = 1)	Not a double-blinded placebo-controlled study; Short study period

2hPG 2-hour postprandial glucose, *BP* blood pressure, *BMI* body mass index, *DBP* diastolic blood pressure, *FIN* fasting plasma insulin, *FPG* Fasting plasma glucose, *HbA1c* glycated hemoglobin, *HC* hip circumferences, *HDL* high-density lipoprotein, *HDL-C* high-density lipoprotein cholesterol, *HOMA-β* homeostatic model assessment β-cell function, *HOMA-IR* homeostatic model assessment insulin resistance, *IGT* Impaired glucose tolerance, *LDL-C* low-density lipoprotein cholesterol, *LVMI* left ventricular mass index, *MBP* mean blood pressure, *OGTT* oral glucose tolerance test, *PPG* postprandial plasma glucose, *SBP* systolic blood pressure, *TC* total cholesterol, *TG* triglyceride, *TO* original heart rate, *WC* waist circumference

Table 3 Risk of bias assessment of the included studies using the Cochrane risk of bias tool

Author, Country, Publication year	Stroke risk factor	Random sequence generation	Allocation concealment	Blinding of participants and personnel	Blinding of outcome assessment	Incomplete outcome data	Selective reporting	Other bias
Lin et al. [18], China, 2004	(Primary) Hypertension	Unclear	Unclear	High risk	Unclear	Low risk	Unclear	Unclear
Li [19], China, 2005	(Primary) Hypertension	Unclear	Unclear	High risk	Unclear	Unclear	Unclear	Unclear
Ye et al. [20], China, 2009	(Primary) Hypertension	Unclear	Unclear	Low risk	Low risk	Unclear	Low risk	Unclear
Zhao et al. [21], China, 2010	(Primary) Hypertension	Unclear	Unclear	Low risk	Unclear	Unclear	Unclear	Unclear
Zhong et al. [22], China, 2011	(Primary) Hypertension	Low risk	High risk	High risk	Unclear	Low risk	Low risk	Unclear
Yang et al. [23], Taiwan, 2012	(Uncontrolled primary) Hypertension	Low risk	Unclear	High risk	Low risk	Unclear	Low risk	High risk
Tong et al. [24], China, 2013	Hypertension	Low risk	High risk	High risk	Low risk	Unclear	Low risk	Unclear
Wu et al. [25], China, 2014	(Primary) Hypertension	Low risk	Low risk	Unclear	Low risk	Low risk	Low risk	Unclear
Li et al. [26], China, 2010	(Isolated systolic) Hypertension	Low risk	Unclear	Low risk	Unclear	High risk	Unclear	Unclear
Chen et al. [27], China, 2012	(Polarized) Hypertension	Low risk	Unclear	High risk	Unclear	Unclear	Unclear	High risk
Gong et al. [28], China, 2010	Hypertension with cardiac damage	Unclear	Unclear	High risk	Unclear	Low risk	Unclear	Unclear
Xu et al. [29], China, 2013	Hypertension, hypertension with diabetes, hypertension with coronary heart disease	Unclear	Unclear	High risk	Unclear	Unclear	Low risk	High risk
Chao et al. [30], China, 2009	Type 2 diabetes	Low risk	Low risk	Low risk	Low risk	Low risk	Low risk	Unclear
Ji et al. [31], China, 2013	Type 2 diabetes	Low risk	Low risk	High risk	Low risk	Low risk	Low risk	Unclear
Tong et al. [32], China, 2013	Type 2 diabetes	Low risk	Unclear	Low risk	Low risk	High risk	Unclear	Unclear
Tu et al. [33], China, 2013	Type 2 diabetes	Low risk	Low risk	High risk	Unclear	Low risk	Low risk	Unclear
Wu & Fan [34], China, 2014	Type 2 diabetes	Unclear	Unclear	High risk	Unclear	Unclear	Unclear	Unclear

Table 3 continued

Author, Country, Publication year	Stroke risk factor	Random sequence generation	Allocation concealment	Blinding of participants and personnel	Blinding of outcome assessment	Incomplete outcome data	Selective reporting	Other bias
Cai et al. [35], China, 2015	Type 2 diabetes	Low risk	Unclear	Low risk	Unclear	Low risk	Low risk	Unclear
Lian et al. [36], China, 2015	Type 2 diabetes	Low risk	Low risk	Low risk	Low risk	Low risk	Low risk	Unclear
Zhang et al. [37], China, 2015	Type 2 diabetes	Low risk	Low risk	High risk	Unclear	Unclear	Low risk	Unclear
Hu et al. [38], China, 2016	Type 2 diabetes	Low risk	High risk	Low risk	Low risk	High risk	Low risk	Unclear
Li et al. [39], China, 2016	Type 2 diabetes	Low risk	Low risk	Low risk	Low risk	Low risk	Low risk	Unclear
Wang et al. [40], China, 1997	Hyperlipidemia	Low risk	Unclear	High risk	Low risk	Low risk	Low risk	Unclear
Yang et al. [41], China, 2006	Hyperlipemia	Unclear	Unclear	Unclear	Unclear	Unclear	Unclear	High risk
Ai et al. [42], China, 2009	Hyperlipemia	High risk	High risk	High risk	High risk	Unclear	Low risk	High risk
Xu et al. [43], China, 2009	Hyperlipemia	Unclear	Unclear	High risk	Unclear	Unclear	Unclear	Unclear
Hu et al. [44], Hong Kong, 2014	Hyperlipemia	Low risk	Low risk	Low risk	Unclear	Low risk	Low risk	High risk
Moriarty et al. [45], USA & China, 2014	Hyperlipemia	Low risk	Low risk	Low risk	Unclear	Low risk	Low risk	Unclear
Heber et al. [46], USA, 1999	Hyperlipidemia	Unclear	Unclear	Low risk	Unclear	Low risk	Low risk	High risk
Lin et al. [47], Taiwan, 2005	Hyperlipidemia	High risk	Unclear	Low risk	Low risk	Low risk	Low risk	High risk
Wei et al. [48], China, 2008	Impaired glucose tolerance	High risk	Unclear	High risk	Unclear	Low risk	Unclear	Unclear
Gao et al. [49], China, 2013	Impaired glucose tolerance	Low risk	Unclear	High risk	Unclear	Low risk	Low risk	Unclear
Fang et al. [50], China, 2014	Impaired glucose tolerance	Unclear	Unclear	High risk	Unclear	Low risk	Low risk	Unclear
Lian et al. [51], China, 2014	Impaired glucose tolerance	Low risk	Low risk	Low risk	Low risk	Low risk	Low risk	Unclear
Huang et al. [52], China, 2016	Impaired glucose tolerance	Low risk	Low risk	High risk	Unclear	Low risk	Low risk	Unclear
Shi et al. [53], China, 2016	Impaired glucose tolerance	Low risk	Unclear	High risk	Unclear	High risk	Low risk	Unclear

Table 3 continued

Author, Country, Publication year	Stroke risk factor	Random sequence generation	Allocation concealment	Blinding of participants and personnel	Blinding of outcome assessment	Incomplete outcome data	Selective reporting	Other bias
Grant et al. [54], Australia, 2013	Impaired glucose tolerance	Low risk	Low risk	Low risk	Low risk	Low risk	Unclear	High risk
Pan et al. [55], China, 2005	Obesity	Low risk	Unclear	Low risk	Unclear	Low risk	Unclear	High risk
Zhou et al. [56], China, 2014	Obesity	Low risk	Unclear	Low risk	Unclear	Unclear	Low risk	Unclear
Lenon et al. [57], Australia, 2012	Obesity	Unclear	Low risk	Low risk	Unclear	Low risk	Low risk	Unclear
Hioki et al. [58], Japan, 2004	Obesity and impaired glucose tolerance	Low risk	High risk	Low risk	Unclear	Unclear	Low risk	High risk
Gao & Hu [59], China, 2006	Type 2 diabetes and hyperlipidemia	Unclear	Unclear	High risk	Unclear	Low risk	Low risk	Unclear
Poppel et al. [60], Netherlands, 2015	Hyperlipidemia and hypertension	High risk	Unclear	Low risk	Unclear	Low risk	Low risk	High risk
Chu et al. [61], China, 2011	Metabolic syndrome	High risk	Unclear	Low risk	Unclear	Low risk	Low risk	Unclear
Chen et al. [62], China, 2013	Hypertension and metabolic syndrome	Low risk	Unclear	Low risk	Unclear	High risk	Low risk	Unclear
Azushima et al. [63], Japan, 2015	Hypertension and obesity	Low risk	Unclear	High risk	High risk	Low risk	Low risk	High risk

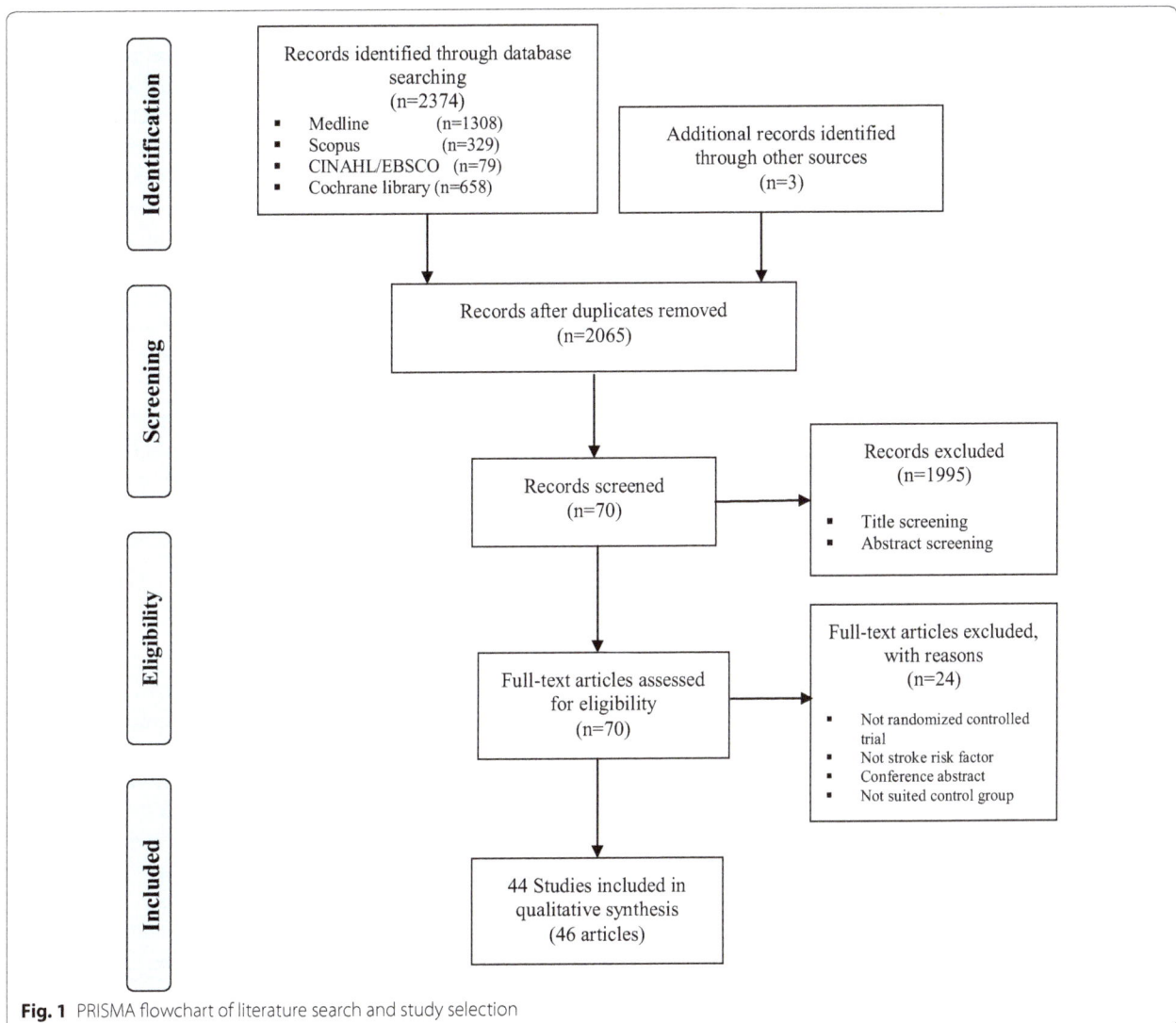

Fig. 1 PRISMA flowchart of literature search and study selection

with regards to the decrease of SBP or DBP amongst the three groups after treatment. *Gouteng* (钩藤) [18, 19, 21, 24, 25, 29] and *Tianma* (天麻) [18, 22, 25–27] were the most frequently used Chinese herbs in the hypertension-focused RCTs included, and all the CHM interventions using *Gouteng* and/or *Tianma* reported significant pre-post effectiveness regarding the decrease of SBP (and/or DBP) level. Also, *Gouteng* was the principal CHM formula constituent amongst four out of six hypertension-focused RCTs presenting between-group effectiveness of the investigated CHM interventions on the decrease of SBP (and/or DBP) levels compared to control interventions [21, 24, 25, 29]. In addition, the sample size of hypertension-focused RCTs ranged from 55 to 219. Six hypertension-focused RCTs did not provide the age and gender profile of the participants in either CHM group

or control group [20, 22, 23, 26, 27, 29]. The duration of the hypertension-focused trials ranged from 2 weeks to 24 months, with the majority of trials conducted between 4 and 12 weeks.

Eight hypertension-focused RCTs reported safety-related information and no deaths were noted [18, 19, 21, 23, 26–29]. One trial reported five cases of serious side effects of the 'CHM plus biomedicine' intervention group [29]. One trial (sample: 55) reported 13 mild side effects in the 'CHM plus biomedicine' intervention group and 15 in the 'placebo plus biomedicine' control group [23]. Only two of the papers reporting results from hypertension-focused RCTs listed any study limitations including small sample size and short study period [23, 24]. As for risk of bias in the hypertension-focused RCTs, three papers provided information on the allocation concealment [22, 24,

25] and four on the blinding of outcome assessment [20, 23–25]. Additionally, only three trials reported double-blinding of participants and personnel involved [20, 21, 26].

Diabetes
All of the 10 included diabetes-focused RCTs were focusing upon patients diagnosed with Type 2 diabetes mellitus and all these RCTs were conducted in China [30–39]. Amongst the 10 RCTs examining the efficacy of CHM on controlling the glucose level of patients with diabetes, four RCTs compared 'CHM' intervention to 'placebo' [32], 'CHM plus biomedicine' intervention to 'placebo plus biomedicine' intervention [39], and further, 'CHM plus lifestyle' intervention to 'placebo plus lifestyle' intervention [30, 35]. These four trials indicated more significant decreased glucose level [e.g. fasting plasma glucose (FPG), 2-hour postprandial glucose (2hPG), glycated hemoglobin (HbA1c)] by using CHM products when compared to the placebos after treatment, while this significant between-group variance in the decrease of glucose level showed no statistical significance when both CHM interventions and placebos were used concurrently with biomedicine or lifestyle intervention. Also amongst these 10 diabetes-focused RCTs, 'CHM plus biomedicine' intervention was compared to 'biomedicine' intervention, showing a more significant decrease of insulin usage by the CHM plus biomedicine treatment after treatment [34]. Also, after treatment, 'CHM, biomedicine plus lifestyle' interventions were found to achieve a more significant decrease of FPG, HbA1c, or hypoglycemia when compared to either 'biomedicine plus lifestyle' intervention [31, 37] or 'placebo, biomedicine plus lifestyle' intervention [36, 38]. Of the nine diabetes-focused RCTs providing CHM formulas, Huanglian (黄连) was the most common Chinese herb [30, 32–34, 36], followed by Ginseng (人参) [33, 34, 36, 37], Shanzhuyu (山茱萸) [34, 36, 37], Dahuang (大黄) [32, 34, 37], and Huangqi (黄芪) [30, 34, 37]. The CHM interventions examined in three out of five diabetes-focused RCTs, showing significant between-group effectiveness on the decrease of glucose level, indicated that the combination of these five commonly used Chinese herbs played a vital role for the efficacy of type 2 diabetes management [34, 36, 37]. All diabetes-focused RCTs defined inclusion criteria of diabetes based on different FPG, 2hPG, and/or HbA1c levels, and all the tested CHM products used in these RCTs were different. The sample size of the diabetes-focused RCTs ranged from 43 to 627. Only one RCT provided the age and gender profile of participants in the CHM and control groups [35]. The duration of the trials ranged from 2 weeks to 12 months, with the majority of trials conducted between 3–12 months.

Only two diabetes-focused RCTs failed to report safety-related information and no death were noted [34, 36]. The side effects of CHM products reported in the diabetes-focused RCTs are generally moderate, such as constipation, gastrointestinal disorders, and urinary tract infection. However, three diabetes-focused RCTs showed that CHM interventions caused slightly abnormal liver and kidney function after 3, 6, and 12 months, respectively [31, 32, 39]. Six diabetes-focused RCTs have specified their study limitations, with a short study period being the most common issue, followed by small sample size and no/short follow-up period [32, 33, 35, 36, 38, 39]. As for risk of bias of the diabetes-focused RCTs, one trial failed to use the random sequence generation method [34], three trials did not report information on allocation concealment [32, 34, 35], four trials failed to apply a double-blinding method [31, 33, 34, 37], and four trials did not provide details on the blinding outcome assessment [33–35, 37].

Hyperlipidemia
Half of the eight RCTs on CHM for the treatment of hyperlipidemia originated from China [40–43]. Amongst the hyperlipidemia-focused RCTs, two compared 'CHM' interventions with 'biomedicine' interventions [42, 43], two compared different 'CHM' interventions [40, 41], two compared 'CHM' interventions with 'placebos' [44, 45] and two compared 'CHM plus lifestyle' interventions with 'placebo plus lifestyle' interventions [46, 47]. Although the inclusion criteria of people with hyperlipidemia shown in the included hyperlipidemia-focused RCTs are limited to the total cholesterol (TC), triglyceride (TG), low-density lipoprotein cholesterol (LDL-C), high-density lipoprotein cholesterol (HDL-C), and/or body mass index (BMI) levels, the threshold value of these indices are diverse across the RCTs. It is worth noting that Monascus purpureus rice preparation (Xuezhikang capsule in Chinese) of which the main ingredient is red yeast rice, was tested in four hyperlipidemia-focused RCTs [40, 45–47]. The effects of the red yeast rice products are not consistent across these four RCTs. When the 'red yeast rice product plus lifestyle' intervention was compared with 'placebo plus lifestyle' intervention, a more significant decrease of TC and LDL-C was found in the red yeast rice product group after treatment. However, there was no significant improvement in TC or LDL-C amongst those receiving the red yeast rice product alone when compared to placebo alone. Amongst the rest four hyperlipidemia-focused RCTs, Danshen (丹参) [41–43], Juemingzi (决明子) [41–43], Zexie (泽泻) [41, 43, 44], and/or Shanzha (山楂) [41, 43, 44] were the main constituents of the CHM formulas examined and three of these trials reported the significant between-group

effectiveness of the investigated CHM interventions on the decrease of TC, LDL-C, and/or TG levels [41, 43, 44] compared to control interventions. The sample size of the hyperlipidemia-focused RCTs ranged from 40 to 446. Only two hyperlipidemia-focused RCTs did not provide the age and gender profile of the participants in CHM and control groups [42, 46]. The duration of the trials ranged from 6 weeks to 12 months while one trial did not specify the study period.

All hyperlipidemia-focused RCTs reported safety-related information and no deaths were noted. Three trials specified their side effects in the CHM intervention groups, including heartburn/flatulence [40], diarrhea [42], and stomach upset [40, 44]. Three hyperlipidemia-focused RCTs reported their study limitations including small sample size, lack of balanced baseline data between the CHM and control groups and no record of the participants' dietary control [44, 45, 47]. As for risk of bias of the hyperlipidemia-focused RCTs, five trials did not use the random sequence generation method [41–43, 46, 47], only two trials specified the appropriate allocation concealment [44, 45], and six trials failed to employ the blinding of outcome assessment [41–46].

Impaired glucose tolerance
The seven RCTs on CHM for the treatment of IGT originated from China (n = 6) [48–53] and Australia (n = 1) [54]. Amongst the IGT-focused RCTs, one compared 'CHM' with 'placebo' [54], five compared 'CHM plus lifestyle' interventions with 'lifestyle' interventions alone [48–50, 52, 53], and one compared 'CHM plus lifestyle' intervention with 'placebo plus lifestyle' intervention [51]. The inclusion criteria regarding the 2hPG level remain stable (7.8–11.0 mmol/l) while the FPG level is either <7.0 or >7.0 mmol/l across all the IGT-focused RCTs. Additionally, all the tested CHM products within the IGT-focused RCTs are different. Despite the variation in the inclusion criteria and CHM products, the results on the effects of CHM interventions are consistent throughout all IGT-focused trials. Specifically, more people with IGT reversed to normal in the CHM group (range 19.1–63.1%) compared to those in the control group (range 3.1–46.6%) and less people with IGT progressed to Type 2 diabetes in the CHM group (range 6.2–22.2%) compared to those in the control group (range 15.3–43.9%). Of the six IGT-focused RCTs with detailed CHM formulas, five reported the significant between-group effectiveness of the investigated CHM interventions regarding the decrease of FPG, 2hPG, and/or HbA1c levels compared to control interventions [48, 49, 52–54] and *Huanglian* (黄连) and *Gegen* (葛根) were the only Chinese herbs both included in these five IGT-focused trials. The sample size of the IGT-focused RCTs ranged from 61 to 514,

and all these RCTs provided the age and gender profile of participants in the CHM and control groups (897 males, 939 females, mean age 53 years with the range from 47 to 60 years). The duration of the IGT-focused trials ranged from 3 to 12 months.

All IGT-focused RCTs reported safety-related information and no deaths were noted. The most common side effects reported in the CHM groups were dizziness, gastrointestinal reactions, and abdominal distension. Almost all IGT-related RCTs provided information on their study limitations including a short study period and short follow-up period as well as small sample size. As for risk of bias of the IGT-focused RCTs, three trials provided information about the allocation concealment [51, 52, 54], two trials provided details on the blinding of outcome assessment [51, 54], and two trials reported double-blinding of participants and personnel [51, 54].

Obesity
Two RCTs on CHM for the treatment of obesity originated from China [55, 56] and one from Australia [57]. The three obesity-focused trials compared three different CHM products with their placebos. BMI is the key indicator of the inclusion criteria of all obesity-focused RCTs included. However, the threshold value of BMI was set differently across these trials. Amongst the obesity-focused RCTs, CHM products all showed more decrease of body weight than placebos after treatment. *Green tea* (绿茶) [55, 57] and *Juemingzi* (决明子) [56, 57] were the Chinese herbs included in two CHM formulas amongst these three obesity-focused trials. The sample size of the obesity-focused RCTs ranged from 78 to 134 and all these RCTs provided the age and gender profile of participants in the CHM and placebo groups. There were 115 males and 214 females across all the obesity-focused RCTs with a mean age of 40 years, ranging from 39 to 41 years. The duration of the obesity-focused trials ranged from 7 weeks to 6 months.

All obesity-focused RCTs reported safety-related information and no death were noted. CHM interventions were reported more side effects than the placebos, including nausea, headache, and skin rash. One obesity-focused RCT indicated the study limitations including short study period, no follow-up period, and no true placebo group [56]. As for risk of bias of the obesity-focused RCTs, all trials reported the double-blinding of participants and personnel while these trials failed to provide any details of the blinding of outcome assessment.

Combined stroke risk factors
Six RCTs exploring the efficacy of CHM on one or more of the stroke risk factors were identified in the systematic review. Specifically, one trial examined the 'CHM

plus lifestyle' intervention for the treatment of 'IGT and obesity' compared to 'placebo plus lifestyle' intervention, showing significant efficacy on both IGT and obesity before and after treatment and a significant effect on obesity control between groups after treatment [58]; Two trials examined the 'CHM plus biomedicine' interventions for the treatment of 'diabetes and hyperlipidemia' and 'hypertension and hyperlipidemia' compared to the 'biomedicine' intervention [59] and 'placebo plus biomedicine' intervention [60], respectively—both of these studies found similar effect on the combined stroke risk factors between groups after treatment. Moreover, three trials examined the 'CHM, biomedicine plus lifestyle' interventions for the treatment of 'metabolic syndrome' [61], 'hypertension and metabolic syndrome' [62], and 'hypertension and obesity' [63] compared to the 'biomedicine plus lifestyle' interventions with or without placebo, respectively, indicating significant effects on all included stroke risk factors by the CHM interventions compared to the control groups after treatment. Except the *Bofu-tsusho-san* (防风通圣散) used in two trials, all the other CHM interventions involved exploring a combination of multiple stroke risk factors were different and therefore it is unable to report the commonly used Chinese herbs which are vital for the efficacy of combined stroke risk factors across these six RCTs. The sample size of the RCTs focused upon combined stroke risk factors ranged from 20 to 106, and two of these RCTs failed to provide the age and gender profile of participants in the CHM and control groups [58, 60]. The duration of the RCTs exploring the combined stroke risk factors ranged from 4 to 6 months.

All RCTs focusing upon combined stroke risk factors reported safety-related information and no deaths were noted. Five out of these six RCTs reported that side effects only occurred in the CHM group [58, 60–63] including headache, dizziness, gastrointestinal reactions, and skin allergy. Only two RCTs focusing upon combined stroke risk factors identified their study limitations [60, 63], including failure to double-blind the RCT, short study period and carry-over effect. As for risk of bias of the RCTs focusing upon combined stroke risk factors, no trial reported appropriate allocation concealment and blinding of outcome assessment, and two trials were found to have a high risk of bias regarding the random sequence generation [60, 61].

Discussion

This paper reports the first comprehensive systematic review of the literature concerning the use of CHM amongst people at greatest risk(s) of stroke. A number of significant findings from our review are important for future evidence-based planning and priority setting for research in stroke prevention.

Our analyses show some positive efficacy and safety evidence of varied CHM interventions in lowering high blood pressure, high blood glucose, high cholesterol, high body BMI and a combination of multiple stroke risk factors. Importantly, our findings indicate that, compared to biomedicine alone/lifestyle modification alone/biomedicine plus lifestyle intervention, CHM monotherapy may be not sufficient enough for people to obtain their treatment goals when treating hypertension, diabetes, and hyperlipidemia, while an intervention of CHM as a supplement to biomedicine and/or a lifestyle intervention is more effective in lowering the levels of SBP/DBP, glucose, BMI, TC, 2hPG, and/or HbA1c. These findings from our review are in line with previous systematic reviews on CHM for cardiovascular diseases [12–14]. In addition, the evidence reported in the papers included with regards to the successful reversion from elevated blood glucose level to normal by using CHM interventions suggests that some CHM products, in combination with a lifestyle intervention, could be considered a potential effective therapeutic regimen for IGT, and these findings are consistent with a Cochrane review on CHM for IGT published in 2009 [13]. Although many RCTs identified in our review demonstrate the therapeutic benefits of CHM in people with a number of stroke risk factors, there is a lack of replicable evidence on CHM use in combined stroke risk factors. It is worth noting that a CHM product (red yeast rice preparation), a medicinal food [64], has been used several times not only for the management of hypertension but also for hyperlipidemia. However, the control interventions of all RCTs examining the efficacy of this rice preparation are different. Therefore, no trial included in our review paper has tested exactly the same CHM and control interventions for the treatment of any stroke risk factor(s).

Our findings show a large variation in the sample size and study period across the included RCTs. The potential risks of bias have been reported in the domains of allocation concealment, the blinding of participants and personnel, and/or the blinding of outcome assessment in the included RCTs. Most included trials have reported their safety information. No serious adverse events were noted although some studies showed some moderate side effects in the CHM groups.

Stroke risk factors vary by ethnic groups and such disparities may influence the etiology of stroke and the implementation of stroke prevention programs [65]. Nevertheless, the majority of studies on CHM use for stroke risk factors included in this review were conducted in China on Chinese populations. As such, the results shown in our review paper may not always be directly applicable to populations at risk of stroke in other countries beyond China. Furthermore, CHM is often composed of a number of herbs and is prescribed based on the unique Chinese medicine theory—syndrome differentiation. The replicability of these trial designs without Chinese medicine practitioners is therefore difficult.

There are some limitations to our systematic review that should be mentioned. Generalisability of the results from this systematic review is limited. Meanwhile, the overall 'unclear' reporting of research methodology in the included RCTs may limit the quality of the results reported in this review. In addition, our review was restricted to English peer-reviewed journal articles.

Conclusion

Although the findings in this systematic review with regards to the effect of CHM for stroke modifiable risk factors should be interpreted with caution, the potential therapeutic benefits of CHM as a treatment—particularly in combination with biomedicine and/or lifestyle intervention—for different stroke risk factors needs to be further examined by conducting rigorous trials. Future research should be designed and implemented with adequate sample size, detailed reporting of the allocation concealment method, sufficient application of double-blinding with an adequate placebo and blinding of outcome assessment, and long-term follow-up in different countries. Moreover, it is important for future research on this topic to pay attention to potential drug-herb interactions as a major safety issue in trial design when participants need to take one or more co-administered biomedicine as well as CHM products.

Abbreviations

2hPG: 2-hour postprandial glucose; BMI: body mass index; BP: blood pressure; CHM: Chinese herbal medicine; DBP: diastolic blood pressure; FIN: fasting plasma insulin; FPG: fasting plasma glucose; HbA1c: glycated hemoglobin; HC: hip circumferences; HDL: high-density lipoprotein; HDL-C: high-density lipoprotein cholesterol; HOMA-β: homeostatic model assessment β-cell function; HOMA-IR: homeostatic model assessment insulin resistance; IGT: impaired glucose tolerance; LDL-C: low-density lipoprotein cholesterol; LVMI: left ventricular mass index; MBP: mean blood pressure; OGTT: oral glucose tolerance test; PPG: postprandial plasma glucose; RCT: randomized controlled trial; SBP: systolic blood pressure; TC: total cholesterol; TG: triglyceride; TIA: transient ischaemic attack; TO: original heart rate; WC: waist circumference.

Authors' contributions
DS designed the study. WP, CF and JF conducted the literature search. WP and RL extracted and interpreted the data. WP drafted the manuscript and prepared tables and figures. JA and DS contributed to the critical revisions of the manuscript. All authors read and approved the final manuscript.

Author details
[1] Australian Research Centre in Complementary and Integrative Medicine (ARCCIM), University of Technology Sydney, Ultimo, NSW, Australia. [2] Centre for Cardiovascular and Chronic Care, University of Technology Sydney, Ultimo, NSW, Australia. [3] Australian Research Centre in Complementary and Integrative Medicine (ARCCIM), Faculty of Health, University of Technology Sydney, Level 8, Building 10, 235-253 Jones St, Ultimo, NSW 2007, Australia.

Acknowledgements
Not applicable.

Competing interests
The authors declare that they have no competing interests.

Funding
This systematic review was funded by the Nancy and Vic Allen Stroke Prevention Fund.

References

1. Kim J, Fann DY, Seet RC, Jo DG, Mattson MP, Arumugam TV. Phytochemicals in ischemic stroke. Neuromol Med. 2016;18:283–305.
2. Mukherjee D, Patil CG. Epidemiology and the global burden of stroke. World Neurosurg. 2011;76:S85–90.
3. Feigin VL, Roth GA, Naghavi M, Parmar P, Krishnamurthi R, Chugh S, et al. Global burden of stroke and risk factors in 188 countries, during 1990–2013: a systematic analysis for the Global Burden of Disease Study 2013. Lancet Neurol. 2016;15:913–24.
4. Holloway RG, Benesch C, Rush SR. Stroke prevention: narrowing the evidence-practice gap. Neurology. 2000;54:1899–906.
5. Straus SE, Majumdar SR, McAlister FA. New evidence for stroke prevention: scientific review. JAMA. 2002;288:1388–95.
6. Collaboration Blood Pressure Lowering Treatment Trialists'. Effects of ACE inhibitors, calcium antagonists, and other blood-pressure-lowering drugs: results of prospectively designed overviews of randomised trials. Lancet. 2000;356:1955–64.
7. Goldstein LB, Adams R, Alberts MJ, Appel LJ, Brass LM, Bushnell CD, et al. Primary prevention of ischemic stroke: a guideline from the American heart association/American stroke association stroke council: cosponsored by the atherosclerotic peripheral vascular disease interdisciplinary working group; cardiovascular nursing council; clinical cardiology council; nutrition, physical activity, and metabolism council; and the quality of care and outcomes research interdisciplinary working group: The American academy of neurology affirms the value of this guideline. Stroke. 2006;37:1583–633.
8. Wang J, Xiong X. Outcome measures of Chinese herbal medicine for hypertension: an overview of systematic reviews. Evid Based Complement Alternat Med. 2012;2012:7.
9. Hu J, Zhang J, Zhao W, Zhang Y, Zhang L, Shang H. Cochrane systematic reviews of Chinese herbal medicines: an overview. PLoS ONE. 2011;6:e28696.
10. National Center for Complementary and Integrative Health. Traditional Chinese medicine: in depth. 2013. https://nccih.nih.gov/health/whatiscam/chinesemed.htm. Accessed Oct 2013.
11. Tachjian A, Maria V, Jahangir A. Use of herbal products and potential interactions in patients with cardiovascular diseases. J Am Coll Cardiol. 2010;55:515–25.
12. Liu JP, Zhang M, Wang WY, Grimsgaard S. Chinese herbal medicines for type 2 diabetes mellitus. Cochrane Database Syst Rev. 2004;3:CD003642.
13. Grant SJ, Bensoussan A, Chang D, Kiat H, Klupp NL, Liu JP, et al. Chinese herbal medicines for people with impaired glucose tolerance or impaired fasting blood glucose. Cochrane Database Syst Rev. 2009;4:CD006690.
14. Liu ZL, Li GQ, Bensoussan A, Kiat H, Chan K, Liu JP. Chinese herbal medicines for hypertriglyceridaemia. Cochrane Database Syst Rev. 2013;6:CD009560.

15. Tong X, Dong L, Chen L, Zhen Z. Treatment of diabetes using traditional Chinese medicine: past, present and future. Am J Chin Med. 2012;40:877–86.

16. Sui Y, Zhao H, Wong V, Brown N, Li X, Kwan A, et al. A systematic review on use of Chinese medicine and acupuncture for treatment of obesity. Obes Rev. 2012;13:409–30.

17. Higgins JP, Altman DG, Gøtzsche PC, Jüni P, Moher D, Oxman AD, et al. The Cochrane Collaboration's tool for assessing risk of bias in randomised trials. BMJ. 2011;343:d5928.

18. Lin Z, Xing Z, Cai C, Tan H, Zhang C. Effects of tianma gouteng decoction on the plasma endothelin of patients with primary hypertension of hyperactivity of the liver yang. Chin J Clin Rehabil. 2004;27:5992–3.

19. Li Y. A clinical study on haunglian fire-purging mixture in treatment of 46 cases of primary hypertension. J Tradit Chin Med. 2005;25:29–33.

20. Ye P, Wu C, Sheng L, Li H. Potential protective effect of long-term therapy with Xuezhikang on left ventricular diastolic function in patients with essential hypertension. J Altern Complement Med. 2009;15:719–25.

21. Zhao Y, Liu Y, Guan Y, Liu N. Effect of Yinian Jiangya Yin on primary hypertension in early stage—a clinical observations on 40 patients. J Tradit Chin Med. 2010;30:171–5.

22. Zhong G, Chen M, Luo Y, Xiang L, Xie Q, Li Y, et al. Effect of Chinese herbal medicine for calming Gan (肝) and suppressing hyperactive yang on arterial elasticity function and circadian rhythm of blood pressure in patients with essential hypertension. Chin J Integr Med. 2011;17:414–20.

23. Yang T, Wei J, Lee M, Chen C, Ueng K. A randomized, double-blind, placebo-controlled study to evaluate the efficacy and tolerability of Fufang Danshen (Salvia miltiorrhiza) as add-on antihypertensive therapy in Taiwanese patients with uncontrolled hypertension. Phytother Res. 2012;26:291–8.

24. Tong X, Lian F, Zhou Q, Xu L, Ji H, Xu G, et al. A prospective multicenter clinical trial of Chinese herbal formula JZQG (Jiangzhuoqinggan) for hypertension. Am J Chin Med. 2013;41:33–42.

25. Wu C, Zhang J, Zhao Y, Chen J, Liu Y. Chinese herbal medicine bushen qinggan formula for blood pressure variability and endothelial injury in hypertensive patients: a randomized controlled pilot clinical trial. Evid Based Complement Alternat Med. 2014;2014:7.

26. Li H, Liu L, Zhao W, Liu J, Yao M, Han Y, et al. Traditional Chinese versus integrative treatment in elderly patients with isolated systolic hypertension: a multicenter, randomized, double-blind controlled trial. J Integr Med. 2010;8:410–6.

27. Chen SL, Liu XY, Xu WM, Mei WY, Chen XL. Clinical study of Western medicine combined with Chinese medicine based on syndrome differentiation in the patients with polarized hypertension. Chin J Integr Med. 2012;18:746–51.

28. Gong C, Huang SL, Huang JF, Zhang ZF, Luo M, Zhao Y, et al. Effects of combined therapy of Xuezhikang Capsule and Valsartan on hypertensive left ventricular hypertrophy and heart rate turbulence. Chin J Integr Med. 2010;16:114–8.

29. Xu Y, Yan H, Yao MJ, Ma J, Jia JM, Ruan FX, et al. Cardioankle vascular index evaluations revealed that cotreatment of ARB Antihypertension medication with traditional Chinese medicine improved arterial functionality. J Cardiovasc Pharmacol. 2013;61:355–60.

30. Chao M, Zou D, Zhang Y, Chen Y, Wang M, Wu H, et al. Improving insulin resistance with traditional Chinese medicine in type 2 diabetic patients. Endocrine. 2009;36:268–74.

31. Ji L, Tong X, Wang H, Tian H, Zhou H, Zhang L, et al. Efficacy and safety of traditional chinese medicine for diabetes: a double-blind, randomised, controlled trial. PLoS ONE. 2013;8:e56703.

32. Tong XL, Wu ST, Lian FM, Zhao M, Zhou SP, Chen XY, et al. The safety and effectiveness of TM81, a Chinese herbal medicine, in the treatment of type 2 diabetes: a randomized double-blind placebo-controlled trial. Diabetes Obes Metab. 2013;15:448–54.

33. Tu X, Xie C, Wang F, Chen Q, Zuo Z, Zhang Q, et al. Fructus Mume formula in the treatment of type 2 diabetes mellitus: A randomized controlled pilot trial. Evid Based Complement Alternat Med. 2013;2013:8.

34. Wu Q, Fan H. The research for the clinical curative effect through combing traditional Chinese medicine with insulin to cure diabetes. Pak J Pharm Sci. 2014;27:1057–61.

35. Cai H, Liu F, Zuo P, Huang G, Song Z, Wang T, et al. Practical application of antidiabetic efficacy of Lycium barbarum polysaccharide in patients with type 2 diabetes. Med Chem. 2015;11:383–90.

36. Lian F, Tian J, Chen X, Li Z, Piao C, Guo J, et al. The efficacy and safety of Chinese herbal medicine Jinlida as add-on medication in type 2 diabetes patients ineffectively managed by metformin monotherapy: a double-blind, randomized, placebo-controlled, multicenter trial. PLoS ONE. 2015;10:e0130550.

37. Zhang X, Liu Y, Xiong D, Xie C. Insulin combined with Chinese medicine improves glycemic outcome through multiple pathways in patients with type 2 diabetes mellitus. J Diabetes Investig. 2015;6:708–15.

38. Hu Y, Zhou X, Liu P, Wang B, Duan D, Guo D. A comparison study of metformin only therapy and metformin combined with Chinese medicine jianyutangkang therapy in patients with type 2 diabetes: a randomized placebo-controlled double-blind study. Complement Ther Med. 2016;24:13–8.

39. Li M, Huang X, Ye H, Chen Y, Yu J, Yang J, et al. Randomized, double-blinded, double-dummy, active-controlled, and multiple-dose clinical study comparing the efficacy and safety of Mulberry Twig (Ramulus Mori, Sangzhi) Alkaloid Tablet and Acarbose in individuals with type 2 diabetes mellitus. Evid Based Complement Alternat Med. 2016;2016:8.

40. Wang J, Lu Z, Chi J, Wang W, Su M, Kou W, et al. Multicenter clinical trial of the serum lipid-lowering effects of a Monascus purpureus (red yeast) rice preparation from traditional Chinese medicine. Curr Ther Res. 1997;58:964–78.

41. Yang H, Han L, Sheng T, He Q, Liang J. Effects of replenishing qi, promoting blood circulation and resolving phlegm on vascular endothelial function and blood coagulation system in senile patients with hyperlipemia. J Tradit Chin Med. 2006;26:120–4.

42. Ai J, Zhao L, Lu Y, Cai B, Zhang Y, Yang B. A randomized, multicentre, open-label, parallel-group trial to compare the efficacy and safety profile of daming capsule in patients with hypercholesterolemia. Phytother Res. 2009;23:1039–42.

43. Xu CF, Lin XR, Wang YK. Clinical observation on hyperlipemia treated with antihyperlipidemic decoction. J Tradit Chin Med. 2009;29:121–4.

44. Hu M, Zeng W, Tomlinson B. Evaluation of a Crataegus-based multiherb formula for dyslipidemia: a randomized, double-blind, placebo-controlled clinical trial. Evid Based Complement Alternat Med. 2014;2014:365742.

45. Moriarty PM, Roth EM, Karns A, Ye P, Zhao SP, Liao Y, et al. Effects of Xuezhikang in patients with dyslipidemia: a multicenter, randomized, placebo-controlled study. J Clin Lipidol. 2014;8:568–75.

46. Heber D, Yip I, Ashley JM, Elashoff DA, Elashoff RM, Go VL. Cholesterol-lowering effects of a proprietary Chinese red-yeast-rice dietary supplement. Am J Clin Nutr. 1999;69:231–6.

47. Lin C, Li T, Lai M. Efficacy and safety of Monascus purpureus Went rice in subjects with hyperlipidemia. Eur J Endocrinol. 2005;153:679–86.

48. Wei Y, Hong YZ, Ye X. Effect of Tang No.1 granule in treating patients with impaired glucose tolerance. Chin J Integr Med. 2008;14:298–302.

49. Gao Y, Zhou H, Zhao H, Feng X, Feng J, Li Y, et al. Clinical research of traditional Chinese medical intervention on impaired glucose tolerance. Am J Chin Med. 2013;41:21–32.

50. Fang Z, Zhao J, Shi G, Shu Y, Ni Y, Wang H, et al. Shenzhu Tiaopi granule combined with lifestyle intervention therapy for impaired glucose tolerance: a randomized controlled trial. Complement Ther Med. 2014;22:842–50.

51. Lian F, Li G, Chen X, Wang X, Piao C, Wang J, et al. Chinese herbal medicine Tianqi reduces progression from impaired glucose tolerance to diabetes: a double-blind, randomized, placebo-controlled, multicenter trial. J Clin Endocrinol Metab. 2014;99:648–55.

52. Huang Y, Yang Q, Wang H, Xu Y, Peng W, Jiang Y. Long-term clinical effect of Tangyiping Granules (糖异平颗粒) on patients with impaired glucose tolerance. Chin J Integr Med. 2016;22:653–9.

53. Shi Y, Liu W, Zhang X, Su W, Chen N, Lu S, et al. Effect of Chinese herbal medicine Jinlida granule in treatment of patients with impaired glucose tolerance. Chin Med J. 2016;129:2281–6.

54. Grant SJ, Chang DH, Liu J, Wong V, Kiat H, Bensoussan A. Chinese herbal medicine for impaired glucose tolerance: a randomized placebo controlled trial. BMC Complement Altern Med. 2013;13:104.

55. Pan L, Li D, Lei M, Zhang L, Zhou L. Preparation-containing node of Lotus Rhizome, green tea and Panax notoginseng for obese adults. Chin J Clin Rehabil. 2005;15:231–3.

56. Zhou Q, Chang B, Chen X, Zhou S, Zhen Z, Zhang L, et al. Chinese herbal medicine for obesity: a randomized, double-blinded, multicenter, prospective trial. Am J Chin Med. 2014;42:1345–56.

57. Lenon GB, Li KX, Chang Y-H, Yang AW, Da Costa C, Li CG, et al. Efficacy and safety of a Chinese herbal medicine formula (RCM-104) in the management of simple obesity: a randomized, placebo-controlled clinical trial. Evid Based Complement Alternat Med. 2012;2012:435702.

58. Hioki C, Yoshimoto K, Yoshida T. Efficacy of bofu-tsusho-san, an oriental herbal medicine, in obese Japanese women with impaired glucose tolerance. Clin Exp Pharmacol Physiol. 2004;31:614–9.

59. Gao F, Hu XF. Effect of Taizhi'an capsule combined with Simvastatin on hyperlipidemia in diabetic patients. Chin J Integr Med. 2006;12:24–8.

60. Poppel PC, Breedveld P, Abbink EJ, Roelofs H, Heerde W, Smits P, et al. Salvia miltiorrhiza root water-extract (Danshen) has no beneficial effect on cardiovascular risk factors. a randomized double-blind cross-over trial. PLoS ONE. 2015;10:e0128695.

61. Chu SL, Fu H, Yang JX, Liu GX, Dou P, Zhang L, et al. A randomized double-blind placebo-controlled study of Pu'er tea extract on the regulation of

metabolic syndrome. Chin J Integr Med. 2011;17:492–8.

62. Chen Y, Fu DY, He YM, Fu XD, Xu YQ, Liu Y, et al. Effects of Chinese herbal medicine Yiqi Huaju Formula on hypertensive patients with metabolic syndrome: a randomized, placebo-controlled trial. J Integr Med. 2013;11:184–94.

63. Azushima K, Tamura K, Haku S, Wakui H, Kanaoka T, Ohsawa M, et al. Effects of the oriental herbal medicine Bofu-tsusho-san in obesity hypertension: a multicenter, randomized, parallel-group controlled trial (ATH-D-14-01021.R2). Atherosclerosis. 2015;240:297–304.

64. Lee C, Jan M, Yu M, Lin C, Wei J, Shih H. Relationship between adiponectin and leptin, and blood lipids in hyperlipidemia patients treated with red yeast rice. Forsch Komplementmed. 2013;20:197–203.

65. Heuschmann PU, Grieve AP, Toschke AM, Rudd AG, Wolfe CD. Ethnic group disparities in 10-year trends in stroke incidence and vascular risk factors. Stroke. 2008;39:2204–10.

9

Effects of Huang Bai (*Phellodendri Cortex*) on bone growth and pubertal development in adolescent female rats

Sun Haeng Lee[1,2], Hyun Jeong Lee[3], Sung Hyun Lee[4], Young-Sik Kim[3], Donghun Lee[3], Jiu Chun[1], Jin Yong Lee[1,2], Hocheol Kim[3*] and Gyu Tae Chang[1,5*] (iD)

Abstract

Background: To evaluate the effects of Huang Bai (*Phellodendron amurense*) on growth and maturation in adolescent female rats.

Methods: Female Sprague–Dawley rats (28 days old; n = 72) were divided into six daily treatment groups: control (distilled water), Huang Bai (100 and 300 mg/kg), recombinant human GH (rhGH; 20 μg/kg), estradiol (1 μg/kg), and triptorelin (100 μg). Body weight, food intake, and vaginal opening were measured daily from postnatal day (PND) 28 to PND 43. Tetracycline (20 mg/kg) was injected on PND 41. After sacrifice on PND 43, the ovaries and uterus were weighed, and the tibias were fixed in 4% paraformaldehyde. Decalcified and dehydrated tibias were sectioned at a thickness of 40 μm, and sectioned tissues were examined with a fluorescence microscope. Insulin-like growth factor (IGF)-1 and bone morphogenetic protein (BMP)-2 were detected using immunohistochemistry.

Results: Relative to controls, body weight was higher in the triptorelin group. Bone growth rate increased in the Huang Bai 100 mg/kg (354.00 ± 31.1 μm/day), rhGH (367.10 ± 27.11 μm/day), and triptorelin (374.50 ± 25.37 μm/day) groups. Expression of IGF-1 and BMP-2 in the hypertrophic zone was higher in all experimental groups. Vaginal opening occurred earlier in the estradiol group (PND 33.58 ± 1.62) than in controls and later in the triptorelin group (PND > 43). Ovarian and uterine weights were lower in the oestradiol and triptorelin groups. However, Huang Bai had nonsignificant effects on vaginal opening and the weights of ovaries and the uterus.

Conclusions: Huang Bai stimulated bone growth by upregulating IGF-1 and BMP-2 in the growth plate. However, it had no effect on pubertal development.

Keywords: Huang Bai, Bone growth, Insulin-like growth factor-1, Bone morphogenetic protein-2, Vaginal opening, Ovarian weight, Uterine weight

Background

Longitudinal bone growth occurs through elongation of the growth plate, a cartilage layer between the epiphysis and metaphysis [1, 2]. The growth plate consists of three distinct zones: the resting, proliferative, and hypertrophic zones. Chondrocytes in the growth plate are differentiated from the top of the resting zone to the bottom of the hypertrophic zone, and the middle proliferative zone is the major location for chondrocyte proliferation for bone elongation [2, 3]. Growth and differentiation of the growth plate are regulated by growth hormone (GH) and cell-signalling polypeptides such as insulin-like growth factor (IGF)-1 and bone morphogenetic protein (BMP)-2 [4]. The bone growth rate and expression of IGF-1 and BMP-2 are useful indicators of growth.

Reproductive maturation requires activation of the hypothalamic–pituitary–gonadal (HPG) axis. Pulsatile

*Correspondence: hckim@khu.ac.kr; gtchang@khu.ac.kr
[3] Department of Herbal Pharmacology, College of Korean Medicine, Kyung Hee University, Seoul 02447, Republic of Korea
[5] Department of Pediatrics of Korean Medicine, Kyung Hee University Hospital at Gangdong, Dongnam-ro 892, Gangdong-gu, Seoul 05278, Republic of Korea
Full list of author information is available at the end of the article

gonadotropin-releasing hormone (GnRH) from the hypothalamus stimulates luteinizing hormone (LH) and follicle-stimulating hormone (FSH) release from the pituitary [5]. LH and FSH stimulate gonadal growth and maturation for the biosynthesis of gametes and sex hormones [6]. Pubertal onset in female rats has been traditionally identified by estrogen-mediated vaginal opening, observed as a visible hole in the membranous coating of the vaginal orifice [7]. In addition, uterotropic assays including ovarian and uterine weight are considered gold standards for identifying estrogenic activity in rats [8]. Vaginal opening and the weight of ovaries and uterus are helpful indicators of pubertal development.

Huang Bai has been used to treat diarrhoea, jaundice, leucorrhoea, stranguria, and swelling of the knee and foot by clearing heat and drying dampness; sores, burns, and eczema by purging fire and detoxifying; and fever by clearing deficiency heat [9]. In our previous in vitro study, Huang Bai promoted GH mRNA and protein in pituitary cells and inhibited GnRH mRNA expression in hypothalamus cells [10]. However, the growth-promoting and maturation-inhibiting effects of Huang Bai were not identified based on that in vivo study.

The present study explored the effects of Huang Bai on growth and pubertal development in adolescent female Sprague–Dawley rats. Huang Bai was compared with recombinant human growth hormone (rhGH; positive control for growth promotion), estradiol (negative control for maturational cessation), and triptorelin (positive control for maturational cessation). The effect on growth was measured based on the daily bone growth rate and expression of BMP-2 and IGF-1 in the tibial growth plate. The effect on pubertal maturation was measured based on vaginal opening and ovarian and uterine weight.

Methods

The minimum standards of reporting checklist (Additional file 1) contains details of the experimental design, statistics, and resources used in this study.

Sample preparation

The cortex of *Phellodendron amurense* (Huang Bai) was imported from Sichuan, China (Kyung Hee Herb Pharm.; Gangwon, Republic of Korea). A total of 400 g of dried Huang Bai was extracted with 4000 mL of 100 °C distilled water (DW) for 3 h with a reflux heater. The extracted fluid was filtered with filter paper (Hyundai Micro Co.; Seoul, Republic of Korea), after which the filtered fluid was evaporated to a volume < 2000 mL using a rotary evaporator (Sunileyela Co.; Gyeonggi, Republic of Korea), and lyophilised using a freeze-dryer (OperonTM; Seoul, Republic of Korea). The powder was stored at − 20 °C. The yield of freeze-dried Huang Bai was approximately 10.4%.

The quantitative authentication of Huang Bai was performed using a Waters instrument (Milford, MA, USA) equipped with a Waters 1525 pump, Waters 2707 autosampler, and a Waters 2998 PDA detector with a Sunfire™ Octadecyl silyl silica C18 column (particle size, 5 μm; 250 × 4.6 mm). The column was equilibrated with 0.1% phosphoric acid (solvent A) and acetonitrile (solvent B) at a flow rate of 1.0 mL/min. The column was eluted as follows: 0–60 min, 0% solvent B; 60–67 min, 100% solvent B; 67–72 min, 0% solvent B. The high-performance liquid chromatogram of Huang Bai is shown in Fig. 1. Huang Bai contained one representative component: 24.36 mg/g berberine chloride.

Animals

A total of 72 intact 21-day-old female Sprague–Dawley rats were purchased from Samtako Co. (Gyeonggi,

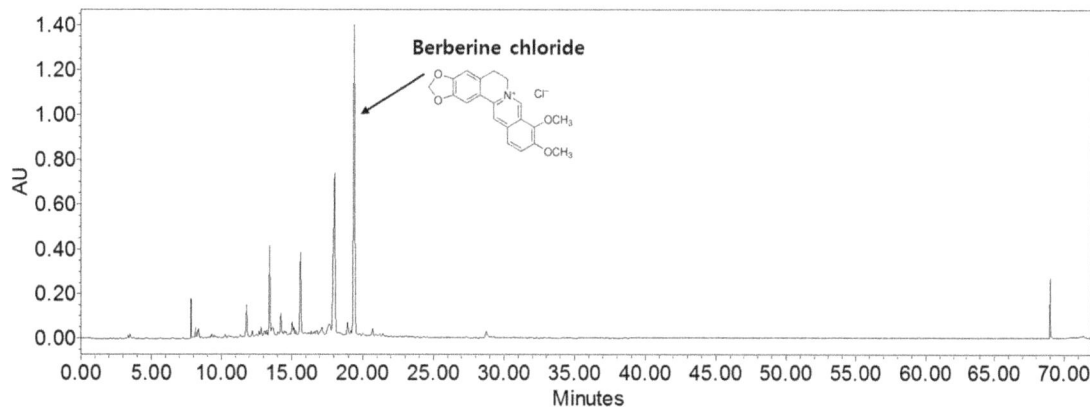

Fig. 1 High-performance liquid chromatography of Huang Bai

Republic of Korea). The sample size was based on recent experiments conducted in our laboratory [11]. The rats were divided into four body weight groups (30–40, 40–50, 50–60, and 60–70 g). They were marked on the tail and housed four per cage under controlled temperature (23 ± 2 °C), humidity (55 ± 10%), and lighting (lights on from 7 a.m. to 7 p.m.) with free access to food and water intake. After 1 week of acclimatisation, the 28-day-old rats, weighing 75 ± 10 g, were administered their respective treatments. All experimental procedures were performed according to the animal care guidelines of Kyung Hee University's Institutional Animal Care and Use Committee [Protocol Number KHUASP(SE)-15-052].

Treatments
The 18 cages were randomly allocated into six groups (three cages per group) according to the treatment regimen. The DW (12 rats) and Huang Bai (100 and 300 mg/kg; 12 rats each) groups were orally administered twice daily at 7 a.m. and 7 p.m. at 10.0 mL/kg. The rhGH (20 µg/kg; 12 rats) (LG Life Science; Seoul, Republic of Korea) [12] and 17β-estradiol (1 µg/kg; 12 rats) (Sigma-Aldrich; MO, USA) [13] groups were administered subcutaneous injections once daily at 7 a.m. at 1.0 mL/kg. A fixed dose and volume of triptorelin (100 µg/0.4 mL; 12 rats) (Ferring AG; Baarermatte, Switzerland) was intraperitoneally injected once daily at 7 a.m. [14].

Body weights of animals, food intake per cage, and vaginal opening were measured daily, and treatments were continued from postnatal day (PND) 28 to PND 43. On PND 41, all animals received an intraperitoneal injection of tetracycline hydrochloride (20 mg/kg, Sigma-Aldrich) in 5.0 mL/kg saline for the fluorescent dye under ultraviolet illumination. On PND 43, all rats were sacrificed under anaesthesia. The ovaries and uterus were dissected with the cervix attached, and trimmed free of fat. The wet weights were then obtained. The tibias were dissected free of the soft tissue, and the bones were immediately fixed in 4% paraformaldehyde.

Measurement of longitudinal bone growth rate
Fixed tibias were decalcified by immersion in 50 mM ethylene diamine tetra acetic acid solution (Sigma-Aldrich) for 2 d. Decalcified bones were dehydrated by immersion in 30% sucrose (Sigma-Aldrich) for 1 day. Dehydrated bones were sectioned longitudinally at a thickness of 40 µm with a sliding microtome (Leica CM1860; Berlin, Germany). Sections of bone tissue were mounted on gelatinised glass slides and photographed with a fluorescence microscope (Olympus; Tokyo, Japan). The longitudinal bone length between the fluorescent line formed by tetracycline and the epiphyseal end line of the growth plate was measured by two blinded investigators (SHL

and YSK) using Image J software (National Institutes of Health; MD, USA). The longitudinal bone growth rate was calculated as the measured length divided by the time between tetracycline injection and death.

Immunohistochemistry for expression of IGF-1 and BMP-2
Dehydrated tibia sections were rinsed twice in 0.1 M phosphate buffer saline (PBS) for 15 min and incubated with 1% triton X-100 (Sigma-Aldrich) and 0.5% bovine serum albumin (BSA, Sigma-Aldrich) mixed in PBS for 10 min at room temperature. The samples were then washed twice in PBS/BSA for 15 min and incubated with 1:200 rabbit IGF-1 primary antibody or 1:200 goat BMP-2 primary antibody (Santa Cruz Biotechnology; TX, USA) overnight at room temperature in a humid chamber. After 24 h, sections were washed twice in PBS/BSA for 15 min and incubated with 1:200 biotinylated anti-goat secondary antibody (Vector Laboratories; CA, USA) or 1:200 biotinylated anti-rabbit secondary antibody (Jackson Immuno Research Laboratories; PA, USA) for 60 min. After being washed twice with PBS/BSA for 15 min, the sections were incubated with 1:100 avidin-biotinperoxidase complex (Vectastain ABC Kit; Vector Laboratories) for 60 min at room temperature. After two washings with 0.1 M phosphate buffer for 15 min, the sections were stained with 0.05% 3,3-diaminobenzidine solution containing hydrogen peroxidase in PBS. Samples were checked for suitable staining with a microscope, and then the reaction was stopped by washing with PBS for 5 min. The samples were then dehydrated with 50, 75, 95, and 100% ethanol and xylene in order. Dehydrated sections were mounted on glass slides with permount medium solution (Fisher Scientific; NJ, USA). When the sections fell off the slides, we immediately reattached them using soft brushes. Finally, the sections were photographed with a microscope. The percentage of labelled chondrocytes was calculated by counting stained and total chondrocytes in two parallel columns using Image J software [3].

Statistical analysis
Data are expressed as the mean ± standard deviation (SD) and were analysed using the Student's t-test (GraphPad Software, Inc.; CA, USA). P-values < 0.05 were considered statistically significant.

Results
Body weight and food intake
From PND 28 to PND 43, body weight gains and food intake of the control, Huang Bai 100 and 300 mg/kg, rhGH, 17β-estradiol, and triptorelin groups were compared (Table 1). There were no statistically significant differences in body weight between any treatment group and the control group ($P > 0.05$), except the triptorelin

Table 1 Body weight and daily food intake gains (g) for 15 days in female adolescent rats

	Control	HB100	HB300	rhGH	Estradiol	Triptorelin
BW gain	66.96 ± 4.45	65.04 ± 7.14	67.18 ± 10.91	72.25 ± 8.34	64.04 ± 8.91	82.46 ± 5.52
P-value	–	0.44	0.95	0.07	0.32	< 0.001***
DFI gain	13.50 ± 5.27	14.83 ± 2.75	13.25 ± 0.35	16.17 ± 7.11	17.17 ± 1.76	28.33 ± 7.97
P-value	–	0.72	0.95	0.63	0.32	0.05

Control DW, HB100 Huang Bai (100 mg/kg), HB300 Huang Bai (300 mg/kg), rhGH recombinant human growth hormone (20 µg/kg), Estradiol 17β-estradiol (1 µg/kg), Triptorelin triptorelin (100 µg), BW body weight, DFI daily food intake

Each value is the mean ± SD of 12 rats except HB300 (11 rats). *** $P < 0.001$ compared to controls

group ($P < 0.001$). There were no statistically significant differences in food intake between any treatment group and the control group ($P > 0.05$).

Longitudinal bone growth rate
The longitudinal bone growth rate of the control, Huang Bai 100 and 300 mg/kg, rhGH, estradiol, and triptorelin groups were 323.80 ± 34.55, 354.00 ± 31.1 µm/day ($P = 0.043$), 342.60 ± 28.91 µm/day ($P = 0.195$), 367.10 ± 27.11 µm/day ($P = 0.005$), 335.10 ± 23.12 µm/day ($P = 0.360$), and 374.50 ± 25.37 µm/day ($P = 0.002$), respectively. Longitudinal bone growth rates of the Huang Bai 100 mg/kg, rhGH, and triptorelin groups were significantly higher than that of the control group (Fig. 2).

Expression of IGF-1 and BMP-2
IGF-1 and BMP-2 in the resting, proliferative, and hypertrophic zones of the tibial growth plate were detected using immunohistochemical methods. IGF-1 and BMP-2 showed higher levels of expression in the hypertrophic zone in all experimental groups than in that of the control group. The triptorelin group showed a slightly higher expression level of IGF-1 and BMP-2 in the proliferative

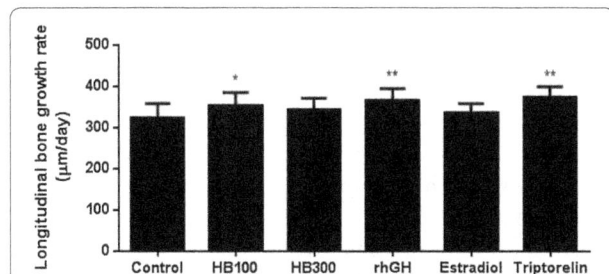

Fig. 2 The daily longitudinal bone growth rate was calculated from the 2-day longitudinal growth plate length. Each value is shown as the mean ± SD for 12 rats, except HB300 (11 rats). Statistical analysis: * $P < 0.05$, ** $P < 0.01$ compared to control (DW–administrated group). HB100: Huang Bai (100 mg/kg, p.o.), HB300: Huang Bai (300 mg/kg, p.o.), rhGH: recombinant human growth hormone (20 µg/kg, s.c.), estradiol: 17β-estradiol (1 µg/kg, s.c.), triptorelin: triptorelin (100 µg, i.p.)

zone compared with the control group. Huang Bai had higher expression levels of IGF-1 and BMP-2 than the control, but lower levels than the rhGH, estradiol and triptorelin groups (Figs. 3, 4).

Vaginal opening
The percent incidence of vaginal opening in each group is shown in Fig. 5. All rats in the triptorelin group and one rat in the Huang Bai 300 mg/kg group did not show vaginal opening, whereas all rats of the control, Huang Bai 100 mg/kg, rhGH, and estradiol groups showed vaginal opening prior to sacrifice. The vaginal opening days of the control, Huang Bai 100 and 300 mg/kg, rhGH, estradiol, and triptorelin groups were 34.17 ± 1.95, 34.50 ± 2.47 ($P = 0.717$), > 35.09 ± 3.51 (no vaginal opening in one rat), 33.58 ± 1.62 ($P = 0.434$), 31.58 ± 1.24 ($P < 0.001$), and > 43 (no vaginal opening in any rat), respectively. The estradiol group showed significantly earlier vaginal opening, and the vaginal opening days of the Huang Bai and rhGH groups were not significantly different from that of the control group.

Ovarian and uterine weight
The ovarian weights and indices of the control, Huang Bai 100 and 300 mg/kg, rhGH, estradiol, and triptorelin groups are described in Table 2. Ovarian indices were calculated as ovarian weight (g) per kg body weight. Ovarian weights of the estradiol and triptorelin groups were significantly lower than those of the control group ($P < 0.001$).

The uterine weights and indices of each group are described in Table 3. Uterine indices were calculated as uterine weight (g) per body weight (kg). Uterine weights of the estradiol (P < 0.01) and triptorelin (P < 0.001) groups were also significantly lower than those of the control group.

The ovarian and uterine indices of both the estradiol group and the triptorelin group were significantly lower than those of the control group, with $P < 0.01$ and $P < 0.001$, respectively (Fig. 6).

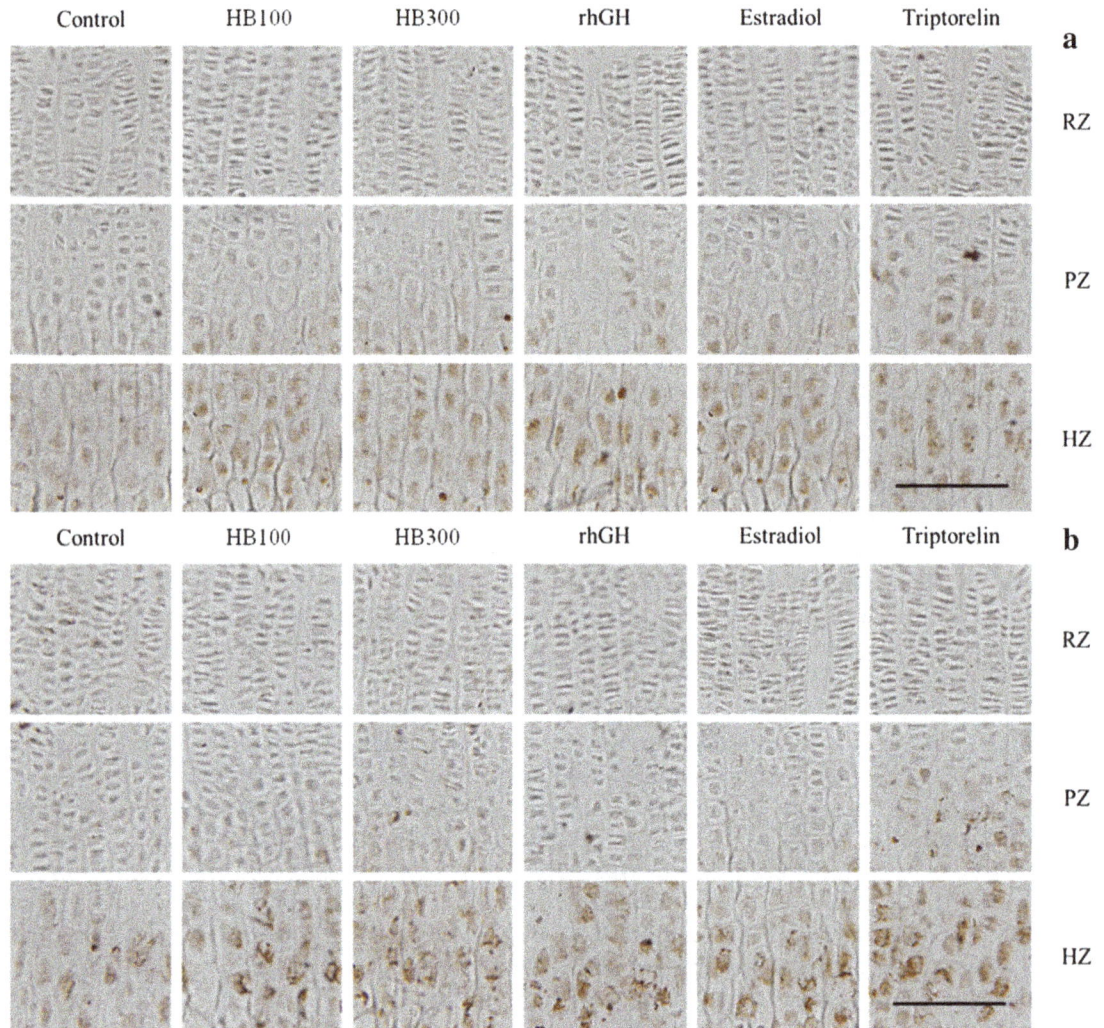

Fig. 3 IGF-1 **a** and BMP-2 **b** in the growth plate was detected using immunohistochemistry. Control: DW, HB100: Huang Bai (100 mg/kg, p.o.), HB300: Huang Bai (300 mg/kg, p.o.), rhGH: recombinant human growth hormone (20 μg/kg, s.c.), estradiol: 17β-estradiol (1 μg/kg, s.c.), triptorelin: triptorelin (100 μg, i.p.). RZ: resting zone, PZ: proliferative zone, HZ: hypertrophic zone. Scale bar = 100 μm

Discussion

Sprague–Dawley rats are commonly used in growth and reproductive experiments because of their outbred genetic background and the availability of a large volume of historical health data for many age points [15]. In this study, the effects of 100 and 300 mg/kg Huang Bai on growth and pubertal maturation were compared with those of rhGH, estradiol, and triptorelin. These two concentrations of Huang Bai were converted from the conventional daily dose of 0.5 and 1.5 g in 30 kg children. The rhGH stimulates bone growth and weight gain in a dose-dependent manner in rats [16]. Estradiol increases wet weight, volume, and the uterine epithelium in immature female rats

[17]. Triptorelin upregulates pituitary GnRH receptors and serum gonadotropins in low doses, while inhibiting GnRH receptors and gonadotropins at high doses in rats [18]. In this experiment, a rat in the Huang Bai 300 mg/kg group showed body weight decrease after PND 40 due to intestinal obstruction (identified postmortem). Therefore, the rat was excluded from our analyses.

Huang Bai did not stimulate weight gain; most daily weights and food intake levels were not significantly different from the control. However, triptorelin did stimulate weight gain. This may be an adverse event of GnRH agonists, which partially cause adiposity [19] and excessive weight gain [20].

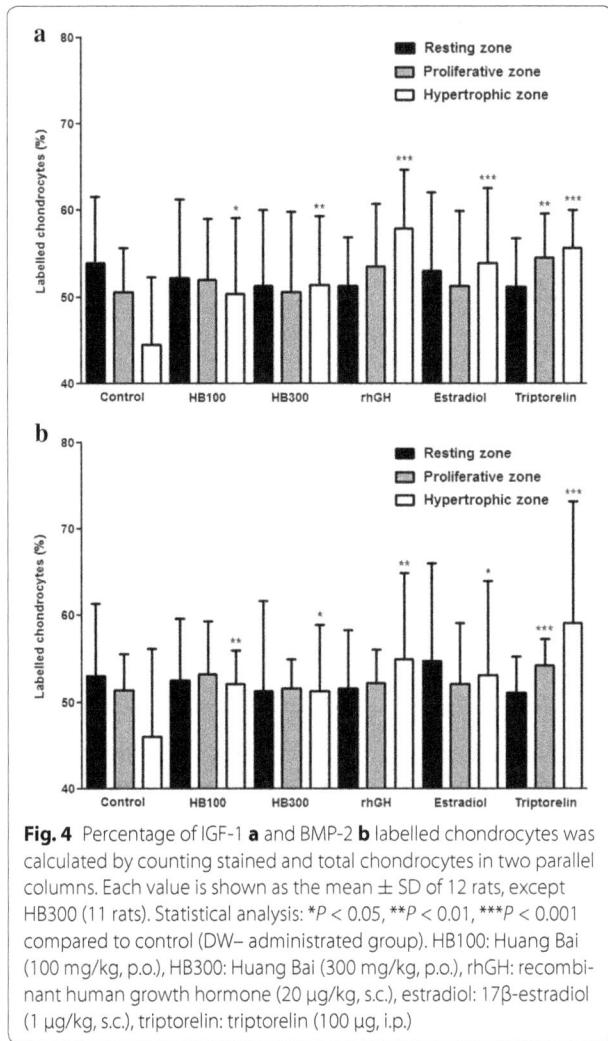

Fig. 4 Percentage of IGF-1 **a** and BMP-2 **b** labelled chondrocytes was calculated by counting stained and total chondrocytes in two parallel columns. Each value is shown as the mean ± SD of 12 rats, except HB300 (11 rats). Statistical analysis: *$P < 0.05$, **$P < 0.01$, ***$P < 0.001$ compared to control (DW– administrated group). HB100: Huang Bai (100 mg/kg, p.o.), HB300: Huang Bai (300 mg/kg, p.o.), rhGH: recombinant human growth hormone (20 µg/kg, s.c.), estradiol: 17β-estradiol (1 µg/kg, s.c.), triptorelin: triptorelin (100 µg, i.p.)

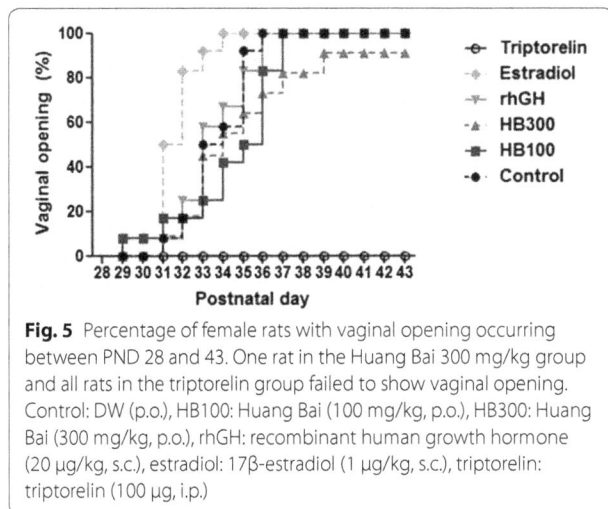

Fig. 5 Percentage of female rats with vaginal opening occurring between PND 28 and 43. One rat in the Huang Bai 300 mg/kg group and all rats in the triptorelin group failed to show vaginal opening. Control: DW (p.o.), HB100: Huang Bai (100 mg/kg, p.o.), HB300: Huang Bai (300 mg/kg, p.o.), rhGH: recombinant human growth hormone (20 µg/kg, s.c.), estradiol: 17β-estradiol (1 µg/kg, s.c.), triptorelin: triptorelin (100 µg, i.p.)

The 100 mg/kg of Huang Bai, rhGH, and triptorelin significantly increased the bone growth rate, by 9.3, 13.4, and 15.7%, respectively, compared to the control. However, 300 mg/kg of Huang Bai had a lower growth effect than 100 mg/kg. Huang Bai has a bitter taste, and the theory of "bitter/cold medicines damage the spleen and stomach" suggests that this bitter-tasting herb may cause anorexia, dyspepsia, or gastric motility disorder. In a previous study, Huang Bai decreased the secretion of gastric juice, increased the pH of gastric juice, and decreased activation of pepsin in rats [21]. In this study, one rat from the 300 mg/kg Huang Bai group had an intestinal obstruction. The lower growth effect of the higher dose Huang Bai may be due to its increased burden on the gastrointestinal tract. Further studies are required to determine the appropriate dose and preparation process for Huang Bai so as to reduce the burden on the gastrointestinal tract. The triptorelin group showed the highest bone growth rate, but this result may have been due to confounding effects of the significant weight gain in this group.

IGF-1 and BMP-2 were highly expressed in the hypertrophic zone following Huang Bai administration, reflecting the proliferation of chondrocytes. IGF-1 regulates cell differentiation, proliferation, and maturation through autocrine and paracrine activity [2], and BMP-2 regulates growth plate chondrogenesis and induces ectopic bone formation and skeletal development [22, 23]. BMP-2 also modulates mitogenic IGF-1 action of chondrocytes in the epiphyseal plate [4]. Huang Bai stimulated chondrocyte proliferation and ectopic bone elongation by increasing IGF-1 and BMP-2 expression in the growth plate. The longitudinal bone growth rate, and IGF-1 and BMP-2 expression in the growth plate indicate that Huang Bai stimulated ectopic skeletal growth by promoting chondrocyte differentiation. This result is in agreement with the GH3 cell study showing that Huang Bai increased GH mRNA and protein expression in pituitary cells [10].

Huang Bai delayed vaginal opening in a dose-dependent manner, but differences from the control were not significant. Further studies using other doses or rats with precocious puberty are required because herbal prescriptions including Huang Bai have been associated with delayed vaginal opening in precocious puberty rats [24–28]. In contrast, vaginal opening day of the estradiol and triptorelin groups was significantly different from that for the control group. The estradiol group showed earlier vaginal opening, and no rats in the triptorelin group showed vaginal opening.

Huang Bai did not affect hypertrophy of the ovaries and uterus, although herbal prescriptions that include Huang

Table 2 Ovarian weight (g) and index (g/kg) at postnatal day 43 in female adolescent rats

	Control	HB100	HB300	rhGH	Estradiol	Triptorelin
Ovarian weight	0.10 ± 0.01	0.10 ± 0.03	0.09 ± 0.02	0.09 ± 0.02	0.07 ± 0.01	0.03 ± 0.01
P-value	–	1.000	0.612	0.431	< 0.001***	< 0.001***
Ovarian index	0.66 ± 0.08	0.69 ± 0.24	0.64 ± 0.16	0.61 ± 0.15	0.54 ± 0.11	0.17 ± 0.08
P-value	–	0.791	0.659	0.300	0.004**	< 0.001***

Control DW, HB100 Huang Bai (100 mg/kg), HB300 Huang Bai (300 mg/kg), rhGH recombinant human growth hormone (20 µg/kg), Estradiol 17β-estradiol (1 µg/kg), Triptorelin triptorelin (100 µg)

Each value is the mean ± SD of 12 rats except HB300 (11 rats). ** $P < 0.01$, *** $P < 0.001$ compared to controls

Table 3 Uterine weight (g) and index (g/kg) at postnatal day 43 in female adolescent rats

	Control	HB100	HB300	rhGH	Estradiol	Triptorelin
Uterine weight	0.39 ± 0.09	0.37 ± 0.14	0.38 ± 0.17	0.39 ± 0.12	0.29 ± 0.05	0.06 ± 0.02
P-value	–	0.663	0.838	0.923	0.002**	< 0.001***
Uterine index	2.76 ± 0.61	2.70 ± 1.04	2.69 ± 1.14	2.67 ± 0.80	2.13 ± 0.42	0.41 ± 0.13
P-value	–	0.863	0.857	0.785	0.008**	< 0.001***

Control DW, HB100 Huang Bai (100 mg/kg), HB300 Huang Bai (300 mg/kg), rhGH recombinant human growth hormone (20 µg/kg), Estradiol 17β-estradiol (1 µg/kg), Triptorelin triptorelin (100 µg)

Each value is the mean ± SD of 12 rats except HB300 (11 rats). ** $P < 0.01$, *** $P < 0.001$ compared to controls

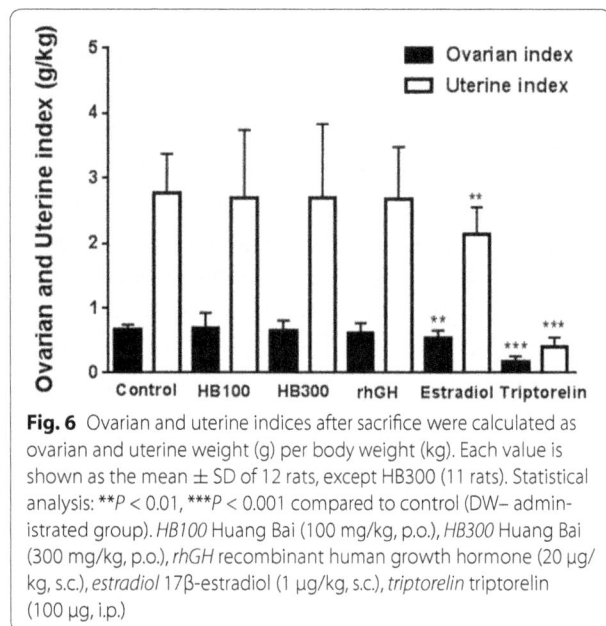

Fig. 6 Ovarian and uterine indices after sacrifice were calculated as ovarian and uterine weight (g) per body weight (kg). Each value is shown as the mean ± SD of 12 rats, except HB300 (11 rats). Statistical analysis: **$P < 0.01$, ***$P < 0.001$ compared to control (DW– administrated group). HB100 Huang Bai (100 mg/kg, p.o.), HB300 Huang Bai (300 mg/kg, p.o.), rhGH recombinant human growth hormone (20 µg/ kg, s.c.), estradiol 17β-estradiol (1 µg/kg, s.c.), triptorelin triptorelin (100 µg, i.p.)

with normal oestrus cycles [31]. Long-term estradiol or triptorelin administration may change the oestrus cycle of rats from normal to a persistent cycle of oestrus and dioestrus.

Results for vaginal opening and ovary and uterus indices indicate that Huang Bai did not inhibit pubertal maturation in the female rat, although it inhibited GnRH mRNA expression in the hypothalamus [10]. The difference between these in vitro results and multiple studies of herbal mixture may be explained by insufficient gastrointestinal absorption, the blood–brain barrier, or other confounding factors of the HPG axis. Further studies are required to explore these discordances.

Conclusions

Huang Bai stimulates longitudinal bone growth and chondrocyte proliferation by upregulating BMP-2 and IGF-1 expression in the growth plate. However, it has no effects on pubertal onset and estrogenic activity. Treatment with rhGH, which promotes growth, is generally safe in children but is associated with pseudotumor cerebri [32], slipped capital femoral epiphysis [33], progression of scoliosis [34], and/or the development of GH antibodies [35]. Huang Bai may be an alternative treatment for stimulating bone growth without affecting pubertal process.

Bai have been associated with lower ovarian weight [29] and with lower ovary and uterus indices [30] in intact rats. In contrast, wet weight and ovary and uterus indices were significantly lower in the estradiol and triptorelin groups than in the control group. In a previous study, ovarian and uterine weights of persistent oestrus- or dioestrus-cycle rats were lower than those of rats

Abbreviations
BMP: bone morphogenetic protein; BSA: bovine serum albumin; FSH: follicle-stimulating hormone; GH: growth hormone; GnRH: gonadotropin-releasing hormone; HPG: hypothalamic–pituitary–gonadal; IGF: insulin-like growth factor; LH: luteinizing hormone; PBS: phosphate-buffered saline; PND: postnatal day; rhGH: recombinant human growth hormone; SD: standard deviation.

Authors' contributions
SHaL carried out the experiments and drafted the manuscript; HJL provided major technical support for the experiments; SHyL and YSK analysed the data and revised the experimental protocol, DL developed the experimental protocol and revised the manuscript; JC and JYL revised the experimental protocol and the manuscript; and HK and GTC approved the overall experimental design. All authors read and approved the final manuscript.

Author details
[1] Department of Clinical Korean Medicine, Graduate School, Kyung Hee University, Seoul 02447, Republic of Korea. [2] Department of Pediatrics of Korean Medicine, Kyung Hee University Korean Medicine Hospital, Kyung Hee University Medical Center, Seoul 02447, Republic of Korea. [3] Department of Herbal Pharmacology, College of Korean Medicine, Kyung Hee University, Seoul 02447, Republic of Korea. [4] Korea Institute of Science and Technology for Eastern Medicine (KISTEM), NeuMed Inc., Seoul 02440, Republic of Korea. [5] Department of Pediatrics of Korean Medicine, Kyung Hee University Hospital at Gangdong, Dongnam-ro 892, Gangdong-gu, Seoul 05278, Republic of Korea.

Acknowledgements
This study was supported by a grant of the Korean Health Technology R & D Project, Ministry of Health & Welfare, Korea (HI14C0976).

Competing interests
The authors declare that they have no competing interests.

Consent for publication
Not applicable.

Funding
None.

References
1. Kim MY, Park Y, Pandit NR, Kim J, Song M, Park J, Choi HY, Kim H. The herbal formula HT042 induces longitudinal bone growth in adolescent female rats. J Med Food. 2010;13:1376–84.
2. Lee SH, Kim JY, Kim H, Park SK, Kim CY, Chung SY, Chang GT. *Amomum villosum* induces longitudinal bone growth in adolescent female rats. J Tradit Chin Med. 2012;32:453–8.
3. Kim JY, Lee JI, Song M, Lee D, Song J, Kim SY, Park J, Choi HY, Kim H. Effects of Eucommia ulmoides extract on longitudinal bone growth rate in adolescent female rats. Phytother Res. 2015;29:148–53.
4. Takahashi T, Morris EA, Trippel SB. Bone morphogenetic protein-2 and -9 regulate the interaction of insulin-like growth factor-I with growth plate chondrocytes. Int J Mol Med. 2007;20:53–7.
5. Dunkel L, Quinton R. Transition in endocrinology: induction of puberty. Eur J Endocrinol. 2014;170:R229–39.
6. Ellison PT, Reiches MW, Shattuck-Faegre H, Breakey A, Konecna M, Urlacher S, Wobber V. Puberty as a life history transition. Ann Hum Biol. 2012;39:352–60.
7. Buck Louis GM, Gray LE Jr, Marcus M, Ojeda SR, Pescovitz OH, Witchel SF, Sippell W, Abbott DH, Soto A, Tyl RW, et al. Environmental factors and puberty timing: expert panel research needs. Pediatrics. 2008;121(Suppl 3):S192–207.
8. Padilla-Banks E, Jefferson WN, Newbold RR. The immature mouse is a suitable model for detection of estrogenicity in the uterotropic bioassay. Environ Health Perspect. 2001;109:821–6.
9. Seo BI, Kwon DY, Choi HY, Lee JH, Oh MS, Bu YM. Medicinal herbology. Seoul: Younglim-Sa; 2012.
10. Lee SH, Kwak SC, Kim DK, Park SW, Kim HS, Kim YS, Lee D, Lee JW, Lee CG, Lee HK, et al. Effects of Huang Bai (Phellodendri Cortex) and Three Other Herbs on GnRH and GH Levels in GT1-7 and GH3 Cells. Evid Based Complement Alternat Med. 2016;2016:9389028.
11. Lee D, Kim YS, Song J, Kim HS, Lee HJ, Guo H, Kim H. Effects of *Phlomis umbrosa* root on longitudinal bone growth rate in adolescent female rats. Molecules. 2016;21:461.
12. Kim MY, Kim JY, Lim D, Lee D, Kim Y, Chang GT, Choi HY, Kim H. Skeletal growth and IGF levels in rats after HT042 treatment. Phytother Res. 2012;26:1771–8.
13. Naciff JM, Overmann GJ, Torontali SM, Carr GJ, Tiesman JP, Richardson BD, Daston GP. Gene expression profile induced by 17 alpha-ethynyl estradiol in the prepubertal female reproductive system of the rat. Toxicol Sci. 2003;72:314–30.
14. Roth CL, Neu C, Jarry H, Schoenau E. Different effects of agonistic vs. antagonistic gnrh-analogues (triptorelin vs. cetrorelix) on bone modeling and remodeling in peripubertal female rats. Exp Clin Endocrinol Diabetes. 2005;113:451–6.
15. Lewis EM, Barnett JF Jr, Freshwater L, Hoberman AM, Christian MS. Sexual maturation data for Crl Sprague–Dawley rats: criteria and confounding factors. Drug Chem Toxicol. 2002;25:437–58.
16. Kwak MJ, Park HJ, Nam MH, Kwon OS, Park SY, Lee SY, Kim MJ, Kim SJ, Paik KH, Jin DK. Comparative study of the effects of different growth hormone doses on growth and spatial performance of hypophysectomized rats. J Korean Med Sci. 2009;24:729–36.
17. Uslu U, Sandal S, Cumbul A, Yildiz S, Aydin M, Yilmaz B. Evaluation of estrogenic effects of polychlorinated biphenyls and organochlorinated pesticides using immature rat uterotrophic assay. Hum Exp Toxicol. 2013;32:476–82.
18. Roth C, Schricker M, Lakomek M, Strege A, Heiden I, Luft H, Munzel U, Wuttke W, Jarry H. Autoregulation of the gonadotropin-releasing hormone (GnRH) system during puberty: effects of antagonistic versus agonistic GnRH analogs in a female rat model. J Endocrinol. 2001;169:361–71.
19. Paterson WF, McNeill E, Young D, Donaldson MD. Auxological outcome and time to menarche following long-acting goserelin therapy in girls with central precocious or early puberty. Clin Endocrinol (Oxf). 2004;61:626–34.
20. Isaac H, Patel L, Meyer S, Hall CM, Cusick C, Price DA, Clayton PE. Efficacy of a monthly compared to 3-monthly depot GnRH analogue (goserelin) in the treatment of children with central precocious puberty. Horm Res. 2007;68:157–63.
21. Lian L, Jia TZ. Effects on mice and rats' gastrointestinal function of *Phellodendron amurense* and its different processed products. Chin Arch Tradit Chin Med. 2008;26:499–501.
22. Otani H, Otsuka F, Takeda M, Mukai T, Terasaka T, Miyoshi T, Inagaki K, Suzuki J, Ogura T, Lawson MA, Makino H. Regulation of GNRH production by estrogen and bone morphogenetic proteins in GT1-7 hypothalamic cells. J Endocrinol. 2009;203:87–97.
23. Yeom M, Kim SH, Lee B, Zhang X, Lee H, Hahm DH, Sohn Y, Lee H. Effects of laser acupuncture on longitudinal bone growth in adolescent rats. Evid Based Complement Alternat Med. 2013;2013:424587.
24. Chen Q, Dai FW, Shao GM, Sa XY. Relative study on the regulation of children anti-premature granule on model SD rats' estradiol. J Zhejiang Chin Med Univ. 2011;35:226–33.
25. Dai FW. Establishment and evaluation of danazol-induced SD rat model

for precocious puberty. Veterinary Medicine, Zhejiang University; 2009.

26. Sun Y. Characteristic of hypothalamic Kiss-1 GPR54 expression in the pubertal development of precocious female rats and the effects of nourishing yin removing fire Chinese herb mixture on the Kiss-1 GPR54 expression. Integrative Medicine: Fudan Univ; 2007.

27. Tian Z, Zhao H, Sun Y, Cai D, Chen B. Evaluation of the true precocious puberty rats induced by neonatal administration of Danazol: therapeutic effects of nourishing "Yin"-Removing "Fire" Chinese herb mixture. Reprod Biol Endocrinol. 2005;3:38.

28. Ye J. Effect of Kangzao granules to Kiss-1 GPR54 mRNA gene expression on female rats with precocious puberty and its clinical research. Pediatrics, Nanjing University of Chinese Medicine; 2011.

29. Qiao LL, Cai DP. Effects of Chinese herbal medicine for nourishing yin and purging fire on mRNA and protein expression of estrogen receptor, insulin growth factor-I and aromatase in uterine and ovary of adolescent rats. Acta Univ Traditionis Medicalis Sinensis Pharmacologiaeque Shanghai. 2009;23:62–5.

30. He L, Li P, Gou S. Effects of compound Rehmannia decoction combined with recombinant human growth hormone on sex development of pubertal female rats. Acta Univ Tradit Med Sinensis Pharmacol Shanghai.

2010;24:74–8.

31. Aihara M, Kobayashi H, Kimura T, Hayashi S, Kato J. Changes in uterine estrogen receptor concentrations in persistent estrous and persistent diestrous rats. Endocrinol Jpn. 1988;35:57–70.

32. Youngster I, Rachmiel R, Pinhas-Hamiel O, Bistritzer T, Zuckerman-Levin N, de Vries L, Naugolny L, Eyal O, Braunstein R, Rachmiel M. Treatment with recombinant human growth hormone during childhood is associated with increased intraocular pressure. J Pediatr. 2012;161:1116–9.

33. Darendeliler F, Karagiannis G, Wilton P. Headache, idiopathic intracranial hypertension and slipped capital femoral epiphysis during growth hormone treatment: a safety update from the KIGS database. Horm Res. 2007;68(Suppl 5):41–7.

34. Blethen SL, Allen DB, Graves D, August G, Moshang T, Rosenfeld R. Safety of recombinant deoxyribonucleic acid-derived growth hormone: the national cooperative growth study experience. J Clin Endocrinol Metab. 1996;81:1704–10.

35. Meazza C, Schaab M, Pagani S, Calcaterra V, Bozzola E, Kratzsch J, Bozzola M. Development of antibodies against growth hormone (GH) during rhGH therapy in a girl with idiopathic GH deficiency: a case report. J Pediatr Endocrinol Metab. 2013;26:785–8.

10

Anticancer activities and mechanisms of heat-clearing and detoxicating traditional Chinese herbal medicine

Yulin Zhang[†], Yeer Liang[†] and Chengwei He[*] [iD]

Abstract

In traditional Chinese medicine (TCM) theory, pathogenic heat and toxins, which are akin to the inflammatory factors, are the causes of cancer and could promote its virulent development. Therefore, heat-clearing and detoxicating (HCD) herbs are essential components of TCM formulas for cancer treatment. An increasing interest has been focused on the study of HCD herbs and accumulated evidences have shown that HCD herbs or HCD herbs-based formulas exhibited remarkable anticancer effects when used alone or combined with other therapeutic approaches. Some of the HCD herb-derived products have been tested in clinical trials. Studies revealed that extracts or pure compounds of the HCD herbs showed a broad anticancer spectrum against both solid and hematologic malignancies without significant toxic effects. Notably, some HCD herbs or formulas could strongly enhance the anticancer activities of chemo- or radio-therapy and alleviate their side effects. The anticancer activities of HCD herb exacts or the pure compounds were reported to be through multiple cellular or molecular mechanisms, such as induction of cancer cell apoptosis, differentiation and cell cycle arrest, inhibition of cancer cell growth, invasion and metastasis, and inhibition of tumor angiogenesis. In this review, we provide comprehensive analysis and summary of research progress and future prospects in this field to facilitate the further study and application of HCD herbs.

Keywords: Traditional Chinese medicine, Heat-clearing and detoxicating herbs, Anticancer, cellular and molecular mechanisms

Background

Cancers have been becoming one of the top killers worldwide. There were approximately 14.1 million new cancer cases and 8.2 million deaths from cancers in the world in 2012 according to the WHO statistics. Cancer still viciously scares people more than any other diseases despite substantial development of cancer diagnosis and treatment has been made. The majority of cancer patients are often diagnosed after the cancer has reached a terminal stage, at which chemotherapy is largely relied on. Although chemotherapy may temporarily slow tumor growth, they often lose the effectiveness as the cancer cells develop drug resistant. Some remedies may not be suitable for long-term use due to severe side effects. Thus, it is important to develop novel effective and safe approaches for cancer treatment. Comparing to modern Western medicine, traditional Chinese medicine (TCM) comprises a particularly safe and effective strategy in the treatment of cancer. In TCM theory, disequilibrium between Yin and Yang and blockage of meridian and viscera caused by interior (long time stress, anxiety, depress, overwork, improper lifestyle, etc.) and exterior factors (physical and chemical hazards) leads to stasis of Chi (vital energy), blood, dampness and phlegm, where the pathogenic heat and toxins, which are similar to the factors that cause prominent inflammation, are generated and promote occurrence and development of cancer eventually after these long-lasting malfunctions. Therefore, heat-clearing and detoxicating (HCD) herbs,

*Correspondence: chengweihe@umac.mo
[†]Yulin Zhang and Yeer Liang contributed equally to this work
State Key Laboratory of Quality Research in Chinese Medicine, Institute of Chinese Medical Sciences, University of Macau, N22-7038, Avenida da Universidade, Taipa, Macao 999078, China

Chi-regulating herbs, circulation-enhancing herbs, dampness and phlegm-resolving herbs are often used to treat cancers in TCM. HCD herbs are mostly cold in nature and bitter in taste and commonly used to clear away heat, purge fire, dry dampness and cool blood, and relieve toxins. Since pathogenic heat and toxins are more directly related to cancer, HCD herbs or formulas play a predominant role in cancer management by TCM. This review aims to summarize the representative anticancer HCD herbs and formulas, with emphasis on discussing the anticancer activities and the molecular mechanisms.

Representative anticancer HCD herbs

The following representative anticancer HCD herbs are discussed in details: *Scutellariae* Radix (Huang Qin), *Coptidis* Rhizome (Huang Lian), *Artemisiae annuae* Herba (Qing Hao), *Hedyotis diffusa* (Bai Hua She She Cao), *Rabdosiae rubescentis* Herba (Dong Ling Cao), and *Scutellariae barbatae* Herba (Ban Zhi Lian), which are very commonly prescribed HCD herbs in the anticancer TCM formulas and have been extensively studied.

Scutellariae Radix

Scutellariae Radix (SR) is the dried root of *Scutellaria baicalensis* Georgi of the Lamiaceae family. SR is traditionally used to clear away pathogenic heat and activate blood circulation to remove stasis. Clinically, SR has long been used to treat pneumonia, jaundice, hypertension, dysentery and intestinal catarrh, pyogenic infection, etc. It is often prescribed in combination with other herbs in TCM formulas, such as Huang Qin Tang, Huang Qin Shao Yao Tang, and Huang Qin Mu Dan Tang. The most abundant compounds in SR are flavonoids, of which baicalein, baicalin, wogonoside and wogonin (Fig. 1a–d) showed strong anticancer activities.

Baicalein, the major flavone in SR, exhibited multiple pharmacological activities, such as anti-hepatotoxicity, anti-viral, anti-inflammation, and anticancer. Baicalein was reported to have anticancer activity against a wide spectrum of cancers [1], including esophagus, gastric, colorectal, pancreatic, lung, breast, ovarian, prostate and skin cancers [2, 3]. The anticancer activity of baicalein was through multiple mechanisms, e.g. suppressing hyperproliferation, inflammation, and metastasis, inducing apoptosis, etc. [3, 4], in which the PI3K/Akt and p38 pathways were engaged [5].

Wogonin, another flavone derived from SR, was proved to be effective in anticancer both in vitro and in mouse models, through inducing apoptosis, cell cycle arrest, and differentiation of cancer cells, inhibiting angiogenesis of tumor, and reversing drug resistance. Polier et al. reported that wogonin specifically inhibited the activity of cyclin-dependent kinase 9 (CDK9) and down-regulated the short-lived anti-apoptotic protein myeloid cell leukemia 1 (Mcl-1), which resulted in apoptosis in cancer cells [6]. Wogonin also induced nasopharyngeal carcinoma (NPC) cell apoptosis via inhibiting the activity of glycogen synthase kinase 3β (GSK-3β), a multifunctional serine/threonine kinase that was reported to inhibit apoptosis, and down-regulating the expression of ΔNp63, a survival factor in NPC cells [7]. In addition, wogonin inhibited tumor angiogenesis by promoting the degradation of hypoxia-inducible factors α (HIF-1α) via increasing its prolyl hydroxylation [8]. Acquired drug resistance is a serious problem in cancer treatment. Wogonin could reverse drug resistance in MCF-7/DOX cells through inhibiting the cell survival factors nuclear factor erythroid 2-related factor 2 (Nrf2) and heme oxygenase-1 (HO-1) [9]. Notably, wogonin significantly potentiated etoposide-induced apoptosis by impairing the function of P-glycoprotein and then increased cellular content of etoposide in HL-60 cells [10]. This synergistic effects were also observed when combination with fluorouracil in human gastric model. The synergistic anticancer activity of wogonin could be due to its pro-apoptotic effect and downregulation of NF-κB [11]. Furthermore, wogonin preferentially killed cancer cells instead of influence on normal cells. Based on these researches, *Scutellariae radix* and its effective constituents may serve as a clinically potential therapeutic agents against aggressive malignancies.

Coptidis Rhizoma

Coptidis Rhizoma (CR) is the dried rhizome of *Coptis Chinese Franch.* of the Ranunculaceae family. The properties of CR are: extremely bitter and cold in nature, very strong in clearing heat and dampness, and detoxication. CR is commonly used in China for the treatment of gastroenteritis, liver disease, hypertension, and other inflammatory diseases accompanied by high fever. CR or its components were found to be beneficial for a wide range of diseases, such as diarrhea, pressure-overload induced cardiac hypertrophy, hypercholesterolemia, atherosclerosis, Alzheimer's disease, and diabetes mellitus. Interestingly, our studies and others demonstrated that CR extract exhibited strong anticancer effects in vitro and in vivo used alone or combined with chemotherapeutic drugs [12–14]. CR extract significantly inhibited tumor growth and colony formation of gastric, colon, and breast cancer cells. Breast cancer cells were particularly sensitive to CR. The growth inhibition was associated with suppression of cyclin B1 protein, which resulted in complete inhibition of CDC2 kinase activity and cell cycle arrest at G_2 phase [15]. Iizuka and his colleagues reported that the aqueous extract of CR exhibited inhibitory effect on the proliferation of esophageal cancer cells and arrested the cells at G_0/G_1 phase [16]. CR

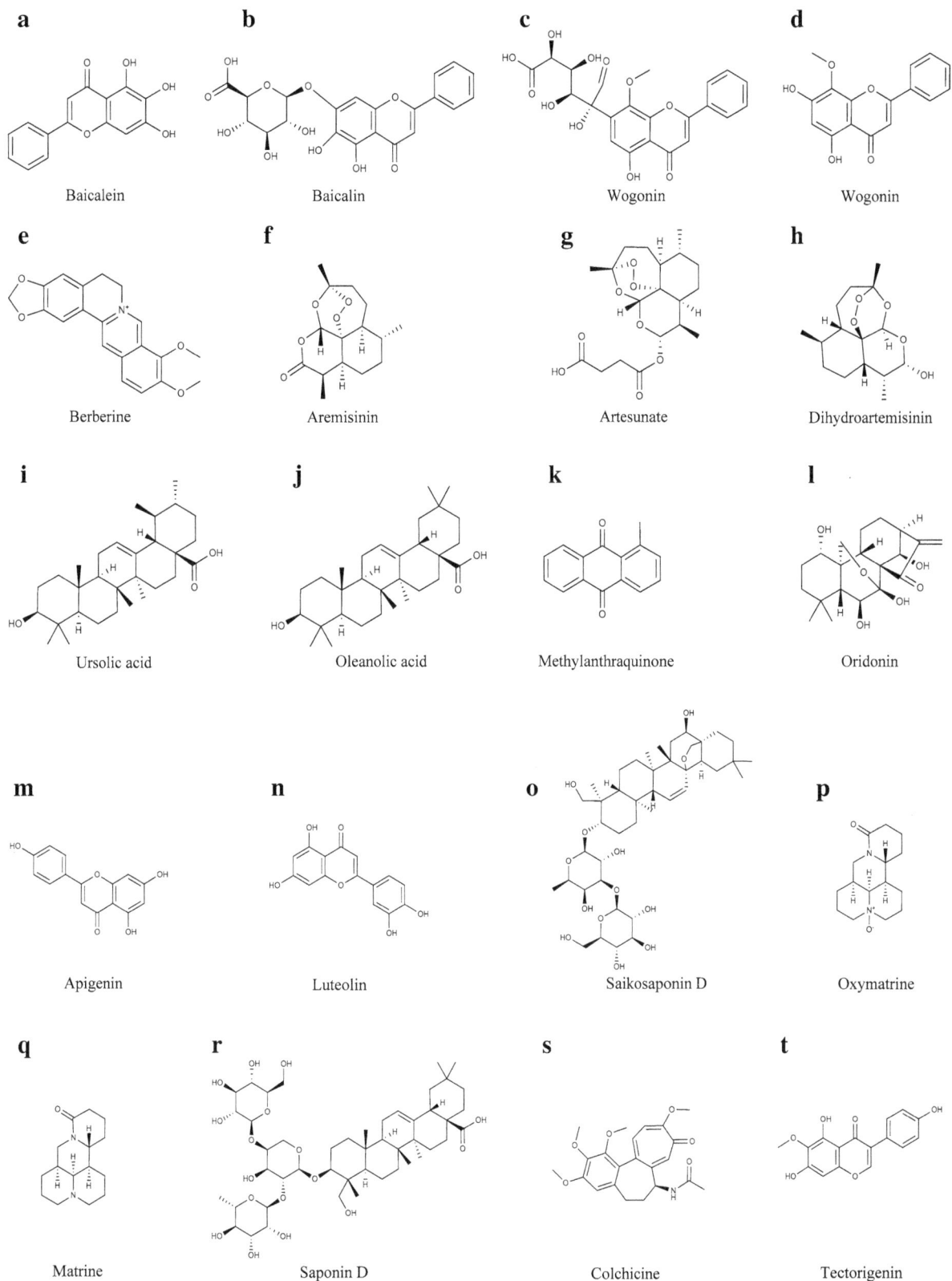

Fig. 1 Chemical structures of major anticancer compounds in the representative HCD herbs

supplementation significantly attenuated weight loss in tumor-bearing nude mice without changing food intake or tumor growth, and maintained good nutritional status in these mice. The anti-cachectic effect was accompanied by significantly reduced interleukin 6 (IL-6) expression [17].

The most abundant compounds in CR are alkaloids, of which berberine (Fig. 1e) is the most important active compound, with its dry weight consisting of up to 7.1 mg/100 mg of CR [18]. Recent data have shown that berberine was applied in treating inflammation, cancer, colitis, diabetes, high blood cholesterol etc. [19]. Considerable attention has been drawn to berberine since its prominent anticancer activity including tongue squamous cancer, esophageal cancer, hepatocelluar cancer, breast cancer, lung cancer, gastric cancer, ovarian cancer, renal cancer, nasopharyngeal cancer and Wilms' tumor [20]. Berberine has been proved to be a heat-clearing and detoxifying compound which acts on diverse cancer cell types through various mechanisms. For the treatment of colorectal cancer, berberine was mainly involved in inducing apoptosis and restraining inflammation, inhibiting tumor growth, inactivating Wnt/β-catenin signaling, promoting the generation of ROS, inhibiting arylamine N-acetyltransferase (NAT) activity and cyclooxygenase 2 (COX-2) expression [21]. Interestingly, berberine significantly reduced the familial adenomatous polyposis patients' polyp size through inhibition of Wnt signaling, suggesting an application in the prevention of colon cancer [22]. Berberine also suppresses the invasive and metastasis of nasopharyngeal carcinoma (NPC) by inhibiting the activation of Signal Transducer and Activator of Transcription 3 (STAT3), a key mediator to trigger tumor-promoting inflammation [23]. The similar actions were observed in lung cancer, of which cell proliferation and tumor spheroid formation were suppressed by berberine [24]. Notably, berberine exhibits selective cytotoxicity against cancer cells instead of normal hepatocytes [25]. In human breast cancer cells, berberine induces apoptosis through a mitochondrial dependent pathway by increasing the Bax/Bcl-2 protein ratio, activating caspases and inducing poly (ADP-ribose) polymerase (PARP) cleavage [26]. The induction of interferon β and tumor necrosis factor (TNF) α in cancer cells is responsible for the anti-breast cancer activity of berberine [13]. Furthermore, berberine significantly enhanced the anticancer effect of estrogen receptor (ER) antagonists on ER positive breast cancer cells through down-regulating the expression of cancer related genes, such as epidermal growth factor receptor (EGFR), human epidermal growth factor receptor 2 (HER2), and bcl-2 [14]. Improvement of the chemo- and radio-sensitivity of tumors by herbs indicates another strategy of treatment in cancer therapy.

Anticancer efficacy was significantly enhanced when combining berberine with granted chemotherapeutic agents such as vincristine or 2-deoxy-D-glucose in certain cancer cells [27]. Combined with γ radiation, berberine exhibited pro-apoptotic effect in hepatocellular carcinoma cells [28]. The chemosensitization of berberine was showed in colon cancer cells while the radiosensitization was obtained in esophageal squamous carcinoma cells, human nasopharyngeal carcinoma cells, and breast carcinoma cells [29, 30]. It's important to note that berberine has so poor bioavailability that it can hardly be an independent anti-tumor agent [31]. Nevertheless, berberine could be a promising adjuvant to chemotherapy and radiotherapy of a wide range of cancers.

Artemisiae annuae Herba

Artemisiae annuae Herba (AAH) is the dried aerial part of *Artemisia annua* L. of the Compositae family. It was initially used for treating fevers in TCM, and was then renowned to be an antimalarial herb. Recent studies indicated that AAH showed high potential anticancer activities [32].

The most abundant compounds in AAH are sesquiterpene lactones, of which artemisinin (Fig. 1f) is the most active compound. Artemisinin has a broad range of biological activities, such as anti-viral, anti-fungal, anti-parasitic, anti-inflammation, and anticancer. The anticancer activities of artemisinin include anti-proliferation, anti-angiogenesis, anti-invasion, anti-metastasis and cytotoxicity [33]. Artemisinin and its derivatives, such as artesunate (Fig. 1g) and dihydroartemisinin (DHA) (Fig. 1h), exhibit potential anticancer effects on various types of cancer cells, including breast cancer, leukemia, ovarian cancer, hematoma, prostate cancer, colon cancer, gastric cancer, melanoma and lung cancer [34]. Artemisinin was reported to inhibit angiogenesis through down-regulating the expression of vascular endothelial growth factor (VEGF), a key angiogenesis stimulator, in in vitro and in vivo assays [35]. Artemisinin induced a strong stringent G1 cell cycle arrest in prostate cancer cells, human breast cancer cells and nasopharyngeal cancer cells by down-regulating the expression of CDK2, CDK4, cyclin E, cyclin D1 and E2F1, and increasing the expression of p16 (also known as cyclin-dependent kinase inhibitor 2A) [36]. DHA treatment caused cervical cancer cell growth inhibition via upregulation of Raf kinase inhibitor protein (RKIP) and downregulation of bcl-2 [37]. Artemisinin can alter apoptosis-related protein expression which may further inhibit cell proliferation and induce apoptosis. Artemisinin downregulated IGF-IR expression and inhibited the growth of MCF-7 breast tumor cell xenografts in nude mice [38]. Moreover, the inhibition of Bcl-2 family, activation of Bax and release of cytochrome c in human colon cancer cells illuminate the pro-apoptotic mechanisms of artemisinin [39]. Artemisinin may also be a potential anti-metasta-sis agent against melanoma cells and hepatocarcinoma cells by reducing MMP2 level [40]. A more recent report revealed that DHA activates the autophagy program by suppressing the nuclear translocation of NF-κB [41]. In vivo experiments showed that oral administration of artemisinin at 50 mg/kg/day decreased tumor growth [40]. The toxicity of artemisinin remains a challenge for its development in the clinical application. In addition to possessing cytotoxicity in various tumors, artemisinin shows slight neurotoxicity and may cause drug resistance in vivo [33]. Besides, artemisinin and its derivatives produce synergistic anticancer effects in combination with other chemotherapeutic drugs. For instance, DHA sensitized human ovarian cancer cells to carboplatin therapy and synergistically enhanced the anticancer effect of gemcitabine on human lung cancer cells [42, 43].

Hedyotis diffusa

Hedyotis diffusa (HD) is the dried whole plant of genus Saxifraga of the *Rubiaceae* family. As a well-known traditional Chinese folk medicine, it frequently appears in Chinese medicinal formulas and has long been used for heat-clearing, detoxification, promotion of blood circulation and removal of blood stasis [44]. Accumulating evidences indicate that HD possesses anticancer, antioxidative, hepatoprotective, neuroprotective, anti-inflammatory, anti-mutagenesis and immunoregulatory activities [45]. It is applied in the treatment of inflammation-related diseases, such as appendicitis, bronchitis and urethritis. Pharmacological studies propose that HD performs vital roles in the treatment of solid tumors, including liver, lung, colon, and other cancers [46]. Both organic and aqueous extracts of HD exhibit remarkable anticancer activities. The methanol extracts of HD can suppress cancer cell proliferation and induce apoptosis, which involve many tumor-related genes and proteins (e.g. TNF-α, IL-1, NF-κB, Fas, AP-1, Bcl-2, Bcl-xL) [45]. The ethanol extracts inhibit angiogenesis and induce mitochondrion-dependent apoptosis through PI3K/Akt and XIAP pathways [47]. The aqueous extracts inhibited HepG2 cell growth and enhanced the anticancer activity of 5-fluorouracil via suppressing CDK2-E2F1 activity [48].

Phytochemistry studies show that it contains components with anticancer activities, including anthraquinones, flavones, hemiterpenes, polyphenols, organic acids and polysaccharides [49], of which ursolic acid (Fig. 1i) and oleanolic acid (Fig. 1j) are two major anticancer compounds [46]. Ursolic acid demonstrated effective in anti-leukemia, which involves diverse biological functions, such as inhibition of cell growth, induction of cell differentiation and apoptosis [50]. The associated mechanisms include inactivation of protein kinase B (PKB), activation of c-Jun N-terminal kinases (JNK) and extracellular signal-regulated kinase (ERK) pathways, intracellular Ca^{2+} release, etc. Ursolic acid also exhibits therapeutic potential in the treatment of hormone refractory and androgen-sensitive prostate cancer through induction of cancer cell apoptosis via activation of JNK-induced Bcl-2 phosphorylation and degradation [51]. Methylanthraquinone (Fig. 1k), another active compound from HD, shows multiple anticancer effects on many cancer types. It induced apoptosis in human breast cancer MCF-7 cells by increasing intracellular calcium levels, activating JNK, calpain, and eventually caspases 4, 9, 7 [52]. Methylanthraquinone also caused apoptosis in human leukemic U937 cells by decreasing phospho-ERK1/2 and increasing phospho-p38 MAPKs [53]. Taking together, accumulating evidences indicates the therapeutic potential of HD or its components in treating various cancers.

Rabdosiae rubescentis Herba

Rabdosiae rubescentis Herba (RRH) is the dried aerial part of genus *Rabdosia rubescens* (Hemsl.) Hara of the Lamiaceae family. RRH, or Dong Ling Cao in Chinese, which means "ice grass" due to its strong heat-clearing and detoxifying properties, is a well-known HCD herb possessing several biological activities, such as anti-bacteria, anti-parasites, anti-inflammation, and anticancer [54].

The chemical components of RRH are relatively complex, mainly including monoterpenes, sesquiterpene, diterpene and tripenoids. Oridonin (Fig. 1l), a tetracyclic terpenoid compound, is the main active component purified from RRH [55]. In recent years, increasing attention has been gained on oridonin due to its remarkable growth inhibition and apoptosis induction activities in cancer cells. In vitro and in vivo studies showed that oridonin induced apoptosis in cells derived from a variety of cancers, including hepatocellular carcinoma, breast cancer, skin cancer, colorectal cancer, gallbladder cancer, gastric cancer, pancreatic cancer and osteoma [56]. Notably, oridonin has less cytotoxicity to normal cells such as fibroblasts and lymphoid cells [56]. Oridonin could arrest cell cycle at the G2/M phase in hepatocarcinoma HepG2 cells by upregulating serine-threonine kinase receptor-associated protein, heat shock 70 kDa protein 1, stress-induced phosphoprotein 1, etc. [57]. Oridonin also drastically suppresses tumor invasion and metastasis in vitro via regulating the integrin β1/FAK pathway and decreasing the expression of MMPs in MDA-MB-231 cells in vitro [58]. A study on cervical cancer found that oridonin induced the apoptosis of cancer cells through PI3K/Akt pathway [59]. In another study on gastric cancer indicated that the mechanism of oridonin-induced apoptosis involved Apaf-1, cytochrome c and caspase-3 signaling pathway [60]. Accumulating studies have shown an enhanced anticancer effect when oridonin was combined with imatinib in Ph^+ acute lymphoblastic leukemia cells. The results showed that oridonin inhibited the activations of LYN (one of SRC family kinases) and ABL and their downstream Raf/MEK/ERK, Akt/mTOR, and STAT5 pathways, decreased Bcl-2/Bax ratio and then induced apoptosis in Ph^+ ALL cells [61]. In addition, some recent studies suggested that oridonin could also inhibit the proliferation of tumor cells by increasing the autophagy of tumor cells [62]. Current research on pancreatic cancer cells indicated that oridonin could induce apoptosis via p53- and caspase-dependent induction of p38 MAPK [63]. Meanwhile, apoptosis, autophagy and loss of the mitochondrial transmembrane potential have been observed in lung cancer cell line A549 treated with oridonin [64]. Therefore, oridonin is supposed to be a promising compound for chemotherapy.

Scutellariae barbatae Herba

Scutellariae barbatae Herba (SBH) is the dried whole plant of genus *Scutellaria barbata* D. Don of the Lamiaceae family. SBH contains several flavonoids, alkaloids, polysaccharides, and steroids [65]. The extracts of SBH exhibited significant anticancer activities in several human cancers such as colon cancer, leukemia, hepatoma, skin cancer, breast cancer and chorioepithelioma [66]. Despite the distinguished success of this herb in treating cancer, the precise molecular mechanisms still remain to be investigated. Studies revealed that ethanol extract of SBH (ESBH) could induce apoptosis, inhibit proliferation and angiogenesis in colon cancer [67]. Administration of ESBH remarkably increased the levels of pro-apoptotic Bax/Bcl-2 ratio and the expression of suppressor gene p21, whereas decreased the expression of pro-proliferative genes Cyclin D1 and CDK4 [67]. Further studies on benign smooth muscle cell tumor model demonstrated that SBH could induce differentiation and apoptosis in uterine smooth muscle cells [68]. In addition, SBH showed well-validated chemopreventive activity at stages of initiation, promotion, and progression of cancer [69]. Increasing evidences have also revealed that the combination therapy of SBH with other commonly prescribed chemotherapeutic agents could considerably inhibit the growth of carcinoma both in vitro and in vivo [70]. Although the active anticancer constituents have not been identified, flavonoids in SBH have become the focus of researches, since this kind of compounds strongly inhibited cancer cell proliferation, induced mitochondria-dependent apoptosis, and inhibited tumor angiogenesis [65]. Nevertheless, more efforts are required to investigate the active compounds in SBH to facilitate the research and development of this promising anticancer herb.

Summary of the major active compounds and their actions

The chemical structures of major anticancer compounds in the representative HCD herbs are shown in Fig. 1. The anticancer activities and their mechanisms of the major compounds in the above-discussed and other typical HCD herbs are summarized in Table 1. The anticancer compounds in HCD herbs are comprised of various types of chemicals, including, but not limiting to, alkaloids (e.g. berberine, matrine and colchicine), flavonoids (e.g. baicalein, wogonin, luteolin, apigenin and tectorigenin), terpenoids (e.g. oridonin, ursolic acid, oleanolic acid, artemisinin and saikogenin), anthraquinones, polyphenols, organic acids (e.g. ursolic acid and oleanolic acid), polysaccharides, saponins (e.g. saikosaponin and pulsatilla saponins), etc. Studies indicated that the active compounds from HCD herbs exhibited multifarious anticancer activities, such as inhibition of proliferation, invasion, metastasis, inflammation, and angiogenesis, induction of differentiation, apoptosis and cell cycle arrest, antioxidation, and modulation of immune function (Fig. 2). The versatile anticancer effects of these compounds are also indicated by the potency against a broad spectrum of cancer types, both various solid tumors and hematopoietic malignancies. HCD herbs are primarily characterized by the heat-clearing and detoxicating properties in TCM theory, which correlate with their antioxidant activity. Indeed, most, if not all, compounds from HCD herbs are antioxidants, such as berberine, matrine, baicalein, polyphenols and polysaccharides. Since tumors frequently exhibit high levels of oxidative stress [71], a general disturbance of redox balance in cancer cells by HCD herbal compounds may contribute to their multifarious anticancer effects. In addition, these compounds could regulate a wide range of signaling pathways, kinase activity and gene expression, which are involved in cell proliferation, cell cycle, apoptosis, invasion, metastasis, etc. However, the anticancer potential and detailed molecular mechanisms of the compounds remain to be further elucidated.

The representative anticancer formulas containing HCD herbs

Cocktails of medicines are usually applied to treat complex syndromes or diseases, like cancers and cardiovascular diseases. Similarly, single herb is seldom used in TCM, of which formulas with combination of various herbs are much more often prescribed on the basis of individual conditions according to TCM theory. Cancers often exhibit excessive heat and toxin. Therefore, one or more HCD herbs are the major components in anticancer TCM formulas. In recent

Table 1 The major active components, anticancer effects and mechanisms of HCD herbs

HCD herbs	Major anticancer compounds	Cancer types (cell lines)	Cellular effects	Molecular mechanisms	References
Scutellariae Radix	Baicalein, wogonin	Esophageal squamous cell carcinoma (EC-109), glioma (U87MG, U251MG, C6, U251), colon cancer (HCT116), bladder cancer (TSGH8301, BFTC905, RT4, T24, HT1376), breast cancer (T47D, MCF-7, SK-BR-3, MDA-MB-231, SKBR3), leukemia (CEM), pancreatic carcinoma (Colo-357), hepatocellular carcinoma (HepG2, SK-HEP-1), Hodgkin's lymphoma (L1236), melanoma (SK-MEL-37), nasopharyngeal carcinoma (NPC-TW076, NPC-TW039)	Inhibiting proliferation, invasion, migration and angiogenesis, inducing apoptosis and differentiation	↑MMP2, ↓MMP9, ↑TIMP1, ↑TIMP2, ↓p38, ↑PI3K/AKT, ↓NF-κB, ↑PPAR γ, ↓CDC2-survivin, ↓Wnt, ↓CDK9, ↓HIF-1α, ↓VEGF, ↑GSK3β/β-catenin, ↓ΔNp63, ↑cleaved PARP, ↑caspase-3, ↑caspase-7, ↑p21	[3–11, 22, 29]
Coptidis Rhizoma	Berberine	Breast cancer (MCF7, MDA-MB-468), gastric cancer (MKN-74), colon cancer (HCT116, SW480, SW620, DLD-1, KM12, KM12SM, KM12L4A,), esophageal cancer (YES-1, YES-2, YES-3, YES-4, YES-5, YES-6), nasopharyngeal carcinoma (5-8F, C666-1), kidney cancer (G401), bladder cancer (T24), hepatocellular carcinoma (HepG2)	Inhibiting proliferation, invasion, migration and angiogenesis, inducing apoptosis, cell cycle arrest at G0/G1 phase and mitochondrial membrane damage, increasing ROS	↑IFN-β, ↑TNF-α, ↓Cyclin B1, ↓CDC2, ↓Ezrin, ↑p27, ↑p21, ↑Cyclin E, ↑AMPK, ↑WTX, ↓GSK3β/β-catenin, ↓JNK/p38, ↓Wnt, ↓STAT3, ↑caspase-8, ↑caspase-3, ↓Bid, ↑Bax/Bcl-2, ↑Fas, ↑cleaved PARP, ↓NAT, ↓COX-2, ↑TRAIL, ↑VEGF	[13–16, 19–31]
Artemisiae annuae Herba	Artemisinin	Leukemia (HL-60, NB4), ovarian cancer (HO-8910), prostate cancer (LNCaP), breast cancer (MCF-7), nasopharyngeal carcinoma (CNE-1, CNE-2), hepatocellular carcinoma (HepG2, SMMC-7721), melanoma (A375P, A375M), myeloma (RPMI 8226), colon cancer (HCT16), cervical cancer (HeLa, Caski)	Inhibiting proliferation, invasion, migration and angiogenesis, Inducing apoptosis, cell cycle arrest at G1 phase and mitochondrial dysfunction, increasing ROS	↑MAPKs, ↓p38MAPK, ↓VEGF, ↓KDR, ↓CDK2, ↓CDK4, ↓Cyclin E, ↓Cyclin D1, ↓E2F1, ↑BMI-1, ↑RKIP, ↓Bcl-2, ↑Bax, ↑caspase-3, ↓IGF-IR, ↓MMP2, ↑TIMP2, ↓αvβ3, ↓NF-κB	[34–43]
Hedyotis diffusa	Ursolic acid, methylanthraquinone	Histiocytic lymphoma (U937), leukemia (HL-60, colon cancer (HT-29), melanoma (B16-F10), lung cancer (A549), breast cancer (MCF-7), prostate cancer (LNCaP, Tsu-Pr1, MDA-MB-453, DU-145, cervical cancer (C-33A, U14), sarcoma (S180), hepatocellular carcinoma (HepG2, H22, SMMC-7721)	Inhibiting proliferation, migration and angiogenesis, inducing differentiation, apoptosis, cell cycle arrest at G0/G1, S or G2/M phases, DNA fragmentation and mitochondrial dysfunction	↑interferon-γ, ↑TNF-α, ↑IL-1, ↓NF-κB, ↑Fas, ↑p53, ↑p21/Cip1, ↓p27/kip1, ↓caspase-3, ↑caspase-9, ↑AP-1, ↓Bcl-2, ↑Bax, ↓STAT3, ↓cyclin D, ↓cyclin D1, ↓cyclin D2, ↓cyclin E, ↓CDK4, ↓CDK2, ↓E2F1, ↑Fas-L, ↑TRAIL, ↑MAPK/ERK, ↓JNK, ↑PI3K, ↑p21/WAF1, ↑CDKN1A, ↓Cyclin A2, ↓Cyclin B1, ↓ODC1, ↓VEGF-α, ↑HSP 70, ↑P16, ↓pim-1, ↓rel, ↓ras, ↓fos, ↓myc, ↑IFN-γ	[45–51, 53]
Rabdosiae rubescentis Herba	Oridonin	Hepatocellular carcinoma (HepG2), gallbladder carcinoma (SGC996, NOZ), breast cancer (MCF-7, MDA-MB-231), cervical cancer (HeLa), histiocytic lymphoma (U937), pancreatic cancer (SW1990)	Inhibiting proliferation, migration and invasion, inducing apoptosis, autophagy, DNA damage and cell cycle arrest at S and G2/M phases, increasing ROS	↑Hsp70-1, ↑STAP, ↑TCTP, ↑Sti1, ↑PPase, ↑hnRNP-1, ↑HP1 β, ↑GlyRS, ↓NF-κB, ↑Bax/Bcl-2, ↓caspase-3, ↑caspase-9, ↑cleaved PARP, ↓IKKα, ↓IKKβ, ↓mTOR, ↑Fas, ↑PPAR-γ, ↓MMP2/MMP9, ↓Integrin β, ↓FAK, ↓Akt, ↓FOXO, ↓GSK3, ↓ERK, ↓IL-1β, ↑Beclin-1, ↑LC3 II/I, ↑Atg4B, ↓p38 MAPK, ↑p53, ↑p21	[53, 56, 57, 59–64]

Table 1 continued

HCD herbs	Major anticancer compounds	Cancer types (cell lines)	Cellular effects	Molecular mechanisms	References
Scutellariae barbatae Herba	Apigenin, luteolin	Hepatocellular carcinoma (MHCC97H), colon cancer (HT-29), leukemia (LM-1, LM-2), cervical cancer (HeLa)	Inhibiting proliferation and invasion, inducing apoptosis, differentiation and cell cycle arrest at G1 phase	↓MMP-2, ↓MMP-9, ↑TIMP-1, ↑TIMP-2, ↑ACTA2, ↑Calponin, ↑p27, ↓Cyclin D1, ↓CDK4, ↑p21, ↑Bax/Bcl-2, ↓STAT3, ↓ERK1/2, ↓p38, ↑Smac, ↑Apaf-1, ↑caspase-9, ↑caspase-3, ↓IGF-1, ↑cytochrome c	[65–70]
Bupleuri Radix	Saikosaponin D	Cervical cancer (HeLa), breast cancer (MCF-7), prostate cancer (PC3), lung cancer (H1299, LLC-1, A549), hepatocellular carcinoma (HepG2, Hep3B), gastric adenocarcinoma (MK-1), cervical cancer (HeLa), melanoma (B16F10), leukemia (P-388), oral epidermoid carcinoma (KB)	Inhibiting proliferation, invasion, metastasis, and angiogenesis, inducing apoptosis, autophagic cell death, cell cycle arrest at G1, or G2/M phases	↑ERK1/2, ↑caspase-3, ↑caspase-9, ↑caspase-7, ↑cleaved PARP, ↑AMPK, ↑mTOR, ↑p27, ↓p53, p21/WAF1, ↑Fas/APO-1, ↑mFasL, ↑sFasL, ↑Bax, ↓IKB-α, ↓NF-κB, ↓Bcl-XL, ↓SERCA Ca²⁺ pump, ↑[Ca²⁺]ᵢ, ↓telomerase, ↑tubulin polymerization	[91–93]
Sophorae flavescentis Radix	Matrine	Hepatocellular carcinoma (H22, S180, SMMC-7721, HepG2, Hep-7402), breast cancer (MA737, MKN45, SGC-70901, MDA-MB-231), gastric cancer (SGC-7901), melanoma (A375, SK-MEL-2, M21, B16-F10), cervical cancer (HeLa), leukemia (K-562), glioma (C6), lung cancer (A549, NCI-H460), ovarian cancer (SK-OV-3), central nervous system cancer (XF498), pulmonary adenoma (SPC-A-1), esophagus cancer (Eca-109), colon cancer (SW1116, HCT-15), osteosarcoma (UMR-108, MNNG/HOS), pancreatic cancer (PANC-1), leukemia (U937, HL-60), adenoid cystic carcinoma (ACC-M), retinoblastoma (Y79, WERI-RB1, SO-RB50), nasopharynx cancer (TW03)	Inhibiting proliferation, adhesion, invasion, metastasis and angiogenesis, inducing apoptosis, autophagy, differentiation and cell cycle arrest at G0/G1 or G2 phases, modulating immune function	↑Beclin 1, ↑Bax, ↓Bcl-2, ↑caspase-8, ↑caspase-3, ↑caspase-9, ↑AKT, ↓NF-κB, ↓IκBα, ↓p65, ↓ERK1/2, ↓JNK, ↓p38 MAPK, ↓TNFαI, ↓IKB-α, ↓p65, ↓ERK1/2, ↑E2F1, ↓Rb, ↑Apaf-1, ↓MMP-9, ↓MMP-2, ↓AKT, ↓EGF, ↓VEGF, ↓VEGF2, ↓VEGFR1, ↑Fas, ↑FasL, ↑p21, ↑p27, ↓Cyclin D1, ↓Cyclin E, ↓hTERT	[94, 95]
Pulsatillae Radix	Pulsatilla saponin A, D, H	Gastric cancer (MKN-45, MKN-28, AGS), colon cancer (HT-29, LoVo), hepatocellular carcinoma (Huh-7, HepG2)	Inducing DNA damage and apoptosis	↑Caspase-3, ↑cleaved PARP, ↑Bax, ↓c-Met, ↓AKT, ↓mTOR, ↓p70S6K, ↓HIF-1α, ↓VEGF	[96, 97]
Cremastrae pseudobulbus, Pleiones pseudobulbus	Colchicine	Hepatocellular carcinoma (HCC24/KMUH, HCC38/KMUH)	Inhibit proliferation interacting with tubulin	↑AKAP12, ↑TGF-β2, ↑MX1	[98, 99]
Belamcandae Rhizoma	Tectorigenin	Hepatocellular carcinoma (HepG2), lung cancer (LLC), sarcoma (S180), prostate cancer (LNCaP)	Inhibiting the proliferation and angiogenesis, inducing apoptosis, differentiation and mitochondrial dysfunction, increasing ROS	↑Caspase-3, ↑caspase-9, ↓PDEF, ↓PSA, ↓IGF-1, ↑TIMP-3, ↑cytochrome c, ↑[Ca²⁺]ᵢ	[100, 101]

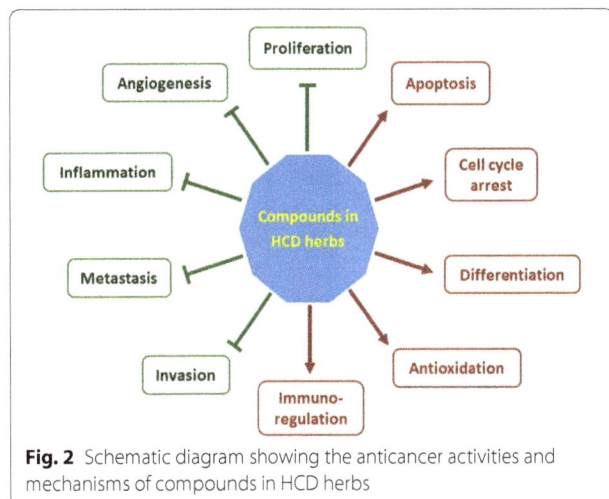

Fig. 2 Schematic diagram showing the anticancer activities and mechanisms of compounds in HCD herbs

years, the application of TCM prescriptions in the treatment of various malignant tumors has obtained encouraging outcomes, at least partially owing to that multiple components can act on multiple targets and exert synergistic therapeutic efficacies. In particular, apart from traditional decoction and oral administration methods, advanced pharmaceutical technologies are used in TCM formula preparations with distinctive advantages and features, including tablets, pills, capsules, injections, powder, liquids, etc. [72]. The following representative anticancer formulas containing HCD herbs are discussed in details, including Yanshu Injection, Huanglian Jiedu Tang, Jiedu Xiaozheng Yin and PHY906. Some others are listed in Table 2.

Yanshu Injection

Yanshu Injection (YSI), also named Fu Fang Ku Shen injection, consists of two herbs: *Sophorae flavescentis* Radix (SFR, or Ku Shen) and *Smilacis glabrae* Rhizoma (SGR, or Tu Fu Ling) with the ratio of 7 to 3. Both of them belong to heat-clearing and detoxifying herbs. SFR is commonly used for the treatment of viral hepatitis, cancer, enteritis, viral myocarditis, arrhythmia, skin diseases, etc. The major anticancer compounds in SFR are oxymatrine (Fig. 1p) and matrine (Fig. 1q), which have been approved for the treatment of cancers by the Chinese State Food and Drug Administration (SFDA) [73]. The compounds showed broad spectrum of anticancer activities including stomach, esophagus, liver, colon, lung, cervix, ovary, and breast cancers, through multiple mechanisms, such as inhibiting cancer cell proliferation, inducing apoptosis and autophagy, modulating immune response, reducing cancer cell adhesion, invasion and migration [73]. SGR is widely used both in food supplementary and health care, owing to its properties of heat-clearing and detoxication. Studies reported its

therapeutic potential for the treatment of rheumatoid arthritis, inflammation, liver injury, hyperinsulinemia and cancer [74]. Crude extraction of SGR as well as its pure compounds including astilbin, 5-*O*-caffeoylshikimic acid and taxifolin, could promote cancer cell apoptosis and block cancer cell adhesion, invasion and migration by inhibiting transforming growth factor beta 1 (TGF-β1) signaling pathway. YSI was reported to be able to directly inhibit gastric cancer cell proliferation and block the experimental gastric carcinogenesis by preventing carcinogen-induced oxidative damage and improving immune function [75]. However, YSI was mostly applied in combination with chemotherapy or radiotherapy in cancer treatment. Studies showed that YSI plus transcatheter arterial chemoembolization (TACE) could synergistically enhance the therapeutic effects of TACE, alleviate the adverse responses of radiotherapy and chemotherapy, improve the patients' life quality, and reduce the cancer recurrence [76].

Huanglian Jiedu Tang

Huanglian Jiedu Tang (HJT), a classic herbal formula, consists of four herbs: *Coptis* Rhizome (Huang Lian), *Phellodendri chinensis* Cortex (Huang Bai), *Scutellariae* Radix (Huang Qin), and *Gardeniae* Fructus (Zhi Zi), with equal proportion. In this prescription, the first three herbs listed above have the roles of purging fire and removing toxin, and function as monarch, minister and assistant in the formula, respectively. The decoction, previously acting as an anti-inflammatory agent, is widely used for treating dermatitis, gastritis, liver injuries, and bleeding of the intestines and uterus [77]. HJT has been extensively used in TCM practice even though their mechanisms of action remain unclear. It was reported that HJT could effectively cause hepatoma cell cycle arrest by upregulating the inactive form of Cdc2 and Cdc25, and downregulating the levels of Bcl-2 and Bcl-xL. Moreover, HJT exerted antitumor effect through increasing the expression of Bax and Bak and decreasing the expression of Bcl-2 and Bcl-xL via inhibition of the NF-κB activity, and consequently inducing the mitochondria-dependent apoptosis in hepatoma cells [78]. HJT could inhibit primary myeloma cell proliferation and survival, and induce the cell apoptosis via a mitochondria-mediated pathway. Further studies revealed that *Scutellaria* Radix and one of its major compounds baicalein were responsible for the anticancer effect of HJT on myeloma [79]. Experiments were conducted on evaluating the preventive effect of oral administration of HJT on stomatitis and diarrhea induced by cytotoxic drugs in patients with acute leukemia. It was found that the incidence of mucositis and diarrhea was apparently lower than the control group [80]. In addition,

Table 2 Anticancer effects and mechanisms of HCD herb-containing formulas

HCD formulas	Components	Cancer types (cell lines)	Cellular effects	Molecular mechanisms	References
Yanshu Injection	*Sophorae flavescentis Radix, Smilacis glabrae Rhizoma*	Hepatocellular carcinoma (HepG2), breast cancer (MDA-MB-231), bladder cancer (T24)	Inhibiting proliferation, adhesion, invasion, migration and metastasis inducing apoptosis and autophagy, modulating immune response	↓TGF-β1, ↓TGFBR1	[73–76]
Huanglian Jiedu Tang	*Coptidis rhizome, Phellodendri chinensis Cortex, Scutellariae Radix, and Gardeniae Fructus*	Hepatocellular carcinoma (HepG2, PLC/PRF/5), myeloma (U266, NOP-2, AMO1, ILKM2)	Inhibiting proliferation, inducing apoptosis and cycle arrest	↑p-Cdc2, ↑p-Cdc25C, ↓Cdc2, ↓Cdc25C, ↓Cyclin A, ↓Cyclin B1, ↑Bak, ↓Bcl-2, ↓Bcl-XL, ↑IKB-α, ↓NF-κB, ↓IL-6, ↓XIAP, ↑caspase-3, ↑caspase-9	[78–81]
Jiedu Xiaozheng Yin	*Hedyotis diffusa Willd, Cremastrae pseudobulbus, Pleiones pseudobulbus, Prunellae Spica and Sophorae flavescentis Radix*	Hepatocellular carcinoma (HepG2, PLC/PRF/5, Huh7)	Inhibiting proliferation, inducing apoptosis, cycle arrest at G0/G1 phase and loss of plasma membrane asymmetry, decreasing mitochondrial membrane potential	↑Cyclin D, ↑Cyclin E, ↓C-myc, ↓Cyclin D1, ↓PCNA, ↓Bmi1, ↑p16, ↑caspase-3, ↑caspase-9, ↑Bax/Bcl-2	[19, 82–84]
PHY906	*Scutellariae Radix, Glycyrrhizae Radix Et Rhizoma, Jujubae Fructus, Paeoniae Radix Alba*	Hepatocellular carcinoma (HepG2)	Inducing apoptosis	↑FasL, ↑FasR, ↑hMCP1, ↑AMPKα-T172-P, ↑ULK1-S555-P, ↑ERK1/2-P	[86–89]
Feiji Recipe	*Astragali Radix, Glehniae Radix, Ophiopogonis Radix, Asparagi Radix, Poria, Ligustri Lucidi Fructus, Selaginella doederleinii Hieron, Coicis semen, Salivae Chinensis Herba, Epimedii Folium, Trichosanthis Pericarpium, Paris polyphylla Smith var. chinensis (Franch.) Hara, Ranunculus ternatus, Pinelliae Rhizoma, Cremastrae Pseudobulbus, Arisaematis Rhizoma Preparatum, Houttuyniae Herba, and Prunellae Spica*	Lung cancer (LLC)	Inhibiting proliferation, intervening immune escape	↓CD4+CD2+Tr, ↓VEGF, ↓Scd44V6, ↓TGR-β1, ↓IL-10	[102, 103]
YiQi ChuTan Recipe	*Panacis Quinquefolii Radix, Ophiopogonis Radix, Phellodendri Chinensis Cortex, Cremastrae Pseudobulbus, Stephaniae Tetrandrae Radix, Pinelliae Rhizoma, Gynostemma pentaphyllum (Thunb) Makino, and Hominis Placenta*	Lung cancer (A549, LLC)	Inhibiting proliferation and metastasis, reversing EMT	↓GRP78, ↓smad2/3, ↓SRC/MAPK, ↑Caspase-4, ↑DNA-PK, ↓Hspd1, ↓PH, ↓PDI, ↓EG433182, ↓HSPA 5 precursor, ↓HSPA 9, ↓PP1, ↓PRDX-1, ↓PRDX-6	[104–106]
Jianpi Yangzheng Xiaozheng Recipe	*Codonopsis Radix, Atractylodis Macrocephalae Rhizoma, Poria, Dioscoreae Rhizoma, Coicis semen, Citri Reticulatae Pericarpium, Aucklandiae Radix, Angelicae Sinensis Radix, Paeoniae Radix Alba, Smilacis Chinae Rhizoma, Salivae Chinensis Herba, and Glycyrrhizae Radix Rhizoma Praeparata Cum Melle*	Gastric cancer (MGC-803)	Inducing apoptosis and autophagy	↑Bax, ↓Bcl-2, ↓cyclin D1, ↓cyclin D2, ↓cyclin D3, ↑Fas, ↓procaspase-3, ↓procaspase-8, ↓procaspase-9, ↑cleaved-PARP, ↑Beclin-1, ↑LC3 II	[107]
Fuzheng Qingjie Recipe	*Astragali Radix, Ligustri Lucidi Fructus, Ganoderma, Dioscoreae Rhizoma, Prunellae Spica and Hedyotis diffusa Willd*	Hepatocellular carcinoma (HepG2)	Inducing apoptosis	↑caspase-9, ↑caspase-3, ↑P38 MAPK, ↑Bax, ↓Bcl-2	[108]
Baihe Recipe	*Solanum lyratum Thunb, Hedyotis diffusa Willd, Agrimoniae Herba, Codonopsis Radix, and Poria,*	Gastric cancer (BGC-823)	Inhibiting proliferation and metastasis	↓VEGF, ↓p53	[109]
Weikangfu Granule	*Curcumae Radix, Astragali Radix, Glycyrrhizae Radix Et Rhizoma, and Poria*	Sarcoma (S180)	Inducing apoptosis and cell cycle arrest at G0/G1 phase, modulating immune response	↑p53, ↑Bax, ↓Bcl-2	[110, 111]

HJT shows remarkable chemopreventive effect with low toxicity on colon cancer by inhibiting COX-2, which is involved in the production of prostanoids that could promote inflammation and tumorigenesis, but not COX-1, a constitutively expressed enzyme for normal functions of many organs [81], indicating the advantages of HJT over non-steroidal anti-inflammatory drugs, which inhibit both COX-1 and COX-2.

Jiedu Xiaozheng Yin

Jiedu Xiaozheng Yin (JXY), an anticancer decoction of TCM possessing heat-clearing and detoxification properties, consists of *Hedyotis diffusa* (Bai Hua She She Cao), *Cremastrae pseudobulbus Pleiones pseudobulbus* (Shan Ci Gu), *Prunellae* Spica (Xia Ku Cao) and *Sophorae flavescentis* Radix (Ku Shen). The formula exerted growth inhibitory effect on HepG2 hepatocarcinoma cells in a dose-dependent manner via increasing the expression of G1-related cyclins D and E [82]. However, the constituents that responsible for the antitumor effects are still largely unknown. In vitro experiments indicated that JXY inhibited the proliferation of gastric carcinoma cell line and promoted apoptosis via mitochondrial pathway in the hepatic carcinoma cancer cells. The ethanol extract of JXY (EE-JXY) decreases the viability of human umbilical vein endothelial cells and the tube formation capacity. Moreover, EE-JXY inhibits angiogenesis in chick chorioallantoic membrane and decreases microvessel density in the xenograft tumor. Further results demonstrated that JXY inhibited angiogenesis by downregulating VEGF-A and VEGFR-2 expression [19]. Recent studies reported that ethyl acetate extraction of JXY significantly inhibited hepatoma cell growth both in vitro and in the mouse xenograft model through arresting cancer cells at G0/G1 phase, inhibiting angiogenesis, and inducing cancer cell apoptosis, which may involve the suppression of the Bmi1 and Wnt/β-catenin signaling pathways [83]. A clinical study was conducted on hepatic carcinoma in III stage patients treated with JXY for 7 days before operation and Fuzheng Yiliu recipe after operation for 2 years. The results demonstrated that administration of compound Chinese herbal medicines in peri-operational period significantly decreased the recurrence rate, improved patients' immune function and increased the cumulative survival rate [84].

PHY906

PHY906, derived from a famous TCM formula called Huang Qin Tang, is composed of four herbs: *Scutellariae* Radix (Huang Qin), *Glycyrrhizae* Radix Et Rhizoma (Gan Cao), *Jujubae Fructus* (Da Zao), *and Paeoniae Radix Alba* (Shao Yao), with a ratio of 3:2:2:2. Huang Qin Tang has been used for more than 1000 years in TCM in treating various gastrointestinal discomfort, such as abdominal cramps, vomiting, diarrhea and nausea [85]. Although PHY906 alone has little antitumor effect, it was developed to be an effective TCM recipe for the relief of gastrointestinal toxicity and improvement of the antitumor efficacy of chemotherapeutic drugs, which has been proven both in preclinical animal models and in clinical studies. In a phase I clinical study, it was found that PHY906 could increase the therapeutic outcomes of capecitabine by reducing side effects such as diarrhea in patients with advanced pancreatic cancer, colon cancer, cholangiocarcinoma, or esophageal cancer [86]. In a phase II study, combination administration of PHY906 and capecitabine for patients with advanced pancreatic cancer resulted in a well tolerate and response of the treatment and improved indices of quality of life, including fatigue, loss of appetite, nausea, impaired sense of well-being, and diarrhea [87]. Studies revealed that PHY906 possessed a wide range of pharmacological activities due to its multiple components and mechanisms, including inhibitory activities on multi-drug resistant protein (MDR) and CYP450 which could result in enhancement of cellular uptake of chemotherapeutic agents, inhibitory activities on NF-κB and matrix metalloproteases which could inhibit angiogenesis and enhance the antitumor effect of chemotherapeutic agents, and inhibition of tachykinin NK-1, opiate δ receptors and acetylcholine esterase which may contribute to the improvement of quality of life [88]. Although PHY906 does not directly protect the initial impairment of intestine caused by irinotecan, it can effectively ameliorate inflammatory responses through inhibiting multiple inflammation related targets, including TNF-α-induced NF-κB-mediated transcriptional activity and COX-2 and iNOS enzyme activity. In addition, PHY906 remarkably promotes the recovery of damaged intestinal mucosa by increasing the proliferation of progenitor or stem cells and the growth of the crypts through potentiating Wnt/β-catenin signaling activity [89]. This suggests that herbal medicines with multiple components and molecular targets could be promising in future drug discovery and development for the potential management of complicated diseases.

Conclusions and perspectives

Organisms, at either cellular, organ, or organismal levels, are complex systems featuring redundant networks, self-organization and adaptation to the environment. Similarly, malignant cancers evolve to be a complex system with highly genetic diversity and enormous capability of adaptation to selective pressure [90]. Chinese medicinal herbs and the person-based formulas contain hundreds even thousands of compounds, which may regulate the activities or expression of a broad spectrum of proteins.

In this regard, Chinese herbal medicine might be a promising approach for the management of multifactorial chronic diseases including cancers. Since the accumulation of heat and toxins plays a key role in the occurrence and development of cancers according to TCM theory, HCD herbs are commonly prescribed in TCM formulas for the treatment of cancer. Increasing evidences have shown that decoction or components of HCD herbs or HCD herbs-containing formulas exhibited favorable anticancer effects directly or through enhancing the activities of chemotherapeutic drugs. However, huge efforts still need to be deployed in this field to bring the most potentials of HCD herbs for cancer treatment, including (1) further evaluation of anticancer efficacy of HCD herbs and formulas, particularly using xenograft animal tumor models; (2) further identification of major component(s) in HCD herbs responsible for the anticancer activity since many of them still have not been identified; (3) investigation of the underlying molecular mechanisms for the anticancer effects of HCD herbs and formulas, particular using cutting-edge technologies for complex sample analysis, e.g. proteomics and metabolomics approaches, since herbs or formulas may have complex mechanisms of action; (4) studies on the adjuvant anticancer activity of HCD herbs and formulas, e.g. sensitizing cancer cells to chemo- or radiotherapy, reversing multidrug resistance, reducing chemotherapy side effects, etc.; (5) studies on the acute and chronic toxicity of HCD herbs extracts and the purified components are also highly demanded. In summary, HCD herbs, formulas and the purified components have highly potential to be developed as anticancer agents used alone or in combination with other therapeutic methods.

Abbreviations

AATG4B: autophagy related 4 homolog B; ACTA2: smooth muscle alpha (α)-2 actin; AKAP12: A-kinase anchor protein 12; AMPK: AMP-activated protein kinase; AP-1: activator protein 1; $[Ca^{2+}]_i$: intracellular calcium; CCNA2: cyclin A2; CDC: cyclin-dependent kinases; COX-2: cyclooxygenase 2; CREB: cAMP response element-binding protein; DNA-PK: DNA-dependent protein kinase; ERK: extracellular signal-regulated kinases; FAK: focal adhesion kinase; FasL: Fas ligand; FOXO: forkhead box O proteins; GlyRS: glycyl-tRNA synthetase; GRP78: glucose-regulated protein 78; GSK3β: glycogen synthase kinase 3β; HCD: heat-clearing and detoxicating; HIF-1α: hypoxia-inducible factor 1α; hMCP1: human monocyte chemoattractant protein-1; hnRNP-1: heterogeneous nuclear ribonucleoprotein 1; HP1: heterochromatin protein 1; HSP 70: heat shock protein 70; hTERT: human telomerase reverse transcriptase; IFN: interferons; IGF-1: insulin-like growth factor 1; IGF-IR: type 1 IGF receptor; IKB: IκB; IKK: IκB kinases; IL-1β: interleukin 1β; JNK: c-Jun N-terminal kinases; KDR: kinase insert domain receptor; LC3: microtubule-associated protein 1A/1B-light chain 3; MAPK: mitogen-activated protein kinases; mFasL: membrane-bound FasL; MMP: matrix metalloproteinases; mTOR: mechanistic target of rapamycin protein; MX1: an interferon-induced GTP-binding protein; NAT: N-acyltransferases; NF-κB: nuclear factor-κB; ODC1: ornithine decarboxylase 1; p70S6K: p70S6 kinase; PARP: poly (ADP-ribose) polymerase; p-Cdc: phosphorylated CDC; PCNA: proliferating cell nuclear antigen; PDEF: prostate-derived Ets transcription factor; PDI: protein disulfide isomerase; PI3K: phosphoinositide 3-kinase; PP1: protein phosphatase 1; PPAR γ: peroxisome proliferator-activated receptor γ; PPase: protein Phosphatase; PRDX: peroxiredoxins; PSA: prostate-specific antigen; Rb: retinoblastoma protein; RKIP: Raf kinase inhibitor protein; sFasL: soluble form of FasL; STAP: stellate cell activation-associated protein; STAT3: signal transducer and activator of transcription 3; TCM: traditional Chinese medicine; TCTP: translationally controlled tumor protein; TGFBR1: transforming growth factor β receptor 1; TIMP: metallopeptidase inhibitors; TNF-α: tumor necrosis factor α; TRAIL: TNF-related apoptosis-inducing ligand; ULK1: Unc-51 like autophagy activating kinase 1; VEGF: vascular endothelial growth factor; WTX: Wilms tumor gene on X chromosome; XIAP: X-linked inhibitor of apoptosis protein.

Authors' contributions

CH supervised the study. YZ, YL and CH collected and analyzed the data and wrote the paper. All authors read and approved the final manuscript.

Acknowledgements

Not applicable.

Competing interests

The authors declare that they have no competing interests.

Funding

Macao Science and Technology Development Fund (041/2016/A), the Research Fund of the University of Macau (MYRG107(Y1-L3)-ICMS13-HCW and MYRG2015-00081-ICMS-QRCM).

References

1. Zhang ZN, Lv JR, Lei XM, Li SY, Zhang Y, Meng LH, Xue RL, Li ZF. Baicalein reduces the invasion of glioma cells via reducing the activity of p38 signaling pathway. PLoS ONE. 2014;9(2):e90318.
2. Zhang HB, Lu P, Guo QY, Zhang ZH, Meng XY. Baicalein induces apoptosis in esophageal squamous cell carcinoma cells through modulation of the PI3K/Akt pathway. Oncol Lett. 2013;5(2):722–8.
3. Ma GZ, Liu CH, Wei B, Qiao J, Lu T, Wei HC, Chen HD, He CD. Baicalein inhibits DMBA/TPA-induced skin tumorigenesis in mice by modulating proliferation, apoptosis, and inflammation. Inflammation. 2013;36(2):457–67.
4. Kim DH, Hossain MA, Kang YJ, Jang JY, Lee YJ, Im E, Yoon JH, Kim HS, Chung HY, Kim ND. Baicalein, an active component of Scutellaria baicalensis Georgi, induces apoptosis in human colon cancer cells and prevents AOM/DSS-induced colon cancer in mice. Int J Oncol. 2013;43(5):1652–8.
5. Chao JI, Su WC, Liu HF. Baicalein induces cancer cell death and proliferation retardation by the inhibition of CDC2 kinase and survivin associated with opposite role of p38 mitogen-activated protein kinase and AKT. Mol Cancer Ther. 2007;6(11):3039–48.
6. Polier G, Ding J, Konkimalla BV, Eick D, Ribeiro N, Kohler R, Giaisi M, Efferth T, Desaubry L, Krammer PH, et al. Wogonin and related natural flavones are inhibitors of CDK9 that induce apoptosis in cancer cells by transcriptional suppression of Mcl-1. Cell Death Dis. 2011;2:e182.
7. Chow SE, Chang YL, Chuang SF, Wang JS. Wogonin induced apoptosis in human nasopharyngeal carcinoma cells by targeting GSK-3beta and DeltaNp63. Cancer Chemother Pharmacol. 2011;68(4):835–45.
8. Song X, Yao J, Wang F, Zhou M, Zhou Y, Wang H, Wei L, Zhao L, Li Z, Lu N, et al. Wogonin inhibits tumor angiogenesis via degradation of HIF-1alpha protein. Toxicol Appl Pharmacol. 2013;271(2):144–55.

9. Zhong Y, Zhang FY, Sun ZY, Zhou W, Li ZY, You QD, Guo QL, Hu R. Drug resistance associates with activation of Nrf2 in MCF-7/DOX cells, and wogonin reverses it by down-regulating NRF2-mediated cellular defense response. Mol Carcinog. 2013;52(10):824–34.

10. Lee E, Enomoto R, Koshiba C, Hirano H. Inhibition of P-glycoprotein by wogonin is involved with the potentiation of etoposide-induced apoptosis in cancer cells. Ann N Y Acad Sci. 2009;1171:132–6.

11. Zhao Q, Wang J, Zou MJ, Hu R, Zhao L, Qiang L, Rong JJ, You QD, Guo QL. Wogonin potentiates the antitumor effects of low dose 5-fluorouracil against gastric cancer through induction of apoptosis by down-regulation of NF-κB and regulation of its metabolism. Toxicol Lett. 2010;197(3):201–10.

12. He C, Rong R, Liu J, Wan J, Zhou K, Kang JX. Effects of Coptis extract combined with chemotherapeutic agents on ROS production, multidrug resistance, and cell growth in A549 human lung cancer cells. Chin Med. 2012;7(1):11.

13. Kang JX, Liu J, Wang J, He C, Li FP. The extract of huanglian, a medicinal herb, induces cell growth arrest and apoptosis by upregulation of interferon-β and TNF-α in human breast cancer cells. Carcinogenesis. 2005;26(11):1934–9.

14. Liu J, He C, Zhou K, Wang J, Kang JX. Coptis extracts enhance the anti-cancer effect of estrogen receptor antagonists on human breast cancer cells. Biochem Biophys Res Commun. 2009;378(2):174–8.

15. Li XK, Motwani M, Tong W, Bornmann W, Schwartz GK. Huanglian, a Chinese herbal extract, inhibits cell growth by suppressing the expression of cyclin B1 and inhibiting CDC2 kinase activity in human cancer cells. Mol Pharmacol. 2000;58(6):1287–93.

16. Iizuka N, Miyamoto K, Okita K, Tangoku A, Hayashi H, Yosino S, Abe T, Morioka T, Hazama S, Oka M. Inhibitory effect of Coptidis rhizoma and berberine on the proliferation of human esophageal cancer cell lines. Cancer Lett. 2000;148(1):19–25.

17. Iizuka N, Hazama S, Yoshimura K, Yoshino S, Tangoku A, Miyamoto K, Okita K, Oka M. Anticachectic effects of the natural herb Coptidis rhizoma and berberine on mice bearing colon 26/clone 20 adenocarcinoma. Int J Cancer. 2002;99(2):286–91.

18. Ong ES, Woo SO, Yong YL. Pressurized liquid extraction of berberine and aristolochic acids in medicinal plants. Chromatogr A. 2000;904(1):57–64.

19. Tang J, Feng Y, Tsao S, Wang N, Curtain R, Wang Y. Berberine and Coptidis rhizoma as novel antineoplastic agents: a review of traditional use and biomedical investigations. J Ethnopharmacol. 2009;126(1):5–17.

20. Marverti G, Ligabue A, Lombardi P, Ferrari S, Monti MG, Frassineti C, Costi MP. Modulation of the expression of folate cycle enzymes and polyamine metabolism by berberine in cisplatin-sensitive and -resistant human ovarian cancer cells. Int J Oncol. 2013;43(4):1269–80.

21. Liu X, Ji Q, Ye NJ, Sui H, Zhou LH, Zhu HR, Fan ZZ, Cai JF, Li Q. Berberine inhibits invasion and metastasis of colorectal cancer cells via COX-2/PGE(2) mediated JAK2/STAT3 signaling pathway. PLoS ONE. 2015;10(5):e0123478.

22. Zhang J, Cao H, Zhang B, Xu X, Ruan H, Yi T, Tan L, Qu R, Song G, Wang B, et al. Berberine potently attenuates intestinal polyps growth in ApcMin mice and familial adenomatous polyposis patients through inhibition of Wnt signalling. J Cell Mol Med. 2013;17(11):1484–93.

23. Tsang CM, Cheung YC, Lui VW, Yip YL, Zhang G, Lin VW, Cheung KC, Feng Y, Tsao SW. Berberine suppresses tumorigenicity and growth of nasopharyngeal carcinoma cells by inhibiting STAT3 activation induced by tumor associated fibroblasts. BMC Cancer. 2013;13:619.

24. Zhu T, Li LL, Xiao GF, Luo QZ, Liu QZ, Yao KT, Xiao GH. Berberine increases doxorubicin sensitivity by suppressing STAT3 in lung cancer. Am J Chin Med. 2015;43(7):1487–502.

25. Hwang JM, Kuo HC, Tseng TH, Liu JY, Chu CY. Berberine induces apoptosis through a mitochondria/caspases pathway in human hepatoma cells. Arch Toxicol. 2006;80(2):62–73.

26. Patil JB, Kim J, Jayaprakasha GK. Berberine induces apoptosis in breast cancer cells (MCF-7) through mitochondrial-dependent pathway. Eur J Pharmacol. 2010;645(1–3):70–8.

27. Fan LX, Liu CM, Gao AH, Zhou YB, Li J. Berberine combined with 2-deoxy-D-glucose synergistically enhances cancer cell proliferation inhibition via energy depletion and unfolded protein response disruption. Biochim Biophys Acta. 2013;1830(11):5175–83.

28. Hur JM, Hyun MS, Lim SY, Lee WY, Kim D. The combination of berberine and irradiation enhances anti-cancer effects via activation of p38 MAPK pathway and ROS generation in human hepatoma cells. J Cell Biochem. 2009;107(5):955–64.

29. Zhang C, Yang X, Zhang Q, Yang B, Xu L, Qin Q, Zhu H, Liu J, Cai J, Tao G, et al. Berberine radiosensitizes human nasopharyngeal carcinoma by suppressing hypoxia-inducible factor-1alpha expression. Acta Oto-Laryngol. 2014;134(2):185–92.

30. Yu M, Tong X, Qi B, Qu H, Dong S, Yu B, Zhang N, Tang N, Wang L, Zhang C. Berberine enhances chemosensitivity to irinotecan in colon cancer via inhibition of NFκB. Mol Med Rep. 2014;9(1):249–54.

31. Tillhon M, Ortiz LMG, Lombardi P, Scovassi AI. Berberine: new perspectives for old remedies. Biochem Pharmacol. 2012;84(10):1260–7.

32. van der Kooy F, Sullivan SE. The complexity of medicinal plants: the traditional Artemisia annua formulation, current status and future perspectives. J Ethnopharmacol. 2013;150(1):1–13.

33. Ho WE, Peh HY, Chan TK, Wong WS. Artemisinins: pharmacological actions beyond anti-malarial. Pharmacol Ther. 2014;142(1):126–39.

34. Efferth T, Sauerbrey A, Olbrich A, Gebhart E, Rauch P, Weber HO, Hengstler JG, Halatsch ME, Volm M, Tew KD, et al. Molecular modes of action of artesunate in tumor cell lines. Mol Pharmacol. 2003;64(2):382–94.

35. Chen HH, Zhou HJ, Wu GD, Lou XE. Inhibitory effects of artesunate on angiogenesis and on expressions of vascular endothelial growth factor and VEGF receptor KDR/flk-1. Pharmacology. 2004;71(1):1–9.

36. Tin AS, Sundar SN, Tran KQ, Park AH, Poindexter KM, Firestone GL. Antiproliferative effects of artemisinin on human breast cancer cells requires the downregulated expression of the E2F1 transcription factor and loss of E2F1-target cell cycle genes. Anticancer Drugs. 2012;23(4):370–9.

37. Hu CJ, Zhou L, Cai Y. Dihydroartemisinin induces apoptosis of cervical cancer cells via upregulation of RKIP and downregulation of bcl-2. Cancer Biol Ther. 2014;15(3):279–88.

38. Dong HY, Wang ZF. Antitumor effects of artesunate on human breast carcinoma MCF-7 cells and IGF-IR expression in nude mice xenografts. Chin J Cancer Res. 2014;26(2):200–7.

39. Riganti C, Doublier S, Viarisio D, Miraglia E, Pescarmona G, Ghigo D, Bosia A. Artemisinin induces doxorubicin resistance in human colon cancer cells via calcium-dependent activation of HIF-1alpha and P-glycoprotein overexpression. Br J Pharmacol. 2009;156(7):1054–66.

40. Weifeng T, Feng S, Xiangji L, Changqing S, Zhiquan Q, Huazhong Z, Peining Y, Yong Y, Mengchao W, Xiaoqing J, et al. Artemisinin inhibits in vitro and in vivo invasion and metastasis of human hepatocellular carcinoma cells. Phytomedicine. 2011;18(2–3):158–62.

41. Hu W, Chen SS, Zhang JL, Lou XE, Zhou HJ. Dihydroartemisinin induces autophagy by suppressing NF-κB activation. Cancer Lett. 2014;343(2):239–48.

42. Chen T, Li M, Zhang R, Wang H. Dihydroartemisinin induces apoptosis and sensitizes human ovarian cancer cells to carboplatin therapy. J Cell Mol Med. 2009;13(7):1358–70.

43. Zhao C, Gao W, Chen T. Synergistic induction of apoptosis in A549 cells by dihydroartemisinin and gemcitabine. Apoptosis. 2014;19(4):668–81.

44. Ishigami SI, Arii S, Furutani M, Niwano M, Harada T, Mizumoto M, Mori A, Onodera H, Imamura M. Predictive value of vascular endothelial growth factor (VEGF) in metastasis and prognosis of human colorectal cancer. Br J Cancer. 1998;78(10):1379–84.

45. Niu Y, Meng QX. Chemical and preclinical studies on Hedyotis diffusa with anticancer potential. J Asian Nat Prod Res. 2013;15(5):550–65.

46. Lee HZ, Bau DT, Kuo CL, Tsai RY, Chen YC, Chang YH. Clarification of the phenotypic characteristics and anti-tumor activity of Hedyotis diffusa. Am J Chin Med. 2011;39(1):201–13.

47. Lin JM, Chen YQ, Wei LH, Chen XZ, Xu W, Hong ZF, Sferra TJ, Peng J. Hedyotis diffusa Willd extract induces apoptosis via activation of the mitochondrion-dependent pathway in human colon carcinoma cells. Int J Oncol. 2010;37(5):1331–8.

48. Chen XZ, Cao ZY, Chen TS, Zhang YQ, Liu ZZ, Su YT, Liao LM, Du J. Water extract of Hedyotis diffusa Willd suppresses proliferation of human HepG2 cells and potentiates the anticancer efficacy of low-dose 5-fluorouracil by inhibiting the CDK2-E2F1 pathway. Oncol Rep. 2012;28(2):742–8.

49. Wang X, Cheng WM, Yao XN, Guo XJ. Qualitative analysis of the chemical constituents in *Hedyotis diffusa* by HPLC-TOF-MS. Nat Prod Res. 2012;26(2):167–72.

50. Gao N, Cheng S, Budhraja A, Gao Z, Chen J, Liu EH, Huang C, Chen D, Yang Z, Liu Q, et al. Ursolic acid induces apoptosis in human leukaemia cells and exhibits anti-leukaemic activity in nude mice through the PKB pathway. Br J Pharmacol. 2012;165(6):1813–26.

51. Zhang YX, Kong CZ, Wang LH, Li JY, Liu XK, Xu B, Xu CL, Sun YH. Ursolic acid overcomes Bcl-2-mediated resistance to apoptosis in prostate cancer cells involving activation of JNK-induced Bcl-2 phosphorylation and degradation. J Cell Biochem. 2010;109(4):764–73.

52. Liu Z, Liu M, Liu M, Li JC. Methylanthraquinone from *Hedyotis diffusa* WILLD induces Ca($^{2+}$)-mediated apoptosis in human breast cancer cells. Toxicol Vitro. 2010;24(1):142–7.

53. Wang N, Li DY, Niu HY, Zhang Y, He P, Wang JH. 2-Hydroxy-3-methylanthraquinone from *Hedyotis diffusa* Willd induces apoptosis in human leukemic U937 cells through modulation of MAPK pathways. Arch Pharm Res. 2013;36(6):752–8.

54. Sun HD, Huang SX, Han QB. Diterpenoids from *Isodon* species and their biological activities. Nat Prod Rep. 2006;23(5):673–98.

55. Liu HM, Yan XB, Kiuchi F, Liu ZZ. A new diterpene glycoside from *Rabdosia rubescens*. Chem Pharm Bull. 2000;48(1):148–9.

56. Bao RF, Shu YJ, Wu XS, Weng H, Ding Q, Cao Y, Li ML, Mu JS, Wu WG, Ding QC, et al. Oridonin induces apoptosis and cell cycle arrest of gallbladder cancer cells via the mitochondrial pathway. BMC Cancer. 2014;14:217.

57. Wang H, Ye Y, Pan SY, Zhu GY, Li YW, Fong DW, Yu ZL. Proteomic identification of proteins involved in the anticancer activities of oridonin in HepG2 cells. Phytomedicine. 2011;18(2–3):163–9.

58. Wang S, Zhong Z, Wan J, Tan W, Wu G, Chen M, Wang Y. Oridonin induces apoptosis, inhibits migration and invasion on highly-metastatic human breast cancer cells. Am J Chin Med. 2013;41(1):177–96.

59. Hu HZ, Yang YB, Xu XD, Shen HW, Shu YM, Ren Z, Li XM, Shen HM, Zeng HT. Oridonin induces apoptosis via PI3K/Akt pathway in cervical carcinoma HeLa cell line. Acta Pharmacol Sin. 2007;28(11):1819–26.

60. Sun KW, Ma YY, Guan TP, Xia YJ, Shao CM, Chen LG, Ren YJ, Yao HB, Yang Q, He XJ. Oridonin induces apoptosis in gastric cancer through Apaf-1, cytochrome c and caspase-3 signaling pathway. World J Gastroenterol. 2012;18(48):7166–74.

61. Zhu M, Hong D, Bao Y, Wang C, Pan W. Oridonin induces the apoptosis of metastatic hepatocellular carcinoma cells via a mitochondrial pathway. Oncol Lett. 2013;6(5):1502–6.

62. Zang LH, Xu Q, Ye YC, Li X, Liu YQ, Tashiro S, Onodera S, Ikejima T. Autophagy enhanced phagocytosis of apoptotic cells by oridonin-treated human histocytic lymphoma U937 cells. Arch Biochem Biophys. 2012;518(1):31–41.

63. Bu HQ, Liu DL, Wei WT, Chen L, Huang H, Li Y, Cui JH. Oridonin induces apoptosis in SW1990 pancreatic cancer cells via p53-and caspase-dependent induction of p38 MAPK. Oncol Rep. 2014;31(2):975–82.

64. Liu Y, Liu JH, Chai K, Tashiro SI, Onodera S, Ikejima T. Inhibition of c-Met promoted apoptosis, autophagy and loss of the mitochondrial transmembrane potential in oridonin-induced A549 lung cancer cells. J Pharm Pharmacol. 2013;65(11):1622–42.

65. Dai ZJ, Lu WF, Gao J, Kang HF, Ma YG, Zhang SQ, Diao Y, Lin S, Wang XJ, Wu WY. Anti-angiogenic effect of the total flavonoids in *Scutellaria barbata* D. Don. BMC Complement Altern Med. 2013;13:150.

66. Dai ZJ, Wang BF, Lu WF, Wang ZD, Ma XB, Min WL, Kang HF, Wang XJ, Wu WY. Total flavonoids of *Scutellaria barbata* inhibit invasion of hepatocarcinoma via MMP/TIMP in vitro. Molecules. 2013;18(1):934–50.

67. Lin JM, Chen YQ, Cai QY, Wei LH, Zhan YZ, Shen A, Sferra TJ, Peng J. *Scutellaria barbata* D Don inhibits colorectal cancer growth via suppression of multiple signaling pathways. Integr Cancer Ther. 2014;13(3):240–8.

68. Lee TK, Lee YJ, Kim DI, Kim HM, Chang YC, Kim CH. Pharmacological activity in growth inhibition and apoptosis of cultured human leiomyomal cells of tropical plant *Scutellaria barbata* D. Don (Lamiaceae). Environ Toxicol Pharmacol. 2006;21(1):70–9.

69. Suh SJ, Yoon JW, Lee TK, Jin UH, Kim SL, Kim MS, Kwon DY, Lee YC, Kim CH. Chemoprevention of *Scutellaria bardata* on human cancer cells and tumorigenesis in skin cancer. Phytother Res. 2007;21(2):135–41.

70. Xu HL, Yu JM, Sun Y, Xu XN, Li L, Xue M, Du GH. *Scutellaria barbata* D. Don extract synergizes the antitumor effects of low dose 5-fluorouracil through induction of apoptosis and metabolism. Phytomedicine. 2013;20(10):897–903.

71. Trachootham D, Alexandre J, Huang P. Targeting cancer cells by ROS-mediated mechanisms: a radical therapeutic approach? Nat Rev Drug Discov. 2009;8(7):579–91.

72. Qi FH, Li AY, Inagaki Y, Gao JJ, Li JJ, Kokudo N, Li XK, Tang W. Chinese herbal medicines as adjuvant treatment during chemo- or radio-therapy for cancer. Biosci Trends. 2010;4(6):297–307.

73. Wang ZY, Li GS, Huang HX. Clinical observation on treatment of 75 mid-late stage cancer patients with yanshu injection. Chin J Integr Med. 2006;26(8):681–4.

74. She T, Zhao C, Feng J, Wang L, Qu L, Fang K, Cai S, Shou C. Sarsaparilla (*Smilax glabra* Rhizome) extract inhibits migration and invasion of cancer cells by suppressing TGF-β1 pathway. PLoS ONE. 2015;10(3):e0118287.

75. Zhou SK, Zhang RL, Xu YF, Bi TN. Antioxidant and immunity activities of Fufang Kushen injection liquid. Molecules. 2012;17(6):6481–90.

76. Wei R, Yang DY, Jiang WZ, Dai YY, Wan LY, Yang Z. Efficacy of Yanshu injection (a compound Chinese traditional medicine) combined with concurrent radiochemotherapy in patients with stage III nasopharyngeal carcinoma. Chin J Oncol. 2011;33(5):391–4.

77. Lin LT, Wu SJ, Lin CC. The anticancer properties and apoptosis-inducing mechanisms of cinnamaldehyde and the herbal prescription Huang-Lian-Jie-Du-Tang (Huang Lian Jie Du Tang) in human hepatoma cells. J Tradit Complement Med. 2013;3(4):227–33.

78. Hsu YL, Kuo PL, Tzeng TF, Sung SC, Yen MH, Lin LT, Lin CC. Huang-lian-jie-du-tang, a traditional Chinese medicine prescription, induces cell-cycle arrest and apoptosis in human liver cancer cells in vitro and in vivo. J Gastroenterol Hepatol. 2008;23(7):E290–9.

79. Ma Z, Otsuyama K, Liu SQ, Abroun S, Ishikawa H, Tsuyama N, Obata M, Li FJ, Zheng X, Maki Y, et al. Baicalein, a component of *Scutellaria* radix from Huang-Lian-Jie-Du-Tang (HLJDT), leads to suppression of proliferation and induction of apoptosis in human myeloma cells. Blood. 2005;105(8):3312–8.

80. Yuki F, Kawaguchi T, Hazemoto K, Asou N. Preventive effects of oren-gedoku-to on mucositis caused by anticancer agents in patients with acute leukemia. Gan To Kagaku Ryoho. 2003;30(9):1303–7.

81. Fukutake M, Miura N, Yamamoto M, Fukuda K, Iijima O, Ishikawa H, Kubo M, Okada M, Komatsu Y, Sasaki H, et al. Suppressive effect of the herbal medicine Oren-gedoku-to on cyclooxygenase-2 activity and azoxymethane-induced aberrant crypt foci development in rats. Cancer Lett. 2000;157(1):9–14.

82. Cao ZY, Lin W, Huang ZR, Chen XZ, Zhao JY, Zheng LP, Ye HZ, Liu ZZ, Liao LM, Du J. Ethyl acetate extraction from a Chinese herbal formula, Jiedu Xiaozheng Yin, inhibits the proliferation of hepatocellular carcinoma cells via induction of G0/G1 phase arrest in vivo and in vitro. Int J Oncol. 2013;42(1):202–10.

83. Chen XZ, Cao ZY, Li JN, Hu HX, Zhang YQ, Huang YM, Liu ZZ, Hu D, Liao LM, Du J. Ethyl acetate extract from Jiedu Xiaozheng Yin inhibits the proliferation of human hepatocellular carcinoma cells by suppressing polycomb gene product Bmi1 and Wnt/beta-catenin signaling. Oncol Rep. 2014;32(6):2710–8.

84. Chen LW, Lin J, Chen W, Zhang W. Effect of Chinese herbal medicine on patients with primary hepatic carcinoma in III stage during perioperational period: a report of 42 cases. Chin J Integr Med. 2005;25(9):832–4.

85. Tilton R, Paiva AA, Guan JQ, Marathe R, Jiang Z, van Eyndhoven W, Bjoraker J, Prusoff Z, Wang H, Liu SH, et al. A comprehensive platform for quality control of botanical drugs (PhytomicsQC): a case study of Huangqin Tang (HQT) and PHY906. Chin Med. 2010;5:30.

86. Saif MW, Lansigan F, Ruta S, Lamb L, Mezes M, Elligers K, Grant N, Jiang ZL, Liu SH, Cheng YC. Phase I study of the botanical formulation PHY906 with capecitabine in advanced pancreatic and other gastrointestinal malignancies. Phytomedicine. 2010;17(3–4):161–9.

87. Saif MW, Li J, Lamb L, Kaley K, Elligers K, Jiang ZL, Bussom S, Liu SH, Cheng YC. First-in-human phase II trial of the botanical formulation PHY906 with capecitabine as second-line therapy in patients with advanced pancreatic cancer. Cancer Chemother Pharmacol. 2014;73(2):373–80.

88. Yen Y, So S, Rose M, Saif MW, Chu E, Liu SH, Foo A, Jiang Z, Su T, Cheng YC. Phase I/II study of PHY906/capecitabine in advanced hepatocellular carcinoma. Anticancer Res. 2009;29(10):4083–92.

89. Lam W, Bussom S, Guan F, Jiang Z, Zhang W, Gullen EA, Liu SH, Cheng YC. The four-herb Chinese medicine PHY906 reduces chemotherapy-induced gastrointestinal toxicity. Sci Transl Med. 2010;2(45):45ra59.

90. Greaves M, Maley CC. Clonal evolution in cancer. Nature. 2012;481(7381):306–13.

91. Hsu YL, Kuo PL, Chiang LC, Lin CC. Involvement of p53, nuclear factor kappaB and Fas/Fas ligand in induction of apoptosis and cell cycle arrest by saikosaponin d in human hepatoma cell lines. Cancer Lett. 2004;213(2):213–21.

92. Ashour ML, Wink M. Genus *Bupleurum*: a review of its phytochemistry, pharmacology and modes of action. J Pharm Pharmacol. 2011;63(3):305–21.

93. Zhu BH, Pu R, Zhang GP, Li MY, Wang LT, Yuan JK. Effect of Saikosaponins-d on reversing malignant phenotype of HepG2 cells in vitro. Chin J Hepatol. 2011;19(10):764–7.

94. Zhang JQ, Li YM, Liu T, He WT, Chen YT, Chen XH, Li X, Zhou WC, Yi JF, Ren ZJ. Antitumor effect of matrine in human hepatoma G2 cells by inducing apoptosis and autophagy. World J Gastroenterol. 2010;16(34):4281–90.

95. Jiang H, Hou C, Zhang S, Xie H, Zhou W, Jin Q, Cheng X, Qian R, Zhang X. Matrine upregulates the cell cycle protein E2F-1 and triggers apoptosis via the mitochondrial pathway in K562 cells. Eur J Pharmacol. 2007;559(2–3):98–108.

96. Hong SW, Jung KH, Lee HS, Son MK, Yan HH, Kang NS, Lee J, Hong SS. SB365, Pulsatilla saponin D, targets c-Met and exerts antiangiogenic and antitumor activities. Carcinogenesis. 2013;34(9):2156–69.

97. Zhang Y, Bao J, Wang K, Jia X, Zhang C, Huang B, Chen M, Wan JB, Su H, Wang Y, et al. Pulsatilla saponin D inhibits autophagic flux and synergistically enhances the anticancer activity of chemotherapeutic agents against hela cells. Am J Chin Med. 2015;43(8):1657–70.

98. Bhattacharyya B, Panda D, Gupta S, Banerjee M. Anti-mitotic activity of colchicine and the structural basis for its interaction with tubulin. Med Res Rev. 2008;28(1):155–83.

99. Lin ZY, Wu CC, Chuang YH, Chuang WL. Anti-cancer mechanisms of clinically acceptable colchicine concentrations on hepatocellular carcinoma. Life Sci. 2013;93(8):323–8.

100. Jiang CP, Ding H, Shi DH, Wang YR, Li EG, Wu JH. Pro-apoptotic effects of tectorigenin on human hepatocellular carcinoma HepG2 cells. World J Gastroenterol. 2012;18(15):1753–64.

101. Jung SH, Lee YS, Lee S, Lim SS, Kim YS, Ohuchi K, Shin KH. Anti-angiogenic and anti-tumor activities of isoflavonoids from the rhizomes of *Belamcanda chinensis*. Planta Med. 2003;69(7):617–22.

102. Huang YS, Shi ZM. Intervention effect of Feiji Recipe on immune escape of lung cancer. Chin J Integr Med. 2007;27(6):501–4.

103. Bi L, Jin S, Zheng Z, Wang Q, Jiao Y, You J, Li HG, Tian JH. Inhibitory effect of Feiji recipe on ido induced immune escape on the murine model of Lewis lung carcinoma. Chin J Integr Med. 2016;36(1):69–74.

104. Li S, Wang SM, Yang YB, Liu QO. Effect of Viqi Chutan Recipe on caspase-4 and DNA-PK of cell apoptosis approach in transplanted lung cancer A549 cells in nude mice. J Chin Mater Med. 2015;38(6):1247–50.

105. Wang SM, Lin LZ, Zhou JX, Xiong SQ, Zhou DH. Effects of Yiqi Chutan Tang on the proteome in Lewis lung cancer in mice. Asian Pac J Cancer Prev. 2011;12(7):1665–9.

106. Chen CM, Sun LL, Fang RM, Lin LZ. YiQi ChuTan recipe inhibits epithelial mesenchymal transition of A549 cells under hypoxia. Cell Mol Biol. 2016;62(1):10–5.

107. Wu J, Liu SL, Zhang XX, Chen M, Zou X. Effect of Jianpi Yangzheng Xiaozheng recipe on apoptosis and autophagy of subcutaneous transplanted tumor in nude mice: an experimental study on mechanism. Chin J Integr Med. 2015;35(9):1113–8.

108. Chen XZ, Li JN, Zhang YQ, Cao ZY, Liu ZZ, Wang SQ, Liao LM, Du J. Fuzheng Qingjie recipe induces apoptosis in HepG2 cells via P38 MAPK activation and the mitochondria-dependent apoptotic pathway. Mol Med Rep. 2014;9(6):2381–7.

109. Dong ZP, Hu ZQ, Peng W, Shu ZJ, Cao YM, Lu L. Effects of Baihe recipe on expressions of vascular endothelial growth factor and p53 proteins in tumor tissues of nude mice bearing orthotopically transplanted gastric carcinoma BGC-823. Chin J Integr Med. 2009;7(5):458–62.

110. Nie X, Shi B, Ding Y, Tao W. Antitumor and immunomodulatory effects of weikangfu granule compound in tumor-bearing mice. Curr Ther Res Clin Exp. 2006;67(2):138–50.

111. Nie XH, Shi BJ, Tao WY. Inhibitory effect of Weikangfu recipe on growth of mouse S180 tumor and its apoptotic induction. China J Chin Mater Med. 2006;31(17):1457–60.

11

Chemical compositions, chromatographic fingerprints and antioxidant activities of Citri Exocarpium Rubrum (*Juhong*)

Yang Zhao[1,2], Chun-Pin Kao[3], Chi-Ren Liao[1], Kun-Chang Wu[1], Xin Zhou[2], Yu-Ling Ho[4*] and Yuan-Shiun Chang[1,5*] (ORCID)

Abstract

Background: Citri Exocarpium Rubrum (CER), which is known as *Juhong* in Chinese, is the dried exocarp of *Citrus reticulata* Blanco and its cultivars (Fam. Rutaceae) and is currently used in Chinese medicine to protect the stomach and eliminate *dampness* and phlegm. The main aim of this study was to develop a high-performance liquid chromatography ultraviolet mass spectrometry (HPLC-UV-MS) method for determining the chemical compositions and fingerprint of CER. We also evaluated the antioxidant properties of CER based on its 2,2-diphenyl-1-picrylhydrazyl (DPPH) free radical scavenging activity, ferric ion reducing antioxidant power (FRAP) and trolox equivalent antioxidant capacity (TEAC) assays.

Methods: Ten CER samples were collected from Hong Kong and mainland China. Each CER sample was extracted using an ultrasonic extraction method. Chromatographic separation was achieved using a conventional Dikma Inspire C18 column with photo diode array detection (190–400 nm). Hesperidin, nobiletin and tangeretin were quantified based on the UV signal observed at 330 nm. The column was eluted with a mobile phase consisting of water and acetonitrile (15–55%) over 55 min. Fingerprints combined with similarity and principal component analyses were used to classify the herbs. The DPPH free radical scavenging activity, FRAP and ABTS properties of the different CER samples were assayed. Bivariate correlation analysis was performed to investigate the correlation between the characteristic peaks and their antioxidant capacities.

Results: Limit of detection (LOD), limit of quantification (LOQ), linearity, inter-day precision, intra-day precision, repeatability, stability and recovery of the developed method were validated, and the method was subsequently used to determine the contents of hesperidin, nobiletin and tangeretin, and to acquire the fingerprints of the CER samples. Seventeen characteristic peaks were found in the fingerprints, and eleven of them were identified. Bivariate correlation analysis revealed correlations between the characteristic peaks and the antioxidant activities of the samples.

Conclusion: An HPLC-UV-MS method was developed and validated after a detailed investigation on extraction of chemical compounds from CER using different solvents and extraction times. None of the peaks was correlated with the DPPH free radical scavenging activity or ferric reducing capacity. Most of the peaks were correlated well with the ABTS radical scavenging capacity.

*Correspondence: elaine@sunrise.hk.edu.tw; yschang@mail.cmu.edu.tw
[1] Department of Chinese Pharmaceutical Sciences and Chinese Medicine Resources, College of Biopharmaceutical and Food Sciences, China Medical University, Taichung 40402, Taiwan
[4] Department of Nursing, Hungkuang University, Taichung 43302, Taiwan
Full list of author information is available at the end of the article

Background

Citri Exocarpium Rubrum (CER), which is known as *Juhong* in Chinese, is the dried exocarp of *Citrus reticulata* Blanco and its cultivars (Fam. Rutaceae), and this material is used in Chinese medicine to protect the stomach and eliminate *dampness* and phlegm [1]. CER has been reported to exhibit antioxidant activity [2] and induce apoptosis in human lung cancer cells [3]. Hesperidin, nobiletin and tangeretin are the main bioactive components of CER, and these compounds have been reported to have several properties, e.g. including antioxidant [4], anti-inflammatory [5] and anticancer activities [5, 6]. However, hesperidin is the only one of these compounds currently described as a chemical marker for quality assessment of CER in the 2015 edition of the Chinese Pharmacopoeia [1], which stipulates that the content of the marker should not be less than 1.7%. Several quantitative quality control methods have been reported for CER and CER-related commercial products [7–9]. However, the quality of herbal materials cannot be thoroughly or accurately evaluated based on the quantification of one or two chemical components. Fingerprinting analysis, which represents a much more accurate form of quality control analysis has therefore been introduced and accepted by the World Health Organization (WHO) as an effective strategy for assessing the quality of herbal medicines [10–13].

The aim of this study was to develop a high-performance liquid chromatography ultraviolet mass spectrometry (HPLC-UV-MS) method to determine the hesperidin, nobiletin and tangeretin contents in different CER samples, as well as developing a deeper understanding of the chemical profiles of these materials. Similarity and principal component analyses (PCA) were also performed based on the contents of hesperidin, nobiletin and tangeretin, as well as the PA/W (peak area divided by sample weight) values of the 17 characteristic peaks. The antioxidant activities of the CER samples were evaluated and subjected to a fingerprint-efficacy correlation process.

Methods

Chemicals, solvents and herbal materials

Hesperidin, nobiletin and tangeretin were purchased from Shanghai R & D Center for Standardization of Traditional Chinese Medicines (China). LC-grade methanol and acetonitrile were purchased from the branch company of Merck in Taipei, Taiwan. Purified water was prepared with Milli-Q system (Millipore, Milford, MA, USA). All other reagents used in the present study were of analytical grade. Ten batches of CER herbal materials were collected from Hong Kong and mainland China, which were marked as L-CER-01–L-CER-04 (from local

in Hong Kong) and CER-01–CER-06 (from mainland China). All the samples were authenticated by professor Yuan-Shiun Chang and the specimens have been deposited in Department of Chinese Pharmaceutical Sciences and Chinese Medicine Resources, School of Pharmacy, China Medical University.

Preparation of herbal materials and reference compounds

CER samples were dried in a shade place and were ground into fine powder (20 mesh) using a grinder with a knife blade. Two hundred milligrams of each CER powder was carefully weighed into a tube. Methanol (20 mL) was then added into the tube. Each sample was then extracted using an ultrasonic cleaner (Delta DC400H) at a frequency of 40 kHz at 25 °C for 30 min. The extract was centrifuged (UX-17414-21 Cole-Parmer™ MS-3400 Variable Speed Clinical Centrifuge, USA) for 10 min at $2000 \times g$ and the supernatant was then transferred into a volumetric flask. The procedure was repeated for one more time and the supernatants were combined. The final volume was made up to 50 mL with methanol which was then filtered through a 0.45 μm PVDF syringe filter (VWR Scientific, Seattle, WA) for analysis.

The reference compounds of hesperidin, nobiletin and tangeretin were weighed and dissolved in methanol at 499.2, 11.94 and 5.0288 mg/L (stock solutions), respectively. The stock solutions were then diluted to 31.20–499.20 mg/L for hesperidin, 0.75–11.94 mg/L for nobiletin and 0.31–5.03 mg/L for tangeretin, respectively for establishment of calibration curves. An aliquot of 10 μL of each solution was used for HPLC and HPLC-ESI-MS analyses.

HPLC analysis

HPLC analyses were performed on a Waters 2695 HPLC system (Waters Corporation, USA) equipped with Waters 2998 photodiode array detector (PDA), Waters e2695 separations module and column heater module. A Dikma Inspire, C18 column (250 mm × 4.6 mm i.d., 5 μm) was used. The mobile phase consisted of water (A) and acetonitrile (B). The optimized elution conditions were as follow: 0–10 min, 15–20% B; 10–25 min, 20% B; 25–35 min, 20–40%; 35–55 min, 40–55%. The flow rate was 1 mL/min and the injection volume was 10 μL. UV spectra were acquired from 190 to 400 nm. The autosampler and column compartment were maintained at 25 and 35 °C, respectively.

HPLC-ESI-MS analysis

HPLC-ESI-MS analyses were performed on a TSQ Quantum Access Max Triple Stage Quadrupole Mass Spectrometer (Thermo Fisher Scientific Inc., Waltham, MA, USA) with an Accela 1250 UHPLC system equipped with an Accela 1250 PDA detector, an Accela HTC PAL autosampler, and an Accela 1250 binary pump. The column and elution conditions used were the same as that described in the section, "HPLC analysis", except that the flow rate was set at 0.20 mL/min with a split ratio. Ultra-high pure helium (He) and high purity nitrogen (N_2) were used as collision gas and nebulizer, respectively. The optimized parameters in negative/positive ion modes were as follows: ion spray voltage, -2.5 kV/3.5 kV; auxiliary gas, 40 arbitrary units; sheath gas, 15 arbitrary units; capillary temperature, 350 °C; vaporizer temperature, 300 °C; capillary offset, -30 V/30 V. Spectra were recorded in the range of m/z 100–1500 for full scan data, meanwhile, the normalized collision energy was tested from 25 to 45% for MS^2 data with dependent scan.

Antioxidant activities
DPPH assay
The DPPH free radical-scavenging activity of each sample was assayed according to published articles [14–16] with minor modifications. In brief, a 0.3 mM solution of methanolic DPPH was freshly prepared. An aliquot (50 μL) of each sample (with appropriate enrichment or dilution if necessary) was added to 150 μL of methanolic DPPH solution to initiate the reaction. Discolorations were measured at 517 nm after reaction for 30 min at room temperature in the dark. Measurements were performed in triplicate. The %DPPH quenched was calculated according to the following equation:

% DPPH quenched

$$= (A_{control} - A_{sample}) \times 100/A_{control} - A_{blank}$$

where $A_{control}$, A_{sample}, and A_{blank} represent the absorbance of the control, the selected antioxidant sample at certain concentration, and the blank, respectively, measured at 517 nm. EC_{50} values calculated denote the concentration of a sample required to decrease the absorbance by 50%. The antioxidant capacity was expressed as μmol butylated hydroxytoluene (BHT) equivalents/gram of dried CER sample.

FRAP assay
The ability to reduce ferric ions was measured based on the methods reported in previous papers [16, 17] with minor revisions. Briefly, 30 μL of each sample (with appropriate enrichment or dilution if necessary) was added to 200 μL of FRAP reagent (10 parts of 300 mM sodium acetate buffer at pH 3.6, 1 part of 10.0 mM 2,4,6-tripyridyl-s-triazine (TPTZ) solution, and 1 part of 20.0 mM $FeCl_3 \cdot 6H_2O$ solution), and the reaction mixture was placed at room temperature for 5 min. Fresh working solutions of $FeSO_4 \cdot 7H_2O$ were used for calibration. The antioxidant capacity of reducing ferric ions of each

sample was expressed as μ mol Fe^{2+} equivalents per gram of dried CER sample.

TEAC assay
The ABTS free radical-scavenging activity of each sample was assayed according to the method described in published papers [16, 18] with minor modifications. A mixture (1:1, v/v) of ABTS (7.0 mM) and potassium persulfate (6 mM) was allowed to react overnight at room temperature in the dark to form radical cation $ABTS^+$. The mixture was then diluted with water to reach absorbance values between 1.0 and 1.5 at 731 nm (constant initial absorbance values must be used for standard and samples) as working solution. An aliquot (50 μL) of each sample (with appropriate enrichment or dilution if necessary) was mixed with the working solution (150 μL), and the decrease of absorbance was measured at 731 nm after 10 min. EC_{50} values calculated denote the concentration of a sample required to decrease the absorbance by 50%. The antioxidant capacity was expressed as μmol BHT equivalents/gram of dried CER sample.

Data analysis
Similarity analysis
Similarity values of the chromatographic fingerprints obtained from CER samples were calculated using the following two formulas:

$$\text{Correlation coefficient} = \frac{\sum_{i=1}^{n} (X_i - \bar{X}_i)(Y_i - \bar{Y}_i)}{\sqrt{\sum_{i=1}^{n} (X_i - \bar{X}_i)^2 (Y_i - \bar{Y}_i)^2}}$$

$$\text{Angle cosin} = \frac{\sum_{i=1}^{n} X_i Y_i}{\sqrt{\sum_{i=1}^{n} X_i^2} \sqrt{\sum_{i=1}^{n} Y_i^2}}$$

where, X_i and Y_i represented the peak area of the characteristic peak in each sample and the peak area of the characteristic peak in reference fingerprint generated, respectively.

Principal component analysis (PCA)
The data obtained from chromatographic fingerprints were analyzed with Solo (Eigenvector Research, Inc.,Wenatchee, WA). Normalize (2-Norm, length = 1) and mean center were used for data reprocessing before PCA was performed.

One-way ANOVA and correlation analyses
Differences in mean values of antioxidant assays for different CER samples were obtained by one-way ANOVA. Pearson r correlation coefficients between the peak areas of the seventeen characteristic peaks and their

antioxidant capacities were calculated by SPSS software (version 17.0, IBM Corporation, USA). P values less than 0.05 were considered statistically significant.

Results and discussion

Optimization of extraction method

The extraction solvents were optimized taking the extraction efficiency of hesperidin, nobiletin and tangeretin as indexes. Methanol, 50% methanol, ethanol and 50% ethanol were investigated with ultrasonic extraction at room temperature. The powder of CER (0.2 g) was extracted with 20 mL of different solvents for twice (30 min for once). As a result, the contents of the three analytes obtained by methanol were the highest compared with the values obtained from other solvents. Furthermore, the three analytes were almost extracted completely (>99%) for the second time (Additional files 1 and 2).

Optimization of chromatographic conditions

Different mobile phase systems, methanol–water and acetonitrile–water elution systems were tested to obtain sharp and symmetrical peaks. Good resolution, baseline, sharp and symmetrical peaks were obtained by acetonitrile–water system. Two other columns (Grace Alltima C18 and Waters XBridge Shield RP18) were screened before Dikma Inspire, C18 column (250 mm × 4.6 mm

i.d., 5 µm) was finally selected as the column of choice (Additional file 3). PDA full scan (190–400 nm) was used to acquire all the main peaks and finally 330 nm was selected as detection wavelength. Representative chromatographic fingerprints obtained from CER-01 and L-CER-04 were shown in Fig. 1, in which characteristic peaks were marked as 1–17. Different column temperatures at 20, 25, 30 and 35 °C were also investigated. Although chromatograms detected at different temperatures didn't show obvious differences, 35 °C was selected as the preferable one to minimize the influences from fluctuating room temperature on the chromatograms. In the process of gradient optimization, gradient time, gradient procedure and initial composition of the mobile phase were taken into consideration. Eventually, the gradient procedure was finalized, as described in "HPLC analysis" section.

Validation of quantitative analytical method

The HPLC method was validated by defining its limit of detection (LOD), limit of quantification (LOQ), linearity, inter-day precision, intra-day precision, repeatability, stability and recovery characteristics.

Calibration curves were plotted based on a linear regression analysis of the integrated peak areas (y) versus the concentrations (x, mg/L) of hesperidin, nobiletin

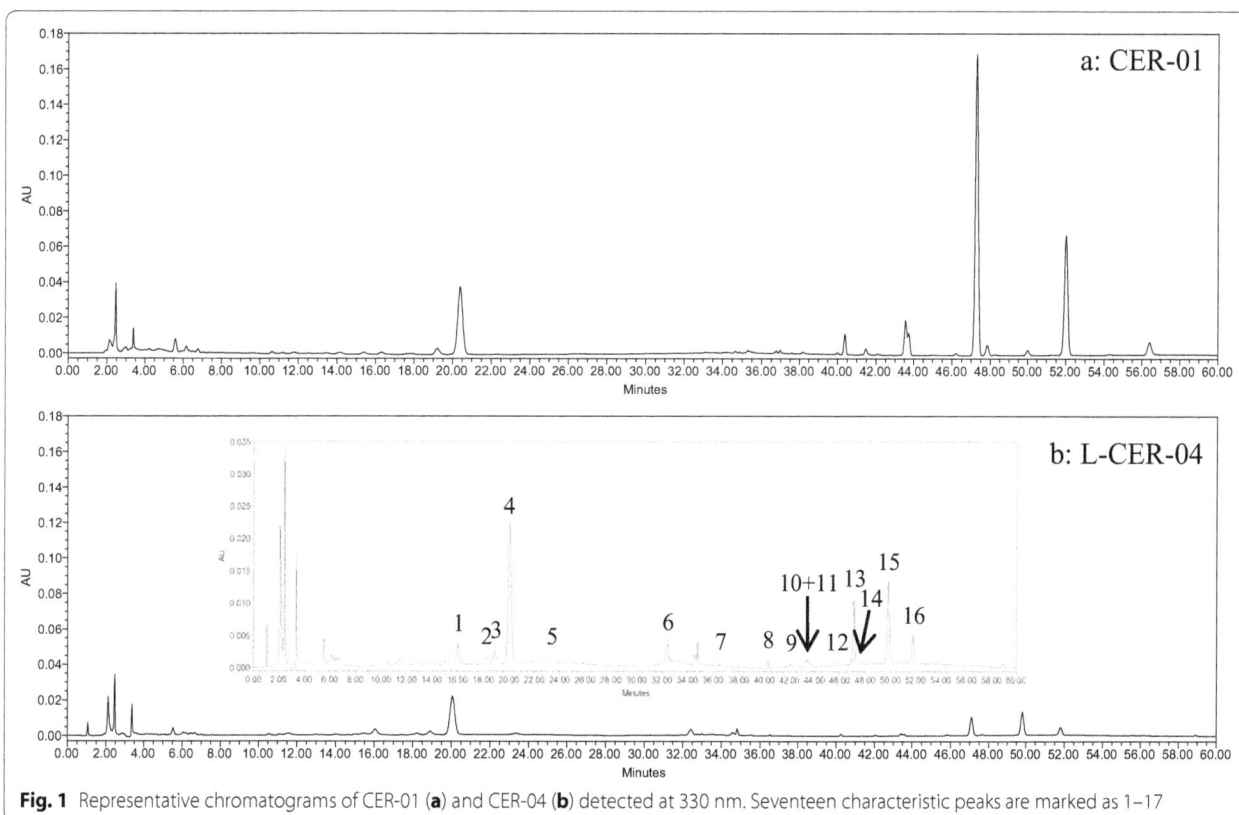

Fig. 1 Representative chromatograms of CER-01 (**a**) and CER-04 (**b**) detected at 330 nm. Seventeen characteristic peaks are marked as 1–17

and tangeretin at five different levels. The LOD and LOQ values were determined amongst the baseline noise for all three of the analytes under the optimized chromatographic conditions according to the International Union of Pure and Applied Chemistry (IUPAC) definition. The LOD values were determined as the concentration of each analyte required to generate a signal with a single-to-noise (S/N) ratio of 3:1, whereas the LOQ was defined as the concentration of each analyte required to generate a signal with an S/N ratio of 10:1. The regression equations, correlation coefficients, linear ranges, LODs and LOQs for hesperidin, nobiletin and tangeretin are shown in Table 1. The correlation coefficients (R^2) of hesperidin, nobiletin and tangeretin were greater than 0.99, indicating good linearity.

Intra- and inter-day variations were chosen to determine the precision of our newly developed method. For the intra-day variability test, one of the mixed standard solutions (hesperidin, 124.80 mg/mL; nobiletin, 2.99 mg/mL; tangeretin, 1.26 mg/mL) was analyzed five times within 1 day, whereas one of the mixed standard solutions was examined in triplicate on a daily basis for three consecutive days for the inter-day variability test. Repeatability was evaluated by analyzing five different working solutions prepared from the same sample (L-CER-01). The stability of the method was determined by the repeated analysis of the same sample solution at different times during a 24 h period of storage at room temperature. The RSD values for the retention times and peak

areas of hesperidin, nobiletin and tangeretin were taken as the measurements of precision and stability. The RSDs of the retention times and contents (mg/g) were taken as the measurements of repeatability. All of the RSD values for the retention times and peak areas (or contents) were found to be less than 2.00 and 3.00%, respectively (Table 2).

The recovery of our newly developed method was determined using spiked CER samples. A small portion (0.2 g) of L-CER-04 was individually spiked with 7.0056 mg of hesperidin, 0.1393 mg of nobiletin and 0.0467 mg of tangeretin. Five replicate samples were extracted and analyzed according to the procedures described above. As shown in Table 3, the mean recoveries (n = 5) of hesperidin, nobiletin and tangeretin were 104.92% ± 0.67, 95.87 ± 0.72 and 96.58 ± 2.08, respectively.

Validation of the chromatographic fingerprinting method

The chromatographic fingerprinting method was validated for its inter- and intra-day precisions, repeatability and stability. The inter-day precision was evaluated by running five consecutive injections of the same test sample within 1 day. The intra-day precision was evaluated by analyzing the same test sample in triplicate each day for 3 consecutive days. The repeatability of the method was examined by determining five different solutions prepared from the same botanical sample (L-CER-04). The stability was examined by analyzing the same sample

Table 1 Regression data, LODs and LOQs for the three analytes assayed in HPLC-UV chromatograms

Analyte	Calibration curve[a]	R^2	Linear range (mg/L)	LOD[b] (ng/mL)	LOQ[c] (ng/mL)
1	$y = 3.0149x - 21.812$	0.9994	31.20–499.20	418.8	128.6
2	$y = 41.396x - 4.1898$	0.9995	0.75–11.94	6.8	24.7
3	$y = 50.822x + 3.2433$	0.9996	0.31–5.03	12.0	40.8

1 Hesperidin, *2* Nobiletin, *3* Tangeretin

[a] y is the peak area in UV chromatograms detected in 330 nm, x is the concentration (mg/L) of the analyte

[b] LOD refers to the limit of detection, s/n = 3

[c] LOQ refers to the limit of quantification, s/n = 10

Table 2 Results of precision, repeatability and stability of the three analytes, expressed as RSD (%)

Analyte	Precision				Repeatability (n = 5)		Stability (n = 6)	
	Intra-day RSD (%) (n = 5)		Inter-day RSD (%) (n = 9)		RSD (%)		RSD (%)	
	t_R^a	PA[b]	t_R	PA	t_R	Contents (mg/g)	t_R	PA
1	0.32	0.39	1.39	2.98	0.52	0.94	1.08	1.65
2	0.42	0.44	1.76	1.31	0.07	1.08	0.72	2.71
3	0.47	0.49	1.65	1.69	0.07	0.88	1.53	1.34

1 Hesperidin, *2* Nobiletin, *3* Tangeretin

[a] Refers to retention time

[b] Refers to peak area

Table 3 Recoveries of the three analytes using L-CER-04 as tested sample

Analytes	Sample weight (g)	Original (mg)	Added (mg)	Found (mg)	Recovery (%)	Mean recovery ± SD
1	0.2029	6.9687	7.0056	14.3330	105.12	104.92 ± 0.67
	0.2014	6.9172	7.0056	14.3097	105.52	
	0.2023	6.9481	7.0056	14.2179	103.77	
	0.2013	6.9137	7.0056	14.2663	104.95	
	0.2065	7.0923	7.0056	14.4638	105.22	
2	0.2029	0.1416	0.1393	0.2745	95.41	95.87 ± 0.72
	0.2014	0.1405	0.1393	0.2738	95.71	
	0.2023	0.1411	0.1393	0.2748	95.97	
	0.2013	0.1404	0.1393	0.2756	97.06	
	0.2065	0.1441	0.1393	0.2767	95.22	
3	0.2029	0.0557	0.0467	0.1009	96.91	
	0.2014	0.0556	0.0467	0.1008	96.65	
	0.2023	0.0547	0.0467	0.1006	98.14	96.58 ± 2.08
	0.2013	0.0546	0.0467	0.1005	98.13	
	0.2065	0.0568	0.0467	0.1003	93.06	

1 Hesperidin, *2* Nobiletin, *3* Tangeretin

solution at different time points (0, 2, 4, 8, 16 and 24 h). The results of these experiments expressed in two forms, including (1) the RSDs of the relative retention times (RRT) and relative peak areas (RPA) of each characteristic peak relative to the reference peak (nobiletin); and (2) the similarity values for the chromatographic fingerprints of the different samples relative to the reference values, which were calculated using the formulas discussed in the "Data analysis" section. The RSD values were all less than 5%, whereas the similarity values were all greater than 0.99, indicating that our newly developed chromatographic fingerprinting method is satisfactory for the analysis of the samples.

Quantitative determination of hesperidin, nobiletin and tangeretin contents of the CER samples

Our newly developed HPLC-UV method was used to quantify the different amounts of hesperidin, nobiletin and tangeretin in several different batches of CER. Calibration curves were generated for these compounds using reference compound and used to calculate the hesperidin, nobiletin and tangeretin contents in different samples (Table 4).

The contents of hesperidin, nobiletin and tangeretin in different samples varied from 23.8 to 79.6 mg/g, 0.587 to 15.7 mg/g and 0.222 to 6.03 mg/g, respectively. The differences in contents of hesperidin in different CER samples were small, whereas the differences in contents of nobiletin and tangeretin changed considerably.

All of the CER samples collected from mainland China were found to have higher hesperidin, nobiletin and tangeretin contents than those collected locally from Hong Kong. CER-01 had the highest content of hesperidin between all the samples tested in the current study at 79.6 mg/g, whereas CER-04 had the highest contents of nobiletin and tangeretin at 15.7 and 6.03 mg/g, respectively. The lowest content of hesperidin was found in L-CER-01 at 23.8 mg/g, whereas the lowest contents of nobiletin and tangeretin were both found in L-CER-03 at 0.588 and 0.222 mg/g, respectively.

Assignment of the characteristic peaks

Figure 1 shows the 17 characteristic peaks detected at 330 nm in the CER-01 and L-CER-04 samples. The structures responsible for these peaks were identified based on their MS and MS^2 behaviors and a comparison of these data with those in the literature (Table 5). The MS conditions were optimized and the data were collected in the negative and positive ESI modes.

Peak 2 had a retention time of 18.3 min and a UV absorption maximum of 282 nm. Although this compound did not give intense mass ions in the negative or positive ionization mode, it was unequivocally identified as naringin based on a comparison of its absorption wavelength and retention time data with those of the reference compound. The identity of this peak was further confirmed by the addition of a standard solution of naringin to the CER extract.

Peak 4 had a retention time of 20.1 min and a UV absorption maximum at 283 nm. MS analysis in the negative ionization mode revealed $[M–H]^-$ and $[2M–H]^-$ ions with an m/z values of 609 and 1219. The fragmentation pattern of the former of these two ions was studied by MS^2 analysis, which revealed a series of product ions

Table 4 Contents (mg/g dry weight, mean ± SD) of hesperidin, nobiletin and tangeretin in different CER samples

Sample no.	Content (mg/g dry weight) (Mean ± SD)			Moisture content (%)
	Hesperidin	Nobiletin	Tangeretin	
L-CER-01	23.7940 ± 0.4782	0.9882 ± 0.0047	0.5086 ± 0.0034	11.86
L-CER-02	48.9356 ± 0.1245	0.8221 ± 0.0121	0.3308 ± 0.0024	11.99
L-CER-03	39.3195 ± 0.2017	0.5771 ± 0.0109	0.2155 ± 0.0055	13.39
L-CER-04	42.6070 ± 0.5382	0.7187 ± 0.0109	0.3069 ± 0.0049	8.14
CER-01	79.5846 ± 0.5380	14.6451 ± 0.0889	5.6522 ± 0.0329	9.33
CER-02	73.2414 ± 0.5380	14.6177 ± 0.6494	5.5453 ± 0.2511	9.60
CER-03	71.6286 ± 0.0907	14.9612 ± 0.0022	5.7574 ± 0.0011	9.20
CER-04	73.7426 ± 0.2926	15.6881 ± 0.0637	6.0309 ± 0.0244	8.39
CER-05	41.2002 ± 0.2510	2.3286 ± 0.0193	1.2122 ± 0.0103	7.96
CER-06	39.7620 ± 0.0302	6.2006 ± 0.0090	4.0030 ± 0.0051	11.58

with m/z values of 301 [M-Rutinosyl–H]$^-$, 286 [M-Rutinosyl–CH$_3$–H]$^-$, 257 [M-Rutinosyl–CO$_2$–H]$^-$, 242 [M-Rutinosyl–CO$_2$–CH$_3$–H]$^-$ and 134 [M-Rutinosyl–CO$_2$–CH$_3$–C$_6$H$_4$O$_2$–H]$^-$. MS analysis of peak 4 in the positive ionization mode revealed a series of protonated molecular ion peaks with m/z values of 611 [M+H]$^+$, 1243 [2M+Na]$^+$, 465 [M-Rhamnosyl+H]$^+$ and 303 [M-Rutinosyl+H]$^+$. The MS^2 fragmentation of the first of these four peaks gave six fragment ions with m/z values of 303 [M-Rutinosyl+H]$^+$, 285 [M-Rutinosyl–H$_2$O+H]$^+$, 270 [M-Rutinosyl–H$_2$O–CH$_3$+H]$^+$, 195 [M-Rutinosyl–C$_6$H$_4$O$_2$+H]$^+$ and 177 [M-Rutinosyl–C$_6$H$_4$O$_2$–H$_2$O+H]$^+$. This peak was unequivocally identified as hesperidin based on a comparison of its MS data with the data from the reference compound and the literature [7, 19].

Peak 5 had a retention time of 23.3 min and a UV absorption maximum of 283 nm. MS analysis in the negative ionization mode gave a peak with an m/z value of 609 [M–H]$^-$. In contrast, analysis in the positive ionization mode gave four peaks with m/z values of 611 [M+H]$^+$, 633 [M+Na]$^+$, 465 [M-Rhamnosyl+H]$^+$ and 303 [M-Rutinosyl+H]$^+$. The peak was identified as neohesperidin.

Peak 10 gave a retention time of 43.6 min with UV absorption maxima at 214, 241 and 330 nm. MS analysis in the negative ion mode did not give a major mass ion signal. In contrast, MS analysis in the positive ion mode revealed several mass ions with m/z values of 373 [M+H]$^+$, 395 [M+Na]$^+$, 767 [2M+Na]$^+$, 358 [M–CH$_3$+H]$^+$, 343 [M–CH$_2$O+H]$^+$ and 312 [M–H$_2$O–CO–CH$_3$+H]$^+$. The first of these peaks was subjected to MS^2 fragmentation analysis, which resulted in three fragment ions with m/z values of 343 [M–CH$_2$O+H]$^+$, 312 [M–H$_2$O–CO–CH$_3$+H]$^+$ and 297 [M–H$_2$O–CO–CH$_2$O+H]$^+$. This peak was identified as sinensetin based on a comparison of its MS data with the data from the

literature [20, 21]. Peak 11 co-eluted with peak 10 with a retention time of 43.73 min and UV absorption maxima at 270, 295 and 341 nm. In a similar manner to peak 10, MS analysis of peak 11 in the negative ion mode revealed no major peak. However, MS analysis in the positive ion mode revealed a molecular ion peak with an m/z value of 343 [M+H]$^+$ along with several other ions with m/z values of 707 [2M+Na]$^+$, 328 [M–CH$_3$+H]$^+$, 313 [M–CH$_2$O+H]$^+$ and 285 [M–CH$_2$O–CO+H]$^+$. The molecular ion peak with an m/z value of 343 was subjected to MS^2 analysis, which resulted in two major daughter ions with m/z values of 313 [M–CH$_2$O+H]$^+$ and 285 [M–CH$_2$O–CO+H]$^+$. This peak was identified as tetramethyl-O-isoscutellarein by comparing its MS data with those from the literature [20].

Peak 12 eluted with a retention time of 46.3 min and gave two UV absorption maxima at 208 and 336 nm. MS analysis in the negative ion mode did not reveal any major peaks, whereas analysis in positive ion mode revealed two protonated molecular ion peaks with m/z values of 403 [M+H]$^+$ and 373 [M–CH$_2$O+H]$^+$. The former of these two peaks was subjected to MS^2 fragmentation analysis, which revealed several fragment ions with m/z values of 373 [M–CH$_2$O+H]$^+$, 388 [M–CH$_3$+H]$^+$, 355 [M–CH$_2$O–H$_2$O+H]$^+$ and 327 [M–CH$_2$O–H$_2$O–CO+H]$^+$. A comparing of these data with the data from a reference compound and the literature [21] revealed that this peak was hexamethoxyflavone.

Peak 13 eluted with a retention time of 47.1 min and gave a UV absorption maximum of 333 nm. MS analysis in the negative ion mode revealed no obvious peak, whereas analysis in the positive ion mode revealed a protonated molecular ion with an m/z value of 403 [M+H]$^+$, as well as two other peaks with m/z values of 388 [M–CH$_3$+H]$^+$ and 373 [M–CH$_2$O+H]$^+$. MS^2 fragmentation analysis of the protonated molecular ion peak with an m/z value of 403 revealed several daughter peaks with

Table 5 Assignment of the characteristic peaks

No.	RT (min)	UV (nm)	MS in neg. mode	MS in pos. mode	MS^2 in neg. mode	MS^2 in pos. mode	Assignment	References
1	15.2	283	/	/	/	/	Unknown	/
2	18.3	282	/	/	/	/	Naringin	/
3	19.2	253, 347	607 [M–H]$^-$	609 [M+H]$^+$ 631 [M+Na]$^+$ 463 [M-Rhamnosyl+H]$^+$ 301 [M-Rutinosyl+H]$^+$	299 [M-Rutinosyl–H]$^-$	301 [M-Rutinosyl+H]$^+$	Unknown	/
4	20.1	283	609 [M–H]$^-$ 1219 [2M–H]$^-$	611 [M+H]$^+$ 1243 [2M+Na]$^+$ 465 [M-Rhamnosyl+H]$^+$ 303 [M-Rutinosyl+H]$^+$	301 [M-Rutinosyl–H]$^-$ 286 [M-Rutinosyl-CH$_3$-H]$^-$ 257 [M-Rutinosyl-CO$_2$-H]$^-$ 242 [M-Rutinosyl-CO$_2$-CH$_3$-H]$^-$ 134 [M-Rutinosyl-CO$_2$-CH$_3$-C$_6$H$_4$O$_2$-H]$^-$	303 [M-Rutinosyl+H]$^+$ 285 [M-Rutinosyl-H$_2$O+H]$^+$ 270 [M-Rutinosyl-H$_2$O-CH$_3$+H]$^+$ 195 [M-Rutinosyl-C$_6$H$_4$O$_2$+H]$^+$ 177 [M-Rutinosyl-C$_6$H$_4$O$_2$-H$_2$O+H]$^+$	Hesperidin	[7, 19]
5	23.3	283	609 [M–H]$^-$	611 [M+H]$^+$ 633 [M+Na]$^+$ 465 [M-Rhamnosyl+H]$^+$ 303 [M-Rutinosyl+H]$^+$	/	/	Neohesperidin	/
6	32.4	254, 347	723 [M–H]$^-$ 695 [M-CO-H]$^-$	725 [M+H]$^+$ 747 [M+Na]$^+$	417 [M-306–H]$^-$	419 [M-306+H]$^+$	Unknown	/
7	36.5	210, 257, 342	/	/	/	/	Unknown	/
8	40.3	203, 269, 345	/	373 [M+H]$^+$ 395 [M+Na]$^+$ 358 [M–CH$_3$+H]$^+$ 343 [M–CH$_2$O+H]$^+$	/	343 [M–CH$_2$O+H]$^+$	Unknown	/
9	42.2	206, 253, 270, 355	/	403 [M+H]$^+$ 425 [M+Na]$^+$ 388 [M–CH$_3$+H]$^+$ 373 [M–CH$_2$O+H]$^+$	/	373 [M–CH$_2$O+H]$^+$	Unknown	/
10	43.6	214, 241, 330	/	373 [M+H]$^+$ 395 [M+Na]$^+$ 767 [2M+Na]$^+$ 358 [M–CH$_3$+H]$^+$ 343 [M–CH$_2$O+H]$^+$ 312 [M–H$_2$O–CO–CH$_3$+H]$^+$	/	343 [M–CH$_2$O+H]$^+$ 312 [M–H$_2$O–CO–CH$_3$+H]$^+$ 297 [M–H$_2$O–CO–CH$_2$O+H]$^+$	Sinensetin	[20, 21]
11	43.7	270, 295, 341	/	343 [M+H]$^+$ 707 [2M+Na]$^+$	/	313 [M–CH$_2$O+H]$^+$ 285 [M–CH$_2$O–CO+H]$^+$	Tetramethyl-O-isoscutellarein	[20]

Table 5 continued

No.	RT (min)	UV (nm)	MS in neg. mode	MS in pos. mode	MS² in neg. mode	MS² in pos. mode	Assignment	References
				328 [M–CH₃+H]⁺				
				313 [M–CH₂O+H]⁺				
				285 [M–CH₂O–CO+H]⁺				
12	46.3	208, 336	/	403 [M+H]⁺	/	388 [M–CH₃+H]⁺	Hexamethoxyflavone	[21]
				373 [M–CH₂O+H]⁺		373 [M–CH₂O+H]⁺		
						355 [M–CH₂O–H₂O+H]⁺		
						327 [M–CH₂O–H₂O–CO+H]⁺		
13	47.1	333	/	403 [M+H]⁺	/	388 [M–CH₃+H]⁺	Nobiletin	[7, 20, 22]
				388 [M-CH₃+H]⁺		373 [M–CH₂O+H]⁺		
				373 [M-CH₂O+H]⁺		343 [M–2CH₂O+H]⁺		
						313 [M–3CH₂O+H]⁺		
						283 [M–4CH₂O+H]⁺		
						239 [M–C₁₀H₁₂O₂+H]⁺		
						211 [M–C₁₀H₁₂O₂–CO+H]⁺		
14	47.7	266, 322	/	343 [M+H]⁺	/	313 [M–CH₂O+H]⁺	Tetramethyl-O-scutellarein	[20]
				365 [M+Na]⁺		299 [M–CO₂+H]⁺		
				328 [M-CH₃+H]⁺				
				313 [M-CH₂O+H]⁺				
15	50.1	253, 343	/	433 [M+H]⁺	/	403 [M–CH₂O+H]⁺	3,5,6,7,8,3',4'-Heptamethoxyflavone	[7, 20]
				455 [M+Na]⁺		373 [M–2CH₂O+H]⁺		
				496 [M+Na+CH₃CN]⁺		345 [M–2CH₂O–CO+H]⁺		
				418 [M-CH₃+H]⁺				
				403 [M-CH₂O+H]⁺				
16	51.8	270, 323	/	373 [M+H]⁺	/	343 [M–CH₂O+H]⁺	Tangeretin	[7, 20, 22]
				395 [M+Na]⁺		283 [M–3CH₂O+H]⁺		
				358 [M-CH₃+H]⁺		312 [M–CH₃–H₂O–CO+H]⁺		
17	56.5	203, 254, 282, 341	/	389 [M+H]⁺	/	374 [M–CH₃+H]⁺	5-Hydroxy-6,7,8,3',4'-pentamethoxyflavone	[7]
				411 [M+Na]⁺		359 [M–CH₂O+H]⁺		
				374 [M-CH₃+H]⁺				
				359 [M-CH₂O+H]⁺				

m/z values of 373 [M–CH₂O+H]⁺, 388 [M–CH₃+H]⁺, 343 [M–2CH₂O+H]⁺, 313 [M–3CH₂O+H]⁺, 283 [M–4CH₂O+H]⁺, 239 [M–C₁₀H₁₂O₂+H]⁺ and 211 [M–C₁₀H₁₂O₂–CO+H]⁺. A comparison of these data with those obtained from a reference compound and the literature [7, 20, 22] revealed that this peak was nobiletin.

Peak 14 eluted with a retention time of 47.7 min and gave two UV absorption maxima at 266 and 322 nm. MS analysis in the negative ion mode did not reveal any

major peak, whereas analysis in the positive ion mode gave several peaks with m/z values of 343 [M+H]⁺, 365 [M+Na]⁺, 328 [M–CH₃+H]⁺ and 313 [M–CH₂O+H]⁺. The peak with an m/z value of 343 [M+H]⁺ was subjected to MS² fragmentation analysis and gave two daughter ions with m/z values of 313 [M–CH₂O+H]⁺ and 299 [M–CO₂+H]⁺. This peak was identified as tetramethyl-O-scutellarein based on a comparison of its data with those described in the literature [20].

Table 6 Similarity values of each sample compared to the reference fingerprint generated

Sample no.	Similarity			
	Correlation coefficient		Angle cosin	
	Mean[a]	Median[b]	Mean	Median
L-CER-01	0.2414	0.1666	0.4666	0.4017
L-CER-02	0.4443	0.5450	0.5903	0.6573
L-CER-03	0.4422	0.5300	0.6050	0.6599
L-CER-04	0.4327	0.5146	0.6124	0.6602
CER-01	0.8866	0.7544	0.9126	0.8247
CER-02	0.8873	0.7536	0.9140	0.8251
CER-03	0.8856	0.7535	0.9116	0.8238
CER-04	0.8853	0.7562	0.9116	0.8257
CER-05	0.7290	0.8199	0.8180	0.8767
CER-06	0.7193	0.7427	0.7929	0.8098

[a] The reference fingerprint was generated with mean values of the samples

[b] The reference fingerprint was generated with median vales of the samples

Peak 15 gave a retention time of 50.1 min and two UV absorption maxima at 253 and 343 nm. MS analysis in the negative ion mode revealed no major ions. However, MS analysis in the positive ion mode revealed five peaks with m/z values of 433 $[M+H]^+$, 455 $[M+Na]^+$, 496 $[M+Na+CH_3CN]^+$, 418 $[M-CH_3+H]^+$ and 403 $[M-CH_2O+H]^+$. The peak with an m/z value of 433 $[M+H]^+$ was subjected to MS^2 analysis, resulting in three major daughter ions with m/z values of 403 $[M-CH_2O+H]^+$, 373 $[M-2CH_2O+H]^+$ and 345 $[M-2CH_2O-CO+H]^+$. This peak was tentatively identified as 3,5,6,7,8,3',4'-heptamethoxyflavone based on a comparison with data from the literature [7, 20].

Peak 16 eluted with a retention time of 51.8 min and two UV absorption maxima at 270 and 323 nm. MS analysis in the negative ion mode revealed no major peaks, whereas analysis in the positive ion mode revealed three major peaks with m/z values of 373 $[M+H]^+$, 395 $[M+Na]^+$ and 358 $[M-CH_3+H]^+$. The protonated molecular ion with an m/z value of 373 $[M+H]^+$ was subjected to MS^2 fragmentation analysis, which resulted in three daughter peaks with m/z values of 343 $[M-CH_2O+H]^+$, 283 $[M-3CH_2O+H]^+$ and 312 $[M-CH_3-H_2O-CO+H]^+$. This peak was identified as tangeretin based on a comparison of these data with those reported in the literature [7, 20, 22], as well as the data obtained from the reference compounds.

Peak 17 gave a retention time of 56.5 min with four UV absorption maxima at 203, 254, 282 and 343 nm. No major peaks were observed by MS analysis in the negative ion mode, whereas analysis in the positive ion mode revealed four peaks with m/z values of 389 $[M+H]^+$, 411 $[M+Na]^+$, 374 $[M-CH_3+H]^+$ and 359 $[M-CH_2O+H]^+$. The peak with an m/z value of 389 $[M+H]^+$ was subjected to MS^2 fragmentation analysis, resulting in two daughter ions with m/z values of 359 $[M-CH_2O+H]^+$ and 374 $[M-CH_3+H]^+$. This peak was tentatively identified as 5-hydroxy-6,7,8,3',4'-pentamethoxyflavone based on a comparison of these data with the data from the literature [7].

Peak 1 eluted with a retention time of 15.2 min and a UV absorption maximum of 283 nm. Peak 7 had a retention time of 36.5 min and three UV absorption maxima at 210, 257 and 342 nm. However, neither of these two peaks gave any major ions when they were analyzed by MS in the negative and positive ionization modes.

Peak 3 had a retention time of 19.2 min with two UV absorption maxima at 253 and 347 nm. MS analysis in the negative ion mode revealed a deprotonated molecular ion peak with an m/z value of 607 $[M-H]^-$. The subsequent fragmentation of this peak by MS^2 analysis resulted in a daughter peak with an m/z value of 299 $[M-Rutinosyl-H]^-$. MS analysis in the positive ion mode resulted in four major peaks with m/z values of 609 $[M+H]^+$, 631 $[M+Na]^+$, 463 $[M-Rhamnosyl+H]^+$ and 301 $[M-Rutinosyl+H]^+$. MS^2 fragmentation analysis of the first of these four peaks resulted in a daughter ion with an m/z value of 301 $[M-Rutinosyl+H]^+$.

Peak 6 eluted with a retention time of 32.4 min and two UV absorption maxima at 254 and 347 nm. Analysis in negative ion mode revealed two peaks with m/z values of 732 $[M-H]^-$ and 695 $[M-CO-H]^-$. The subsequent fragmentation of the former of these two peaks by MS^2 analysis gave a daughter ion with an m/z value of 417 $[M-306-H]^-$. MS analysis in the positive ion mode resulted in two peaks with m/z values of 725 $[M+H]^+$ and 747 $[M+Na]^+$. The MS^2 fragmentation of the former of these two peaks resulted in a daughter peak with an m/z value of 419 $[M-306+H]^+$.

Peak 8 had a retention time of 40.3 min and gave three UV absorption maxima at 203, 269 and 345 nm. MS analysis in the negative ion mode did not reveal any major peaks, whereas analysis in the positive ion mode gave four peaks with m/z values of 373 $[M+H]^+$, 395 $[M+Na]^+$, 358 $[M-CH_3+H]^+$ and 343 $[M-CH_2O+H]^+$. The first of these four peaks was subjected to MS^2 analysis, which resulted in a major daughter peak with an m/z value of 343 $[M-CH_2O+H]^+$.

Peak 9 had a retention time of 42.2 min with four UV absorption maxima at 206, 253, 270 and 355 nm. MS analysis in the negative ionization mode revealed major peaks whereas analysis in the positive ion mode revealed four peaks with m/z values of 403 $[M+H]^+$, 425 $[M+Na]^+$, 388 $[M-CH_3+H]^+$ and 373 $[M-CH_2O+H]^+$. The peak observed with an m/z value of 403 $[M+H]^+$ was subjected to MS^2 fragmentation analysis, resulting in a daughter peak with an m/z value of 373 $[M-CH_2O+H]^+$.

Despite of best efforts, we were unable to identify peaks 1, 3, 6–9.

Fingerprinting and chemometrics

In this study, all the CER samples were compared with the corresponding reference samples (generated from all the CER samples) based on their calculated similarity values (Table 6). We also performed PCA based on the contents of three specific analytes, as well as the PA/W values of the remaining 14 characteristic peaks. This operation can be thought of as revealing the internal structure of the data in a way that explains the variance of the samples.

Fingerprinting analysis was conducted using the 17 characteristic peaks shown in the overlapped chromatograms (Fig. 2). These peaks were used as variables to calculate the similarity values. The results of this process showed that the similarity values of the L-CER samples (0.24–0.66) were lower than those of the CER samples (0.72–0.91), indicating that the chemical profiles of the CER samples were similar to that of the reference fingerprint. Based on the contents and PA/W values of the different samples, we determined that the hesperidin, nobiletin and tangeretin contents of the L-CER samples were lower than those of the CER samples. Furthermore, the CER samples contained 10–30 times as much nobiletin and tangeretin as the L-CER samples. Peaks 1, 6 and 7 were not detected in most of the CER samples, however, they were found to be particularly prominent in the L-CER samples. None of the L-CER samples contained a signal corresponding to peak 17 (5-hydroxy-6,7,8,3′,4′-pentamethoxyflavone), which

was found in all the CER samples. Although all of the L-CER samples purchased in pharmacies in Hong Kong were actually imported from mainland China, they all showed considerable differences in the chemical profiles. For example, the hesperidin contents of the CER samples were around two times higher than those of the L-CER samples. Further work should therefore be conducted to determine whether these differences in the chemical compositions of the samples could lead to differences in their efficacies in clinical practice.

In this study, the variables for each sample in the PCA consisted of their hesperidin, nobiletin and tangeretin contents, as well as the PA/W values of the remaining 14 characteristic peaks. The resulting data were exported to Excel (Microsoft, Inc., Belleview, WA, USA) to form a two-dimensional matrix (10 samples versus 17 variables), which cumulatively accounted for 94.31 of the total variance, based on which PCA scores plot (Fig. 3) was generated. CER-01, CER-02, CER-03, CER-04 and CER-06 were tightly clustered to the left of the plot, with PC1 scores around −0.6. L-CER-02, L-CER-03 and L-CER-04 were tightly clustered in the lower right of the plot with high PC2 scores. CER-05 was the only CER sample to be found at some distance from the other CER samples, although it was close to the L-CER samples. L-CER-01 was positioned in the upper right of the plot and far away from all of the other samples giving it the highest PC2 score. The loading plot of a variable on a PC generally reflects the extent to which that variable contributes to the PC, and how well the PC accounts for variations in the variable over the data points. The loading results also described the relationships between different variables.

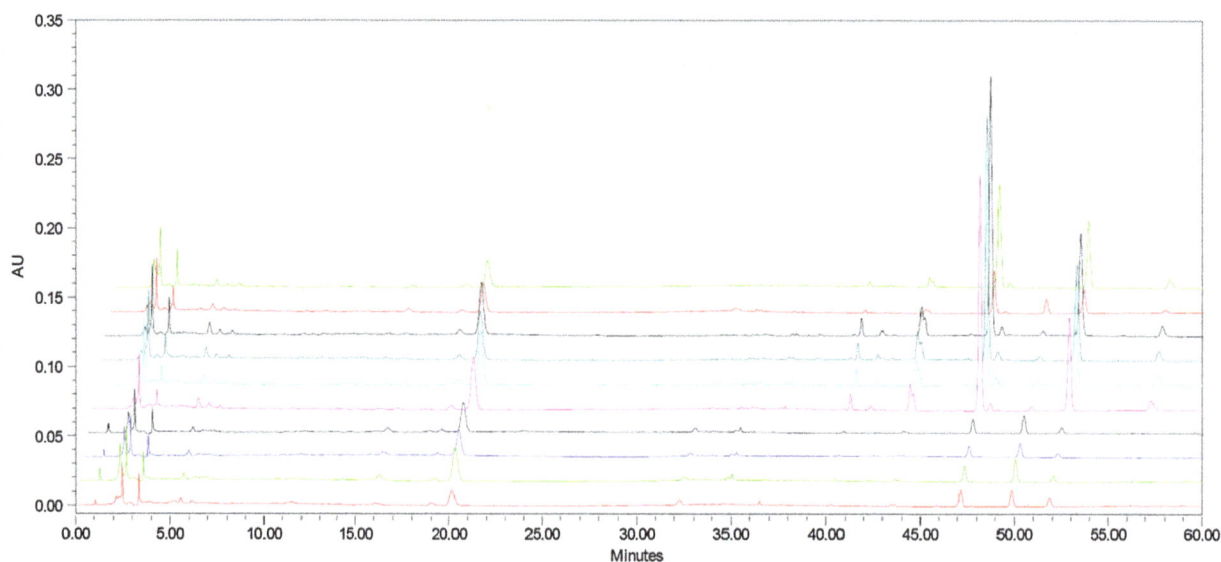

Fig. 2 Overlapped chromatographic fingerprints of the testes CER samples

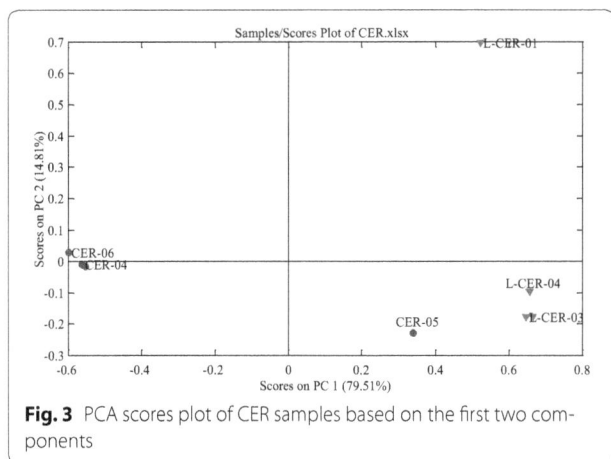

Fig. 3 PCA scores plot of CER samples based on the first two components

PC1 loadings plot indicated that peak 8, peaks 10 and 11 (sinensetin and tetramethyl-O-isoscutellarein), peak 14 (tetramethyl-O-scutellarein) and peak 17 (5-hydroxy-6,7,8,3',4'-pentamethoxyflavone) had made a negative contribution to the positions of the samples tested in PC1. In contrast, peak 1, peak 5 (neohesperidin), peak 6 and peak 15 (3,5,6,7,8,3',4'-heptamethoxyflavone) had made a positive contribution to PC1. In other words, samples with higher contents or PA/W values of peak 8, peaks 10 and 11 (sinensetin and tetramethyl-O-isoscutellarein), peak 14 (tetramethyl-O-scutellarein) and peak 17 (5-hydroxy-6,7,8,3',4'-pentamethoxyflavone) would be positioned to the left of the scores plot. Meanwhile, samples with higher contents or PA/W values of peak 1, peak 5 (neohesperidin), peaks 6 and 15 (3,5,6,7,8,3',4'-heptamethoxyflavone) would be positioned to the right of the scores plot. In this study, CER-01, CER-02, CER-03, CER-04 and CER-06 had high PA/W values for peak 8, peak 10 + 11 (sinensetin and tetramethyl-O-isoscutellarein), peak 14 (tetramethyl-O-scutellarein) and peak 17 (5-hydroxy-6,7,8,3',4'-pentamethoxyflavone), and were consequently positioned to the left of the scores plot. In contrast, all of the L-CER samples had high PA/W values for peak 5 (neohesperidin), peak 6 and peak 15 (3,5,6,7,8,3',4'-heptamethoxyflavone). The hesperidin, nobiletin and tangeretin contents of CER-05 and the PA/W values of the other characteristic peaks resembled those of the L-CER samples more closely than those of the CER samples.

The loading plot for PC2 showed that peak 1, peak 3, peak 5 (neohesperidin), peak 10 + 11 and peak 15 were having the greatest influence on the samples on the PC2 positions. Peak 5 (neohesperidin) made a positive contribution to the positions, whereas peak 1, peak 3, peak 10 + 11 and peak 15 made a negative contribution to these positions. L-CER-01 had the highest value for peak 5 (neohesperidin) of all of the samples tested in the current study.

Antioxidant activity of CER samples

2,2-Diphenyl-1-picrylhydrazyl (DPPH) assay

The DPPH free radical scavenging activities of the CER samples are shown in Fig. 4a. Each sample was tested at three different concentrations. CER-06 had the highest value at 173.005 μmol butylated hydroxytoluene equivalent (BHTE)/g of dried sample, followed by L-CER-01 at 164.741 μmol BHTE/g of dried sample. L-CER-03 had the lowest value at 68.818 μmol BHTE/g of dried sample, followed by L-CER-02 at 94.372 μmol BHTE/g of dried sample. The EC_{50} values of the samples were calculated and the results are shown in Fig. 4b. Materials with the lowest EC_{50} value exhibited the greatest free radical-scavenging activity. Although the DPPH radical-scavenging activities of all the CER samples tested in the current study were lower than that of BHT, the results showed that the different samples exhibited different radical-scavenging abilities.

Ferric ion reducing antioxidant power (FRAP) assay

The FRAP values (expressed as Fe^{2+} equivalents) were used to determine the ferric reducing activities of the different CER samples (Fig. 5). The values were between 19.887 (L-CER-03) and 43.890 (CER-06) μmol Fe^{2+} equivalents/g of dried CER sample. The value obtained for BHT was the highest of all of the samples tested at 275.01 μmol Fe^{2+} equivalents/g of BHT. The ferric reducing activities of all of the CER samples were less than that of BHT.

Trolox equivalent antioxidant capacity (TEAC) assay

The antioxidant activities of the CER samples were determined using the TEAC method, which gave values in the range of 27.120 to 58.391 μmol BHTE/g of dried sample (Fig. 6a). L-CER-03 showed the highest value of all of the samples tested at 58.391 μmol BHTE/g of dried sample, whereas CER-06 gave the lowest value at 27.120 μmol BHTE/g of dried sample. The EC_{50} values were calculated and the results are displayed in Fig. 6b. The differences in the antioxidant activities of the different CER samples were attributed to differences in their chemical compositions.

Correlation analysis

Pearson r correlation values were calculated using bivariate correlation analysis because we only evaluated 10 CER samples in the present study, and we were therefore unable to determine whether these samples did or did not obey a Gaussian distribution. The results of this analysis are shown in Table 7, where "−" and "+" have been used to represent negative and positive correlations, respectively. Peaks 03, 04, 08, 10, 11, 13, 14, 16 and 17 positively correlated with the ABTS radical scavenging activity,

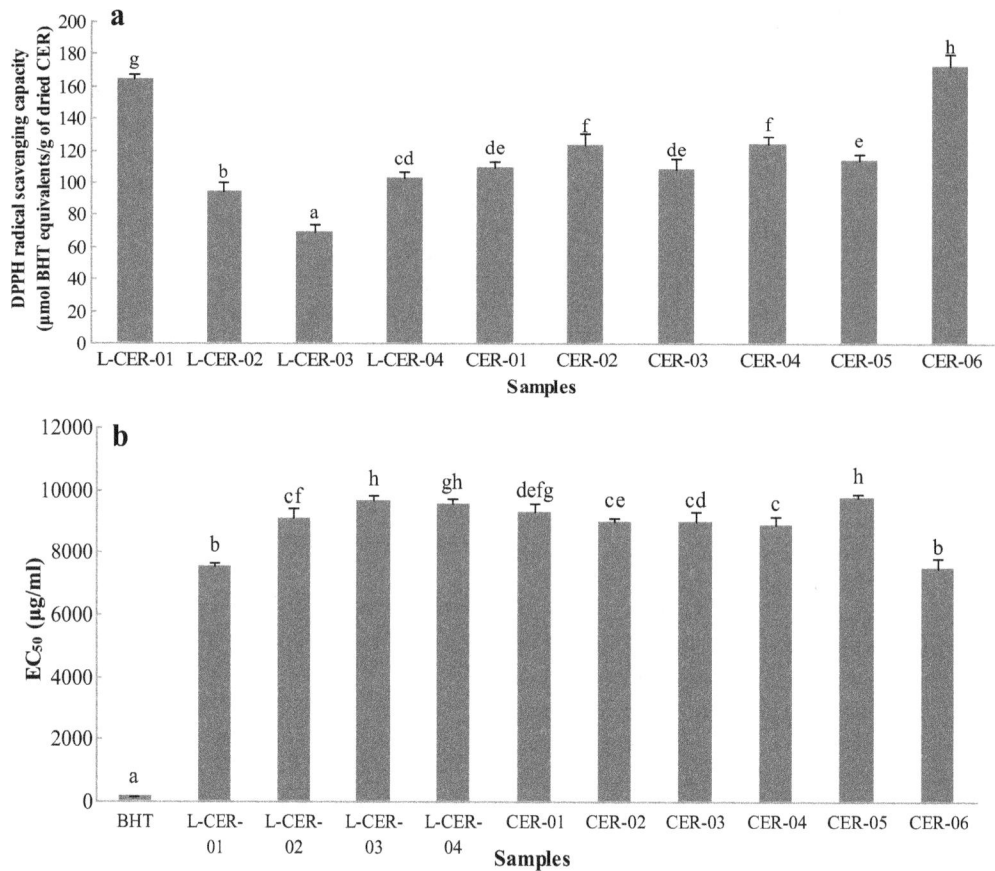

Fig. 4 DPPH radical scavenging capacity of CER samples (**a**) and EC_{50} values of BHT and CER samples (**b**). *Different letters* represent significant differences ($P < 0.05$)

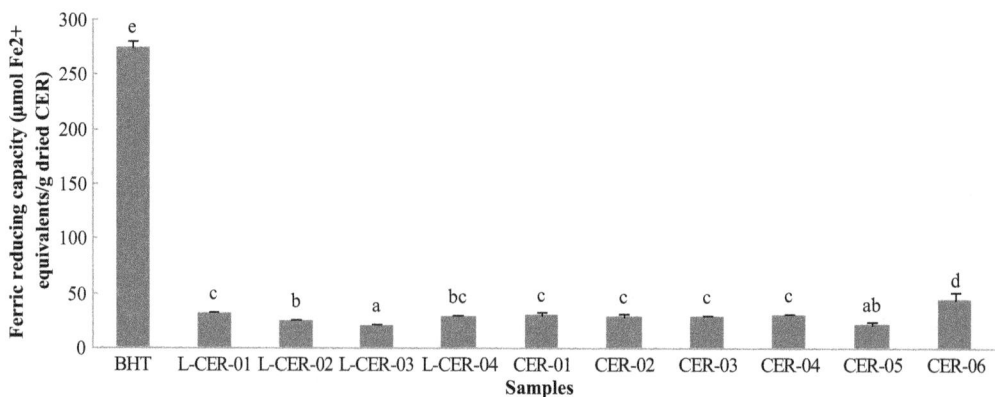

Fig. 5 Ferric reducing capacity of CER samples. The values are expressed as mol Fe^{2+} equivalents per gram of dried CER sample (mean $\pm$ SD). *Different letters* represent significant differences ($P < 0.05$)

whereas peaks 01, 06 and 15 negatively correlated with the ABTS radical scavenging activity. None of the peaks correlated with the DPPH free radical scavenging or ferric reducing activity.

Conclusion

An HPLC-UV-MS method has been developed and validated after a detailed investigation on extraction of chemical compounds from CER using different solvents

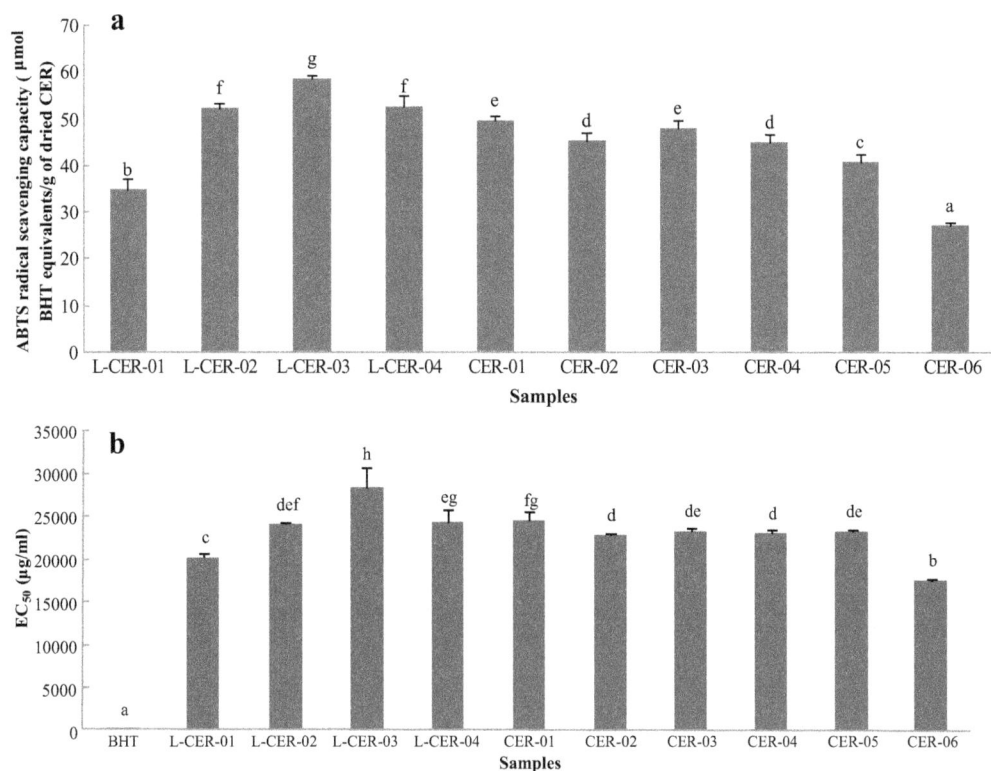

Fig. 6 ABTS radical scavenging capacity of CER samples (**a**) and EC_{50} values of BHT and CER samples (**b**). *Different letters* represent significant differences ($P < 0.05$)

Table 7 Spearman's correlation between the characteristic peaks of each CER sample and its antioxidant capacities

Peak no.	Correlation coefficient		
	DPPH free radical scavenging capacity	Ferric reducing capacity	ABTS radical scavenging capacity
Peak 01	−0.575	0.446	−0.760**
Peak 02	−0.290	0.174	−0.406
Peak 03	0.152	−0.224	0.697**
Peak 04	−0.055	0.079	0.709**
Peak 05	0.138	0.450	−0.510
Peak 06	−0.307	0.533	−0.792**
Peak 07	−0.252	0.511	−0.743
Peak 08	0.527	−0.042	0.952**
Peak 09	−0.115	0.394	0.612
Peak 10 + 11	0.503	−0.030	0.976**
Peak 12	−0.018	0.395	0.638*
Peak 13	0.503	−0.030	0.976**
Peak 14	—	—	0.915**
Peak 15	−0.418	0.697	−0.709*
Peak 16	0.503	−0.030	0.976**
Peak 17	0.550	−0.306	0.932**

* $P < 0.05$

** $P < 0.01$

and extraction times. None of the peaks correlated with the DPPH free radical scavenging activity or ferric reducing capacity. In contrast, most of the peaks correlated well with the ABTS radical scavenging capacity.

Authors' contributions

YLH, YSC and XZ designed the study. YZ, CPK, CRL and KCW performed the experiments. YZ wrote the manuscript. YSC revised the manuscript. All authors read and approved the manuscript.

Author details

[1] Department of Chinese Pharmaceutical Sciences and Chinese Medicine Resources, College of Biopharmaceutical and Food Sciences, China Medical University, Taichung 40402, Taiwan. [2] Key Laboratory for Information System of Mountainous Areas and Protection of Ecological Environment, Guizhou Normal University, Guiyang 550001, China. [3] Department of Nursing, Hsin Sheng College of Medical Care and Management, Taoyuan 32544, Taiwan. [4] Department of Nursing, Hungkuang University, Taichung 43302, Taiwan. [5] Chinese Crude Drug Pharmacy, China Medical University Hospital, Taichung 40402, Taiwan.

Acknowledgements

The authors would like to acknowledge the grant support from Hong Kong Chinese Materia Medica Standard Office, Department of Health, Hong Kong, for this study. (HKCMMS-CMU-Phase VII to YS Chang).

Competing interests

The authors declare that they have no competing interests.

References

1. The State Pharmacopoeia Commission of The People's Republic of China. Pharmacopoeia of the People's Republic of China. Beijing: Chemical Industry Press; 2015. p. 602–3.
2. Yu MW, Lou SN, Chiu EM, Ho CT. Antioxidant activity and effective compounds of immature calamondin peel. Food Chem. 2013;136:1130–5.
3. Xiao H, Yang CS, Li S, Jin H, Ho CT, Patel T. Monodemethylated polymethoxyflavones from sweet orange (Citrus sinensis) peel inhibit growth of human lung cancer cells by apoptosis. Mol Nutr Food Res. 2009;53:398–406.
4. Yi ZB, Yu Y, Liang YZ, Zeng B. In vitro antioxidant and antimicrobial activities of the extract of Pericarpium Citri Reticulatae of new Citrus cultivar and its main flavonoids. LWT-Food Sci Technol. 2008;41:597–603.
5. Manthey JA, Grohmann K, Guthrie N. Biological properties of citrus flavonoids pertaining to cancer and inflammation. Curr Med Chem. 2001;8:135–53.
6. Attaway JA. Citrus juice flavonoids with anticarcinogenic and antitumor properties. Food Phytochem Cancer Prev. 1994;19:240–8.
7. Liu EH, Zhao P, Duan L, Zheng GD, Guo L, Yang H, Li P. Simultaneous determination of six bioactive flavonoids in Citri Reticulatae Pericarpium by rapid resolution liquid chromatography coupled with triple quadrupole electrospray tandem mass spectrometry. Food Chem. 2013;141:3977–83.
8. Zhang J, Gao W, Liu Z, Zhang Z. Identification and simultaneous determination of twelve active components in the methanol extract of traditional medicine Weichang'an Pill by HPLC-DAD-ESI-MS/MS. Iran J Pharm Res. 2013;12:15–24.
9. Yu JW, Deng KY, Peng T, Zhu BY, Liu HY. Simultaneous determination of six ingredients in Huoxiang Zhengqi oral liquid by UPLC. Zhongguo Zhong Yao Za Zhi. 2013;38:2314–7.
10. Zhao Y, Sun JH, Yu LL, Chen P. Chromatographic and mass spectrometric fingerprinting analyses of Angelica sinensis (Oliv.) Diels-derived dietary supplements. Anal Bioanal Chem. 2013;405:4477–85.
11. Zhao Y, Kao CP, Chang YS, Ho YL. Quality assessment on Polygoni Multiflori Caulis using HPLC/UV/MS combined with principle component analysis. Chem Cent J. 2013;7:106.
12. Sun JH, Chen P. Chromatographic fingerprint analysis of yohimbe bark and related dietary supplements using UHPLC/UV/MS. J Pharm Biomed Anal. 2012;61:142–9.
13. Zhao Y, Chen P, Lin LZ, Harnly JM, Yu LL, Li ZW. Tentative identification, quantitation, and principal component analysis of green pu-erh, green, and white teas using UPLC/DAD/MS. Food Chem. 2011;126:1269–77.
14. Cheng ZH, Moore J, Yu LL. High-throughput relative DPPH radical scavenging capacity assay. J Agric Food Chem. 2006;54:7429–36.
15. Yi T, Lo HW, Zhao ZZ, Yu ZL, Yang ZJ, Chen HB. Comparison of the chemical composition and pharmacological effects of the aqueous and ethanolic extracts from a Tibetan "Snow Lotus" (Saussurea laniceps) herb. Molecules. 2012;17:7183–94.
16. Yi T, Chen QL, He XC, So SW, Lo YL, Fan LL, et al. Chemical quantification and antioxidant assay of four active components in Ficus hirta root using UPLC-PAD-MS fingerprinting combined with cluster analysis. Chem Cent J. 2013;7:115.
17. Benzie Iris FF, Strain JJ. The ferric reducing ability of plasma (FRAP) as a measure of "antioxidant powder": the FRAP assay. Anal Biochem. 1996;239:70–6.
18. Stratil P, Klejdus B, Kuban V. Determination of total content of phenolic compounds and their antioxidant activity in vegetables—evaluation of spectrophotometric methods. J Agric Food Chem. 2006;54:607–16.
19. Roowi S, Crozier A. Flavonoids in tropical citrus species. J Agric Food Chem. 2011;59:12217–25.
20. Wang DD, Wang J, Huang XH, Tu Y, Ni KY. Identification of polymethoxylated flavones from green tangerine peel (Pericarpium Citri Reticulatae Viride) by chromatographic and spectroscopic techniques. J Pharm Biomed Anal. 2007;44:63–9.
21. Dugo P, Mondello L, Dugo L, Stancanelli R, Dugo G. LC-MS for the identification of oxygen heterocyclic compounds in citrus essential oils. J Pharm Biomed Anal. 2000;24:147–54.
22. Zhang JY, Zhang Q, Zhang HX, Ma Q, Lu JQ, Qiao YJ. Characterization of polymethoxylated flavonoids (PMFs) in the peels of 'Shatangju' Mandarin (Citrus reticulate Blanco) by online high-performance liquid chromatography coupled to photodiode array detection and electrospray tandem mass spectrometry. J Agric Food Chem. 2012;60:9023–34.

12

Different modulation of *Panax notoginseng* on the absorption profiling of triptolide and tripterine from *Tripterygium wilfordii* in rat intestine

Yiqun Li[1], Huiting Cao[1], Mengzhu Liu[1], Benyong Zhang[1], Xinlong Zhang[2], Donglei Shi[2], Liwei Guo[1], Jinao Duan[1], Xueping Zhou[1], Huaxu Zhu[1*] and Qichun Zhang[1,3*]

Abstract

Background: Compatibility with *Panax notoginseng* (PN) reduced the plasma concentration of triptolide and delayed the T_{max} of *Tripterygium wilfordii* (TW), the sovereign medicine of Qing-Luo Tong-Bi decoction, which hinted the absorption process of triptolide might be involved in decreasing the toxicity in liver and kidney.

Methods: The absorption of triptolide, triptonide, wilforlide and tripterine from monomer, TW, TW-PN, TW-*Caulis Sinomenii* (TW-CS) and Qing-Luo Tong-Bi were analyzed in duodenum, jejunum, ileum and colon of rat via single-pass intestinal perfusion model. An UPLC-MS/MS analysis method was developed to determine the concentration of triptolide, triptonide, wilforlide and tripterine in the inlet and outlet. Then P_{eff}, 10 cm%ABS and K_a were calculated based on the perfusate flux, perfusate volume and candidate chemicals concentration.

Results: The absorption of triptolide, triptonide, wilforlide and tripterine in duodenum, jejunum, ileum and colon was independent of concentration within range of 3–9 μg/mL. The target compounds, triptolide, triptonide, wilforlide and tripterine from the TW extract, showed higher absorption extent and rate than those administrated alone, and compared with the absorption situation of the chemicals of TW extract, the absorption of triptolide, triptonide and wilforlide of the extract of TW-PN, TW-CS and Qing-Luo Tong-Bi were decreased in these intestinal segments. However, PN-promoted tripterine absorption was observed in the intestine.

Conclusions: Modulation of absorption of chemicals in TW by subsidiary herbs may be responsible for reinforcing the actions and neutralizing the adverse effects through compatibility in the formula of Qing-Luo Tong-Bi. PN inhibits the absorption of triptolide of TW and promote the absorption of tripterine.

Keywords: Single-pass intestinal perfusion, Qing-Luo Tong-Bi, Effective permeability

Background

Tripterygium wilfordii (TW), the root of the herb *Tripterygium wilfordii* Hook. F., is a routine and important traditional Chinese herbal medicine, the properties and actions of which are described as dispelling pathogenic wind and removing dampness, promoting blood circulation and freeing meridians, detumescence for suppressing pains, destroying parasites and detoxifying [1, 2]. Clinically, TW is employed primarily to treat disorders associated with autoimmunity and inflammation such as rheumatoid arthritis, systemic lupus erythematosus, nephritis, encephalomyelitis and psoriasis [1, 3, 4]. Due to the narrow therapeutic window and adverse effects such as hepatotoxicity and nephrotoxicity emerge usually during the therapeutic process [5]. Compatibility is the principal protocol of medicines application in traditional

*Correspondence: zhuhx@njucm.edu.cn; zhangqichun@njucm.edu.cn
[1] Jiangsu Collaborative Innovation Center of Chinese Medicinal Resources Industrialization, Nanjing University of Chinese Medicine, Nanjing 210023, China
Full list of author information is available at the end of the article

Chinese medicine, the aim of which is to reinforce the expected curative effect and neutralize the toxicity of sovereign medicine in a prescription [6].

Qing-Luo Tong-Bi (QLTB) decoction is a prevalent formula including TW, *Panax notoginseng* (PN), *Caulis Sinomenii* (CS), *Rehmannia glutinosa* (RG) and *Bombyx batryticatus* (BB) in a proportion of 15:3:15:15:10 from the Rheumatism Department of Jiangsu Province Hospital of Traditional Chinese Medicine (Nanjing, PRC). In the previous investigation [6], PN was shown to significantly block the TW-induced elevation of alanine aminotransferase (ALT), aspartate aminotransferase (AST) and lactate dehydrogenase (LDH) in the rat plasma and ameliorate the histopathological damage of liver. Further pharmacokinetics analysis of triptolide, one of key active components of TW, demonstrated that PN changed the pharmacokinetic process of triptolide. With bare change of the dose in the body, extended T_{max} and decreased C_{max}, one of the possible mechanisms for PN to interfere the pharmacokinetic process of triptolide is proposed to modulate the absorption in intestinal tract. Meanwhile, the absorption of other chemicals from TW is still vague with or without PN.

Absorption is a complex kinetic process described via several in vitro or in vivo models. Single-pass intestinal perfusion (SPIP) technique is a powerful predictive absorption model developed to provide mathematical descriptions of rate and extent of drug absorption in vivo [7]. Unlike the cell model as Caco-2, SPIP has advantage properties of having intact blood supply and the ability to perform a mechanism evaluation of absorption process under controlled and semi conscience conditions. The effective permeability coefficient (P_{eff}) is directly related to the first-order absorption rate process in this model, which is used to estimate the extent of absorption [8]. Moreover, SPIP has been demonstrated to closely correlate to in vivo human data and a useful tool to predict absorption for both passive and carrier-mediated transport [9, 10].

To achieve more comprehensive understanding the absorption properties of TW under combination of the subsidiary herbal medicines, four representative components including triptolide, triptonide, wilforlide and tripterine are adopted to investigate the absorption parameters via SPIP model in rat. UPLC-MS/MS method was also developed to analyse the concentration change of drugs in the intestinal perfusate solution inlet and outlet. The results demonstrate that the absorption of triptolide, triptonide and wilforlide is inhibited in the formulae of TW-PN, TW-SC and QLTB. The influx of tripterine in the intestine is elevated in TW-PN but still decreased in TW-SC. With synergic influence of PN and SC, the absorption of tripterine in QLTB is increased in duodenum and jejunum, and reduced in ileum and colon.

Methods
The Minimum Standards of Reporting Checklist (Additional file 1) contains details of the experimental design, and statistics, and resources used in this study.

Chemicals and reagents
Triptolide (purity: 98%, Batch Number: 111567–200603) and prednisolone (purity: 99.4%, Batch Number: 100153–201004) were purchased from the National Institute for the Control of Pharmaceutical and Biological products (Beijing, China). Triptonide (purity: 98%, Batch Number: 20120720), wilforlide (purity: 98%, Batch Number: 20120720), tripterine (purity: 98%, Batch Number: 20120720) were purchased from Nanjing Zelang Medical Technology Co., Ltd. (Nanjing, China). The chemical structures of triptolide, triptonide, wilforlide and tripterine were shown in Fig. 1. TW was purchased from Xichang Materials Company of Sichuan (Batch Number: 120620), while PN was collected at Bozhou Medicine Company of Anhui (Batch Number: 111208), and all herbal medicine were identified by Dr. Qinan Wu (Department of Pharmacognosy, Nanjing University of Chinese Medicine, Nanjing, China) (College of Pharmacy, Nanjing University of Chinese Medicine, Nanjing, China). Normal saline was purchased from Nanjing Bianzheng Medical Technology Co., Ltd. (Nanjing, China). Acetonitrile and methanol used for UPLC were chromatographic grade (Merck, Darmstadt, Germany). All of the other reagents were analytical grade (Sino Pharm Chemical Reagent Co., Ltd., Shanghai, China). Milli-Q water (Millipore, Bedford, MA, USA) was used throughout the study.

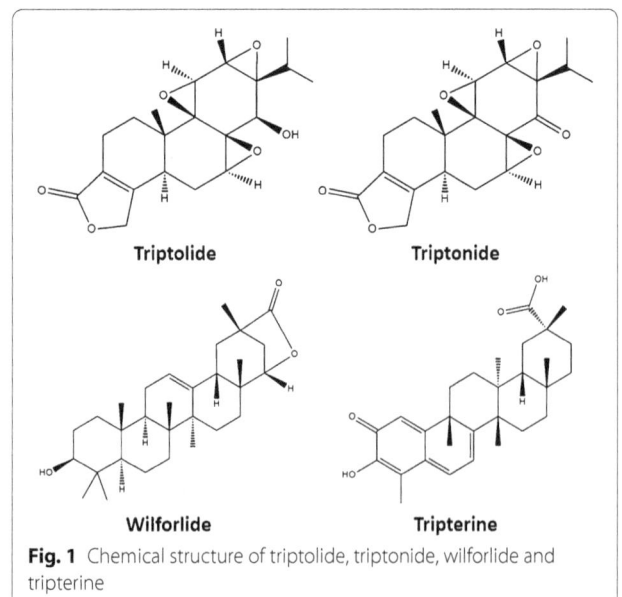

Fig. 1 Chemical structure of triptolide, triptonide, wilforlide and tripterine

Apparatus

These primary apparatus utilized in present research include BT100-1L constant flow peristalsis pump (Longer Pump Co., Ltd.), UPLC AcquityTM system (Waters, USA), Xevo triple quadrupole mass spectrometer (Waters, USA), Electrospray ion source (ESI), Masslynx 4.1 (Waters, USA), Votex Genius 3 vortex mixing equipment (Germany IKA company), Allegra 64 r Centrifuge including a high-speed refrigerated centrifuge (Beckman Coulter, USA), Ultra-pure water system (Millipore, USA), Multifuge X1R refrigerated centrifuge (Thermo, USA), Votex Genius 3 vortex mixing equipment (Germany IKA company), FE20 pH meter (Mettler-Toledo) and CentriVap® centrifugal concentrator (Labconco, USA).

Preparation of the extracts of TW, TW-PN, TW-SC and QLTB

Herb material of TW (3000 g) were crushed to pieces and were extracted with boiling water (1:11, w/v, and then 1:7, w/v) for 1.5 h each time. The filtrates filtered through gauze were merged and evaporated to approximately 150 mL under a vacuum at 65 °C by rotary evaporation. Then, the concentrate of TW was obtained and stored at 4 °C until use. A total of 3600 g of TW-PN with pieces of TW (3000 g) and PN (600 g), TW-SC of 6000 g with pieces of TW (3000 g) and CS (3000 g) and QLTB of 11600 g with pieces of TW (3000 g), PN (600 g), CS (3000 g), RG (3000 g), BB (2000 g) were extracted through the same process of TW product.

Preparation of perfusate

The stock solution of triptolide (100 μg/mL), triptonide (100 μg/mL), wilforlide (500 μg/mL), tripterine (500 μg/mL) and internal standard prednisolone (300 μg/mL) were prepared by dissolving accurately weighed chemical into methanol respectively. The perfusate solutions of these chemicals were prepared by diluting the corresponding stock solutions with HBSS solution (CaCl$_2$, 0.14 g; D-glucose, 4.5 g; NaCl, 9.164 g; HEPES, 5.96 g; KCl, 0.4 g; NaHCO$_3$, 0.37 g; MgSO$_4$·7H$_2$O, 0.245 g; Na$_2$HPO$_4$·12H$_2$O, 0.126 g; KH$_2$PO$_4$, 0.06 g; dissolved in water to 1 L, pH 7.4) to concentrations of 3, 6, 9 μg/mL.

The four extracts of TW, TW-PN, TW-CS and QLTB were freeze-dried into powder and redissolved in HBSS solution to obtain TW, TW-PN, TW-CS and QLTB perfusate solutions and stored at 4 °C until use. The concentrations of triptolide in TW, TW-PN, TW-CS and QLTB working solutions were regulated to 3 μg/mL. All the intestinal perfusate solutions were stored at 4 °C until use.

Animal experiment and samples collection

Male Sprague–Dawley rats (250 ± 15 g) were supplied by Nanjing University of Chinese Medicine Animal Center and kept in a breeding room with temperature of 24 ± 2 °C,

humidity of 55 ± 5%, and 12 h light/dark cycle for 7 days before the experiment. Animal welfare and experimental procedures were strictly in accordance with the Guide for the Care and Use of Laboratory Animals (US National Research Council, 1996). The study protocol and the total number of rat were approved by the Animal Care and Use Committee of Nanjing University of Chinese Medicine. The investigation conformed to the Guide for the Care and Use of Laboratory Animals published by the US National Institutes of Health (NIH Publication No. 85-23, revised 1996). Forty-eight rats were randomized into eight groups (Triptolide, Triptonide, Wilforlide, Tripterine, TW, TW-PN, TW-CS and QLTB, n = 6 for each group).

Rats were fasted for 16 h with free access to water prior to the perfusion study and anesthetized with 10% chloral hydrate solution (3.4 mL/kg, i.p.). A laparotomy was made through a midline incision of about 4 cm to separate the duodenum, jejunum, ileum and colon from the abdominal cavity, and approximate 10 cm of the four intestinal segments were exposed. At both ends of each measured intestinal segments, silicone cannulas were inserted. First, the intestinal lumen was cleaned by normal saline (37 °C) perfusion via the inlet until the effluent from the outlet was judged to be free of feces and clear. The perfusion solution was pumped by peristaltic pump through the intestine at a flow rate of 1.0 mL/min for 10 min. Following that, the perfusion solution through the intestinal lumen was changed to a constant flow rate of 0.2 mL/min for 20 min. After being stable for 30 min, the effluent solution were collected from the outlets of the four intestinal segments during each 10-min period (30–40, 40–50, 50–60, 60–70, 70–80 min) into pre-weighted vials. Then the weight of each perfusion solution was analyzed. During the perfusion operation, these exposed intestines were covered with gauze that had been moistened by frequent applications of warm (37 °C) normal saline, and kept warm by a small lamp placed over the area. At the end of the sampling, animals were euthanized with saturated potassium chloride solution by intracardiac injection, according to protocols of euthanasia in experimental animals. After death, the four segments of intestine were removed for measurements of length and radius (l and r, respectively). Duodenum segment was measured from 1 cm blow the pylorus, jejunum segment was measured from 15 cm blow the pylorus, ileum segment was measured from 20 cm above the cecum and colon segment was measured from 1 cm blow the cecum. The constant length of segment is 10 cm.

Sample preparation

The intestinal perfusion solution samples for UPLC-MS/MS analysis were prepared as follows. The internal standard prednisolone (100 μL, 30 μg/mL) was added to intestinal perfusion solution samples (1.0 mL) in a 10.0 mL centrifuge tube. After vortex with 4 mL ethyl acetate for 3 min, the intestinal perfusion solution samples were centrifuged at 3000 rpm for 10 min and the supernatants was transferred into a new 10.0 mL tube. Then another 4 mL ethyl acetate was added to the residue followed by vortex for 3 min and centrifuged at 3000 rpm for 10 min. The two supernatants were merged and evaporated to dryness by the centrifugal concentrator at 40 °C. The residue was dissolved by 1.0 mL acetonitrile followed by vortex for 3 min and centrifuging at 12,000 rpm for 10 min. At last, 20 μL of the supernatant was injected into the UPLC-MS/MS system for analysis.

UPLC conditions and UPLC-MS/MS analysis

An Agilent Zorbax Eclipse Plus C18 column (2.1 mm × 100 mm, 1.7 μm, Agilent, USA) was employed and the column temperature was kept at 35 °C. Mobile phase A consisted of acetonitrile and mobile phase B was 0.1% formic acid (v/v) in water. The gradient conditions were as follows: 0–1 min, 0–35% A; 1–2 min, 35–85% A; 2–4 min, 85% A; 4–4.8 min, 85–98% A; 4.8–5 min, 98–35% A. The injection volume was 2 μL and the flow rate of 0.4 mL/min.

For MS detection, we used an electrospray ionization source operating in the positive ion mode. The scanning mode we used was multiple reaction monitoring (MRM). The ion source temperature was set at 110 °C. A desolvation gas temperature of 350 °C, a cone gas rate of 50 L/h and a desolvation gas flow of 1000 L/h were used. The capillary voltage and cone voltage were set at 3000 and 40 V, respectively. The collision energy of prednisolone, triptolide, triptonide, wilforlide and tripterine are 40, 40, 40, 38 and 38 eV. Leucine-enkephalin was used as the lockmass in all analyses (m/z 556.2771 for positive ion mode and m/z 554.2615 for negative ion mode) at a concentration of 0.5 μg/mL with a flow rate of 5 μL/min. Data were collected in the centroid mode from m/z 100 to m/z 1000. The m/z of prednisolone, triptolide, triptonide, wilforlide and tripterine are as follows: 358.9/91.06, 360.89/91.07, 360.90/147.10, 451.03/201.07, 455.10/119.14.

Method validation

The methods for quantitative analysis of triptolide, triptonide, wilforlide and tripterine in perfusate samples were validated according to the requirement of biopharmaceutical analysis, which was examined for specificity, linearity, precision, extraction recovery and stability under the UPLC analytical conditions.

The specificity was evaluated by comparing blank perfusate, perfusate mixed by triptolide, triptonide, wilforlide and tripterine, TW perfusate, TW-PN perfusate, TW-CS perfusate, and QLTB perfusate.

The precision was determined from inter-day and intra-day using five sets of quality control (QC) samples and was expressed by the relative standard deviation (RSD %), which was estimated as follows: RSD (%) = (standard deviation (SD)/the observed concentrations of replicate analyses of QC samples (Cobs)) × 100. The QC samples of triptolide, triptonide, wilforlide and tripterine were diluted by those stock solutions in HBSS solution (pH 7.4) to produced three QC samples of each chemical as follows: triptolide (0.5, 1, 3 μg/mL), triptonide (0.5, 1, 2.5 μg/mL), wilforlide (0.2, 1, 2 μg/mL) and tripterine (0.2, 1, 2 μg/mL).

The extraction recoveries were determined by calculating the ratio of triptolide, triptonide, wilforlide and tripterine detected in QC samples against that initial content in HBSS solution.

The stability of the method was evaluated by analyzing QC samples mixed with triptolide, triptonide, wilforlide and tripterine with concentrations of 2.5, 5, 2.5, 5 μg/mL at 37 °C for 0 and 2 h.

Calculation

The absorption parameters of triptolide, triptonide, wilforlide and tripterine were calculated according to the methods as previously described [11, 12].

The effective permeability, P_{eff}, in the SPIP studies was calculated by gravimetric method and the volume of perfusate was corrected and calculated by the following equation (Eq. (1)):

$$P_{eff} = -Q\ln(C_{out}/C_{in} * Q_{out}/Q_{in})/2\pi rl \qquad (1)$$

where Q = constant perfusate flux of the peristaltic pump (0.2 mL/min), C_{out} = outlet drug concentration, C_{in} = inlet drug concentration, Q_{out} = outlet perfusate volume of each intestinal segment during the 10-min period, Q_{in} = inlet perfusate volume of each intestinal segment during the 10-min period, r = radius of every intestinal segment (duodenum, jejunum, ileum, colon), l = actual length of every intestinal segment (duodenum, jejunum, ileum, colon).

The K_a was calculated through the equation below (Eq. (2)):

$$K_a = Q(1 - C_{out}/C_{in})/\pi r^2 l \qquad (2)$$

where Q = constant perfusate flux of the peristaltic pump (0.2 mL/min), C_{out} = outlet drug concentration, C_{in} = inlet drug concentration, r = radius of every intestinal segment (duodenum, jejunum, ileum, colon), l = actual length of every intestinal segment (duodenum, jejunum, ileum, colon).

The percentage of 10 cm intestinal absorption (10 cm%ABS) was calculated through the equation below (Eq. (3)):

$$10 \text{ cm\%ABS} = (1 - Q_{out}/Q_{in} * C_{out}/C_{in}) * 100\% \quad (3)$$

where C_{out} = outlet drug concentration, C_{in} = inlet drug concentration, Q_{out} = outlet perfusate volume of each intestinal segment during the 10-min period, Q_{in} = inlet perfusate volume of each intestinal segment during the 10-min period.

Statistical analysis

The statistical analyses were performed by SPSS 16.0 (SPSS Inc., Chicago, USA). Statistical comparison of 10 cm%ABS was performed using Tukey tests and one-way ANOVA. All values are expressed as mean ± standard deviation. Means were assumed to be statistically significant when $p < 0.05$.

Results

Method validation for the HPLC assay of triptolide, triptonide, wilforlide and tripterine in rat plasma.

The retention times of triptolide, triptonide, wilforlide, tripterine and prednisolone were 1.59, 2.21, 3.63, 3.64 and 1.21 min, respectively. A significant endogenous peak could not be observed in this time-interval when these candidates were detected. Representative HPLC chromatograms are shown in Fig. 2.

The standard calibration curve of triptolide was linear over the range from 0.1 to 10.0 μg/mL with good linearity ($R^2 = 0.9990$), and a typical equation for the calibration curve was $Y = 0.0887X + 0.0026$. The standard calibration curve of triptonide was linear over the range from 0.04 to 10.0 μg/mL with good linearity ($R^2 = 0.9976$), and a typical equation for the calibration curve was $Y = 0.1138X + 0.0108$. The standard calibration curve of wilforlide was linear over the range from 0.02 to 20.0 μg/mL with good linearity ($R^2 = 0.9961$), and a typical equation for the calibration curve was $Y = 0.0232X + 0.0071$. The standard calibration curve of tripterine was linear over the range from 0.02 to 5.0 μg/mL with good linearity ($R^2 = 0.9958$), and a typical equation for the calibration curve was $Y = 8.6242X + 2.9543$.

The method showed good precision with intra-day and inter-day precision. As shown in Table 1 that the analytical precision of triptolide, triptonide, wilforlide and tripterine in intestinal perfusate solutions.

The extraction recoveries of triptolide were 82.75 ± 7.12, 85.36 ± 3.96 and 84.75 ± 4.11% at the concentrations of 0.5, 1.0 and 3.0 μg/mL. The extraction recoveries of triptonide were 78.60 ± 5.20, 74.80 ± 6.76 and 76.40 ± 5.78% at the concentrations of 0.5, 1.0 and 2.5 μg/mL. The extraction recoveries of wilforlide were 77.23 ± 7.04, 82.80 ± 5.86 and 82.68 ± 5.30% at the concentrations of 0.1, 1.0 and 2.0 μg/mL. The extraction recoveries of tripterine were 86.88 ± 7.67, 88.25 ± 4.62

and 84.69 ± 7.54% at the concentrations of 0.1, 1.0 and 2.0 μg/mL.

The stability analysis showed that the ratio of triptolide, triptonide, wilforlide and tripterine follow 2 h at 37 °C were 99.2, 96.86, 98.80 and 97.1% and showed no significant difference between the initial and tested concentrations.

The validated UPLC method was reproducible and reliable for determining triptolide, triptonide, wilforlide and tripterine in intestinal perfusate solutions.

Absorption profiling of triptolide in intestinal tract

To analyze the basic absorption properties of triptolide in the small intestine and colon, the absorption parameters of P_{eff}, 10 cm%ABS and K_a of triptolide at concentration of 3, 6 and 9 μg/mL were determined through SPIP model. As shown in Table 2, increasing the concentration of triptolide in the perfusate didn't result in significant alteration of P_{eff}, 10 cm%ABS and K_a (Table 2). Compared with pure triptolide, the P_{eff}, 10 cm%ABS and K_a of triptolide in TW were enhanced in the whole intestine lumen. Meanwhile, pronounced increasing of P_{eff} and 10 cm%ABS were observed in the colon. Moreover, significantly elevated K_a of triptolide from TW was observed in jejunum and ileum. In TW-containing formulae, all the P_{eff}, 10 cm%ABS and K_a of triptolide were decreased, and among which QLTB showed the maximum influence on the absorption of triptolide followed by TW-PN and TW-SC (Table 3).

Absorption properties of triptonide in intestinal tract

Similar with triptolide, the absorption parameters, P_{eff}, 10 cm%ABS and K_a showed concentration-independent characteristics within range of 3–9 μg/mL, and none significant variation of P_{eff} and 10 cm%ABS was observed among the four intestinal segments, duodenum, jejunum, ileum and colon. But the highest K_a was observed in the duodenum (Table 4). Unlike triptolide, TW did not promote obviously the absorption of triptonide. The P_{eff}, 10 cm%ABS and K_a were pronouncedly reduced in the formulae of TW-PN and QLTB within the lumen of duodenum, jejunum, ileum and colon, and QLTB exerted more influence than TW-PN. Moreover, the K_a of triptonide was down-regulated significantly in the duodenum and jejunum (Table 5).

Absorption properties of wilforlide in intestinal tract

With the enhancement of concentrations in the perfusate, P_{eff}, 10 cm%ABS and K_a of wilforlide were retained constant relatively, which indicated the passive transporting and/or unsaturated active absorption process. The cardinal absorption locations of wilforlide were jejunum and ileum (Table 6). TW elevated wilforlide absorption

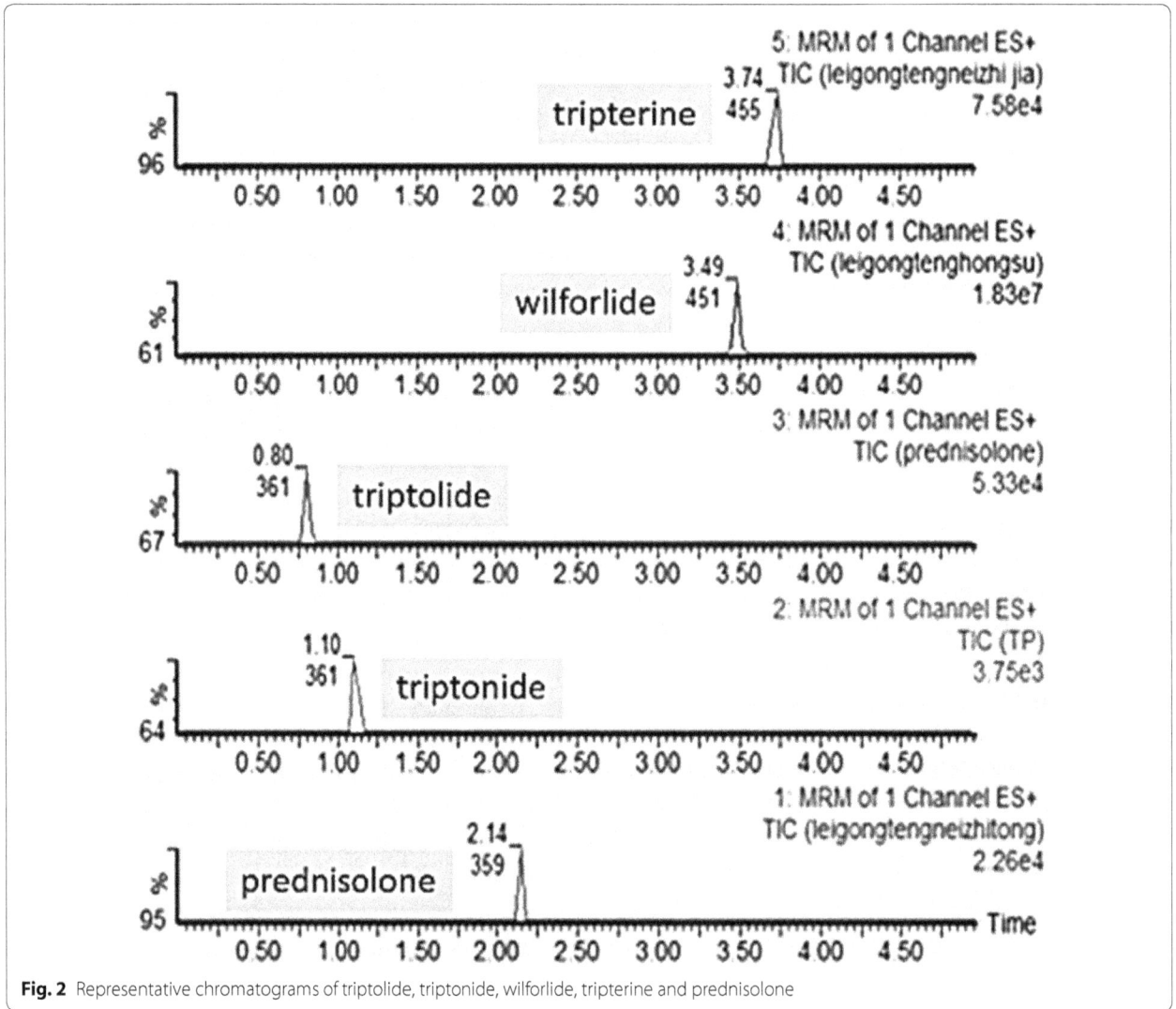

Fig. 2 Representative chromatograms of triptolide, triptonide, wilforlide, tripterine and prednisolone

Table 1 Inter-day and intra-day precision of triptolide, triptonide, wilforlide and tripterine in intestinal perfusate solutions (inter-day n = 6; intra-day n = 6)

Con. (µg/mL)	Triptolide			Triptonide			Wilforlide			Tripterine		
	0.5	1.0	3.0	0.2	1.0	2.0	0.5	1.0	2.5	0.2	1.0	2.0
Inter-day (%)	1.11	0.52	1.62	1.63	0.40	1.27	1.48	0.95	1.11	1.53	0.33	1.14
Intra-day (%)	1.18	0.63	1.80	1.77	0.44	1.35	1.72	1.05	1.25	1.79	0.37	1.47

within the intestinal tract, and significant enhancement of P_{eff} of wilforlide in TW was observed in jejunum and colon.

Both TW-PN and TW-SC decreased the absorption extent and rate of wilforlide, especially in the jejunum, ileum and colon (p < 0.05). However, wilforlide was not detected in QLTB perfusate prepared according to the ratio of herbal medicines (Table 7).

Absorption properties of tripterine in intestinal tract

Sharing the possible same transport process with the above three chemicals, P_{eff}, 10 cm%ABS and K_a of tripterine were independent of concentration in the perfusate. Although tripterine had greater K_a in jejunum and ileum than that in duodenum and colon, minor fluctuation of P_{eff} and 10 cm%ABS between the four intestinal segments (Table 8). As shown in Table 9, TW facilitated the

Table 2 Absorption parameters of triptolide in perfusate solution within duodenum, jejunum, ileum and colon ($\bar{x} \pm s$, n = 6)

Parameters	Con. (μg/mL)	Duodenum	Jejunum	Ileum	Colon
$P_{eff} \times 10^{-3}$	3	5.20 ± 1.72	4.98 ± 1.67	6.46 ± 2.0	6.35 ± 1.28
	6	5.05 ± 1.91	4.85 ± 1.88	6.36 ± 1.92	6.20 ± 1.45
	9	5.14 ± 0.56	4.77 ± 2.21	6.29 ± 2.31	6.36 ± 1.17
10 cm%ABS	3	42.7 ± 1.85	41.3 ± 2.4	47.8 ± 1.64	41.1 ± 3.33
	6	46.5 ± 3.52	41.6 ± 1.28	47.8 ± 1.34	41.8 ± 2.87
	9	45.8 ± 4.03	41.4 ± 1.67	48.4 ± 1.69	41.9 ± 2.88
$K_a \times 10^{-2}$	3	1.79 ± 0.33	1.64 ± 0.39	2.93 ± 0.29	1.81 ± 0.11
	6	1.75 ± 0.29	1.49 ± 0.79	2.86 ± 0.34	1.77 ± 0.23
	9	1.69 ± 0.31	1.53 ± 0.84	2.93 ± 0.24	1.69 ± 0.29

Table 3 Absorption parameters of triptolide of various formulae in perfusate solution within duodenum, jejunum, ileum and colon ($\bar{x} \pm s$, n = 6)

Parameters	Con. (μg/mL)	Duodenum	Jejunum	Ileum	Colon
$P_{eff} \times 10^{-3}$	Triptolide	5.2 ± 1.72	4.98 ± 1.67	6.46 ± 2.0	6.35 ± 1.28
	TW	8.5 ± 3.61	5.54 ± 1.54	7.87 ± 1.68	8.35 ± 1.17[#]
	TW-PN	4.2 ± 1.23*	4.3 ± 0.98	5.9 ± 0.86*	5.36 ± 0.75**
	TW-CS	6.8 ± 2.12	5.4 ± 1.77	6.68 ± 0.9	6.95 ± 0.72*
	QLTB	2.8 ± 0.54**	4.03 ± 1.55	5.28 ± 0.81**	5.73 ± 0.26**
10 cm%ABS	Triptolide	42.7 ± 8.51	41.3 ± 9.1	42.8 ± 6.64	41.1 ± 3.33
	TW	45.6 ± 5.83	42.5 ± 4.3	43.4 ± 2.33	47.8 ± 2.76[##]
	TW-PN	37.38 ± 6.47*	28.9 ± 3.5**	37.9 ± 1.67**	29.9 ± 5.32**
	TW-CS	38.38 ± 4.21*	30.5 ± 7.3**	42.5 ± 2.12	27.9 ± 5.09**
	QLTB	29.9 ± 4.33**	23.1 ± 2.1**	28.4 ± 3.17**	21.5 ± 3.19**
$K_a \times 10^{-2}$	Triptolide	1.79 ± 0.33	1.64 ± 0.39	2.93 ± 0.29	1.81 ± 0.11
	TW	1.83 ± 0.82	2.63 ± 0.47[##]	2.31 ± 0.30[##]	1.95 ± 0.20
	TW-PN	0.93 ± 0.29*	1.34 ± 0.11**	1.76 ± 0.45*	1.71 ± 0.36
	TW-CS	1.19 ± 0.56	1.11 ± 0.25**	2.18 ± 0.35	1.55 ± 0.26*
	QLTB	1.27 ± 0.395	0.88 ± 0.25**	1.52 ± 0.21**	1.15 ± 0.22**

[#] $p < 0.05$, [##] $p < 0.01$, compared with triptolide; * $p < 0.05$, ** $p < 0.01$, compared with TW

Table 4 Absorption parameters of triptonide in perfusate solution within duodenum, jejunum, ileum and colon ($\bar{x} \pm s$, n = 6)

Parameters	Con. (μg/mL)	Duodenum	Jejunum	Ileum	Colon
$P_{eff} \times 10^{-3}$	3	11.6 ± 2.95	8.77 ± 1.47	9.34 ± 2.92	8.40 ± 1.94
	6	10.9 ± 3.55	8.92 ± 0.97	9.72 ± 2.41	8.52 ± 1.78
	9	12.3 ± 2.31	8.84 ± 0.96	9.81 ± 3.44	8.32 ± 1.18
10 cm%ABS	3	46.1 ± 2.89	44.9 ± 3.67	44.5 ± 3.31	45.6 ± 3.76
	6	43.9 ± 4.52	46.4 ± 2.49	43.8 ± 3.21	46.5 ± 3.07
	9	44.7 ± 3.78	46.1 ± 2.98	45.4 ± 1.99	45.7 ± 3.76
$K_a \times 10^{-2}$	3	5.64 ± 1.22	2.60 ± 0.23	1.15 ± 0.47	1.33 ± 0.66
	6	5.49 ± 1.42	2.48 ± 0.42	1.08 ± 0.52	1.28 ± 0.57
	9	5.57 ± 1.35	2.55 ± 0.33	1.16 ± 0.38	1.31 ± 0.63

Table 5 **Absorption parameters of triptonide of various formulae in perfusate solution within duodenum, jejunum, ileum and colon ($\bar{x} \pm s$, n = 6)**

Parameters	Con. (μg/mL)	Duodenum	Jejunum	Ileum	Colon
$P_{eff} \times 10^{-3}$	Triptonide	11.6 ± 2.95	8.77 ± 1.47	9.34 ± 2.92	8.40 ± 1.94
	TW	13.3 ± 3.43	8.98 ± 1.26	11.3 ± 3.3	10.4 ± 2.04
	TW-PN	7.86 ± 1.36**	6.12 ± 1.38**	7.05 ± 1.29*	6.6 ± 1.57**
	TW-CS	12.8 ± 1.28	7.68 ± 1.64	9.93 ± 2.73	8.44 ± 1.31
	QLTB	5.55 ± 0.55**	5.48 ± 1.07**	4.75 ± 1.18**	5.22 ± 1.13**
10 cm%ABS	Triptonide	46.1 ± 2.89	44.9 ± 3.67	44.5 ± 3.31	45.6 ± 3.76
	TW	51.2 ± 8.5	46.8 ± 5.76	47.7 ± 7.12	49.7 ± 4.5
	TW-PN	40.4 ± 4.7*	33.6 ± 3.04**	37.0 ± 6.96*	35.9 ± 5.8**
	TW-CS	46.8 ± 5.3	41.3 ± 4.09	44.4 ± 4.18	45.6 ± 3.1
	QLTB	34.0 ± 5.7**	31.9 ± 3.27**	31.1 ± 7.18**	33.8 ± 3.4**
$K_a \times 10^{-2}$	Triptonide	5.64 ± 1.22	2.60 ± 0.23	1.15 ± 0.47	1.33 ± 0.66
	TW	6.03 ± 1.03	2.81 ± 0.18	1.32 ± 0.55	1.53 ± 0.46
	TW-PN	4.51 ± 0.83*	1.86 ± 0.14**	1.47 ± 0.68	0.99 ± 0.33*
	TW-CS	2.9 ± 1.68**	1.46 ± 0.28**	1.23 ± 0.78	1.37 ± 0.49
	QLTB	3.13 ± 1.11**	1.42 ± 0.08**	1.39 ± 0.36	0.70 ± 0.13**

* $p < 0.05$, ** $p < 0.01$, compared with TW

Table 6 **Absorption parameters of wilforlide in perfusate solution within duodenum, jejunum, ileum and colon ($\bar{x} \pm s$, n = 6)**

Parameters	Con. (μg/mL)	Duodenum	Jejunum	Ileum	Colon
$P_{eff} \times 10^{-3}$	3	5.49 ± 2.14	9.57 ± 1.25	12.2 ± 3.14	9.65 ± 1.95
	6	5.25 ± 2.08	9.93 ± 0.78	12.5 ± 2.97	9.35 ± 2.13
	9	5.17 ± 2.69	10.2 ± 1.14	11.7 ± 3.26	10.7 ± 1.89
10 cm%ABS	3	31.3 ± 3.26	37.5 ± 2.47	41.3 ± 3.78	42.1 ± 4.22
	6	29.8 ± 3.89	37.9 ± 2.34	43.1 ± 3.27	45.7 ± 1.63
	9	30.6 ± 2.75	39.5 ± 0.64	40.3 ± 4.26	41.6 ± 4.64
$K_a \times 10^{-2}$	3	1.34 ± 0.55	2.27 ± 0.21	2.53 ± 0.43	1.36 ± 0.12
	6	1.57 ± 0.33	2.21 ± 0.15	2.48 ± 0.56	1.27 ± 0.26
	9	1.44 ± 0.48	2.27 ± 0.20	2.61 ± 0.19	1.14 ± 0.43

absorption of tripterine partly. But significant elevation of absorption extent and rate of tripterine was observed in TW-PN, which demonstrated that PN further augment the effect of TW. However, TW-SC inhibited the absorption of tripterine in the intestine suggested SC dramatically reversed the action of TW on the absorption of tripterine. Interestingly, QLTB demonstrated promotion of tripterine absorption in the duodenum and blockage in the ileum and colon.

Discussion

Oral administration is definitely the most common and convenient route in the therapeutic system of traditional Chinese medicine and natural herb. The absorption extent and rate, namely bioavailability, at which unchanged drug proceeds from the gastrointestinal tract to the system circulation successively passing through the apical membrane of the epithelial cells, pre-hepatic blood vessels, portal vein and liver is the first limiting step of the pharmacokinetic process, which directly influences the peak concentrations of drug and retention time in the body and closely involves in the drug actions and side effect [13, 14]. It's paramount to evaluate the effective bioavailability of screening drug candidates in developing an oral dosage form [15]. Absorption is a complex kinetic process that is dependent on numerous factors including the physiochemical properties of the drug candidates and the physiochemical properties of the gastrointestinal barrier membrane [16]. During the chemicals passing through the gastrointestinal tract, solubility is a critical parameter for absorption since they must be in solution to permeate the intestinal wall, which is influenced by

Table 7 Absorption parameters of wilforlide of various formulae in perfusate solution within duodenum, jejunum, ileum and colon ($\bar{x} \pm s$, n = 6)

Parameters	Con. (µg/mL)	Duodenum	Jejunum	Ileum	Colon
$P_{eff} \times 10^{-3}$	Wilforlide	6.07 ± 2.14	9.57 ± 1.25	12.2 ± 3.14	9.65 ± 1.95
	TW	6.69 ± 1.93	11.6 ± 1.08[#]	14.7 ± 3.51	12.5 ± 1.65[#]
	TW-PN	5.91 ± 1.03	4.41 ± 1.27**	5.46 ± 2.79**	9.9 ± 0.63**
	TW-CS	4.98 ± 1.39	3.89 ± 0.41**	10.6 ± 1.27*	4.77 ± 2.56**
	QLTB	NA	NA	NA	NA
10 cm%ABS	Wilforlide	31.3 ± 3.26	37.5 ± 2.47	41.3 ± 3.78	42.1 ± 4.22
	TW	33.2 ± 7.06	39.8 ± 1.51	43.5 ± 4.44	44.0 ± 3.51
	TW-PN	26.2 ± 5.75	18.2 ± 5.69**	21.4 ± 1.35**	26.0 ± 4.69**
	TW-CS	26.8 ± 5.08	25.6 ± 4.16**	35.6 ± 1.37**	30.7 ± 1.59**
	QLTB	NA	NA	NA	NA
$K_a \times 10^{-2}$	Wilforlide	1.34 ± 0.55	2.27 ± 0.21	2.53 ± 0.43	1.36 ± 0.12
	TW	1.54 ± 0.55	2.39 ± 0.03	2.73 ± 0.35	1.54 ± 0.19
	TW-PN	1.37 ± 0.32	0.92 ± 0.44**	1.18 ± 0.78**	0.83 ± 0.39**
	TW-CS	1.18 ± 0.32*	0.77 ± 0.15**	1.21 ± 0.54**	0.50 ± 0.33**
	QLTB	NA	NA	NA	NA

[#] $p < 0.05$, compared with wilforlide; * $p < 0.05$, ** $p < 0.01$, compared with TW; *NA* none detected

Table 8 Absorption parameters of tripterine in perfusate solution within duodenum, jejunum, ileum and colon ($\bar{x} \pm s$, n = 6)

Parameters	Con. (µg/mL)	Duodenum	Jejunum	Ileum	Colon
$P_{eff} \times 10^{-3}$	3	7.11 ± 3.68	8.72 ± 3.47	9.48 ± 2.91	10.3 ± 1.56
	6	6.93 ± 3.01	9.52 ± 3.28	8.15 ± 3.82	10.8 ± 1.79
	9	9.03 ± 1.35	10.5 ± 1.67	9.13 ± 2.63	8.57 ± 3.75
10 cm%ABS	3	4.76 ± 1.27	4.98 ± 2.46	5.62 ± 1.81	6.34 ± 1.63
	6	4.69 ± 1.46	5.19 ± 1.44	5.34 ± 2.57	5.59 ± 2.34
	9	4.75 ± 0.98	5.09 ± 1.45	5.46 ± 2.24	5.75 ± 1.86
$K_a \times 10^{-2}$	3	1.52 ± 0.41	2.08 ± 0.33	2.62 ± 0.17	1.27 ± 0.19
	6	1.66 ± 0.23	2.12 ± 0.23	2.48 ± 0.45	1.03 ± 0.37
	9	1.44 ± 0.58	2.03 ± 0.45	2.43 ± 0.74	1.19 ± 0.24

the ionization, molecular weight and lipophilicity. Therefore, introducing ionizable groups, reducing molecular size and lipophilicity are the most efficient and frequent strategy used by medicinal chemists to increase the solubility. The pKa of molecules and the pH of gastrointestinal tract jointly govern the solubility. The above mentioned properties are the primarily limiting factors of the passive transport, the driving force of which is the concentration gradient between the two sides of the membrane, allowing chemicals to move from the side of higher concentration to the side of lower concentration without the expenditure of cellular energy. Moreover, the carriers-mediated active transport requires specialized carrier proteins allowing chemicals to cross the membrane against a concentration gradient [17–19]. According to the prescription principal, the oral formulation

of decoction from single or several combinational herbs is the routine remedy regimen carrying some active components through the gastrointestinal tract. Unlike chemical drug candidates, there are no directly artificial modifications of chemical structure in the herbal remedy. Similar with chemical drugs, however, the components of herb are undergoing the permeation process of influx and efflux through the intestinal membrane. The components from the same herb or these compatible ones are responsible for regulating absorption circumstance such as the pH and involved transporters [20].

Component-component interaction is the basic characteristics of the decoction formulation during the absorption process within the gastric and intestinal lumen, at or within the gut wall, as well as within the liver, which leads to the effects of the potentiation or antagonism between

Table 9 Absorption parameters of tripterine of various formulae in perfusate solution within duodenum, jejunum, ileum and colon ($\bar{x} \pm s$, n = 6)

Parameters	Con. (µg/mL)	Duodenum	Jejunum	Ileum	Colon
$P_{eff} \times 10^{-3}$	Tripterine	6.78 ± 3.68	8.72 ± 3.47	9.48 ± 2.91	10.3 ± 1.56
	TW	7.11 ± 2.77	10.7 ± 4.51	11.6 ± 3.01	12.4 ± 3.63
	TW-PN	10.3 ± 1.14*	13.3 ± 4.08	15.2 ± 2.63	9.98 ± 0.21
	TW-CS	3.20 ± 0.49**	3.35 ± 0.78**	5.69 ± 2.12**	3.39 ± 1.15**
	QLTB	11.7 ± 0.82**	11.1 ± 5.3	6.10 ± 3.63*	5.62 ± 3.11**
10 cm%ABS	Tripterine	4.76 ± 1.27	4.98 ± 2.46	5.62 ± 1.81	6.34 ± 1.63
	TW	5.87 ± 1.23	6.27 ± 2.26	7.60 ± 1.17#	7.14 ± 1.63
	TW-PN	6.49 ± 1.91	9.29 ± 0.54**	9.43 ± 0.56**	5.82 ± 1.42
	TW-CS	2.91 ± 0.49**	3.74 ± 0.95*	4.23 ± 2.67*	3.97 ± 1.19**
	QLTB	8.13 ± 0.81**	7.38 ± 1.07	4.84 ± 1.58**	5.65 ± 1.31
$K_a \times 10^{-2}$	Tripterine	1.52 ± 0.41	2.08 ± 0.33	2.62 ± 0.17	1.27 ± 0.19
	TW	1.88 ± 0.38	2.21 ± 0.51	2.91 ± 0.35	1.34 ± 0.54
	TW-PN	2.31 ± 0.83	3.27 ± 0.21**	3.21 ± 0.14	2.52 ± 0.13**
	TW-CS	1.64 ± 0.30	1.22 ± 0.20**	1.39 ± 0.40**	1.54 ± 0.11
	QLTB	2.14 ± 0.30	1.69 ± 0.45	1.86 ± 0.16**	1.66 ± 0.31

# $p < 0.05$, compared with tripterine; * $p < 0.05$, ** $p < 0.01$, compared with TW

them [21–23]. One of the common mechanisms underlying the interaction is the alteration of gastrointestinal pH. The solubility of drug with specific pKa is regulated by the intestinal fluid pH. Basic drugs are more soluble in acidic fluids, and acidic drugs are more soluble in basic fluids. However, drug solubility does not completely ensure absorption because only un-ionized molecules are absorbed. Tannin, one kind of plant polyphenol, is widespread in leaves, roots and fruits of plant, has the ability to change the pH of gastrointestinal tract. Tannic acid is a polymer of gallic acid molecules and glucose, and demonstrates weak acidity due to the numerous phenol groups in the structure. In the decoction of herbal medicine, tannin binds with other components such as alkaloids forming chelation and directly changing the solubility of some active chemicals, which results in failing to permeate the intestinal mucosa [24, 25]. However, acidic chemicals like tannin are verified to inhibit the motility of intestine, which prolong the exposure period and might enhance the absorption [26]. Both TW and PN contain tannin. Another mechanism possibly influencing the absorption of the four components of TW investigated in the present study is ameliorating intestinal blood flow by PN theoretically affecting the absorption of lipophilic compounds. Notoginseng triterpenes from PN shows positive effect on the cerebral hypoxia and myocardial ischemia via dilating the blood vessels [27]. The vasoactive action can still be held on the mesentery. Meanwhile, monomers Rg3 in the notoginseng triterpenes inhibited the P-glycoprotein (P-gp) function and promoted accumulation of rhodamine 123 in drug-resistant

KBV20C cells in a dose-dependent manner [28]. P-gp is an efflux transporter proteins from the ATP-binding cassette family expressing at the lumenal surface of the intestinal epithelium and opposing the absorption by transporting lipophilic compounds out of enterocytes back into the gastrointestinal lumen [29, 30]. Interestingly, some specific substrates of P-gp have affinities to a pivotal metabolism enzyme CYP3A responsible for Phase I oxidative metabolism [31]. Generally, inhibition of CYP3A4/5 results in a minimum threefold increase in the extent of absorption and toxicity of the concomitantly administered agent, but can also result in decreased efficacy of prodrugs needing CYP3A for conversion to active moieties. Notoginseng triterpenes was demonstrated to inhibit the CYP3A in liver, and the action on the CYP3A4/5 in intestine is supposed [32]. However, further investigations are required to suggest which component associated with the toxicity is the substrates of CYP3A4/5.

SPIP is a typical in situ intestinal perfusion model to study absorption rates [10]. Although the animal has been anaesthetized and surgically manipulated, the neural, endocrine, lymphatic, and mesenteric blood supplies are still working and therefore all the transport mechanisms are maintained, which is more advantage than in vitro techniques. Meanwhile, multiple samples may be taken, thus enabling kinetic studies to be performed in situ intestinal perfusion method, data from which at the rat model has been demonstrated to correlate with in vivo human data [33]. Unlike the closed loop intestinal perfusion technique, SPIP is an open loop system that is developed to evaluate the properties of drug absorption with continuous fluid flow through the intestine and provides better control of the hydrodynamics and increased surface area than the closed loop method. Although the P_{eff} values are generally similar obtained from both open and closed loop techniques, SPIP is proven to produce more reproducible absorption rat and lower variance within experiments. Otherwise, what should be considered for the SPIP is the assumption that all drug passes into portal vein, that is drug disappearance reflects drug absorption, may not be valid in some circumstances. The bio-transformations in intestine by the major cytochrome P450 enzymes, CYP3A4/5, is also responsible for the disappearance of in intestinal lumen and significantly reduce oral bioavailability [34, 35]. Then the absorption rate estimated in SPIP should be called disappearance rate. The technique to overcome the shortcoming of SPIP is intestinal perfusion with venous sampling models. Based on the appearance kinetics in pre-hepatic blood, drug absorption through the enterocytes can be quantified through plasma sample analysis, which facilitates quantification of both steady-state disappearance kinetics from the intestinal lumen and concurrent appearance kinetics into pre-hepatic blood. The drug appearance in pre-hepatic blood represents the net levels of absorption into the apical membrane and flux through the enterocyte. For compounds with minimal intestinal first-pass metabolism, the P_{eff} calculated with the disappearance from lumen and then appearance into pre-hepatic blood is similar [36]. Moreover, the experimental operation of SPIP is simpler than the intestinal perfusion with plasma sampling.

P_{eff} is the effective intestinal permeability coefficient and commonly used to estimate the extent of absorption, which is proportional to the first-order absorption rate constant, K_a, and weighted with the surface area and the volume of the intestine [37, 38]. The estimation of P_{eff} may be impacted by several factors such as reperfusion flow rates, intestinal radius, intestinal surface area and the time to reach steady-state conditions. In SPIP model, the most widely used estimate for the rat intestinal radius is 0.18 cm/min. It was maintained 0.2 cm/min in the present study and the length of intestine used to estimate P_{eff} is 10 cm, which make consistent of the radius and surface area of intestine. The value of P_{eff} represents the extent and rate of absorption and also be employed to distinguish the transport process of chemical. With the increasing drug concentration in the perfusate, constant or no significant variation of P_{eff} value demonstrates the passive diffusion, a reduction in P_{eff} suggests saturation of carrier-mediated influx, and an increasing P_{eff} values hints saturation of efflux transporters. In this study, the P_{eff} of triptolide, triptonide, and wilforlide at different

concentration are consistent in the duodenum, jejunum, ileum and colon, respectively. Similar conclusion aroused from tripterine, but in duodenum and jejunum, P_{eff} of tripterine has the increasing tendency (p > 0.05). These four components of TW should be absorbed in the rat intestine through passive diffusion primarily or unsaturated carrier-mediated absorption. Furthermore, no obvious difference of P_{eff} was observed between the small intestine and colon.

Conclusions

In the present investigation, four ingredients were employed to reveal the absorption process of TW in the absence or presence of other herbal materials, which help to understand the basic principle of compatibility as action promotion and toxicity neutralization. In general, these interesting chemicals in TW show quicker absorption rate and greater influx extent than the pure ones, which lead to the increased therapeutic effect and the paralleled adverse reaction as well. For triptolide, triptonide and wilforlide, the combinational formulae decreased their absorption. Synergic action was observed in QLTB, which exhibit the most powerful influence. However, intestinal absorption of tripterine with relative therapeutic window was enhanced in the formula of TW-PN indicated PN promoted TW-derived tripterine influx. But in formula of TW-SC, SC still block the absorption process of tripterine. Opposite-direction of PN and SC finally resulted in the different appearance of tripterine absorption through the four intestinal segments in QLTB as increased in duodenum and jejunum, and decreased in ileum and colon.

In summary, herbal compatibility regulates the intestinal absorption characteristics of TW-containing chemicals, which is responsible for the promoting therapeutic effect and reducing toxicity. In the formula QLTB, PN is the key subsidiary component to support the sovereign medicinal to complete the treatment. As shown in this study, one of pivotal mechanism underlying the positive role of PN and QLTB is modulating the absorption process in the intestinal lumen.

Abbreviations

10 cm%ABS: 10 cm intestinal absorption; CS: *Caulis Sinomenii*; QLTB: Qing-Luo Tong-Bi; QC: quality control; P_{eff}: permeability coefficient; P-gp: P-glycoprotein; PN: *Panax notoginseng*; RSD: relative standard deviation; SD: standard deviation; SPIP: single-pass intestinal perfusion; TW: *Tripterygium wilfordii*; UPLC-MS/MS: ultra-performance liquid-chromatography tandem mass spectrometry; ALT: alanine aminotransferase; AST: aspartate aminotransferase; LDH: lactate dehydrogenase.

Authors' contributions
LWG and XPZ conceived and designed the work. QCZ, HTC, YQL, MZL, BYZ collected the data. QCZ analysed and interpreted the data. QCZ, XLZ, DLS drafted the article. HXZ and JAD revised the article. All authors read and approved the final manuscript.

Author details
[1] Jiangsu Collaborative Innovation Center of Chinese Medicinal Resources Industrialization, Nanjing University of Chinese Medicine, Nanjing 210023, China. [2] Jiangsu Key Laboratory for High Technology Research of TCM Formulae, Nanjing University of Chinese Medicine, Nanjing 210023, China. [3] Department of Pharmacology, School of Pharmacy, Nanjing University of Chinese Medicine, Nanjing 210023, China.

Acknowledgements
Not applicable.

Competing interests
The authors declare that they have no competing interests.

Consent for publication
Not applicable.

Funding
This research was financially supported by the National Natural Science Foundation of China (Project Nos. 81573635; 81072749; 30873450; 30873449; 81573869), Projects Funded by Natural Science Foundation of Jiangsu Province (Project Nos. BK 2012855; BY 2012036), A Project Funded by the Innovation Research Team of Nanjing University of Chinese Medicine; A Project Funded by the Six Talent Project in Jiangsu Province and A Project Funded by the Priority Academic Program Development of Jiangsu Higher Education Institutions (PAPD).

References
1. Li Y, Wang J, Xiao Y, et al. A systems pharmacology approach to investigate the mechanisms of action of *Semen Strychni* and *Tripterygium wilfordii* Hook F for treatment of rheumatoid arthritis. J Ethnopharmacol. 2015;175:301–14.
2. Zhang Y, Xu W, Li H, et al. Therapeutic effects of total alkaloids of *Tripterygium wilfordii* Hook f. on collagen-induced arthritis in rats. J Ethnopharmacol. 2013;145:699–705.
3. Li J, Shen F, Guan C, et al. Activation of Nrf2 protects against triptolide-induced hepatotoxicity. PLoS ONE. 2014;9:e100685.
4. Ma J, Dey M, Yang H, et al. Anti-inflammatory and immunosuppressive compounds from *Tripterygium wilfordii*. Phytochemistry. 2007;68:1172–8.
5. Li XX, Du FY, Liu HX, et al. Investigation of the active components in *Tripterygium wilfordii* leading to its acute hepatotoxicity and nephrotoxicity. J Ethnopharmacol. 2015;162:238–43.
6. Zhang B, Zhang Q, Liu M, et al. Increased involvement of *Panax notoginseng* in the mechanism of decreased hepatotoxicity induced by *Tripterygium wilfordii* in rats. J Ethnopharmacol. 2016;185:243–54.
7. Liang XL, Liao ZG, Zhu JY, et al. The absorption characterization effects and mechanism of *Radix Angelicae dahuricae* extracts on baicalin in *Radix Scutellariae* using in vivo and in vitro absorption models. J Ethnopharmacol. 2012;139:52–7.
8. Fagerholm U, Lindahl A, Lennernas H. Regional intestinal permeability in rats of compounds with different physicochemical properties and transport mechanisms. J Pharm Pharmacol. 1997;49:687–90.
9. Fagerholm U, Johansson M, Lennernas H. Comparison between permeability coefficients in rat and human jejunum. Pharm Res. 1996;13:1336–42.
10. Salphati L, Childers K, Pan L, et al. Evaluation of a single-pass intestinal-perfusion method in rat for the prediction of absorption in man. J Pharm Pharmacol. 2001;53:1007–13.
11. Nie SF, Pan WS, Yang XG, et al. Evaluation of gravimetry in the rat single-pass intestinal perfusion technique. Chin J New Drugs. 2005;14:1176–9.
12. Huang SH, Long XY, Yuan F, et al. Transport of puerarin in rat intestine in situ by modified gravimetry and phenol red assay. J Guangdong Pharm Univ. 2012;28:603–7.
13. Varma MV, Obach RS, Rotter C, et al. Physicochemical space for optimum oral bioavailability: contribution of human intestinal absorption and first-pass elimination. J Med Chem. 2010;53:1098–108.
14. Sugano K, Terada K. Rate- and extent-limiting factors of oral drug absorption: theory and applications. J Pharm Sci. 2015;104:2777–88.
15. Lipinski CA, Lombardo F, Dominy BW, et al. Experimental and computational approaches to estimate solubility and permeability in drug discovery and development settings. Adv Drug Deliv Rev. 2001;46:3–26.
16. Oshima T, Miwa H. Gastrointestinal mucosal barrier function and diseases. J Gastroenterol. 2016;51:768–78.
17. Anzai K, Fukagawa K, Iwakiri R, et al. Increased lipid absorption and transport in the small intestine of zucker obese rats. J Clin Biochem Nutr. 2009;45:82–5.
18. Terato K, Hiramatsu Y, Yoshino Y. Studies on iron absorption. II. Transport mechanism of low molecular iron chelate in rat intestine. Am J Dig Dis. 1973;18:129–34.
19. Mahmud F, Jeon OC, Al-Hilal TA, et al. Absorption mechanism of a physical complex of monomeric insulin and deoxycholyl-L-lysyl-methylester in the small intestine. Mol Pharm. 2015;12:1911–20.
20. Zhai L, Shi J, Xu W, et al. Ex vivo and in situ evaluation of 'dispelling-wind' Chinese medicine herb–drugs on intestinal absorption of chlorogenic acid. Phytother Res. 2015;29:1974–81.
21. Dahan A, Amidon GL. MRP2 mediated drug–drug interaction: indomethacin increases sulfasalazine absorption in the small intestine, potentially decreasing its colonic targeting. Int J Pharm. 2010;386:216–20.
22. Hackam DJ. Guts, germs and glucose: understanding the effects of prematurity on the interaction between bacteria and nutrient absorption across the intestine. Br J Nutr. 2012;108:571–3.
23. Martinez-Montano E, Pena E, Viana MT. Intestinal absorption of amino acids in the Pacific bluefin tuna (*Thunnus orientalis*): in vitro lysine–arginine interaction using the everted intestine system. Fish Physiol Biochem. 2013;39:325–34.
24. Hassan IA, Elzubeir EA, El Tinay AH. Growth and apparent absorption of minerals in broiler chicks fed diets with low or high tannin contents. Trop Anim Health Prod. 2003;35:189–96.
25. Mao X, Wu LF, Zhao HJ, et al. Transport of corilagin, gallic acid, and ellagic acid from Fructus phyllanthi tannin fraction in Caco-2 cell monolayers. Evid Based Complement Altern Med. 2016;2016:9205379.
26. Jamroz D, Wiliczkiewicz A, Skorupinska J, et al. Effect of sweet chestnut tannin (SCT) on the performance, microbial status of intestine and histological characteristics of intestine wall in chickens. Br Poult Sci. 2009;50:687–99.
27. He X, Deng FJ, Ge JW, et al. Effects of total saponins of *Panax notoginseng* on immature neuroblasts in the adult olfactory bulb following global cerebral ischemia/reperfusion. Neural Regen Res. 2015;10:1450–6.
28. Kim SW, Kwon HY, Chi DW, et al. Reversal of P-glycoprotein-mediated multidrug resistance by ginsenoside Rg(3). Biochem Pharmacol. 2003;65:75–82.
29. Drescher S, Glaeser H, Murdter T, et al. P-glycoprotein-mediated intestinal and biliary digoxin transport in humans. Clin Pharmacol Ther.

2003;73:223–31.
30. Murakami T, Takano M. Intestinal efflux transporters and drug absorption. Expert Opin Drug Metab Toxicol. 2008;4:923–39.
31. Wacher VJ, Wu CY, Benet LZ. Overlapping substrate specificities and tissue distribution of cytochrome P450 3A and P-glycoprotein: implications for drug delivery and activity in cancer chemotherapy. Mol Carcinog. 1995;13:129–34.
32. Kuze J, Mutoh T, Takenaka T, et al. Evaluation of animal models for intestinal first-pass metabolism of drug candidates to be metabolized by CYP3A enzymes via in vivo and in vitro oxidation of midazolam and triazolam. Xenobiotica. 2013;43:598–606.
33. Schurgers N, Bijdendijk J, Tukker JJ, et al. Comparison of four experimental techniques for studying drug absorption kinetics in the anesthetized rat in situ. J Pharm Sci. 1986;75:117–9.
34. Takara K, Ohnishi N, Horibe S, et al. Expression profiles of drug-metabo-

lizing enzyme CYP3A and drug efflux transporter multidrug resistance 1 subfamily mRNAS in small intestine. Drug Metab Dispos. 2003;31:1235–9.
35. Van Peer E, Verbueken E, Saad M, et al. Ontogeny of CYP3A and P-glycoprotein in the liver and the small intestine of the Gottingen mini-pig: an immunohistochemical evaluation. Basic Clin Pharmacol Toxicol. 2014;114:387–94.
36. Singhal D, Ho NF, Anderson BD. Absorption and intestinal metabolism of purine dideoxynucleosides and an adenosine deaminase-activated prodrug of 2′,3′-dideoxyinosine in the mesenteric vein cannulated rat ileum. J Pharm Sci. 1998;87:569–77.
37. Suarez-Sharp S, Li M, Duan J, et al. Regulatory experience with in vivo in vitro correlations (IVIVC) in new drug applications. AAPS J. 2016;18:1379–90. https://doi.org/10.1208/s12248-016-9966-2.
38. Lu Y, Kim S, Park K. In vitro-in vivo correlation: perspectives on model development. Int J Pharm. 2011;418:142–8.

13

Danggui Buxue Tang, a simple Chinese formula containing Astragali Radix and Angelicae Sinensis Radix, stimulates the expressions of neurotrophic factors in cultured SH-SY5Y cells

Amy G. W. Gong[1,2], Huai Y. Wang[1], Tina T. X. Dong[1,2], Karl W. K. Tsim[1,2] and Y. Z. Zheng[3*]

Abstract

Background: Danggui Buxue Tang (DBT), a phytoestrogen-enriched Chinese herbal formula, serves as dietary supplement in stimulating the "*Blood*" functions of menopausal women. In traditional Chinese medicine (TCM) theory, "*Blood*" has a strong relationship with brain activities. Previous studies supported that some ingredients of DBT possessed neuronal beneficial functions. Therefore, the neurotrophic function and the mechanistic action of DBT were systematically evaluated in cultured human neuroblastoma SH-SY5Y cells.

Methods: The DBT-triggered protein expressions were analyzed by western blotting, while the transcriptional activities of promoters coding for related genes were revealed by luciferase assays. For mechanistic analysis of DBT, Erk1/2 and its inhibitor U0126 were analyzed.

Results: The application of DBT in cultured neuroblastoma cells showed the efficacies in: (1) up-regulation of nerve growth factor (NGF), brain-derived neurotrophic factor (BDNF) and glial cell line-derived neurotrophic factor (GDNF); (2) activation of transcriptional activities of promoters coding for NGF, BDNF, GDNF; (3) activation of Erk1/2 and CREB; and (4) attenuation of the neurotrophic factor expression by the treatment of an Erk1/2 inhibitor.

Conclusions: Our study supports that MAPK/Erk pathway acts as fundamental role in monitoring DBT-induced expression of neurotrophic factors in cultured human neuroblastoma cell. These results shed light in developing the working mechanism of this ancient herbal decoction for its neuronal function.

Keywords: Danggui Buxue Tang, Neuronal functions, SH-SY5Y cells

Background

Danggui Buxue Tang (DBT), a traditional Chinese medicine (TCM) herbal decoction, includes two common herbs, Astragali Radix (AR) and Angelicae Sinensis Radx (ASR) at the weight ratio of 5 parts to 1 part [1, 2]. DBT was recorded in **Neiwaishang Bianhuo Lun** by Li Dongyuan in AD 1247. Traditionally, DBT is utilized in enriching "*Blood*" and nourishing "*Qi*". Today, DBT is suggested to be taken every day as a remedy for symptoms of menopause [3, 4]. Recent studies have revealed the pharmacological properties of DBT both in vivo and in vitro. In various animal models, the administration of DBT have shown effects in (1) enhancing population of red and white blood cells [5]; (2) stimulating estrogenic properties [6]; (3) increasing bone regeneration [7]; (4) triggering immune responses [8]; and (5) inducing formation of capillaries and blood vessels [9]. In parallel, those efficiencies were re-confirmed in cultured cells [3, 4].

*Correspondence: zhengyuzhong@gmail.com
[3] Department of Biology, Hanshan Normal University, Chaozhou 521041, Guangdong, China
Full list of author information is available at the end of the article

AR, one of the most famous raw materials found in TCM herbal formulae, has abundantly amount of flavonoids, which exhibits similar functions to 17-β-estradiol [1, 2]. Formononetin, ononin, calycosin and calycosin-7-O-β-d-glucoside, the predominant bioactive components found within AR, possessed hematopoietic functions by stimulating protein expressions of hypoxia-inducible factor-1α (HIF-1α) and erythropoietin (EPO) in cultures [10]; the combination of these 4 flavonoids increased the hematological parameters in anemia rat models [11]. Besides, several lines of evidence supported the notion that flavonoids could have beneficial effects in human body on distinct aspects, including anti-tumor growth, anti-oxidation and neuronal beneficial functions [12]. Nevertheless, the possible role of flavonoid-enriched DBT decoction in neuronal function has not been illustrated.

Neurogenesis is a crucial turnover mechanism that rescues the number and survival of neurons. Neurogenesis involves neuronal regeneration, neuronal differentiation and synapse formation. The synthesis and secretion of neurotrophic factors, including nerve growth factor (NGF), brain-derived neurotrophic factor (BDNF) and glial cell line-derived neurotrophic factor (GDNF), are one of the major inducers for neurogenesis: these neurotrophic factors could regulate growth, survival and differentiation of neurons [13]. The MAPK/Erk transduction mechanism responding for external stimulations is activated under stressed condition. The inhibition of MAPK/Erk pathway was capable of stimulating oxidative stress and seizure-like activity in brain [14]. Furthermore, U0126, a MEPK/Erk specific inhibitor, was shown to protect primary cortical cultures against oxidative stress triggered by glutamate or hypoxia, suggesting that the activation of MAPK/Erk transduction plays a crucial role in regulating neuroprotection [15]. Here, we aimed at revealing the potential neuroprotection effects of DBT in cultures. A well-studied human neuroblastoma cell line, SH-SY5Y, was employed here to investigate the induction effect of DBT on neurotrophic factor expression as well as the signaling pathways being involved.

Methods

Raw materials and preparation of DBT formula

Three-year-old *Astragalus membranaceus* var. *mongholicus* (AR) and two-year-old *Angelica sinensis* roots (ASR) were collected. The raw materials were qualified according to analysis listed in China Pharmacopeia, and the microscope identifications were carried by Dr. Tina Dong. In order to produce DBT formula, the amounts of ASR and AR were preciously weighed at 1:5. The herbs were mixed well and then boiled twice in water [1, 2]. Before performing biological assay, the water extract was lyophilized and re-suspended in water at final concentration at 100 mg/mL. All the samples were kept at −80 °C.

Fingerprint chromatograms of DBT

An Agilent 1200 series system (Agilent, Santa Clara, CA), supplied with auto-sampler, binary pump, degasser and thermo-stated column compartment, was involved here for chemical fingerprint analysis. Chromatographic conditions were performed on an Agilent, Eclipse Plus, C_{18} column (4.6 × 250 mm, 5 μm). Here, acetonitrile (as Solvent A) and 0. 1% formic acid (as Solvent B) were utilized as mobile phase, the flow rate was kept as 1.0 mL/min at room temperature. In brief, the chromatographic condition of DBT was shown here: 0–10 min, 15% of solvent A; 10–45 min, 15–50% solvent A; 45–50 min, 50% of solvent A; 50–70 min, 50–80% solvent A. All samples were able to pass through 0.45 μm Millipore syringe filter before injecting for analysis, and 10 μL was injected for HPLC. An ELSD detector and a DAD detector at an absorbance of 254 nm were used [2, 16].

Cell culture

SH-SY5Y cells, a human neuroblastoma line, were purchased from American Type Culture Collection (ATCC, Manassas, VA, USA). In brief, cells were supplied with Dulbecco's modified eagle's medium (DMEM) with 10% fetal bovine serum (FBS), 100 units/mL penicillin and streptomycin in 37 °C incubator. DMEM, FBS and penicillin and streptomycin were obtained from Invitrogen Technologies (Carlsbad, CA, USA).

Luciferase assay

Four promoter constructs were purchased from Addgene (Suite, MA), namely pBDNF-Luc, pGDNF-Luc, pNGF-Luc and pCRE-Luc carrying BDNF, GDNF, NGF, and CRE promoter sequences, respectively. Two hundred nanogram of each plasmid was transfected by Lipofectamine 3000 reagent (Invitrogen) in cultured SH-SY5Y cells. Cultured cells were seeded in 24-well plates at 6×10^4 cell/mL, and then added various concentrations of drugs for 2 days. After drug treatment, the medium was aspirated, and PBS was utilized twice for washing cells. Luciferase lysis buffer was stored at 4 °C, containing 0.2% Triton X-100, 1 mM dithiothreitol (DTT) and 100 mM potassium phosphate, was employed here to lyse cell. Centrifugation at 13,200 rpm for 10 min, and then the supernatant was harvested and used to carry out luciferase assay (Tropix Inc., Bedford, MA, USA). Forskolin (FSK) served as a positive control.

Western blot

The phosphorylations of Erk1/2 and CREB were analyzed here by western blot with using specific antibodies.

Serum-starved were at least 3 h of cultured before drug applications. The cultures were collected immediately in 2× lysis buffer (125 mM Tris–HCl, 2% SDS, 10% glycerol, 200 mM 2-mercaptoethanol, pH 6.8) after drug/inhibitor (U0126, 10 μM)/activator (TPA, 100 nM) applications, and the samples were prepared for SDS-PAGE. After transferring, the membranes were incubated with 1: 5,000 dilutions of anti-phospho-Erk1/2 (Upstate, Lake Placid, NY, USA), 1:5000 dilutions of anti-phospho-CREB (Cell Signaling, Danvers, MA, USA) overnight and incubated at cold room. Before adding secondary antibody, TBST should be employed here for washing membranes 4 times, and each time at 10 min. Lastly, 1:5000 dilutions of horseradish peroxidase (HRP)-conjugated anti-rabbit secondary were incubated at 3 h at room temperature, the immune-complexes were observed by the enhanced chemiluminescence (ECL) method (Amersham Biosciences, Piscataway, NJ, USA). The band intensities were compared on an image analyze tool.

The expression levels of NGF, BDNF and GDNF were analyzed by western blot. In brief, cells were seeded onto 6-well plate, and after 2 days of drug/activators (FSK, 10 μM)/blockers (U0126, 10 μM) treatments, the cultures were washed by PBS twice and harvested in high salt lysis buffer (1 M NaCl, 10 mM HEPES, pH 7.5, 1 mM EDTA, 0.5% Triton X-100). After 10 min of centrifugation at 16,100 rpm, supernatant was kept for further step. Equal amount of sample protein was added by 2× lysis buffer and heated at 95 °C before subjecting to SDS-PAGE. The specific antibodies, i.e. anti-GDNF, BDNF and NGF antibodies (Cell Signaling) were incubated with membranes after transferring at 1:1000 dilutions at cold room for 12 h.

Cell viability assay
MTT was employed for revealing cell viability. In brief, cells were seeded in 96-well plate. Drug treatments for 2 days, the final concentration of 0.5 mg/mL of MTT solution was applied into after 2 h durations, the production of purple crystal was dissolved in DMSO. The optimized absorbance was set at 570 nm.

Statistical analysis and other assays
One-way analysis of variance was utilized for statistical tests. Data were expressed as Mean ± SEM, where $n = 4$–5. The highly significant was labeled as (***) where $p < 0.001$, more significant (**) where $p < 0.01$ and significant (*) where $p < 0.05$ compared with corresponding control group without U0126; (^^^) where $p < 0.001$, more significant (^^) where $p < 0.01$ compared with corresponding FSK or DBT group without U0126, respectively. The Minimum Standards of Reporting Checklist (Additional file 1) contains details of the experimental design, and statistics, and resources used in this study.

Results
Chemical standardization of DBT
Chemical standardization is the critical step for ensuring consistency and repeatability of biological experiments. DBT, prepared according to the optimized condition, was guaranteed the quality by chemical standardization [2, 16]. Chromatographic conditions of DBT were carried out by both ELSD and DAD detectors (Additional file 2), as reported previously [2, 16]. By quality control analysis, 1 g of dried DBT herbal extract, a qualified DBT extracts should consists of 809 μg of ASR-derived ferulic acid and 212 μg of Z-ligustilide, 693 μg of AR-generated calycosin and 164 μg of formononetin.

DBT induces neurotrophic factor expressions
The productions of neurotrophic factors, i.e. NGF, BDNF, GDNF, are essential for neuronal survival, growth and differentiation [17]. The deficiencies of neurotrophic factors could lead to malfunction of the nervous system, resulting in various kinds of neurological disorders. We tested both transcriptional activities and protein expressions of NGF, BDNF, and GDNF in cultured SH-SY5Y cells. Forskolin (FSK), an inducer of cAMP, was shown to induce neurite outgrowths and neurotrophic factor productions [18]. Application of 10 μM of FSK in cultures was employed as a positive control, having ~12- , ~10- and ~15-fold of increase in NGF, BDNF and GDNF protein expressions, respectively (Fig. 1). Before performing the bioassay, MTT assay was performed to ensure the maximal concentration of the herbal extract, and the results indicated that the highest concentration of DBT should be less than 1 mg/mL (Data not shown here). DBT extract (0.5 mg/mL) was added onto SH-SY5Y cultures for 2 days, and it could induce the expressions of neurotrophic factors, i.e. NGF at ~4.5-fold, BDNF at ~fourfold and GDNF at ~sixfold (Fig. 1). The activations of Erk1/2 and CREB were proposed to be the predominant mechanisms for production of neurotrophic factors [17]. In line to this notion, the pre-treatment of Erk1/2 inhibitor, U0126, could attenuate the activation of neurotrophic factors, induced by DBT herbal decoction (Fig. 1).

The transcriptional activities of NGF, BDNF and GDNF were also revealed here. The promoter constructs of neurotrophic factors tagged with luciferase, i.e. pNGF-Luc, pBDNG-Luc and pGDNF-Luc, were employed here. In the transfected SH-SY5Y cells, FSK stimulated the transcriptional activities in a concentration-dependent manner. The highest induction was reached at 20 μM, i.e. ~80-fold for BDNF, ~20-fold for GDNF and ~20-fold for NGF (Fig. 2a). In parallel, the application of DBT

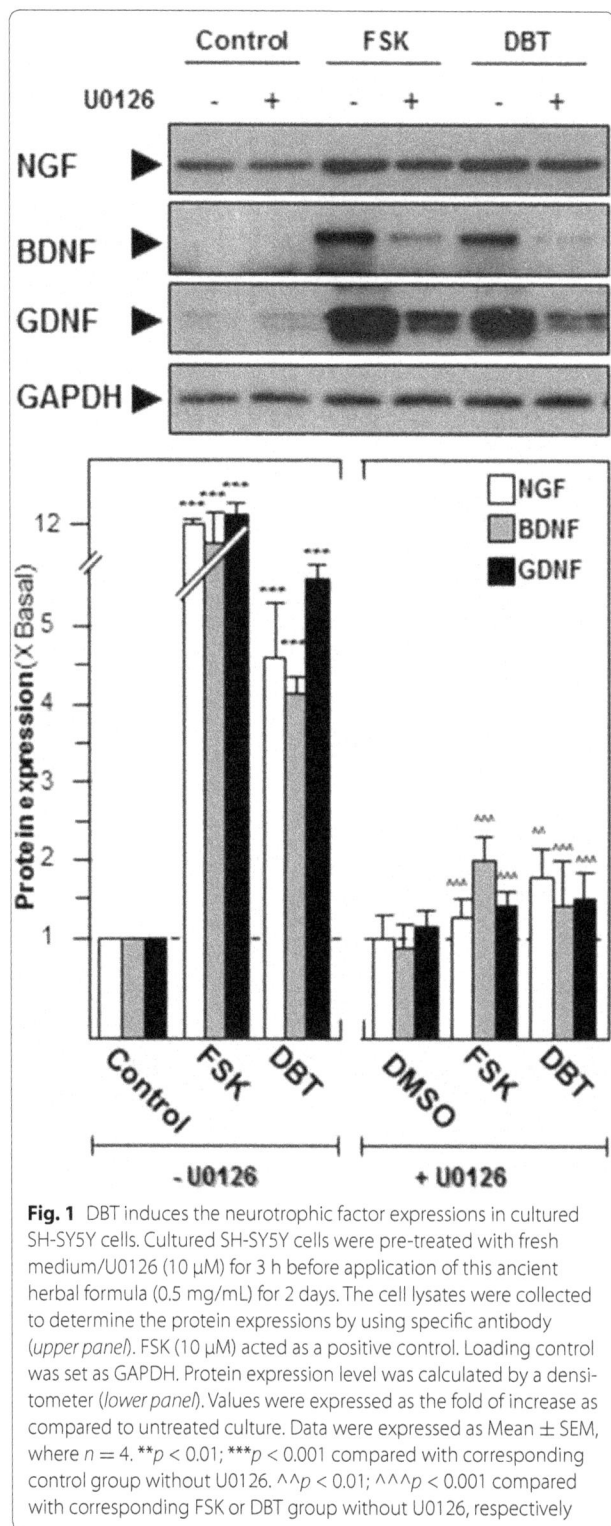

Fig. 1 DBT induces the neurotrophic factor expressions in cultured SH-SY5Y cells. Cultured SH-SY5Y cells were pre-treated with fresh medium/U0126 (10 µM) for 3 h before application of this ancient herbal formula (0.5 mg/mL) for 2 days. The cell lysates were collected to determine the protein expressions by using specific antibody (*upper panel*). FSK (10 µM) acted as a positive control. Loading control was set as GAPDH. Protein expression level was calculated by a densitometer (*lower panel*). Values were expressed as the fold of increase as compared to untreated culture. Data were expressed as Mean ± SEM, where $n = 4$. **$p < 0.01$; ***$p < 0.001$ compared with corresponding control group without U0126. ^^$p < 0.01$; ^^^$p < 0.001$ compared with corresponding FSK or DBT group without U0126, respectively

induced the transcriptional activities of NGF, BDNF and GDNF in a dose-dependent manner; the maximal stimulations were revealed at ~eightfold for NGF, ~3.5-fold for BDNF, ~sixfold for GDNF (Fig. 2b). Again, the

pre-treatment of U0126 suppressed markedly the DBT-induced transcriptional activation of neurotropic factor (Fig. 2b).

DBT induces Erk1/2 and CREB phosphorylation

The stimulations of Erk1/2 and CREB are the predominant mechanism for neurotrophic factor production [17]. In cultured SH-SY5Y cells, application of DBT induced Erk1/2 phosphorylation in a time-dependent manner; the maximal activation was revealed ~13 folds at ~20 min (Fig. 3a). Furthermore, we investigated the downstream signaling of Erk1/2, i.e. the inducer of CREB phosphorylation. Similar to our analysis of Erk1/2 phosphorylation, the treatment of DBT induced CREB phosphorylation in a time-dependent manner: the maximal induction was revealed at 20 min of ~sixfolds of activation (Fig. 3b). TPA, the activator of Erk1/2, and FSK served as a positive control for phosphorylations of Erk1/2 and CREB, respectively (Fig. 3). Here, U0126 was utilized to further specify the cell signaling pathways. In the presence of U0126 (10 µM), the phosphorylations of Erk1/2 and CREB were significantly suppressed in DBT-treated cells (Fig. 4a, b). Moreover, we also tested the transcriptional activity of cyclic AMP responsive element (CRE), a key factor to promote neurogenesis. DBT induced the promoter activation of pCRE-Luc-transfected cells in a concentration-dependent manner with a maximum of ~fivefolds activation at 0.5 mg/mL (Fig. 4c). Nevertheless, the pre-treatment of U0126 significantly attenuated the DBT-stimulated pCRE-Luc transcriptional activities as shown in Fig. 4c.

Discussion

According to TCM theory, the herbal combination was believed to enhance the therapeutic efficacy of single herb via herbal compatibility [19]. Synergistic works among different herbs had been well illustrated in DBT [4]. For example, the boiling AR and ASR together could generate a perfect decoction having the best chemical and biological properties [1, 10]. Traditionally, DBT is prescribed to improve menopausal symptoms [2]. In addition, the efficacies of DBT have been revealed and confirmed in different aspects, i.e. estrogenic effect, bone development, blood enhancement, immune stimulation and cardiovascular function [1, 2, 16]. Here, we proposed a possible function of DBT in the brain.

The neuro-functions of AR and ASR, two herbs making up DBT, had been verified in enhancing memory and in promoting synaptic plasticity [20]. In particular, the flavonoids derived from AR, such as calycosin and formononetin, are regarded as an important and effective constituent within DBT. These flavonoids were shown to be absorbable by cells [10]. Several types of flavonoids

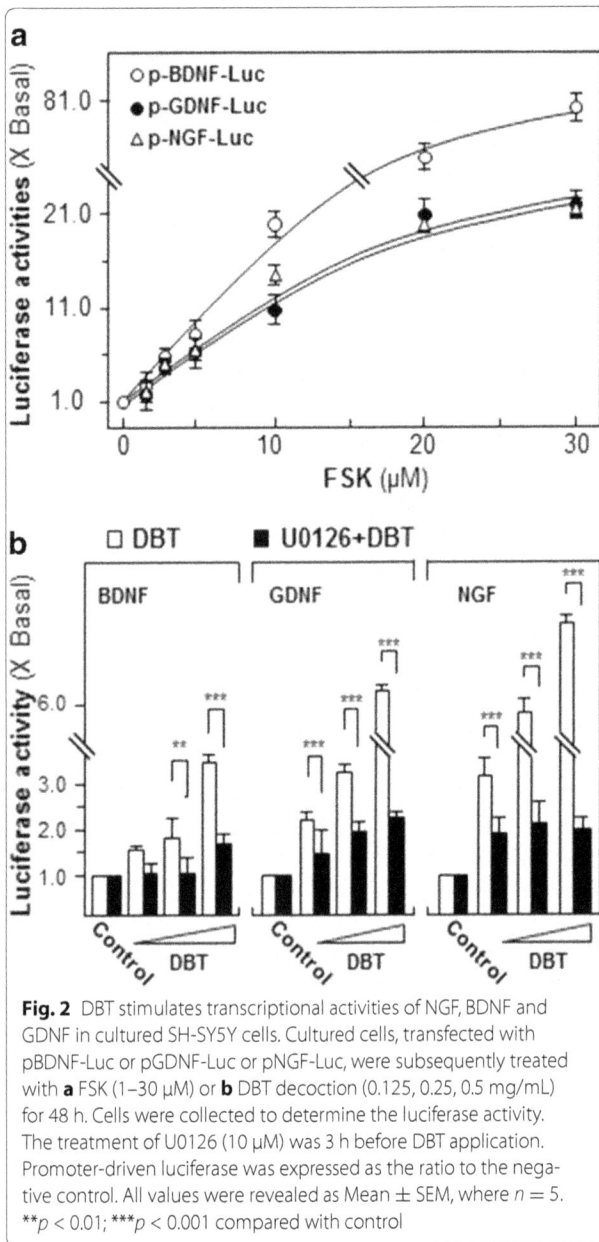

Fig. 2 DBT stimulates transcriptional activities of NGF, BDNF and GDNF in cultured SH-SY5Y cells. Cultured cells, transfected with pBDNF-Luc or pGDNF-Luc or pNGF-Luc, were subsequently treated with **a** FSK (1–30 µM) or **b** DBT decoction (0.125, 0.25, 0.5 mg/mL) for 48 h. Cells were collected to determine the luciferase activity. The treatment of U0126 (10 µM) was 3 h before DBT application. Promoter-driven luciferase was expressed as the ratio to the negative control. All values were revealed as Mean ± SEM, where $n = 5$. **p < 0.01$; ***$p < 0.001$ compared with control

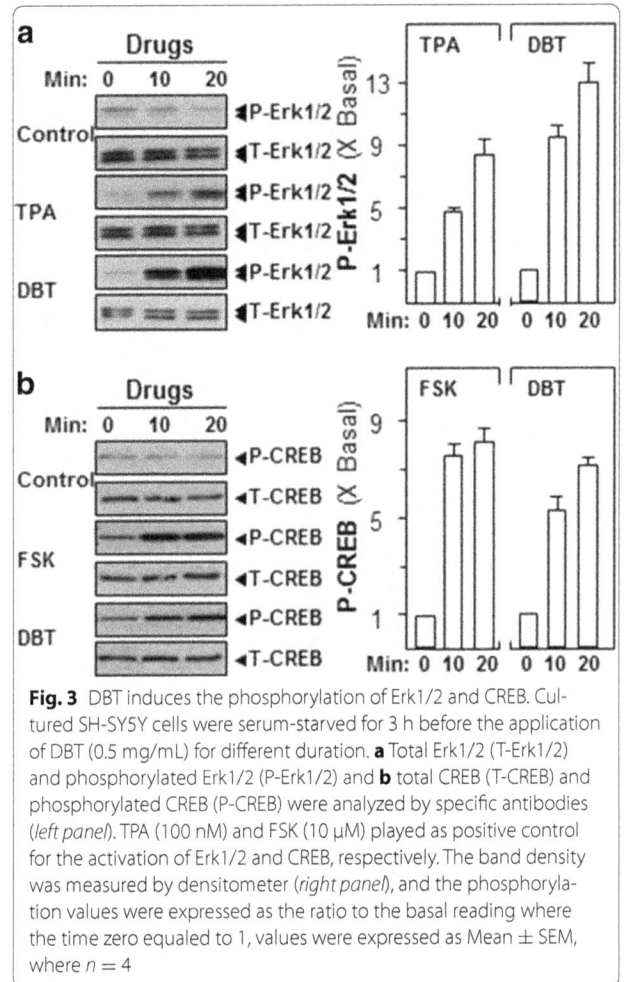

Fig. 3 DBT induces the phosphorylation of Erk1/2 and CREB. Cultured SH-SY5Y cells were serum-starved for 3 h before the application of DBT (0.5 mg/mL) for different duration. **a** Total Erk1/2 (T-Erk1/2) and phosphorylated Erk1/2 (P-Erk1/2) and **b** total CREB (T-CREB) and phosphorylated CREB (P-CREB) were analyzed by specific antibodies (*left panel*). TPA (100 nM) and FSK (10 µM) played as positive control for the activation of Erk1/2 and CREB, respectively. The band density was measured by densitometer (*right panel*), and the phosphorylation values were expressed as the ratio to the basal reading where the time zero equaled to 1, values were expressed as Mean ± SEM, where $n = 4$

are believed to show beneficial effects on neural stem cell for its differentiation and survive. Hesperidin was able to increase survival rate of neural crest cells [20]. Pretreatment of quercetin, a flavonol, was capable to prevent H_2O_2-induced cellular viability [21]. Furthermore, Baicalein, a flavone, was shown to protect neural progenitor cells from irradiation-induced necrotic cell apoptosis by elevating the BDNF-mediated signaling in hippocampus [22]. It also reported that flavonoids, and their known physiologically relevant metabolites, were able to cross the blood–brain barrier using well-established in vitro models, i.e. brain endothelial cell lines and ECV304

monolayers co-cultured with C6 glioma cells [23]. The intake of isoflavonoid-enriched herbal decoction in rat could induce productions of neurotrophic factors, and subsequently the decoction rescued cognitive impairment associated with N-methyl-D-aspartate (NMDA) receptor antagonism [24], promoted hippocampal neurogenesis [25] and attenuated depressive symptoms [26]. Aging and Alzheimer's disease (AD) are characterized by deficiency of learning and memory. The close relationship between AD and aging plays a critical role in elucidating the pathophysiological mechanism in each event, e.g. the involvement of neurotrophic factors in both processes [27]. BDNF is important in neuronal growth and neuronal survival, in particular the effect in synaptic processes of memory. Indeed, a decreased level of proBDNF was shown in mild cognitive impairment (MCI) patients [25]. The intake of NGF in AD patients showed improvements in cognitive functions, as well as a low level of amyloid β in cerebrospinal fluid [28]. Moreover, a reduced level of GDNF led to excess glutamate release

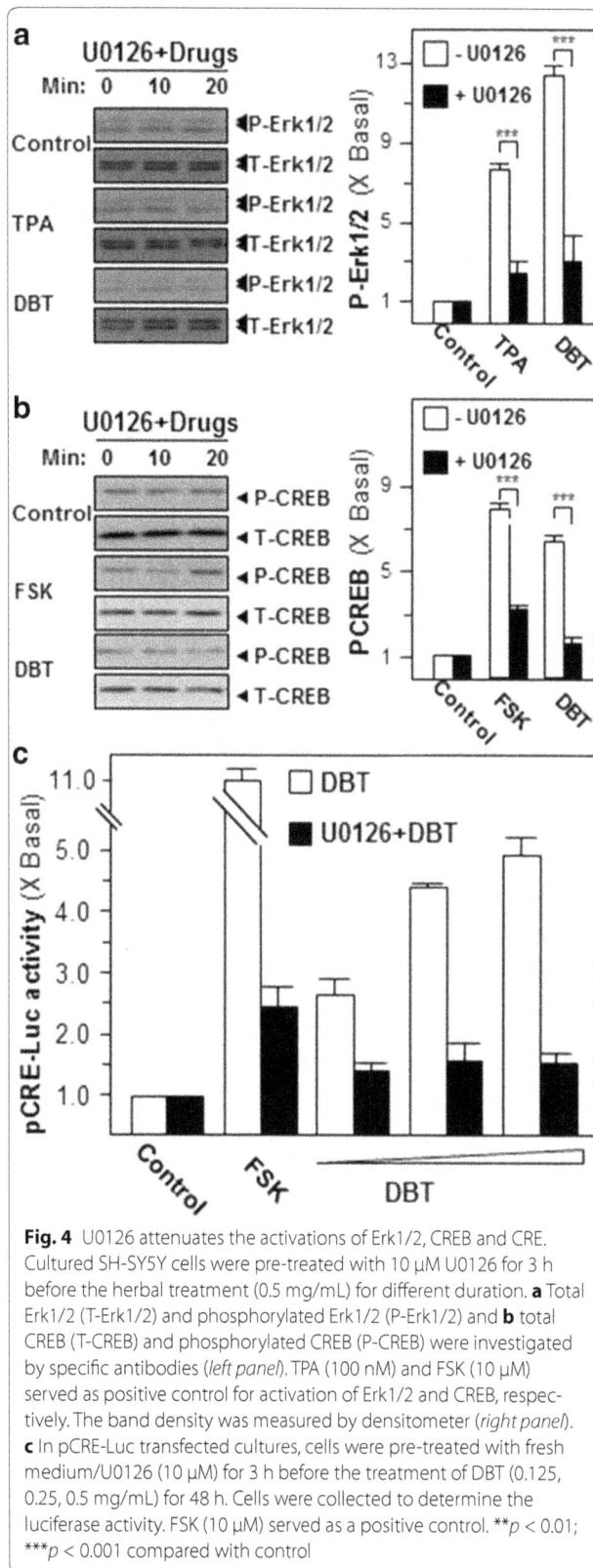

Fig. 4 U0126 attenuates the activations of Erk1/2, CREB and CRE. Cultured SH-SY5Y cells were pre-treated with 10 μM U0126 for 3 h before the herbal treatment (0.5 mg/mL) for different duration. **a** Total Erk1/2 (T-Erk1/2) and phosphorylated Erk1/2 (P-Erk1/2) and **b** total CREB (T-CREB) and phosphorylated CREB (P-CREB) were investigated by specific antibodies (*left panel*). TPA (100 nM) and FSK (10 μM) served as positive control for activation of Erk1/2 and CREB, respectively. The band density was measured by densitometer (*right panel*). **c** In pCRE-Luc transfected cultures, cells were pre-treated with fresh medium/U0126 (10 μM) for 3 h before the treatment of DBT (0.125, 0.25, 0.5 mg/mL) for 48 h. Cells were collected to determine the luciferase activity. FSK (10 μM) served as a positive control. **p < 0.01; ***p < 0.001 compared with control

and deregulation of glutamate transporter-1, which caused the excitotoxicity in nervous system [29].

Neurons are responsible to process and transmit information within human body. MAPK/Erk pathway is a key factor of NMDA receptor signaling transduction in regulating neuronal development, synaptic communications and neuroplasticity. The stimulated MAPK/Erk mechanism is believed to contribute AD pathogenesis via multiple mechanisms, e.g. up-regulation of neuronal apoptosis, transcriptional and translational activations of β- and γ-secretases, and stabilization and phosphorylation of amyloid precursor protein [30]. In fact, the initiation of MAPK/Erk signaling can trigger the activation of cAMP response element binding protein (CREB) [31]. CREB activation is important in gene transcriptions, in particular during the promotion of cell survival [32]. Here, the application of this ancient herbal formula was capable of inducing the activations of Erk and CREB in a time-dependent manner. More importantly, the activations of Erk1/2 and CREB could be blocked by U0126. Thus, we believed that MAPK/Erk might involve in regulating neurotrophic expressions.

Conclusion

We revealed that DBT could up regulate the expressions of neurotrophic factors via MAPK/Erk signaling mechanism. Furthermore, we believed that MAPK/Erk signaling pathway could act as the fundamental role in regulating neuronal functions. Therefore, DBT shed light as health supplements or therapeutic treatments for neurodegenerative diseases, e.g. possible treatment of AD.

Abbreviations

AD: Alzheimer's disease; AR: Astragali Radix; ASR: Angelicae Sinensis Radix; ATCC: American Type Culture Collection; BDNF: brain-derived neurotrophic factor; CRE: cyclic AMP responsive element; DBT: Danggui Buxue Tang; DMEM: Dulbecco's modified Eagle's medium; DTT: dithiothreitol; ECL: enhanced chemiluminescence; FSK: forskolin; GDNF: glial cell line-derived neurotrophic factor; HRP: horseradish peroxidase; MCI: mild cognitive impairment; NGF: nerve growth factor; NMDA: N-methyl-D-aspartate; TCM: traditional Chinese medicine.

Authors' contributions

AGWG designed and performed experiments. HYW and Dong TTXD contributed reagents/materials/analysis. KWKT and YZZ wrote the main manuscript text. All authors reviewed the manuscript. All authors read and approved the final manuscript.

Author details

[1] HKUST Shenzhen Research Institute, Hi-Tech Park, Nanshan, Shenzhen 518000, China. [2] Division of Life Science and Center for Chinese Medicine, The Hong Kong University of Science and Technology, Clear Water Bay, Hong Kong, China. [3] Department of Biology, Hanshan Normal University, Chaozhou 521041, Guangdong, China.

Acknowledgements

Not applicable.

Competing interests

The authors declare that they have no competing interests.

Consent for publication

Not applicable.

Funding

Supported by Hong Kong Research Grants Council Theme-based Research Scheme (T13-607/12R), GRF (662713, M-HKUST604/13), TUYF15SC01, The Hong Kong Jockey Club Charities Trust (HKJCCT12SC01), Foundation of The Awareness of Nature (TAON12SC01), Shenzhen Science and Technology Innovation (JCYJ20160229205726699, JCYJ20160229205812004, JCYJ20160229210027564 and 20170326). NNSF of China (81202907).

References

1. Dong TTX, Zhao KJ, Gao QT, Ji ZN, Zhu TT, Li J, et al. Chemical and biological assessment of a Chinese herbal decoction containing Radix. Astragali and Radix Angelicae Sinensis: determination of drug ratio in having optimized properties. J Agric Food Chem. 2006;54:2767–74.
2. Gong AGW, Li N, Lau KM, Lee PSC, Yan L, Xu ML, et al. Calycosin orchestrates the functions of Danggui Buxue Tang, a Chinese herbal decoction composing of Astragali Radix and Angelica Sinensis Radix: an evaluation by using calycosin-knock out herbal extract. J Ethnopharmacol. 2015;16:150–7.
3. Gao QT, Choi RC, Cheung AW, Zhu JT, Li J, Chu GK, et al. Danggui Buxue Tang—a Chinese herbal decoction activates the phosphorylations of extracellular signal-regulated kinase and estrogen receptor alpha in cultured MCF-7 cells. FEBS Lett. 2007;581:233–40.
4. Lin HQ, Gong AG, Wang HY, Duan R, Dong TT, Zhao KJ, et al. Danggui Buxue Tang (Astragali Radix and Angelicae Sinensis Radix) for menopausal symptoms: a review. J Ethnopharmacol. 2017;199:205–10.
5. Ning L, Chen CX, Jin RM, Wu YP, Zhang HG, Sun CL, et al. Effect of components of dang-gui- bu-xue decoction on hematopenia. Zhongguo Zhong Yao Za Zhi. 2002;27:50–3.
6. Zierau O, Zheng KY, Papke A, Dong TT, Tsim KW, Vollmer G. Functions of Danggui Buxue Tang, a Chinese herbal decoction containing Astragali Radix and Angelicae Sinensis Radix, in uterus and liver are both estrogen receptor-dependent and -independent. Evid Based Complement Alternat Med. 2014. doi:10.1155/2014/438531.
7. Wang WL, Sheu SY, Chen YS, Kao ST, Fu YT, Kuo TF, et al. Enhanced bone tissue regeneration by porous gelatin composites loaded with the Chinese herbal decoction Danggui Buxue Tang. PLoS ONE. 2015;10:e0131999.
8. Yang X, Huang CG, Du SY, Yang SP, Zhang X, Liu JY, et al. Effect of Danggui Buxue Tang on immune-mediated aplastic anemia bone marrow proliferation mice. Phytomedicine. 2014;21:640–6.
9. Lv J, Zhao Z, Chen Y, Wang Q, Tao Y, Yang L, et al. The Chinese herbal decoction Danggui Buxue Tang inhibits angiogenesis in a rat model of liver fibrosis. Evid Based Complement Alternat Med. 2012. doi:10.1155/2012/284963.
10. Zheng KYZ, Choi RC, Guo AJ, Bi CW, Zhu KY, Du CY, et al. The membrane permeability of Astragali Radix-derived formononetin and calycosin is increased by Angelicae Sinensis Radix in Caco-2 cells: a synergistic action of an ancient herbal decoction Danggui Buxue Tang. J Pharm Biomed Anal. 2012;70:671–9.
11. Zhang L, Gong AG, Riaz K, Ho CM, Lin HQ, Dong TT, et al. A novel combination of four flavonoids derived from Astragali Radix relieves the symptoms of cyclophosphamide-induced anemic rats. FEBS Open Bio. 2017;7:318–23.
12. Xu SL, Zhu KY, Bi CW, Yan L, Men SW, Dong TT, et al. Flavonoids, derived from traditional Chinese medicines, show roles in the differentiation of neurons: possible targets in developing health food products. Birth Defects Res C Embryo Today. 2013;99:292–9.
13. Espinet C, Gonzalo H, Fleitas C, Menal MJ, Egea J. Oxidative stress and neurodegenerative diseases: a neurotrophic approach. Curr Drug Targets. 2015;16:20–30.
14. Murray B, Alessandrini A, Cole AJ, Yee AG, Furshpan EJ. Inhibition of the p44/42 MAP kinase pathway protects hippocampal neurons in a cell-culture model of seizure activity. Proc Natl Acad Sci. 1998;95:11975–80.
15. Satoh T, Nakatsuka D, Watanabe Y, Nagata I, Kikuchi H, Namura S. Neuroprotection by MAPK/ERK kinase inhibition with U0126 against oxidative stress in a mouse neuronal cell line and rat primary cultured cortical neurons. Neurosci Lett. 2000;288:163–6.
16. Gong AG, Lau KM, Xu ML, Lin HQ, Dong TT, Zheng KY, et al. The estrogenic properties of Danggui Buxue Tang, a Chinese herbal decoction, are triggered predominantly by calycosin in MCF-7 cells. J Ethnopharmacol. 2016;189:81–9.
17. Yang Q, Feng B, Zhang K, Guo YY, Liu SB, Wu YM, et al. Excessive astrocyte-derived neurotrophin-3 contributes to the abnormal neuronal dendritic development in a mouse model of fragile X syndrome. PLoS Genet. 2012;8:e1003172.
18. Yan L, Xu SL, Zhu KY, Lam KY, Xin G, Maiwulanjiang M, et al. Optimizing the compatibility of paired-herb in an ancient Chinese herbal decoction Kai-Xin-San in activating neurofilament expression in cultured PC12 cells. J Ethnopharmacol. 2015;162:155–62.
19. Pan SY, Chen SB, Dong HG, Yu ZL, Dong JC, Long ZX, et al. New perspectives on Chinese herbal medicine (Zhong-Yao) research and development. Evid Based Complement Alternat Med. 2011. doi:10.1093/ecam/neq056.
20. Tohda C, Tamura T, Matsuyama S, Komatsu K. Promotion of axonal maturation and prevention of memory loss in mice by extracts of *Astragalus mongholicus*. Br J Pharmacol. 2006;149:532–41.
21. Sajad M, Zargan J, Zargar MA, Sharma J, Umar S, Arora R, et al. Quercetin prevents protein nitration and glycolytic block of proliferation in hydrogen peroxide insulted cultured neuronal precursor cells (NPCs): implications on CNS regeneration. Neurotoxicology. 2013;36:24–33.
22. Oh SB, Park HR, Jang YJ, Choi SY, Son TG, Lee J. Baicalein attenuates impaired hippocampal neurogenesis and the neurocognitive deficits induced by ã-ray radiation. Br J Pharmacol. 2013;168:421–31.
23. Youdim KA, Dobbie MS, Kuhnle G, Proteggente AR, Abbott NJ, Rice-Evans C. Interaction between flavonoids and the blood–brain barrier: in vitro studies. J Neurochem. 2003;85:180–92.
24. Guo X, Chen ZH, Wang HL, Liu ZC, Wang XP, Zhou BH, et al. WSKY, a traditional Chinese decoction, rescues cognitive impairment associated with NMDA receptor antagonism by enhancing BDNF/ERK/CREB signaling. Mol Med Rep. 2015;11:2927–34.
25. An L, Zhang YZ, Yu NJ, Liu XM, Zhao N, Yuan L, et al. The total flavonoids extracted from Xiaobuxin-Tang up-regulate the decreased hippocampal neurogenesis and neurotrophic molecules expression in chronically stressed rats. Prog Neuropsychopharmacol Biol Psychiatry. 2008;32:1484–90.
26. Xing H, Zhang K, Zhang R, Shi H, Bi K, Chen X. Anti-depressant-like effect of the water extract of the fixed combination of *Gardenia jasminoides*, *Citrus aurantium* and *Magnolia officinalis* in a rat model of chronic unpredictable mild stress. Phytomedicine. 2015;22:1178–85.
27. Budni J, Bellettini-Santos T, Mina F, Garcez ML, Zugno AI. The involvement of BDNF, NGF and GDNF in aging and Alzheimer's disease. Aging Dis. 2015;6:331–41.
28. Farrand AQ, Gregory RA, Scofield MD, Helke KL, Boger HA. Effects of aging on glutamate neurotransmission in the substantia nigra of GDNF

heterozygous mice. Neurobiol Aging. 2015;36:1569–76.

29. Ferreira D, Westman E, Eyjolfsdottir H, Almqvist P, Lind G, Linderoth B, et al. Brain changes in Alzheimer's disease patients with implanted encapsulated cells releasing nerve growth factor. J. Alzheimers Dis. 2015;43:1059–72.

30. Kim EK, Choi EJ. Pathological roles of MAPK signaling pathways in human diseases. Biochim Biophys Acta. 2010;1802:396–405.

31. Villalba M, Bockaert J, Journot L. Pituitary adenylate cyclase-activating polypeptide (PACAP-38) protects cerebellar granule neurons from apoptosis by activating the mitogen-activated protein kinase (MAP kinase) pathway. J Neurosci. 1997;17:83–90.

32. Cao R, Lee B, Cho HY, Saklayen S, Obrietan K. Photic regulation of the mTOR signaling pathway in the suprachiasmatic circadian clock. Mol Cell Neurosci. 2008;38:312–24.

14

Effects of Bushen Tianjing Recipe in a rat model of tripterygium glycoside-induced premature ovarian failure

Xiaofeng Xu[1], Yong Tan[2], Guorong Jiang[3], Xuanyi Chen[1*], Rensheng Lai[4], Lurong Zhang[3] and Guoqiang Liang[3]

Abstract

Background: Bushen Tianjing Recipe (BTR) is a traditional Chinese herbal medicine that has been prescribed for premature ovarian failure (POF) for decades in China. Nevertheless, little is known regarding its underlying molecular mechanism. In the present study, we investigated the effects of BTR in a tripterygium glycoside (TG)-induced-POF rat model.

Methods: Three doses of BTR were administered via intragastric gavage to adult female Sprague–Dawley (SD) rats with TG-induced POF. After 15 days of treatment, the estrous cycle was examined by vaginal smear analysis. Serum levels of estradiol, follicle-stimulating hormone, progesterone, and testosterone were measured by radioimmunoassay. Histological analysis and assessment of apoptosis were performed after hematoxylin and eosin staining of ovarian tissue sections. The expression of vascular endothelial growth factor (VEGF), vascular endothelial growth factor receptor 2 (VEGFR2), anti-apoptotic factor Bcl-2, and pro-apoptotic factors Bax and caspase 3 in ovaries of animals was examined by an immunohistochemistry process.

Results: BTR not only reverted an abnormal estrous cycle and decreased the ovary index in POF rats but also improved the abnormal secretion of reproductive hormones associated with POF. In addition, treatment with BTR can protect ovaries from TG-induced damage, induce intraovarian expression of VEGF and VEGFR2, and regulate intraovarian expression of apoptosis-related proteins.

Conclusions: Our results show that BTR is effective in the treatment of TG-induced POF rats. Promotion of angiogenesis and anti-apoptosis are most likely to contribute to the effects of BTR against POF.

Keywords: Bushen Tianjing Recipe, Premature ovarian failure, Tripterygium glycoside, Angiogenesis, Apoptosis

Background

Primary hypogonadism is defined as ovarian insufficiency accompanied by a high serum level of follicle stimulating hormone (FSH). In women, one of the most common forms of primary hypogonadism is premature ovarian failure (POF), which is also known as premature menopause [1]. POF occurs in 1% of all women and in 0.1% of women younger than 30 years [2]. It may be caused by either an increased rate of follicle loss, a decreased number of follicles being formed during ovarian development, or follicles unresponsive to hormonal stimulation [3]. The loss of fertility and the clinical effects of hypoestrogenism are the two significant consequences of POF [4], which are manifested by amenorrhea, elevated gonadotropin levels, and an irregular menstrual cycle [5]. Previous studies have regarded POF as a disease with a heterogenous pathogenic background, and the known etiologic factors of POF include genetic abnormalities, autoimmune disease, and environmental insults, as well as iatrogenic impairment following surgery, radiotherapy, and pharmacotherapy [6, 7].

Management of POF essentially involves hormone replacement therapy (HRT), and infertility treatment.

*Correspondence: chenxuanyi1212@sohu.com
[1] Department of Gynecology, Suzhou Hospital Affiliated to Nanjing University of Chinese Medicine, No. 18 Yangsu Road, Gusu District, Suzhou 215009, Jiangsu Province, China
Full list of author information is available at the end of the article

HRT can compensate for the estrogen deficiency in POF patients, consequently relieving their menopausal symptoms [8, 9]. However, concerns have been raised regarding this therapy due to the increased risk of breast cancer, heart attack, and stroke [7]. Therefore, HRT is usually a last resort for POF and the lowest dose for the shortest period of time should be employed [10]. Infertility is a significant issue for most patients suffering from POF. Recently, a number of treatment regimens, including clomiphene, gonadotropins, gonadotropin-releasing hormone (GnRH) agonists, and immunosuppressants, have been used clinically with the aim of restoring fertility [11, 12]. However, these treatment approaches have limited success in improving the likelihood of conception as well as ameliorating menopausal symptoms [13]. Thus, there is still an increasing demand for novel and effective therapeutics for POF.

In recent years, Traditional Chinese Medicine (TCM) has attracted significant attention for the management of female reproductive dysfunctions due to its efficacy, safety, and low cost [14–18]. Bushen Tianjing Recipe (BTR) is a traditional Chinese herbal medicine that has been prescribed for female reproductive disorders including POF for decades in China. Recently, several clinical studies demonstrated the clinical efficacy of BTR. For example, Liang et al. [19] reported that in patients undergoing in vitro fertilization-embryo transfer (IVF-ET), administration of BTR could enhance the quality of oocytes, and increase the sensitivity of ovarian follicles to exogenous gonadotropins. In another randomized clinical trial, the combination of BTR and HRT showed significant therapeutic effects in patients with POF, which was manifested by substantial improvements in clinical symptoms, menstrual states, and serum sex hormones levels [20]. Taken together, these findings provide a rationale for implicating the therapeutic use of BTR in the treatment of POF and other female reproductive disorders. Nevertheless, little is known regarding the underlying molecular mechanism.

BTR contains four components, *Rehmanniae Radix Praeparata*, *Paeoniae Radix Alba*, *Testudinis Carapax et Plastrum*, and *Corni Fructus*. In vitro and in vivo studies have revealed that the major bioactive compounds isolated from these components have ovarian failure-resistant effects or pharmacological activities against gynaecological disorders [21, 22]. More importantly, pro-angiogenic and anti-apoptotic signaling cascades have been implicated in the bioactivities of these compounds [23–26]. Therefore, we hypothesized that the effect of BTR against POF may be mediated through pro-angiogenic and anti-apoptotic mechanisms. To validate this hypothesis, in the present study, we investigated the effects of BTR as well as the underling mechanisms in a tripterygium glycoside (TG)-induced POF rat model.

Methods

The Minimum Standards of Reporting Checklist (Additional file 1) contains details of the experimental design, and statistics, and resources used in this study.

Chemicals and reagents

BTR was provided by Suzhou Chunhui Traditional Chinese Herbal Medicine Factory (Suzhou, China). The components of BTR and their amounts are listed in Table 1. The preparation process of BTR was as described in the following.

All components were mixed in proportion and then decocted with an eightfold quantity of water (volume/weight) twice, for 1.5 h each time. The resultant decoction was filtrated, combined, and concentrated to a relative density of 1.2 g/ml (at 60 °C) under vacuum. The concentrated decoction (i.e., BTR) was stored at 4 °C for future use. According to the Pharmacopoeia of the People's Republic of China (2010 edition) and the Quality Specifications of Chinese Traditional Medicine of Jiangsu Province, high performance liquid chromatogram (HPLC) and thin-layer chromatography (TLC) methods were employed to control the quality of BTR (Table 2; Additional file 2: Figures S1–S4, Table S1).

TG tablets (10 mg) were purchased from Hunan Qianjin Xieli Pharmaceutics Co., Ltd. (Batch No.: 20090102, Zhuzhou, China) and dissolved in sterile distilled water to yield a 50 mg/ml solution. Immunoradioassay kits for rat estradiol (E2) (Catalog No.: B05JFB), progesterone (P) (Catalog No.: B08JFB), FSH (Catalog No.: B03TFB), and testosterone (T) (Catalog No.: B10TLB) were obtained from Beijing Beifang Medical & Bioengineering Co., Ltd. (Beijing, China). Immunohistochemistry (IHC)

Table 1 The components of Bushen Tianjing Recipe

Components	Chinese name	Origin	Amount used (g)
Rehmanniae Radix Praeparata	Shu Di Huang	*Rehmannia glutinosa*	10
Testudinis Carapax et Plastrum	Gui Jia	*Chinemys reevesii*	10
Paeoniae Radix Alba	Bai Shao	*Paeonia lactiflora*	10
Corni Fructus	Shan Yu Rou	*Cornus officinalis*	10

Table 2 Quality evaluation of BTR

Major constituents	Method of determination	Quality specifications
Catalpol	HPLC	>50 mg per 10 g BTR
Paeoniflorin	HPLC	>0.2 g per 10 g BTR
Morroniside	HPLC	>50 mg per 10 g BTR
Testudinis Carapax et Plastrum	TLC	Arginine contained

HPLC high performance liquid chromatogram, *TLC* thin-layer chromatography

Table 3 Drug dose and administration schedule for each group of animals

Group	Drug dose and administration schedule
Control	4 ml 0.9% saline twice daily (9:00 a.m. and 3:00 p.m.), i.g., for 15 days
POF model	TG at 50 mg/kg, i.g. at 9:00 a.m. plus 4 ml 0.9% saline, i.g. at 3:00 p.m., for 15 days
BTR-low	TG at 50 mg/kg, i.g. at 9:00 a.m. plus BTR at 1.88 g/kg, i.g. at 3:00 p.m., for 15 days
BTR-medium	TG at 50 mg/kg, i.g. at 9:00 a.m. plus BTR at 3.75 g/kg, i.g. at 3:00 p.m., for 15 days
BTR-high	TG at 50 mg/kg, i.g. at 9:00 a.m. plus BTR at 7.50 g/kg, i.g. at 3:00 p.m., for 15 days

POF premature ovarian failure, *TG* tripterygium glycoside, *BTR* Bushen Tianjing Recipe, *i.g.* intragastric gavage, *AM* in the morning, *PM* in the afternoon

kits for detection of vascular endothelial growth factor (VEGF) (Catalog No.: LYM00952) and vascular endothelial growth factor receptor-2 (VEGFR2) (Catalog No.: LYM00761) were obtained from Lanzhou Yijian Medical Co., Ltd. (Lanzhou China). IHC kits for Bax (Catalog No.: BA0315-1), Bcl-2 (Catalog No.: BA0412), and caspase-3 (active form, Catalog No.: BA2142) were provided by Wuhan Boster Bio-engineering Co., Ltd. (Wuhan, China).

Animals and POF induction

The protocol of the animal study was approved by the Animal Ethics Committee of Nanjing University of Traditional Chinese Medicine (Nanjing, China) (Approval No. JSSZUSPF/SQ-11). All animal care and treatment were conducted in strict accordance with institutional guidelines. Adult female Sprague–Dawley (SD) rats (weighing 180–220 g, aged 12 weeks) were purchased from Shanghai Slac Laboratory Animal Technology Co., Ltd. (Shanghai, China) and housed in an air-conditioned facility with a room temperature of 25 ± 1 °C, humidity of $50 \pm 5\%$, and a 12-h light/dark cycle. All animals were supplied with food and water ad libitum. Prior to experiments, they were allowed to acclimate to the animal facility for 1 week. Then, vaginal smear analysis was performed every day for 10 days to screen 50 animals with normal estrous cycle (defined as 4–6 days in length) as experimental subjects [27]. The screened animals were randomly divided into the following five groups of ten animals each: the control group, the POF model group, the BTR-low group, the BTR-medium group, and the BTR-high group. Drug dosage and administration schedules for each group of animals are summarized in Table 3. The doses of BTR selected for animals were based on human equivalent doses calculated by the method of Reagan-Shaw et al. [28].

Assessment of estrous cycles and sample collection

During the administration period, the estrous cycle of each animal was examined by vaginal smear analysis according to a previously described method [29]. The length of a cycle was determined as the number of days

between two non-consecutive days during which estrus cytology was observed [30]. The length of estrous cycle $\geq$15 days was defined as cessation of cycle. For each animal, the mean length of estrous cycle was calculated when the number of estrous cycles was $\geq$2. After 15 days of administration, animals with estrous cycles (based on vaginal smear analysis) were sacrificed at the proestrus stage (within 1–5 days after the last administration); while those with cessation of cycle were sacrificed on the day after the last administration. Before sacrifice, blood samples were collected from the femoral artery of the animals. After sacrifice, both ovaries were surgically removed and weighed by an electronic balance. The ovary index for each animal was calculated according to the following formula: ovary index = the wet weight of bilateral ovaries (mg)/body weight (g) × 100%.

Measurement of serum levels of E2, FSH, P, and T

For each animal, the serum levels of E2, FSH, P, and T were measured by γ-radioimmunoassay using commercialized immunoradioassay kits (Beijing Beifang Medical & Bioengineering Co., Ltd.) in accordance with the manufacturer's instructions. Each assay was performed in duplicate and the mean vale was calculated.

Histological analysis

For histochemical analysis, the left ovary of each animal was fixed in 4% neutral buffered paraformaldehyde, embedded in paraffin, and sliced into 3–5 µm sections. The sections were then stained with hematoxylin and eosin (H&E) according to standard protocols. Slides were viewed and photographed under 100× magnification using an Olympus BX-51 microscope (Olympus, Tokyo, Japan). For quantitative assessment of apoptosis, five sections were randomly selected for each rat and photographed at 400×. Subsequently, a total of ten non-overlapping high power fields (HPFs) were randomly chosen from these sections for counting the number of apoptotic granulosa cells. The counting was conducted by two independent analysts who were blinded to the treatment assignment, and the average values were recorded. Then, the average value across all HPFs was calculated for each animal.

Immunohistochemical analysis

IHC analysis was conducted to detect expression levels of VEGF, VEGFR2, Bcl-2, Bax, and caspases 3 in ovarian sections from different treatment groups. Briefly, the right ovary of each animal was fixed in 4% neutral buffered paraformaldehyde solution for 2 h. Then, the fixed samples were dehydrated in gradient alcohol solutions, embedded in paraffin, and cut into 3–5 μm sections. Then, IHC staining was performed using commercialized IHC kits according to the manufacturers' instructions. Finally, the sections were visualized with 3,3′-diaminobenzidine (DAB), counterstained using hematoxylin, and photographed at 100×. For an individual rat, the immunoreactivity of VEGF, VEGFR2, Bcl-2, Bax, and caspases 3 was analyzed in ten random HPFs from five sections and scored using a semi-quantitative scoring system for staining intensity as previously described [31]: 0, no staining; 1, weak staining; 2, moderate staining; and 3, strong staining. Scoring was performed by an experienced pathologist who was blinded to the treatment assignment using an automatic IHC image analysis software (https://imagej.nih.gov/ij/plugins/ihc-toolbox/index.html). Then, the median value across all HPFs was calculated for each animal.

Statistical analysis

Statistical analysis was conducted using SPSS 13.0 software (SPSS Inc., Chicago, IL, USA). All continuous data were tested for normal distribution using the D'Agostino-Pearson omnibus test. Data with normal distribution are presented as mean ± standard deviation (SD). Data with skewed distribution are presented as median and interquartile range (IQR, range from the 25th to the 75th percentile). Statistical differences between means were assessed using one-way analysis of variance (ANOVA), followed by Tukey's post hoc multiple comparison tests. Statistical differences between medians were assessed with the nonparametric Kruskal–Wallis test followed by Dunn's post hoc multiple comparison tests. $P < 0.05$ was considered statistically significant.

Results

BTR reverted abnormal estrous cycle and improved the ovary index in a TG-induced POF rat model

During the experiment, one animal in the POF model group died of unknown causes, and its data were discarded from subsequent analyses. First, we examined the estrous cycle and ovary index of the animals from different groups. After 5 days of TG induction, the POF model group showed a decrease in food intake, locomotor activity, and stimulus response, compared to the control group. For the three BTR-treated groups, however, the food intake of the animals remained unchanged, and no abnormal behavior was observed during the entire course of the experiment. Within 15 days of TG induction, the majority of the animals (6 of 9) in the POF model group displayed cessation of the estrous cycle and the rest showed a significantly longer estrous cycle duration than the control animals ($P < 0.0001$) (Fig. 1a). However, this TG-induced abnormality in the estrous cycle was significantly counteracted by BTR in a dose-dependent manner. Specifically, the animals treated with a high dose of BTR displayed similar estrous cycle duration as the control group.

By the end of treatment, anatomical examination of the ovaries was performed and the ovary index was calculated for each animal in all groups. As shown in Fig. 1b, the ovary index in the POF model group was significantly decreased, compared to the control group ($P = 0.012$). However, this TG-induced decrease in the ovary index could be prevented by different concentrations of BTR in a dose-dependent manner. Taken together, these findings indicate that BTR can revert abnormal estrous cycle and improve the ovary index in a TG-induced POF rat model.

Effect of BTR on serum levels of E2, FSH, P, and T in a TG-induced POF model

Under the POF condition, the ovary fails to function normally in response to appropriate gonadotropin stimulation, and thus doesn't produce normal amounts of sex hormones [7]. Previous studies have reported that POF is associated with a decreased serum level of E2 and increased serum levels of P, FSH, and T [32]. We therefore measured serum levels of E2, FSH, P, and T in the animals from different groups to investigate the effect of BTR on secretion of these reproductive hormones. As shown in Table 4, animals in the POF model group showed a dramatically lower serum level of E2 and considerably higher levels of FSH, P, and T compared with the control group. However, these TG-induced changes were significantly prevented by BTR in a dose-dependent manner, suggesting that BTR can improve the abnormal secretion of reproductive hormones associated with POF.

Effect of BTR on primary and maturing follicles as well as luteal function in TG-induced POF model

POF is manifested by a decrease in the number of developing follicles and consequently affects reproductive activity [33]. Therefore, we performed histological

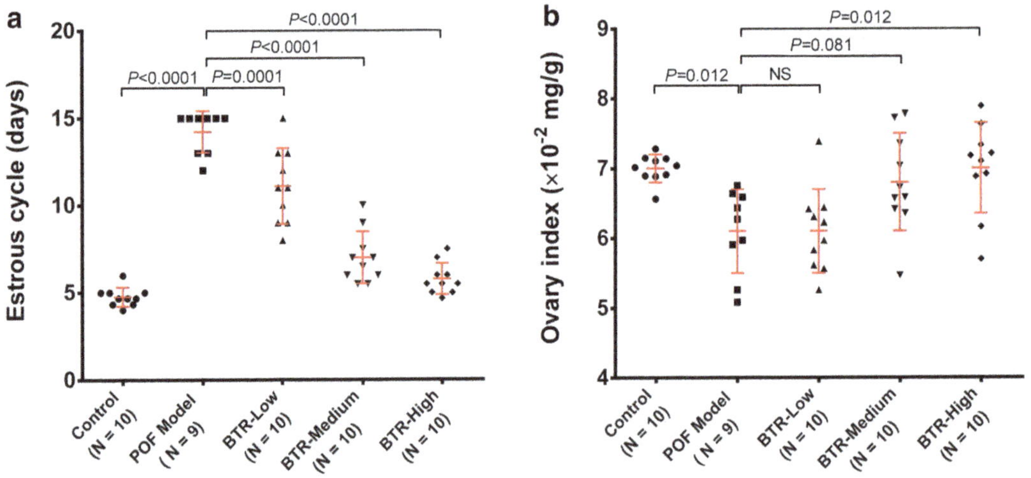

Fig. 1 The length of the estrous cycle (**a**) and ovary index (**b**) in different treatment groups. Each *dot* in **a** and **b** represents the length of estrous cycle during the 15-day administration period and the ovary index at the end of administration for an individual animal, respectively. When the number of estrous cycles ≥ 2, the mean value is presented. *Bars* and *error bars* are means and SD. All statistical analyses were performed using ANOVA followed by Tukey's post hoc test. *NS* not significant

Table 4 Effect of Bushen Tianjing Recipe on serum levels of E2, FSH, P, and T in a TG-induced rat POF model

Group	Number of animals	E2 (pg/ml)[a,b]	FSH (µg/ml)[a,b]	P (ng/ml)[a,b]	T (pg/dl)[a,b]
Control	10	643.9 ± 157.9	2.52 ± 0.59	0.65 ± 0.52	6.97 ± 2.52
POF model	9	355.8 ± 130.6*	8.56 ± 2.13**	0.95 ± 0.21*	21.68 ± 9.61**
BTR-low	10	364.1 ± 79.8	7.85 ± 1.62	0.82 ± 0.18[#]	12.17 ± 3.20[##]
BTR-medium	10	553.1 ± 107.5[##]	3.52 ± 0.75[##]	0.59 ± 0.56[#]	10.60 ± 4.33[##]
BTR-high	10	578.6 ± 129.0[##]	3.57 ± 0.70[##]	0.52 ± 0.15[#]	7.71 ± 1.24[##]

E2 estradiol, *FSH* follicle-stimulating hormone, *P* progesterone, *T* testosterone, *POF* premature ovarian failure, *BTR* Bushen Tianjing Recipe

[a] Data are presented as mean $\pm$ SD

[b] * $P < 0.05$ and ** $P < 0.01$ versus the control group; [#] $P < 0.05$ and [##] $P < 0.01$ versus the POF model group

analyses of ovarian sections to investigate the effect of BTR on primary and growing follicles and luteal function in TG-induced POF model. The H&E stained sections of the control group showed the normal histologic structure of the cortex and medulla with multiple maturing follicles at different stages (Fig. 2a). The corpus luteum could be seen, but neither follicular ovarian cysts nor corpus luteum hematomas were observed. Additionally, no infiltration of inflammatory cells or ovarian fibrosis was found in either the cortex or medulla. In the sections from the POF model group, however, an abnormal histology of the cortex and medulla was observed with a markedly reduced number of primordial and primary follicles, and few developing and mature follicles with degenerated oocytes (Fig. 2b; Additional file 2: Figure S5). In addition, ovarian interstitial fibrosis, as well as regression and necrosis of the corpus luteum accompanied by inflammatory cell infiltration and vessel dilation could be distinguished in the sections. For the three BTR-treated

groups, the sections showed that the TG-induced histopathological changes were significantly alleviated by treatment with BTR (Fig. 2c–e). Specifically, the BTR-medium and -high groups showed almost normal histology comparable to that of the control group.

Effect of BTR on intraovarian expression of VEGF and VEGFR2 in a TG-induced POF rat model

Histologic analyses of the ovarian sections showed morphological changes of vessels in different groups. We therefore performed IHC staining to investigate the effect of BTR on intraovarian expression of two key angiogenic factors, VEGF and VEGFR2, in a TG-induced POF model. As presented in Fig. 3a, samples from the POF model group showed significantly decreased IHC staining intensity, compared to those from the control group; while this decrease was restored by the administration of BTR in a dose-dependent manner. Results of semi-quantitative IHC assessment also confirmed these

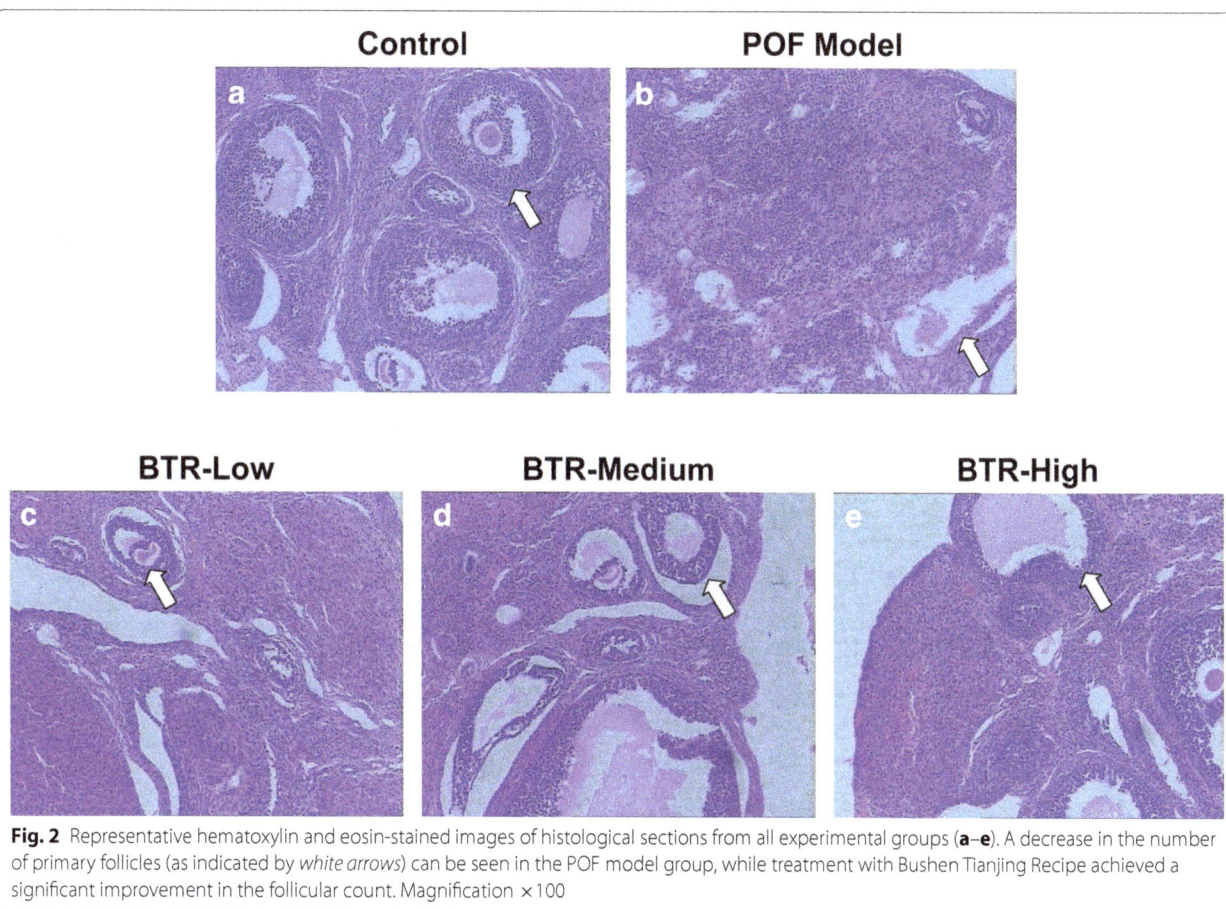

Fig. 2 Representative hematoxylin and eosin-stained images of histological sections from all experimental groups (**a–e**). A decrease in the number of primary follicles (as indicated by *white arrows*) can be seen in the POF model group, while treatment with Bushen Tianjing Recipe achieved a significant improvement in the follicular count. Magnification ×100

findings (Fig. 3b, c). Collectively, these data suggest that TG-induced POF is associated with decreased intraovarian expression of VEGF and VEGFR2, whereas treatment with BTR is able to induce intraovarian expression of both proteins, which may contribute to its effects in TG-induced POF model.

BTR protects granulosa cells from apoptosis in a TG-induced POF rat model

Next, we investigated the protective effect of BTR against apoptosis of granulosa cells in a TG-induced POF rat model. H&E stained ovarian sections from the control group showed that most granulosa cells appeared healthy with no sign of apoptosis (Fig. 4a). In the POF model group, however, some cells were compact and irregularly shaped with smaller and condensed nuclei. In addition, the nuclei of cells in advanced stages of apoptosis were fragmented, resulting in vacuolation and apoptotic bodies. Samples from the BTR-treated groups displayed that the majority of granulosa cells had intact cell membranes and clear nuclei (Fig. 4a), and quantitative analysis indicated that the percentage of apoptotic cells was decreased in all BTR-treated groups, especially in the BTR-high

group (Fig. 4b). These findings suggest that BTR can protect granulosa cells from apoptosis in a TG-induced POF rat model.

In order to further validate the findings of the histological examination, we investigated the effect of BTR on intraovarian expression of several apoptosis-related proteins, Bcl-2, Bax, and caspase-3 in ovarian tissues by IHC staining. As shown in Fig. 5a, samples from the POF model group showed a significantly lower level of Bcl-2 and considerably higher levels of Bax and caspase 3, compared to control ovaries. However, these alterations could be reversed by treatment with BTR in a dose-dependent manner. These findings were also supported by the data of semi-quantitative IHC analysis (Fig. 5b, d), indicating that the effects of BTR treatment may be through regulation of the intraovarian expression of apoptosis-related proteins.

Discussion

POF is a common cause of infertility in women and is characterized by amenorrhea. It is related to the symptoms and metabolic effects of sex steroid deficiency, as well as the emotional sequelae experienced by couples

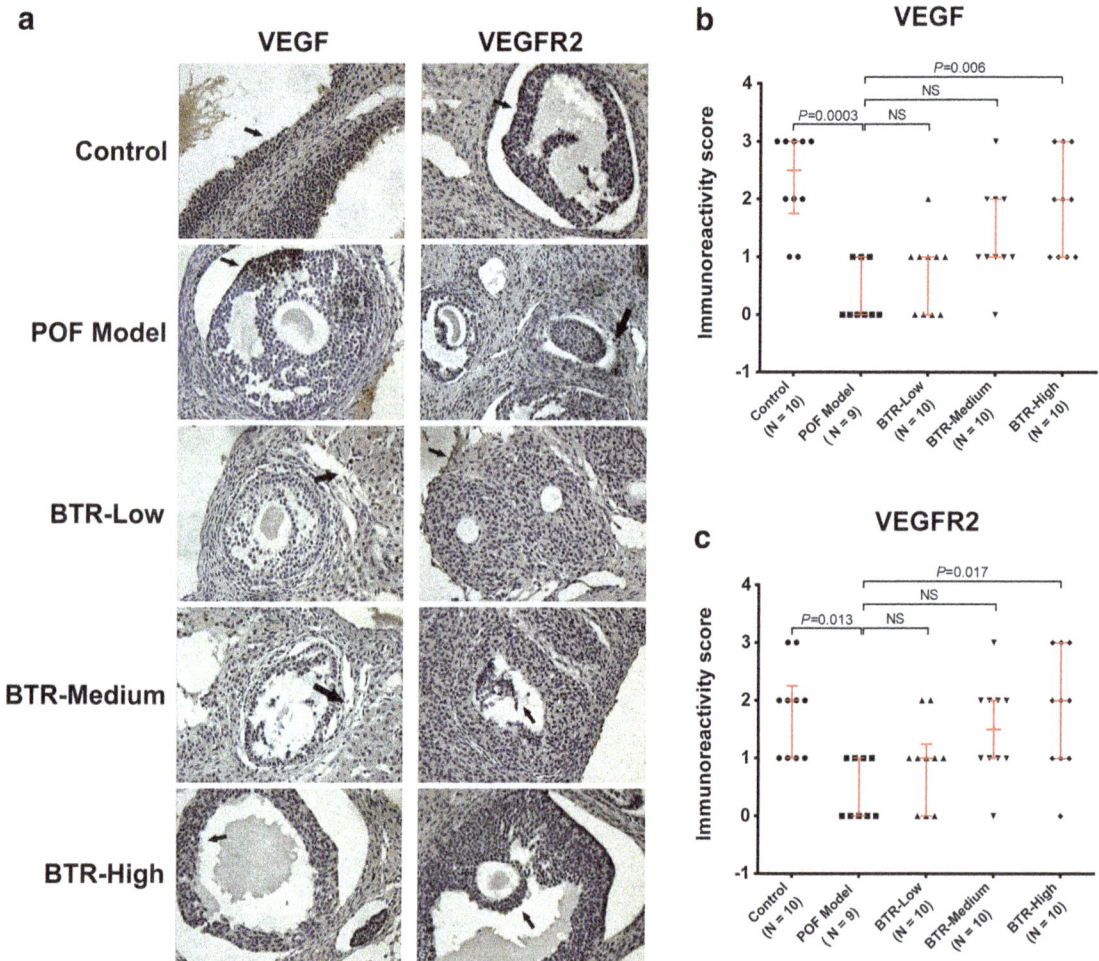

Fig. 3 Representative immunohistochemistry images (**a**) and quantitative analysis (**b, c**) of VEGF and VEGFR2 in histological sections from all experimental groups. Immunostaining (*brown*) are indicated by *black arrows*. For each animal, ten random high power fields (HPFs) from five sections were used for quantitative analysis. Each *dot* in **b** and **c** represents the median value across these HPFs. *Bars* and *error bars* are medians and quartiles, respectively. All statistical analyses were performed using nonparametric Kruskal–Wallis test followed by Dunn's post hoc test. *NS* not significant. Magnification ×100

who have difficulty in conceiving a pregnancy [34]. In addition, POF is associated with risks of cardiovascular disease, osteoporosis, and psychiatric diseases [35–37]. Currently, there are no effective treatments for this disease. Most therapeutic strategies are aimed at relieving the menopausal symptoms, reducing the risk of osteoporosis, and dealing with the loss of fertility [32].

BTR is a TCM formula that has been prescribed by Chinese medicine doctors for decades for the treatment of POF. As compared with other TCM formulas, e.g. Tongmai Dasheng Tablet [38] or Luan-Pao-Prescription [39], BTR only contains four herbs, which may increase safety and reduce treatment cost. In this study, we used a TG-induced POF rat model to investigate the effects of BTR for POF and the underlying mechanisms. TG is

an active component of *Tripterygium wilfordii*, which is widely used to treat autoimmune and inflammatory diseases. However, a long-term use of TG can cause irregular menstruation, amenorrhea and even POF [40]. Therefore, the side effects of TG on female reproductive system can be used to induce a POF animal model. Chen et al. [41] have established a mouse POF model via subcutaneous injection of TG, while TG-induced rat POF model has also been established and widely used for reproductive experimental studies [38, 42]. In the current study, we found that BTR not only reverts an abnormal estrous cycle and a decreased ovary index in this model but also improves the abnormal secretion of reproductive hormones associated with POF. In addition, treatment with BTR can protect ovaries

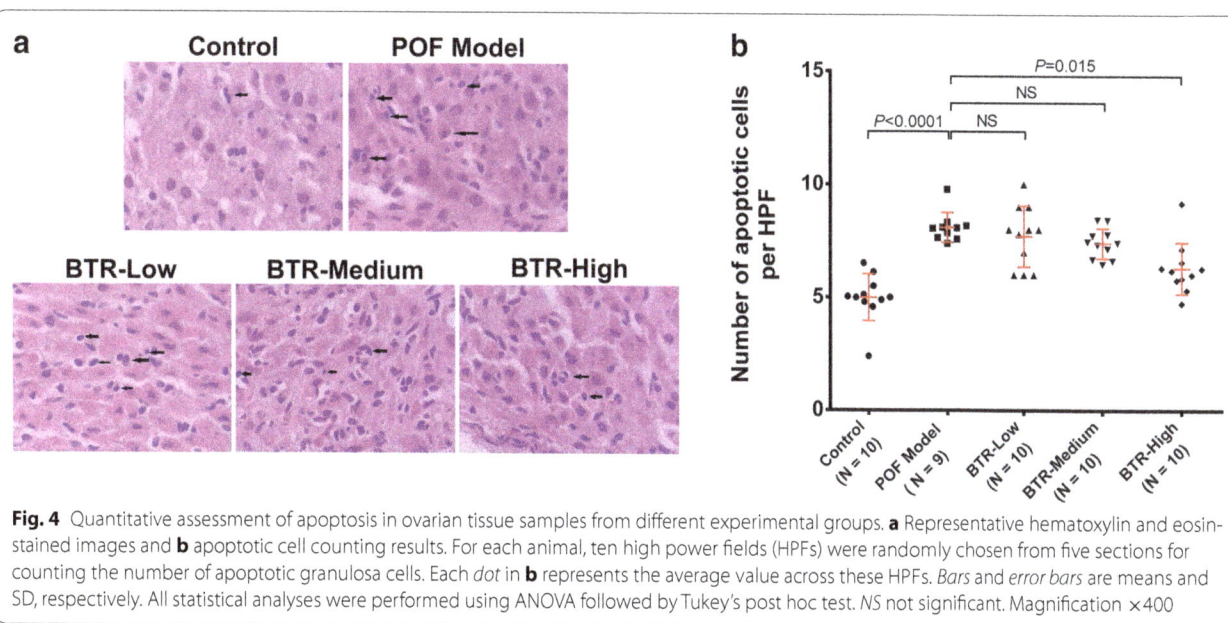

Fig. 4 Quantitative assessment of apoptosis in ovarian tissue samples from different experimental groups. **a** Representative hematoxylin and eosin-stained images and **b** apoptotic cell counting results. For each animal, ten high power fields (HPFs) were randomly chosen from five sections for counting the number of apoptotic granulosa cells. Each *dot* in **b** represents the average value across these HPFs. *Bars* and *error bars* are means and SD, respectively. All statistical analyses were performed using ANOVA followed by Tukey's post hoc test. *NS* not significant. Magnification ×400

from TG-induced damage. Further studies showed that BTR can induce intraovarian expression of VEGF and VEGFR2 and regulate intraovarian expression of apoptosis-related proteins, suggesting that promotion of angiogenesis and anti-apoptosis most likely to contribute to the effects of BTR for POF.

The well-established paradigm of reproduction in mammals holds that the correct formation of the thecal vasculature is necessary to assure a proper nutrition and hormonal supply to the developing follicle [43]. This process involves ovarian angiogenesis and vasculogenesis, which are crucial for folliculogenesis, normal development of the corpus luteum, and maintenance of the function of the mature corpus luteum [44]. When angiogenesis and vasculogenesis are impaired, the ovary becomes hypoxic, which may trigger apoptosis of ovarian cells and follicle atresia, eventually leading to POF [43]. VEGF is considered to be a prime regulator of angiogenesis and vasculogenesis that can induce vascular permeability and promote endothelial cell proliferation, migration, and survival through the interaction with its receptors [45, 46]. The VEGF receptor family consists of three members, VEGFR-1, -2, and -3, of which VEGFR-2 is predominantly involved in mediating the effects of VEGF [47]. Researchers have demonstrated the essential role of VEGF and VEGFR-2 in follicular development, ovulation, and corpus luteum formation [48]. When the intraovarian expression of VEGF and VEGFR-2 is inhibited, follicular development and ovulation may also be suppressed [49]. In this study, TG-induced POF was associated with significantly decreased intraovarian expression of VEGF

and VEGFR-2. However, treatment with BTR restored VEGF and VEGFR-2 levels in a dose-dependent manner. This effect may be due to the angiogenic properties of the active components of BTR.

BTR contains four Chinese medical herbs, of which *Rehmanniae Radix Praeparata* is the major active component; it has been prescribed for wound healing and tissue regeneration in Chinese Traditional Medicine for decades. A recent study has revealed that the aqueous extract of *Rehmanniae Radix Praeparata* is effective in promoting diabetic foot ulcer healing in rats through up-regulation of VEGF expression [23]. Additionally, another component of BTR, *Corni Fructus*, contains active substances such as cornel iridoid glycoside, which can also promote angiogenesis by increasing the expression of VEGF and VEGFR-2 [24]. Therefore, the restoration of VEGF and VEGFR-2 expression by BTR may be attributed to, at least in part, the angiogenic effect of these two herbs.

Previous studies have documented that POF is associated with accelerated follicular atresia, which primarily results from apoptosis of granulosa cells [50, 51]. Apoptosis is a physiological process that maintains the homeostasis of adult tissue. In most adult tissues, the occurrence of apoptosis is proportional to the cell proliferation rate. In the ovary, however, a high rate of follicular cell apoptosis without constant stem cell renewal ultimately leads to reproductive senescence [52]. Under pathological conditions, the balance between pro-apoptotic and anti-apoptotic signals is disrupted, and excessive apoptosis results in ovarian disorders characterized by infertility including polycystic ovary syndrome and POF. Usually,

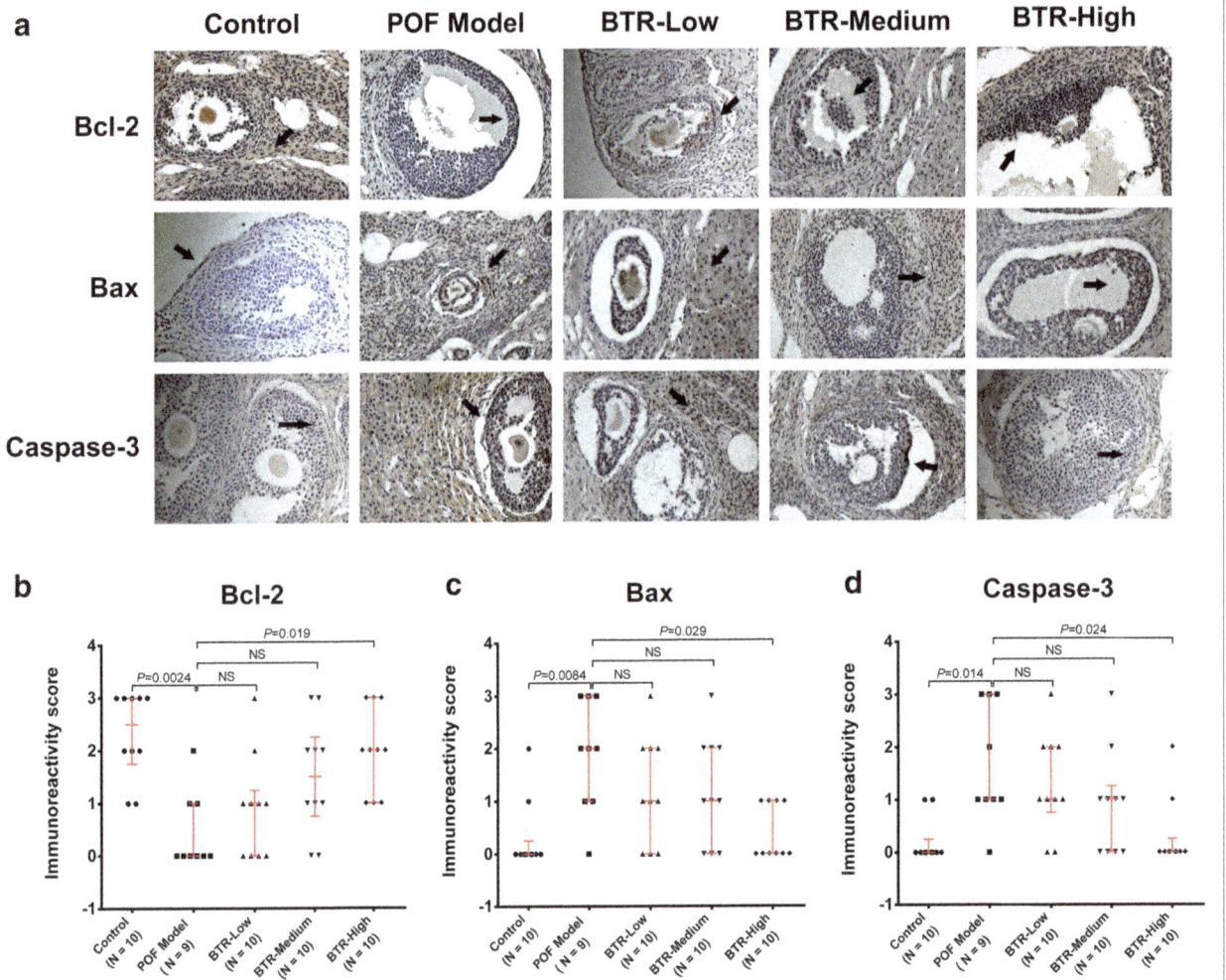

Fig. 5 Representative immunohistochemistry images (**a**) and quantitative analysis (**b**, **c**, **d**) of Bcl-2, Bax, and caspase 3 in histological sections from all experimental groups. Immunostaining (*brown*) are indicated by *black arrows*. For each animal, ten random high power fields (HPFs) from five sections were used for quantitative analysis. Each *dot* in **b** and **c** represents the median value across these HPFs. *Bars* and *error bars* are medians and quartiles, respectively. All statistical analyses were performed using the nonparametric Kruskal–Wallis test followed by Dunn's post hoc test. *NS* not significant. Magnification ×100

apoptosis is a tightly regulated process, which can be initiated via two alternative signaling pathways, the death receptor-mediated "extrinsic apoptotic pathway" and the mitochondrion-mediated "intrinsic apoptotic pathway". The latter is considered to be involved in the POF process [53]. In the mitochondrion-mediated apoptosis pathway, Bax is a pro-apoptotic protein that promotes the release of cytochrome c (Cyt-c) into the cytosol. Following the release, Cyt-c forms a complex with ATP and apoptotic protease activating factor (Apaf-1), subsequently activating caspase 9, and in turn the executioner caspases, including caspase 3. Recent reports have demonstrated that up-regulation of Bax and caspase 3 can be detected in chemotherapy-induced POF animal models [54,

55]. Additionally, as a key anti-apoptotic factor, Bcl-2 is involved in the regulation of caspase activity and its up-regulation can prevent apoptosis of ovarian granulosa cells [56]. In the current study, we found that treatment with BTR could ameliorate TG-induced apoptotic death of ovarian tissues, which was accompanied by down-regulation of Bax and caspase 3 and up-regulation of Bcl-2. This effect may be attributed to the anti-apoptotic activity of the two components of BTR, *Paeoniae Radix Alba* and *Corni Fructus*. Sun et al. [25] found that the aqueous extract of Radix Paeoniae Alba is able to up-regulate Bcl-2 and down-regulate Bax in PC12 cells. Park et al. [26] reported that phenolic compounds isolated from *Corni Fructus* can ameliorates renal damage by reducing renal expression of pro-apoptotic factors such as Bax and Cyt-c. However, as an aqueous extract of four herbs, BTR is of great complexity in ingredients; the major substances responsible for the anti-apoptotic activity and how they exert their signaling functions requires further investigation.

Several limitations should be addressed regarding the current study. First, although TG-induced POF rat model is widely used, it does not fully reflect the pathogenetic process of POF. Therefore, the findings of this study still need to be validated in other POF animal models (e.g. natural aging POF rat model). Second, the results of mechanistic study are still preliminary; additional studies are necessary to elaborate the precise signaling pathways that are involved in the pro-angiogenic and anti-apoptotic effects of BTR. Additionally, it should be noted that there was a great discrepancy with previous literature as to the serum level of E2 in experimental animals [38, 39], which may be due to differences in detection methods or assay kits across the studies. This indicates that the assay of serum E2 level should be carefully optimized in the future.

Conclusion

In summary, the current study shows that BTR is effective for the treatment of TG-induced POF rats. Results of histological and IHC analyses suggest promotion of angiogenesis and anti-apoptosis are the two possible mechanisms accounting for the effects of BTR. These findings provide new insights into the molecular mechanisms whereby BTR improves POF.

Abbreviations

ANOVA: one-way analysis of variance; BTR: Bushen Tianjing Recipe; DAB: 3,3′-diaminobenzidine; E2: estradiol; FSH: follicle-stimulating hormone; GnRH: gonadotropin-releasing hormone; H&E: hematoxylin and eosin; HPFs: high power fields; HRT: hormone replacement therapy; IHC: immunohistochemistry; IQR: interquartile range; P: progesterone; POF: premature ovarian failure; SD: standard deviation; T: testosterone; TCM: Traditional Chinese Medicine; VEGF: vascular endothelial growth factor; VEGFR2: vascular endothelial growth factor receptor 2.

Authors' contributions

XX, YT, GJ, and XC designed the study. XX, YT, and GJ performed the experiments and obtained the data. XX, RL, LZ, and GL performed data analysis. XX, YT, LZ, and GL wrote the manuscript. XC and GJ revised the manuscript. All authors read and approved the final manuscript.

Author details

[1] Department of Gynecology, Suzhou Hospital Affiliated to Nanjing University of Chinese Medicine, No. 18 Yangsu Road, Gusu District, Suzhou 215009, Jiangsu Province, China. [2] Department of Gynecology, The No.1 Clinical Medical College, Nanjing University of Chinese Medicine, No. 138 Xianlin Avenue, Xianlin University City, Nanjing 210046, Jiangsu Province, China. [3] Institute of Traditional Chinese Medicine, Suzhou Hospital Affiliated to Nanjing University of Chinese Medicine, No. 18 Yangsu Road, Gusu District, Suzhou 215009, Jiangsu Province, China. [4] Department of Pathology, Jiangsu Hospital of Traditional Chinese Medicine, No.155 Hanzhong Road, Qinhuai District, Nanjing 210002, Jiangsu Province, China.

Acknowledgements
All authors thank Dr. Robin L. Wulffson for his kind assistance in proofreading this manuscript.

Competing interests
The manufacturer of Bushen Tianjing Recipe did not participate in the study design, data analysis, data interpretation, or writing of the manuscript. The authors declare that they have no competing interests.

Funding
This study was funded by the Graduate Students' Research and Innovation Plan of Jiangsu Provincial Department of Education (No. CX08D-188Z) and the Science and Technology Program of Suzhou Administration of Science and Technology (Nos. SZD0851 and YJS0938).

References
1. Coulam CB, Adamson SC, Annegers JF. Incidence of premature ovarian failure. Obstet Gynecol. 1986;67:604–6.
2. Kokcu A. Premature ovarian failure from current perspective. Gynecol Endocrinol. 2010;26:555–62.
3. Nelson LM. Clinical practice. Primary ovarian insufficiency. N Engl J Med. 2009;360:606–14.
4. Kalantaridou SN, Davis SR, Nelson LM. Premature ovarian failure. Endocrinol Metab Clin N Am. 1998;27:989–1006.
5. Woad KJ, Watkins WJ, Prendergast D, Shelling AN. The genetic basis of premature ovarian failure. Aust N Z J Obstet Gynaecol. 2006;46:242–4.
6. Goswami D, Conway GS. Premature ovarian failure. Hum Reprod Update. 2005;11:391–410.
7. Rebar RW. Premature ovarian failure. Obstet Gynecol. 2009;113:1355–63.
8. Alzubaidi NH, Chapin HL, Vanderhoof VH, Calis KA, Nelson LM. Meeting the needs of young women with secondary amenorrhea and spontaneous premature ovarian failure. Obstet Gynecol. 2002;99:720–5.
9. Welt CK. Primary ovarian insufficiency: a more accurate term for premature ovarian failure. Clin Endocrinol. 2008;68:499–509.
10. Roberts H. Managing the menopause. BMJ. 2007;334:736–41.
11. Wang C, Chen M, Fu F, Huang M. Gonadotropin-releasing hormone analog cotreatment for the preservation of ovarian function during gonadotoxic chemotherapy for breast cancer: a meta-analysis. PLoS ONE. 2013;8:e66360.
12. Badawy A, Elnashar A, El-Ashry M, Shahat M. Gonadotropin-releasing hormone agonists for prevention of chemotherapy-induced ovarian damage: prospective randomized study. Fertil Steril. 2009;91:694–7.
13. Bidet M, Bachelot A, Touraine P. Premature ovarian failure: predictability of intermittent ovarian function and response to ovulation induction agents. Curr Opin Obstet Gynecol. 2008;20:416–20.
14. Beal MW. Women's use of complementary and alternative therapies in reproductive health care. J Nurse Midwifery. 1998;43:224–34.
15. Huang ST, Chen AP. Traditional Chinese medicine and infertility. Curr Opin Obstet Gynecol. 2008;20:211–5.
16. Sze SC, Cheung HP, Ng TB, Zhang ZJ, Wong KL, Wong HK, Hu YM, Yow CM, Tong Y. Effects of Erxian decoction, a Chinese medicinal formulation, on serum lipid profile in a rat model of menopause. Chin Med. 2011;6:40.

17. Mohammad-Alizadeh-Charandabi S, Shahnazi M, Nahaee J, Bayatipayan S. Efficacy of black cohosh (*Cimicifuga racemosa* L.) in treating early symptoms of menopause: a randomized clinical trial. Chin Med. 2013;8:20.

18. Wang S, Tong Y, Ng TB, Lao L, Lam JK, Zhang KY, Zhang ZJ, Sze SC. Network pharmacological identification of active compounds and potential actions of erxian decoction in alleviating menopause-related symptoms. Chin Med. 2015;10:19.

19. Liang Y, Du HL, Chang XF, Zhao SN, Lei LM. Effect of Bushen Tiaojing Recipe on the quality of the oocytes and reproductive hormones in the follicular fluid in IVF-ET patients. Zhongguo Zhong Xi Yi Jie He Za Zhi. 2014;34:911–6.

20. Xu BH, Li MQ, Luo YJ. Treatment of premature ovarian failure patients by Bushen Tiaojing Recipe combined hormone replacement therapy: a clinical observation. Zhongguo Zhong Xi Yi Jie He Za Zhi. 2013;33:1332–5.

21. Wei M, Lu Y, Liu D, Ru W. Ovarian failure-resistant effects of catalpol in aged female rats. Biol Pharm Bull. 2014;37:1444–9.

22. Takeuchi T, Nishii O, Okamura T, Yaginuma T. Effect of paeoniflorin, glycyrrhizin and glycyrrhetic acid on ovarian androgen production. Am J Chin Med. 1991;19:73–8.

23. Lau TW, Lam FF, Lau KM, Chan YW, Lee KM, Sahota DS, Ho YY, Fung KP, Leung PC, Lau CB. Pharmacological investigation on the wound healing effects of Radix Rehmanniae in an animal model of diabetic foot ulcer. J Ethnopharmacol. 2009;123:155–62.

24. Yao RQ, Zhang L, Wang W, Li L. Cornel iridoid glycoside promotes neurogenesis and angiogenesis and improves neurological function after focal cerebral ischemia in rats. Brain Res Bull. 2009;79:69–76.

25. Sun R, Wang K, Wu D, Li X, Ou Y. Protective effect of paeoniflorin against glutamate-induced neurotoxicity in PC12 cells via Bcl-2/Bax signal pathway. Folia Neuropathol. 2012;50:270–6.

26. Park CH, Noh JS, Tanaka T, Yokozawa T. 7-*O*-Galloyl-D-sedoheptulose ameliorates renal damage triggered by reactive oxygen species-sensitive pathway of inflammation and apoptosis. J Pharm Pharmacol. 2012;64:1730–40.

27. Tropp J, Markus EJ. Effects of mild food deprivation on the estrous cycle of rats. Physiol Behav. 2001;73:553–9.

28. Reagan-Shaw S, Nihal M, Ahmad N. Dose translation from animal to human studies revisited. FASEB J. 2008;22:659–61.

29. Westwood FR. The female rat reproductive cycle: a practical histological guide to staging. Toxicol Pathol. 2008;36:375–84.

30. Fraser EJ, Shah NM. Complex chemosensory control of female reproductive behaviors. PLoS ONE. 2014;9:e90368.

31. Bhavina K, Radhika J, Pandian SS. VEGF and eNOS expression in umbilical cord from pregnancy complicated by hypertensive disorder with different severity. Biomed Res Int. 2014;2014:982159.

32. Shelling AN. Premature ovarian failure. Reproduction. 2010;140:633–41.

33. Ebrahimi M, Asbagh FA. Pathogenesis and causes of premature ovarian failure: an update. Int J Fertil Steril. 2011;5:54–65.

34. Kovanci E, Schutt AK. Premature ovarian failure: clinical presentation and treatment. Obstet Gynecol Clin N Am. 2015;42:153–61.

35. Bruning PF, Pit MJ, de Jong-Bakker M, van den Ende A, Hart A, van Enk A. Bone mineral density after adjuvant chemotherapy for premenopausal breast cancer. Br J Cancer. 1990;61:308–10.

36. Carter J, Rowland K, Chi D, Brown C, Abu-Rustum N, Castiel M, Barakat R. Gynecologic cancer treatment and the impact of cancer-related infertility. Gynecol Oncol. 2005;97:90–5.

37. Jeanes H, Newby D, Gray GA. Cardiovascular risk in women: the impact of hormone replacement therapy and prospects for new therapeutic approaches. Expert Opin Pharmacother. 2007;8:279–88.

38. Fu Y, Zhao Z, Wu Y, Wu K, Xu X, Liu Y, Tong C. Therapeutic mechanisms of Tongmai Dasheng Tablet on tripterygium glycosides induced rat model for premature ovarian failure. J Ethnopharmacol. 2012;139:26–33.

39. Jiang B, Sun K, Li M, Wang Y, Zhuang L, Zhang L, Wang Y, Liu X, Wu W, Guan S, et al. Study of Luan-Pao-Prescription on ovarian dysfunction in rats. J Ethnopharmacol. 2012;141:653–8.

40. Chen X, Chen SL. A woman with premature ovarian failure induced by *Tripterygium wilfordii* Hook. f. gives birth to a healthy child. Fertil Steril. 2011;96:e19–21.

41. Chen XY, Gu C, Ma M, Cong Q, Guo T, Ma D, Li B. A mouse model of premature ovarian insufficiency induced by tripterygium glycoside via subcutaneous injection. Int J Clin Exp Pathol. 2014;7:144–51.

42. Su J, Ding L, Cheng J, Yang J, Li X, Yan G, Sun H, Dai J, Hu Y. Transplantation of adipose-derived stem cells combined with collagen scaffolds restores ovarian function in a rat model of premature ovarian insufficiency. Hum Reprod. 2016;31:1075–86.

43. Malamitsi-Puchner A, Sarandakou A, Tziotis J, Stavreus-Evers A, Tzonou A, Landgren BM. Circulating angiogenic factors during periovulation and the luteal phase of normal menstrual cycles. Fertil Steril. 2004;81:1322–7.

44. Stouffer RL, Xu F, Duffy DM. Molecular control of ovulation and luteinization in the primate follicle. Front Biosci. 2007;12:297–307.

45. Araujo VR, Duarte AB, Bruno JB, Pinho Lopes CA, de Figueiredo JR. Importance of vascular endothelial growth factor (VEGF) in ovarian physiology of mammals. Zygote. 2013;21:295–304.

46. Dvorak HF, Nagy JA, Feng D, Brown LF, Dvorak AM. Vascular permeability factor/vascular endothelial growth factor and the significance of microvascular hyperpermeability in angiogenesis. Curr Top Microbiol Immunol. 1999;237:97–132.

47. Lam PM, Haines C. Vascular endothelial growth factor plays more than an angiogenic role in the female reproductive system. Fertil Steril. 2005;84:1775–8.

48. Robinson RS, Woad KJ, Hammond AJ, Laird M, Hunter MG, Mann GE. Angiogenesis and vascular function in the ovary. Reproduction. 2009;138:869–81.

49. Fraser HM. Regulation of the ovarian follicular vasculature. Reprod Biol Endocrinol. 2006;4:18.

50. Fotovati A, Abu-Ali S, Nakayama K, Nakayama KI. Impaired ovarian development and reduced fertility in female mice deficient in Skp2. J Anat. 2011;218:668–77.

51. Zhao XJ, Huang YH, Yu YC, Xin XY. GnRH antagonist cetrorelix inhibits mitochondria-dependent apoptosis triggered by chemotherapy in granulosa cells of rats. Gynecol Oncol. 2010;118:69–75.

52. Hsueh AJ, Billig H, Tsafriri A. Ovarian follicle atresia: a hormonally controlled apoptotic process. Endocr Rev. 1994;15:707–24.

53. Kappeler CJ, Hoyer PB. 4-Vinylcyclohexene diepoxide: a model chemical for ovotoxicity. Syst Biol Reprod Med. 2012;58:57–62.

54. Vujovic S. Aetiology of premature ovarian failure. Menopause Int. 2009;15:72–5.

55. Xia T, Fu Y, Gao H, Zhao Z, Zhao L, Han B. Recovery of ovary function impaired by chemotherapy using Chinese herbal medicine in a rat model. Syst Biol Reprod Med. 2014;60:293–303.

56. Kaipia A, Hsu SY, Hsueh AJ. Expression and function of a proapoptotic Bcl-2 family member Bcl-XL/Bcl-2-associated death promoter (BAD) in rat ovary. Endocrinology. 1997;138:5497–504.

15

Effect of methanol extract of Salviae miltiorrhizae Radix in high-fat diet-induced hyperlipidemic mice

Chiyeon Lim[1†], Sehyun Lim[2†], Byoungho Lee[3], Buyeo Kim[4] and Suin Cho[5*]

Abstract

Background: The dried root of *Salvia miltiorrhiza*, Salviae miltiorrhizae Radix (SR), is one of the most popular medicinal herbs in Asian countries such as China and Korea. In Asian traditional medicine, SR is considered to have a bitter flavor, be slightly cold in nature, and exert therapeutic actions in the heart and liver meridians. Thus, SR has been used to control symptoms related to cardiovascular diseases. Hyperlipidemia is recognized as the main cause of cerebrovascular and heart diseases; consequently, therapeutic strategies for hyperlipidemia have been widely studied. In this study, the effects and molecular targets of methanol extract of SR (SRme) in hyperlipidemic mice were investigated.

Methods: High-fat diet was fed to mice to induce hyperlipidemia, and measurement of blood cholesterol and triglycerides were conducted to evaluate the effect of SRme on hyperlipidemic mice, and gene expression in mice liver was analyzed to identify key molecules which could be potential targets for developing anti-hyperlipidemic herbal medicines.

Results: There was no significant effect on the body weight gain of hyperlipidemic mice, but the triglyceride content in blood was significantly reduced by the administration of SRme to hyperlipidemic mice. Proteins such as minichromosome maintenance (Mcm) family which play a key role in DNA replication were identified as molecular targets in the amelioration of hyperlipidemia.

Conclusions: SRme ameliorated hyperlipidemia in high-fat diet fed mice by inhibiting increase of blood serum level of triglycerides. And several proteins such as Mcm proteins were deduced to be molecular targets in treating hyperlipidemia.

Keywords: Salviae miltiorrhizae Radix, Hyperlipidemia, Cardiovascular diseases

Background

Urbanized living environments and excessive nutritional intake have resulted in the recent increase of various metabolic diseases such as diabetes, hypertension, hyperlipidemia, and cardiovascular diseases [1, 2]. After cancer, cerebrovascular disease and heart disease are the second and third most common causes of death in Korea [3–5].

Hyperlipidemia is recognized as a direct cause of cerebrovascular disease and heart disease; thus, diverse therapeutic strategies for hyperlipidemia have been studied [6]. A direct correlation between diabetes and hyperlipidemia as risk factors has been reported [1, 7, 8]. Indeed, cardiovascular disease is the leading cause of death in diabetic patients, and it is known that 31–34% of diabetic patients also have coronary artery disease [1, 2, 8].

Salviae miltiorrhizae Radix (SR), the dried root of *Salvia miltiorrhiza*, is one of the most popularly used medicinal herbs. Recently, it has received increasing attention for the treatment and prevention of cardiovascular system disorders [9–12]. The major bioactive constituents of SR can be classified into hydrophilic components, such as

*Correspondence: sicho@pusan.ac.kr
†Chiyeon Lim and Sehyun Lim contributed equally to this work
[5] School of Korean Medicine, Yangsan Campus of Pusan National University, Yangsan-si 50612, Republic of Korea
Full list of author information is available at the end of the article

salvianolic acids, and lipophilic components, such as diterpenoid tanshinones [12, 13].

As herbal extracts such as SR contain many kinds of bioactive compounds, and the selection of extraction methods of herbal preparations may affect results of pharmaceutical research of herbal medicines. Thus its extraction process is one of the most important steps in research of herbal resources. Recently, pharmaceutical network studies are conducted to identify the molecular targets which play key role on the effects of herbal medicines. But there are still many unclear data from pharmaceutical network studies due to the diversity of extraction methods on pharmaceutical researches which were used to support the pharmaceutical network studies.

Salviae miltiorrhizae Radix has been reported to affect coronary heart disease [14], ischemia/reperfusion-induced myocardial injury [15], cancer [16], metabolic syndrome [10], Alzheimer's disease [17], and osteoporosis [12]. Several research articles have reported the effects of SR on diet-induced hyperlipidemia in rats; in one study, rats were administered SR extract for 4 weeks, which resulted in a significant decrease in serum lipid levels [18–20]. Recently, we reported the anti-inflammatory and anti-hyperlipidemic effects of SR, which were thought to be mediated through the anti-oxidative effects of the extract [19, 21]. In the above study, we modified a mouse model for hyperlipidemia experimentation, orally administered the herbal extracts mixed with chow for rodents, and determined the appropriate dosages for mice.

As SR exerts various pharmacological activities, it has great potential as a pharmacological agent [12, 15, 18]. In this study, we aimed to confirm the anti-hyperlipidemic effects in mice and to determine the molecular targets of SR.

In order to investigate the effects and the molecular targets of the methanol extract of SR (SRme) in high-fat diet induced hyperlipidemic mice, we monitored changes in body weight and the blood serum contents of total cholesterol, high-density lipoprotein (HDL)-cholesterol, and triglycerides. The extent of accumulation of lipid peroxide owing to lipid metabolism disorder was also evaluated through measurement of malondialdehyde (MDA) level. In addition, after the evaluation of gene expression in hepatic tissues, the target proteins of SRme were identified by using a protein interaction database.

Methods
Animals
Six-week-old male ICR mice (SAMTAKO, Korea), weight 20–25 g, were used for the experiments involving the induction of hyperlipidemia. The mice were adapted to the laboratory environment (room temperature:

24 ± 2 °C; humidity: $55 \pm 5\%$; 12-h light/dark cycle) for a minimum of 1 week with a sufficient supply of solid feed and water. The experimental protocol involving animals was approved by the ethics committee of PNU (Pusan National University; Approval Number PNU-2013-0311). The Minimum Standards of Reporting Checklist (Additional file 1) contains details of the experimental design, statistics, and resources used in this study.

Preparation of SRme
The SR used in this study was purchased from an authorized pharmaceutical company (Gwangmyoung Co., Korea) and authenticated by Dr. Cho (School of Korean Medicine, Pusan National University, Yangsan, Korea). Fingerprinting data of the SR was kindly provided from Gwangmyoung Co., and the data are shown as Additional file 2: Figure S1. A voucher specimen (No. SM14-0611) was deposited in the low temperature room (4 °C) of the laboratory. SR (500 g) was immersed in methanol at room temperature for 5 days; this process was repeated twice and a total of 58.4 g of dry extract was obtained (11.7% yield).

Induction of hyperlipidemia and classification of experimental groups
To induce hyperlipidemia, we fed a high-fat diet to the mice in the control group (HFD) and the SRme-treated group (SRG) for 4 weeks. Mice in the normal group (NOR) were supplied general feed. On the fifth week of the experiment, high-fat diet-fed mice were randomly allocated to HFD and SRG based on body weight. From the fifth week of the experiment, SRG mice, which received a high-fat diet with SRme, and HFD mice, which received a high-fat diet only, were fed for an additional 2 weeks. The rodent chow was custom made by Daol Biotech (Daejeon, Korea). The composition of main ingredients and nutrition facts are given in Tables 1, 2. The schematic design of this study is shown in Fig. 1.

Harvesting liver tissues, preparation for gene expression analysis, and MDA measurement
After the experimental animals were sacrificed, the liver tissue was excised and blood was removed using cold (4 °C) perfusion solution (130 mM NaCl, 5 mM KCl, and 10 mM Tris–HCl, pH 7.4). In order to observe gene expression, total RNA was isolated by using a Qiagen RNeasy Kit (Qiagen Korea Ltd) in accordance with the manufacturer's instructions. An Agilent microarray containing approximately 45,000 oligo-spots (Agilent Technologies Co.) was used for hybridization. In comparison with RNA from NOR mice as a reference, we considered genes that showed a greater than threefold upregulation or downregulation. Gene expression folds based on NOR

Table 1 Experimental groups and compositions of normal and high fat diet

Main ingredients	Diet (g/kg)		
	Normal	High fat	High fat + SRme
Casein	200	200	200
Sucrose	172.8	172.8	172.8
Dextrose	100	100	100
Soybeal oil	–	25	25
Lard[a]	–	177.5	177.5
Cholesterol	–	12.9	12.9
Cholic acid	–	4.3	4.3
SRme	–	–	1

[a] Typical analysis of cholesterol in lard = 0.95 mg/g

Table 2 Gram percentage of main nutrition facts

Compounds	Diet (g%)		
	Normal	High fat	High fat + SRme
Protein	28	28	28
Carbohydrate	25	25	25
Fat	5	24	24
Crude fiber	4	4	4
Mineral mix	5	5	5
Vitamin mix	2	2	2
Water	12	12	12
Total kcal/g	3.5	4.7	4.7

were shown as Additional file 3. Hierarchical clusters of genes were analyzed using a multiple experiment viewer (MeV ver. 4.9, mev.tm4.org) and a functional protein association networks database (STRING, https://string-db.org) was applied for interaction network analysis.

To measure the MDA levels, a Stadie-Riggs microtome (Tomas Co. USA) was used to prepare tissue slices approximately 1-mm wide and 0.3–0.5-mm thick, with a horizontal length and a vertical length of 1 cm each. Phosphoric acid (3 ml) and 0.6% thiobarbituric acid solution were added to the slices and boiled for 60 min. Finally, 1-butanol (4 ml) was added, thoroughly mixed, and centrifuged at $800 \times g$ for 25 min. The absorbance of the supernatant of the mixed solution was measured at 534 and 510 nm.

Blood collection and measurement of blood cholesterol and triglycerides

At the end of the 2-week drug administration period, blood was collected from the mouse abdominal vein. After the collected blood was centrifuged at $5000 \times g$ for 20 min, the supernatant was removed for the measurements of blood cholesterol and triglyceride levels. Serum total cholesterol, HDL-cholesterol, and triglycerides were measured by using measurement kits (FUJIFILM, Japan).

Statistical analysis

To perform the statistical analyses on the experimental material, SigmaPlot ver. 12 (SigmaStat, USA) was used. The experimental results were expressed as the mean ± standard deviation (mean ± SD) and statistical significance between groups was determined by using one-way ANOVA followed by Tukey's post hoc analysis. Values of $P < 0.05$ were considered to be statistically significant.

Results
Effect on body weight

A slight increase in body weight was observed in HFD mice in comparison to that of NOR mice over the 4-week hyperlipidemia induction period, but in the additional

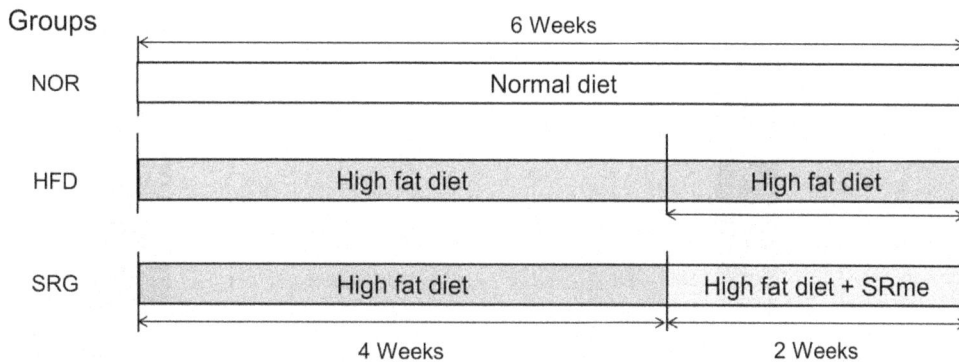

Fig. 1 Design of hyperlipidemia induction. The mice were fed a normal diet or high-fat diet, based on their allocated group, for 6 weeks. SRme mixed with high-fat diet was fed to the mice in the SRme administration group (SRG) for the final 2 weeks. NOR: naive mice (n = 8), HFD: hyperlipidemic mice (n = 8), SRG: SRme-treated hyperlipidemic mice (n = 8)

2-week period, there was no statistically significant difference among the groups (Fig. 2). There was also no difference between the groups in food intake during the experimental periods (data not shown).

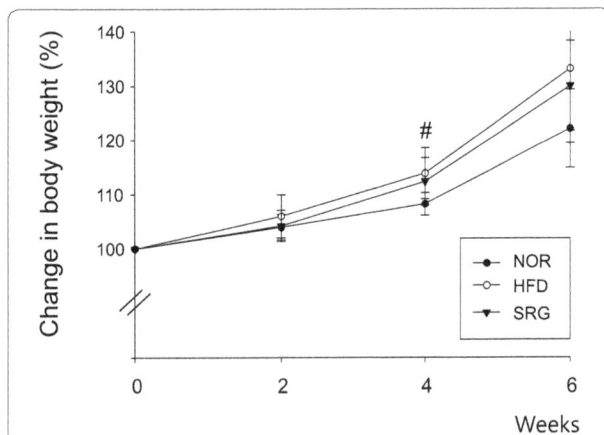

Fig. 2 Effects of SRme on body weight in hyperlipidemic mice. Body weight was measured every 2 weeks. NOR: naive mice (n = 8), HFD: hyperlipidemic mice (n = 8), SRG: SRme-treated hyperlipidemic mice (n = 8). The values are presented as the mean ± SD

Effect on serum lipid content

The total cholesterol content in blood was significantly different between NOR and HFD mice (121.38 ± 16.42 and 162.00 ± 6.09 mg/dl, respectively). However, the total cholesterol content in SRG mice was 142.88 ± 10.80 mg/dl, which was not significantly different from that of HFD mice (Fig. 3a).

The HDL-cholesterol content in mouse blood was not observed to be significantly different in any groups (Fig. 3b).

A statistically significant increase was observed when NOR and HFD mice were compared (83.00 ± 17.56 and 175.88 ± 26.07 mg/dl, respectively). In SRG mice, the value was 117.75 ± 26.26, which was also significantly different from that in HFD mice (Fig. 3c).

Changes in lipid peroxide content in liver tissue

Level of MDA, a lipid peroxide, in mouse liver tissue, showed a significant increase in hyperlipidemic HFD mice in comparison to that in the non-hyperlipidemic NOR mice (188.5 ± 21.3 pmol MDA/mg protein and 112.6 ± 18.3 pmol MDA/mg protein, respectively). However, SRG mice showed no significant change compared with HFD mice (164.6 ± 22.2 pmol MDA/mg protein) (Fig. 4).

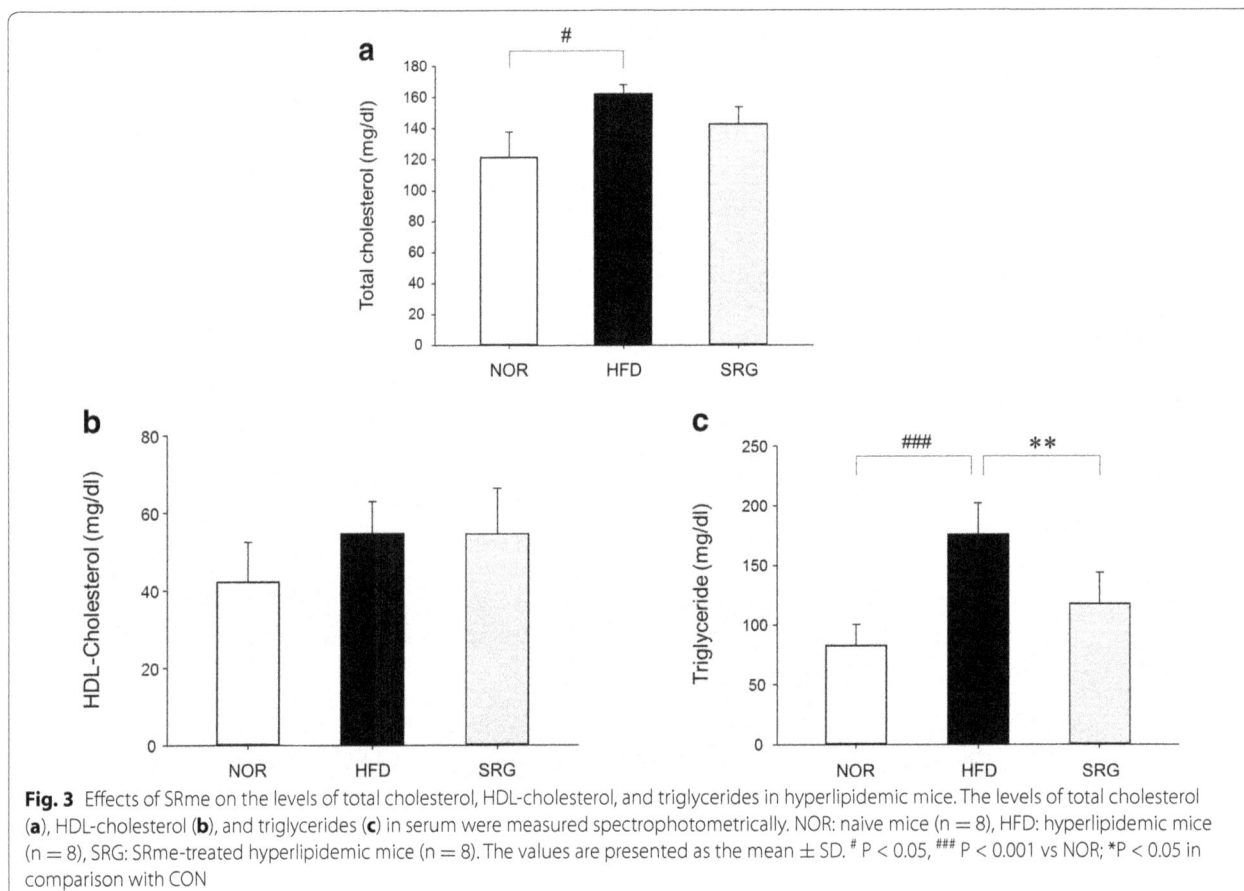

Fig. 3 Effects of SRme on the levels of total cholesterol, HDL-cholesterol, and triglycerides in hyperlipidemic mice. The levels of total cholesterol (**a**), HDL-cholesterol (**b**), and triglycerides (**c**) in serum were measured spectrophotometrically. NOR: naive mice (n = 8), HFD: hyperlipidemic mice (n = 8), SRG: SRme-treated hyperlipidemic mice (n = 8). The values are presented as the mean ± SD. [#] $P < 0.05$, [###] $P < 0.001$ vs NOR; *$P < 0.05$ in comparison with CON

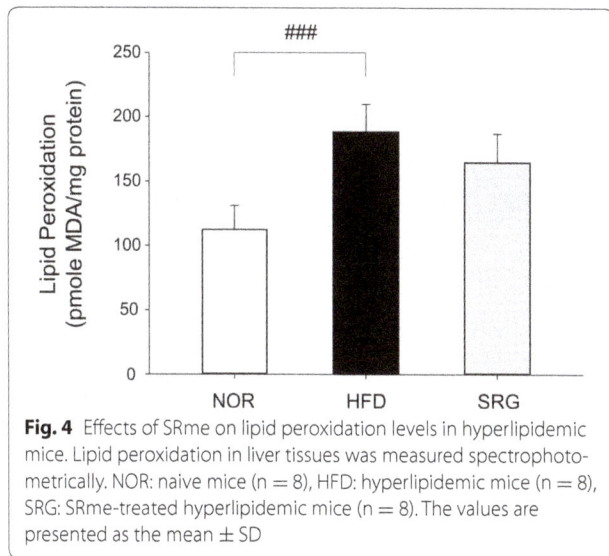

Fig. 4 Effects of SRme on lipid peroxidation levels in hyperlipidemic mice. Lipid peroxidation in liver tissues was measured spectrophotometrically. NOR: naive mice (n = 8), HFD: hyperlipidemic mice (n = 8), SRG: SRme-treated hyperlipidemic mice (n = 8). The values are presented as the mean ± SD

Expression profile of genes

The analysis of the expression pattern of genes in mice liver revealed that a total of 291 genes showed at least threefold change in HFD mice as compared to the values in NOR mice. These changed genes were hierarchically clustered (Additional file 4: Figure S2), as shown in Fig. 5. It is clear that the expression of 291 genes was significantly changed in the livers of hyperlipidemic HFD mice in comparison to that in NOR mice. From the altered genes, we selected 71 genes whose expression was restored by SRme administration, based on hierarchical clustering using MeV software (Fig. 5). The trends in alteration and restoration of the genes are shown in Fig. 6.

By using the STRING database, we assessed functional genomics and explored the predicted interaction networks, which can suggest new directions for future experimental research. In this study, the assessment of 71 genes restored by SRme administration illustrated the changes in pathway activities in liver tissue (Table 3). Pathway analysis suggested that pathways such as DNA replication initiation and DNA helicase activity, and the minichromosome maintenance protein (Mcm) complex had a critical role in the amelioration of hyperlipidemia in mice. Furthermore, the main target proteins with key roles in the aforementioned pathways were identified as Mcm proteins (Fig. 7).

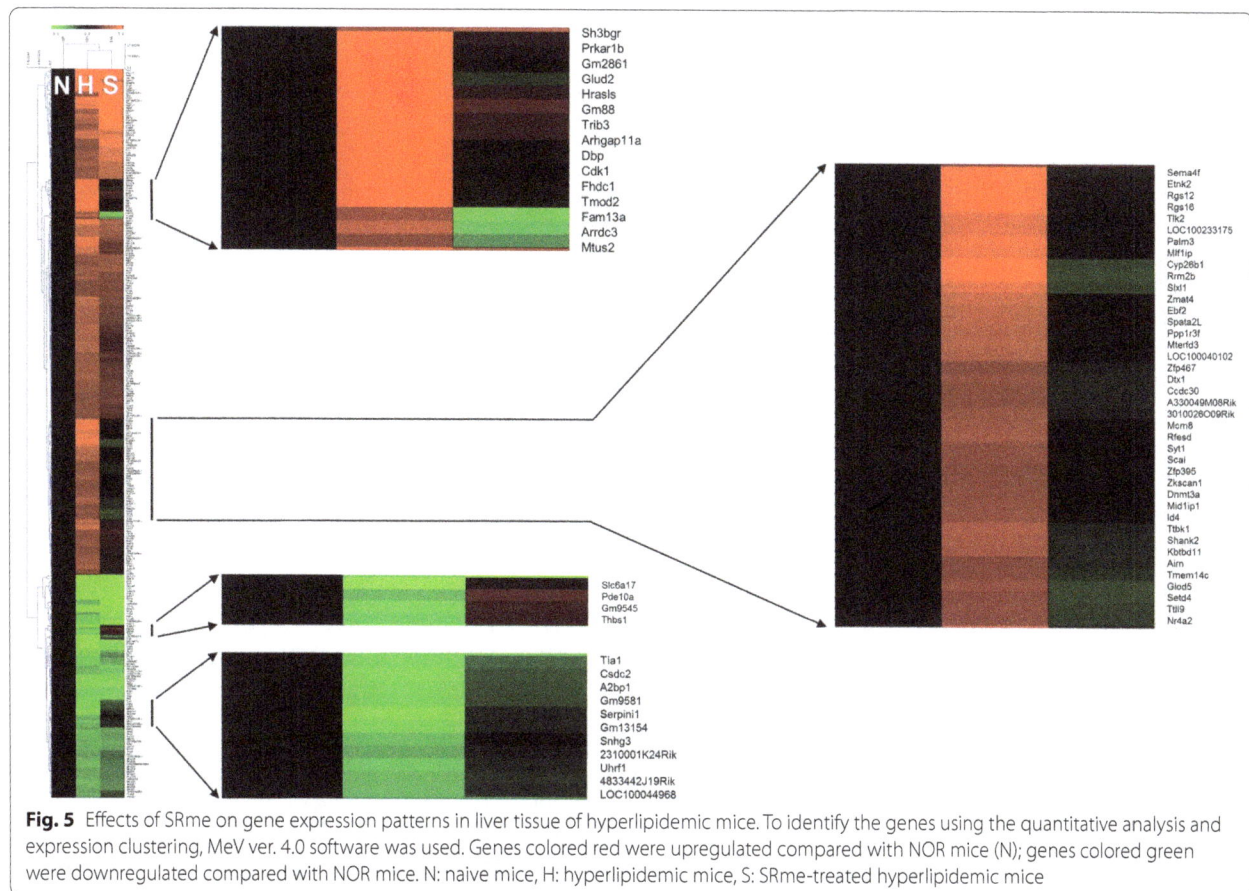

Fig. 5 Effects of SRme on gene expression patterns in liver tissue of hyperlipidemic mice. To identify the genes using the quantitative analysis and expression clustering, MeV ver. 4.0 software was used. Genes colored red were upregulated compared with NOR mice (N); genes colored green were downregulated compared with NOR mice. N: naive mice, H: hyperlipidemic mice, S: SRme-treated hyperlipidemic mice

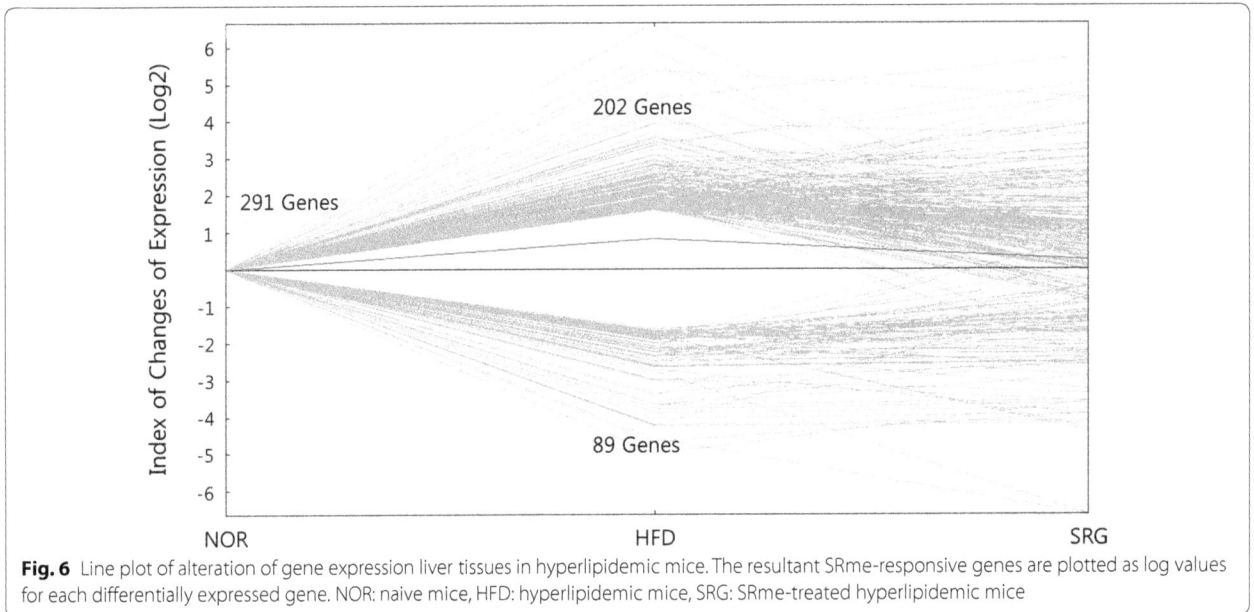

Fig. 6 Line plot of alteration of gene expression liver tissues in hyperlipidemic mice. The resultant SRme-responsive genes are plotted as log values for each differentially expressed gene. NOR: naive mice, HFD: hyperlipidemic mice, SRG: SRme-treated hyperlipidemic mice

Table 3 Functional enrichments in protein network

Pathway ID	Pathway description	Count in gene set	False discovery rate
Biological process (GO)			
GO:0006270	DNA replication initiation	4	0.00262
GO:0006268	DNA unwinding involved in DNA replication	3	0.0227
Molecular function (GO)			
GO:0003678	DNA helicase activity	4	0.00299
GO:0004386	Helicase activity	6	0.00299
GO:0032559	Adenyl ribonucleotide binding	16	0.00299
GO:0036094	Small molecule binding	21	0.00299
GO:0000166	Nucleotide binding	19	0.00685
GO:0004691	cAMP-dependent protein kinase activity	2	0.00951
GO:0004748	Ribonucleoside-diphosphate reductase activity, thioredoxin disulfide as acceptor	2	0.00951
GO:0097367	Carbohydrate derivative binding	18	0.00951
GO:0005524	ATP binding	14	0.0139
GO:0043168	Anion binding	19	0.0149
GO:0051018	Protein kinase A binding	3	0.023
Cellular component (GO)			
GO:0042555	MCM complex	6	2.29e−10
GO:0005952	cAMP-dependent protein kinase complex	3	0.00123
GO:0097362	MCM8-MCM9 complex	2	0.00495
GO:0070033	Synaptobrevin 2-SNAP-25-syntaxin-1a-complexin II complex	2	0.0111
GO:0070032	Synaptobrevin 2-SNAP-25-syntaxin-1a-complexin I complex	2	0.0178

GO terms and pathways associated with differentially expressed genes of liver tissues in hyperlipidemic mice. False discovery rate corrections were calculated using the Benjamini–Hochberg procedure

Discussion

Salviae miltiorrhizae Radix, the dried root of *S. miltiorrhiza*, is one of the most well-known medicinal resources in Asian traditional medicine [10–14, 17]. Many studies have been conducted on SR, which have provided information on its traditional uses [22], chemical constituents [23, 24], and pharmacological effects [15, 25, 26]; however, the identification of molecular targets and specific effects is still required.

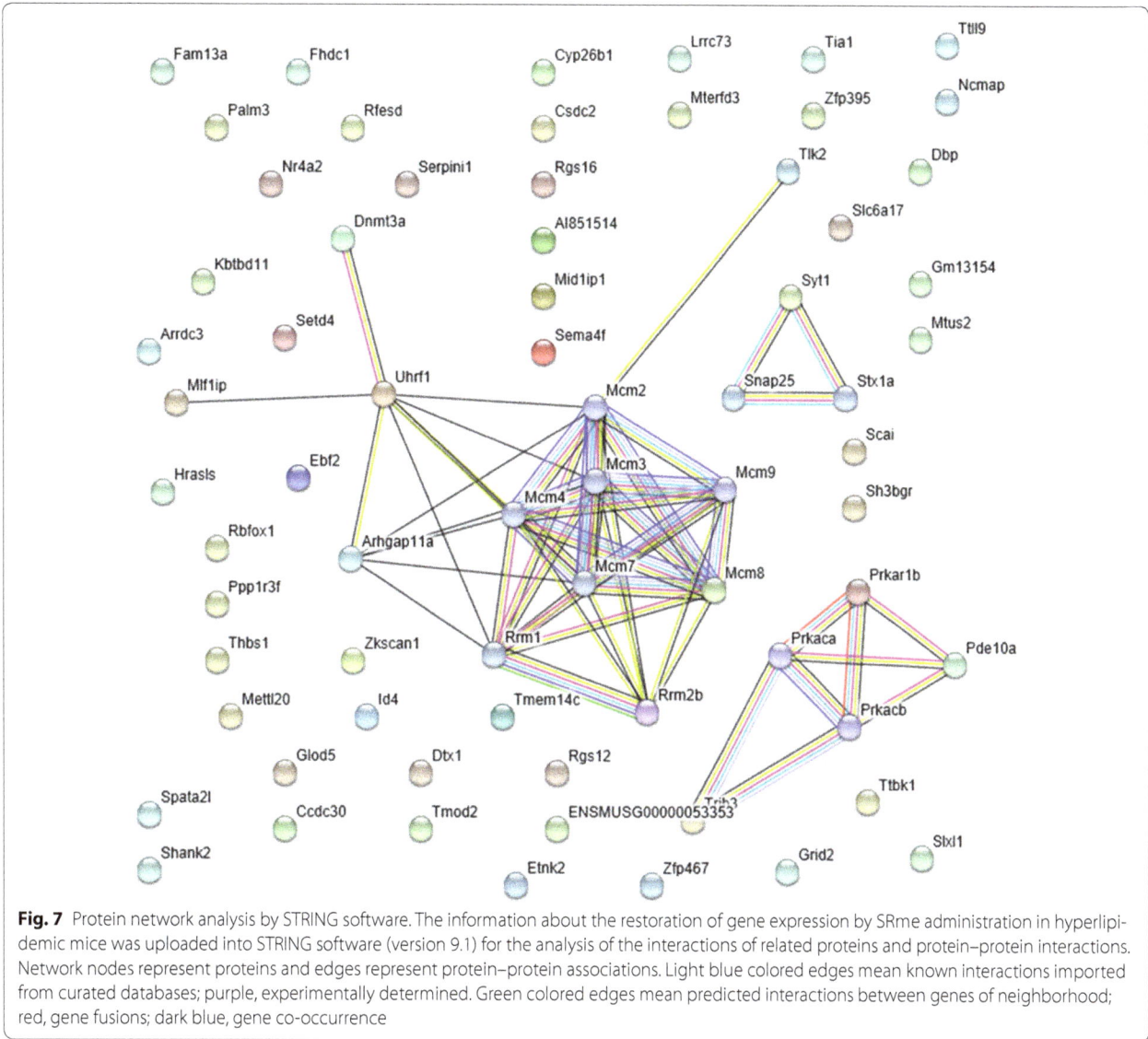

Fig. 7 Protein network analysis by STRING software. The information about the restoration of gene expression by SRme administration in hyperlipidemic mice was uploaded into STRING software (version 9.1) for the analysis of the interactions of related proteins and protein–protein interactions. Network nodes represent proteins and edges represent protein–protein associations. Light blue colored edges mean known interactions imported from curated databases; purple, experimentally determined. Green colored edges mean predicted interactions between genes of neighborhood; red, gene fusions; dark blue, gene co-occurrence

Recently, many researchers conducted studies on tanshinone IIA, one of well-known pharmacologically active components of SR, and demonstrated its involving in intake and efflux of cholesterol, therapeutic potential on cardiovascular diseases such as atherosclerosis [27–30]. Furthermore, tanshinone IIA was reported to have effects stabilizing vulnerable plaques in apolipoprotein-E-deficient (apoE−/−) mice [31].

In Asian traditional medicine, whole plants or mixtures of several plants are used rather than isolated compounds. The aim of this study is to investigate anti-hyperlipidemic effects of SRme in mice model, and deduce molecular target of SRme by evaluation of gene expression in hepatic tissues.

In this study, it was shown that SRme administration significantly decreased triglyceride content without alteration of body weight in mice (Figs. 2, 3c). In our preliminary study, food intake was observed to exclude the possibility that the incorporation of SRme into rodent chow affected food intake and subsequently influenced the changes in body weight and total lipid content in blood. However, it was found that SRme mixed chow did not affect food intake; therefore, it may contribute to the restoration of body weight among the experimental groups of mice. Although the content of MDA was not significantly altered by the administration of SRme, the levels tended to decrease (Fig. 4).

Through the evaluation of hundreds of differentially expressed genes in hyperlipidemic mice, we identified key molecular pathways that play important roles in DNA replication (Table 3); using another database, similar results were observed (Additional file 5: Table S1).

By using a protein network database such as STRING, we identified target proteins, including Mcm proteins, which play a key role in DNA replication (Fig. 7). These results support the data from molecular pathway identification (Table 3). Mcm proteins are known as essential replication initiation factors, and orchestration of the functional interactions between Mcm proteins results in initiation of DNA synthesis in cell cycle [32]. Names of genes which are functionally important in Fig. 7 are provided in Additional file 5: Table S2. One of critical limitations of our study is lack of investigating meaningful relationship between biochemical and genomic data. Furthermore, the currently identified targets of SRme in hyperlipidemic mice are relatively broad, and still not clearly explored. However, based on the present study, we hope the limitation of our study will be overcome through our future researches.

Collectively, the results showed that SRme suppressed hyperlipidemia and the accumulation of triglycerides. In addition, we proposed that the effect of SRme on hyperlipidemia occurred through the restoration of expression of genes and proteins related to DNA replication.

Conclusions

In order to ascertain the influence of SRme in hyperlipidemic HFD mice, the changes in serum lipids and gene expression were observed. There was no significant effect on the body weight gain in hyperlipidemic HFD mice. The blood serum level of triglycerides induced by hyperlipidemia was restored to that of non-hyperlipidemic mice. Mcm proteins were identified as molecular targets that play a key role in the amelioration of hyperlipidemia.

Abbreviations
SR: Salviae miltiorrhizae Radix; SRme: methanol extract of Salviae miltiorrhizae Radix; HDL-cholesterol: high density lipoprotein; MDA: malondialdehyde.

Authors' contributions
CL and SC designed the study. BK and SC performed the experiments. CL and SL conducted the statistical analyses. BL, BK, and SC wrote the manuscript. All authors read and approved the final manuscript.

Author details
[1] College of Medicine, Dongguk University, Ilsandong-gu, Gyeonggi-Do 10326, Republic of Korea. [2] School of Public Health, Far East University, Chungbuk 27601, Republic of Korea. [3] Kyunghee Naseul Korean Medicine Clinic, Bucheon-si, Gyeonggi-do 14548, Republic of Korea. [4] Department of Medical Research, Korea Institute of Oriental Medicine, Daejeon 34054, Republic of Korea. [5] School of Korean Medicine, Yangsan Campus of Pusan National University, Yangsan-si 50612, Republic of Korea.

Acknowledgements
Not applicable.

Competing interests
The authors declare that they have no competing interests.

Funding
Not applicable.

References
1. Bao CD, Sun B, Lan L, Qiao H, Zhang DF, Liu XY, Wang J, Zhao YS. Interaction between family history of diabetes and hyperlipidemia on risk of diabetes in population with normotension in Harbin: a cross-sectional study. Zhonghua Liu Xing Bing Xue Za Zhi. 2017;38(5):611–4.
2. Danese MD, Gleeson M, Griffiths RI, Catterick D, Kutikova L. Methods for estimating costs in patients with hyperlipidemia experiencing their first cardiovascular event in the United Kingdom. J Med Econ. 2017. doi:10.1080/13696998.2017.1345747.
3. Kim MH, Jung-Choi K, Ko H, Song YM. Educational inequality in obesity-related mortality in Korea. J Korean Med Sci. 2017;32(3):386–92.
4. Lee SW, Kim HC, Lee HS, Suh I. Thirty-year trends in mortality from cerebrovascular diseases in Korea. Korean Circ J. 2016;46(4):507–14.
5. Yun JW, Son M. Forecasting cause-specific mortality in Korea up to year 2032. J Korean Med Sci. 2016;31(8):1181–9.
6. Sanders TA, Oakley FR, Miller GJ, Mitropoulos KA, Crook D, Oliver MF. Influence of n−6 versus n−3 polyunsaturated fatty acids in diets low in saturated fatty acids on plasma lipoproteins and hemostatic factors. Arterioscler Thromb Vasc Biol. 1997;17(12):3449–60.
7. Hasanpour Z, Javanmard SH, Gharaaty M, Sadeghi M. Association between serum myeloperoxidase levels and coronary artery disease in patients without diabetes, hypertension, obesity, and hyperlipidemia. Adv Biomed Res. 2016;5:103–9175.
8. Sugai T, Suzuki Y, Yamazaki M, Shimoda K, Mori T, Ozeki Y, Matsuda H, Sugawara N, Yasui-Furukori N, Minami Y, Okamoto K, Sagae T, Someya T. High prevalence of obesity, hypertension, hyperlipidemia, and diabetes mellitus in Japanese outpatients with schizophrenia: a nationwide survey. PLoS ONE. 2016;11(11):e0166429.
9. Ji KT, Chai JD, Xing C, Nan JL, Yang PL, Tang JF. Danshen protects endothelial progenitor cells from oxidized low-density lipoprotein induced impairment. J Zhejiang Univ Sci B. 2010;11(8):618–26.
10. Tan Y, Kamal MA, Wang ZZ, Xiao W, Seale JP, Qu X. Chinese herbal extracts (SK0506) as a potential candidate for the therapy of the metabolic syndrome. Clin Sci (Lond). 2011;120(7):297–305.
11. Wang XW, Guo J, Wang XF, Chen XP, Wen ZY. Effects of cardiotonic pill on RBC rheologic abnormalities in HFD-induced mice and LPL deficient mice. Clin Hemorheol Microcirc. 2008;40(4):281–8.
12. Zhang ZP, You TT, Zou LY, Wu T, Wu Y, Cui L. Effect of Danshen root compound on blood lipid and bone biomechanics in mice with hyperlipemia-induced osteoporosis. Nan Fang Yi Ke Da Xue Xue Bao. 2008;28(9):1550–3.
13. Liu M, Li Y, Chou G, Cheng X, Zhang M, Wang Z. Extraction and ultra-performance liquid chromatography of hydrophilic and lipophilic bioactive components in a Chinese herb Radix Salviae Miltiorrhizae. J Chromatogr A. 2007;1157(1–2):51–5.
14. Gong P, Li Y, Yao C, Guo H, Hwang H, Liu X, Xu Y, Wang X. Literature review of traditional Chinese medicine on the treatment of coronary heart disease in recent 20 years in China. J Altern Complement Med. 2017. doi:10.1089/acm.2016.0420.

15. Mu F, Duan J, Bian H, Yin Y, Zhu Y, Wei G, Guan Y, Wang Y, Guo C, Wen A, Yang Y, Xi M. Cardioprotective effects and mechanism of Radix Salviae Miltiorrhizae and Lignum Dalbergiae odoriferae on rat myocardial ischemia/reperfusion injury. Mol Med Rep. 2017. doi:10.3892/mmr.2017.6821.

16. Shen L, Lou Z, Zhang G, Xu G, Zhang G. Diterpenoid Tanshinones, the extract from Danshen (Radix Salviae Miltiorrhizae) induced apoptosis in nine human cancer cell lines. J Tradit Chin Med. 2016;36(4):514–21.

17. Wang ZY, Liu JG, Li H, Yang HM. Pharmacological effects of active components of chinese herbal medicine in the treatment of alzheimer's disease: a review. Am J Chin Med. 2016;44(8):1525–41.

18. Kim MS, Seo IB, Kim JB. Effects of Salviae Miltiorrhizae Radix on the diet-induced hyperlipidemia in rats. Korean J Orient Physiol Pathol. 2004;18:431–35.

19. Kim H, Kim H, Kim Y, Lee J, Kwon J, Kim Y, Cho S. Effects of Salviae miltiorrhizae Radix (SMR) on serum lipid level in hyperlipidemic rats. Korea J Herbol. 2007;22(4):239.

20. Kim HC, Kim YK. Genome-wide analysis on the effects of Salviae miltiorrhizae Radix in hyperlipidemic mice. J Korean Med Sci Daejeon Univ. 2013;21(2):73–84.

21. Lee SE, Cho S. Anti-inflammatory effects of Salviae miltiorrhizae Radix extract on RAW264.7 cell. via anti-oxidative activities. Korea J Herbol. 2015;30(4):89.

22. Wu JR, Guo WX, Zhang XM, Yang B, Zhang B. Study on medication regularity of grand master of traditional Chinese medicine YAN Zheng-hua's Ostreae Concha-containing prescriptions based on data mining. Zhongguo Zhong Yao Za Zhi. 2014;39(14):2762–6.

23. Pang H, Wu L, Tang Y, Zhou G, Qu C, Duan JA. Chemical analysis of the herbal medicine Salviae miltiorrhizae Radix et Rhizoma (Danshen). Molecules. 2016;21(1):51.

24. Wang FR, Zhang Y, Yang XB, Liu CX, Yang XW, Xu W, Liu JX. Rapid determination of 30 polyphenols in Tongmai formula, a combination of Puerariae Lobatae Radix, Salviae miltiorrhizae Radix et Rhizoma, and Chuanxiong Rhizoma, via liquid chromatography-tandem mass spectrometry. Molecules. 2017;22(4):545. doi:10.3390/molecules22040545.

25. Bu Y, Lee K, Jung HS, Moon SK. Therapeutic effects of traditional herbal medicine on cerebral ischemia: a perspective of vascular protection. Chin J Integr Med. 2013;19(11):804–14.

26. Lu KH, Liu CT, Raghu R, Sheen LY. Therapeutic potential of chinese herbal medicines in alcoholic liver disease. J Tradit Complement Med. 2012;2(2):115–22.

27. Jia LQ, Ni Z, Ying X, Chen WN, Zhu ML, Song N, Ren L, Cao HM, Wang JY, Yang GL. Tanshinone IIA affects the HDL subfractions distribution not serum lipid levels: involving in intake and efflux of cholesterol. Arch Biochem Biophys. 2016;592:50–9.

28. Gao S, Liu Z, Li H, Little PJ, Liu P, Xu S. Cardiovascular actions and therapeutic potential of tanshinone IIA. Atherosclerosis. 2012;220:3–10.

29. Wang B, Ge Z, Cheng Z, Zhao Z. Tanshinone IIA suppresses the progression of atherosclerosis by inhibiting the apoptosis of vascular smooth muscle cells and the proliferation and migration of macrophages induced by ox-LDL. Biol Open. 2017;6:489–95.

30. Fang J, Little PJ, Xu S. Atheroprotective effects and molecular targets of tanshinones derived from herbal medicine danshen. Med Res Rev. 2017. doi:10.1002/med.21438.

31. Zhao D, Tong L, Zhang L, Li H, Wan Y, Zhang T. Tanshinone II A stabilizes vulnerable plaques by suppressing RAGE signaling and NF-κB activation in apolipoprotein-E-deficient mice. Mol Med Rep. 2016;14:4983–90.

32. Tye BK. MCM proteins in DNA replication. Annu Rev Biochem. 1999;68:649–86.

16

Metabolomics approach reveals annual metabolic variation in roots of *Cyathula officinalis* Kuan based on gas chromatography–mass spectrum

Kai Tong[1], Zhao-ling Li[2], Xu Sun[1], Shen Yan[1], Mei-jie Jiang[1], Meng-sheng Deng[1], Ji Chen[1], Jing-wei Li[3] and Meng-liang Tian[1,3]*

Abstract

Background: Herbal quality is strongly influenced by harvest time. It is therefore one of crucial factors that should be well respected by herbal producers when optimizing cultivation techniques, so that to obtain herbal products of high quality. In this work, we paid attention on one of common used Chinese herbals, *Cyathula officinalis* Kuan. According to previous studies, its quality may be related with growth years because of the variation of several main bioactive components in different growth years. However, information about the whole chemical composition is still scarce, which may jointly determine the herbal quality.

Methods: *Cyathula officinalis* samples were collected in 1–4 growth years after sowing. To obtain a global insight on chemical profile of herbs, we applied a metabolomics approach based on gas chromatography–mass spectrum. Analysis of variance, principal component analysis, partial least squares discriminant analysis and hierarchical cluster analysis were combined to explore the significant difference in different growth years.

Results: 166 metabolites were identified by using gas chromatography–mass spectrum method. 63 metabolites showed significant change in different growth years in terms of analysis of variance. Those metabolites then were grouped into 4 classes by hierarchical cluster analysis, characterizing the samples of different growth ages. Samples harvested in the earliest years (1–2) were obviously differ with the latest years (3–4) as reported by principal component analysis. Further, partial least squares discriminant analysis revealed the detail difference in each growth year. Gluconic acid, xylitol, glutaric acid, pipecolinic acid, ribonic acid, mannose, oxalic acid, digalacturonic acid, lactic acid, 2-deoxyerythritol, acetol, 3-hydroxybutyric acid, citramalic acid, *N*-carbamylglutamate, and cellobiose are the main 15 discrimination metabolites between different growth years.

Conclusion: Harvest time should be well considered when producing *C. officinalis*. In order to boost the consistency of herbal quality, *C. officinalis* is recommended to harvest in 4th growth year. The method of GC–MS combined with multivariate analysis was a powerful tool to evaluate the herbal quality.

Keywords: Metabolomics, *Cyathula officinalis*, GC–MS, Harvest time, PCA, PLS-DA, Multivariate analysis, Herbal quality

*Correspondence: 652430882@qq.com
[3] Institute for New Rural Development, Sichuan Agricultural University, 608 Room, No. 1 building, 211 Huiming Road, Wenjiang District, Chengdu City 611130, Sichuan Province, People's Republic of China
Full list of author information is available at the end of the article

Background

Lots of Chinese herbs are recommended to harvest in fixed time period due to the variation of bioactive components during different cultivated years or different sampling seasons, such as *Alpinia oxyphylla* [1], *Hydrastis canadensis* [2], *Salvia miltiorrhizae* [3], *Sphallerocarpus gracilis* [4]. Uncontrolled metabolic variation has risk to decrease the herbal quality, which is contributed by the whole specific chemical profile [5, 6]. Hence, related study about chemical variation in different harvest time is valuable to establish the good agriculture practice (GAP) standards of Chinese traditional herbs in China [7].

As one of the most frequently-used traditional Chinese herbs [8], the roots of *Cyathula officinalis* Kuan have effects on anti inflammation [9], antioxidation [10], immune-enhancing [11], etc. and usually used to treat related diseases such as osteoarthritis [12], rheumatism [13] and chronic bacterial prostatitis [14] when combined with other herbs.

Historically, the cultivated *C. officinalis* is prior to harvest in the 3rd year after sowing by farmers in the main producing areas in China, like Sichuan province, China. However, without authoritative standards and powerful enforcement, herbal producers used to freely gather *C. officinalis* during 2–4 growth years in terms of herbal price fluctuation. Previous studies reported that several main bioactive compounds in *C. officinalis*, such as cyasterone, sengosterone, scoparone, daidzin and purerarin, varied significantly in different growth years [15]. Those results supported that fixed harvest year should be well considered on *C. officinalis* cultivation as one of important quality control factors, with an attempt to boost the consistency of different batches herbs or to obtain herbs with satisfied content of target components.

Recently, many literatures have illustrated that metabolomics approach is an efficient tool to evaluate herbal quality or discriminate easy-confused samples [16, 17]. This "omic" technique [18] provided us more comprehensive insight into the metabolic profile of herbs [19, 20]. Metabolomics approach based on LC–MS has been used to explore chemical difference of *C. officinalis* sampled from different areas [21]. However, besides of several main bioactive components, information about the total chemical composition of *C. officinalis* in different growth years is still scarce. In this study, we investigated the *C. officinalis* with different growth years by the GC–MS metabolomics platform. Analysis of variance (ANOVA), principal component analysis (PCA), partial least squares discriminant analysis (PLS-DA), hierarchical cluster analysis (HCA) data analysis methods were combined to measure annual metabolic variation in roots of *C. officinalis*, with the aim to finally facilitate the quality control of herbs.

Methods

Plant materials

The experimental plants were sowed among four successive years (2011–2014) in Baoxing country, Ya'an city, Sichuan province, China. In March, 2015, they were simultaneously collected. In total, 32 batches of authentic roots of *Cyathula officinalis* Kuan were identified by prof. Meng-liang Tian at College of Agronomy, Sichuan Agricultural University, where we deposited the voucher specimens of *C. officinalis*. All the plant materials were grew in a same farm by QiXiang farmer professional cooperative with same cultivated techniques before this study. We sorted these roots into 4 groups in terms of their growth years. They were labeled group A, group B, group C, and group D, which denoted that they had been grown for 1, 2, 3 and 4 years until sampling. Each group was composed of 8 biological replicates and each replicate was named by a unique sample identifier, which combined with group label and random number, like A1 or D8 (details see in Additional file 1). After washing the roots with pure water, all samples were immediately frozen in liquid N_2 and stored at $-80\,°C$ until processing.

Sample preparation

Samples for HPLC detection were prepared based on Ref. [8] with little modification. 1000 mg dried root powder was accurately weighted and then extract by methyl alcohol (20 ml) in ultrasonic for 30 min. Each sample group contained 8 replicates and each extraction repeated 3 times. Before HPLC analysis, extracting solutions were filtrated by 0.45 μm nylon membrane filter and diluted with equal amount of water.

Samples for GC–MS detection were prepared as follow: 100 mg fresh root tissue of each sample was accurately weighed and mixed with 0.4 ml methanol-chloroform (v/v; 3:1) and vortex for 10 s. 20 μl ribitol (0.2 mg/ml, stock in dH_2O) was added in mixtures as internal standard. Mixtures were homogenized in ball mill (JXFSTPRP-24, Shanghai jinxin industrial development Co., Ltd) for 5 min at 55 Hz, subsequently centrifuged at 12,000 rpm for 15 min at 4 °C. The supernatant (approximately 0.4 ml) was transferred to a new GC/MS glass vial. The extracts were dried in a vacuum concentrator without heating for about 1.5 h. 80 μl methoxymethyl amine salt (dissolved in pyridine, final concentration of 20 mg/ml) was added into dried metabolites, afterwards incubated at 80 °C for 20 min in an oven after mixing and sealing. After that, 100 μl BSTFA (containing 1% TCMS, v/v) was added into each sample and incubated at 70 °C for an hour. When sample cooled to room temperature, 10 μl FAMEs (Standard mixture of fatty acid methyl esters, C8–C16:1 mg/ml; C18–C30:0.5 mg/ml in chloroform) was added to it, and finally mixed well for GC–MS detection.

HPLC parameters

The cyasterone assaying used below parameters: Chromatographic column: Agilent Zorbax Eclipse XDB-C18 (5 μm particles, 4.6 mm × 150 mm). Flow rate: 0.8 ml/min. Temperature: 35 °C. Determine wavelength: 243 nm. Mobile phase: water and acetonitrile. Isocratic elution: 0–20 min, 18% water.

GC–MS detection

Gas chromatography–mass spectrum analysis was performed using an Agilent 7890 gas chromatograph system coupled with a Pegasus HT time-of-flight mass spectrometer. The system utilized a DB-5M Scapillary column coated with 5% diphenyl cross-linked with 95% dimethylpolysiloxane (30 m × 250 μm inner diameter, 0.25 μm film thickness; J&W Scientific, Folsom, CA, USA). A 1 μl aliquot of the analyte was injected in splitless mode. Helium was used as the carrier gas, the front inlet purge flow was 3 ml/min, and the gas flow rate through the column was 20 ml/min. The initial temperature was kept at 50 °C for 1 min, then raised to 330 °C at a rate of 10 °C/min, then kept for 5 min at 330 °C. The injection, transfer line, and ion source temperatures were 280, 280, and 250 °C, respectively. The energy was −70 eV in electron impact mode. The mass spectrometry data were acquired in full-scan mode with the m/z range of 30–600 at a rate of 20 spectra per second after a solvent delay of 366 s. Before statistical analysis, the GC–MS method was validated by internal standard compound (Ribitol), whose standard deviation of retention time was 0.014 (n = 32).

Statistical analysis

Chroma TOF 4.3X software of LECO Corporation and LECO-Fiehn Rtx5 database were used for raw peaks exacting, the data baselines filtering and calibration of the baseline, peak alignment, deconvolution analysis, peak identification and integration of the peak area [22]. The RI (retention time index) method was used in the peak identification, and the RI tolerance was 5000. Metabolite data were normalized by dividing each peak area value by the area of internal standard (Ribitol). After that, the data were log10 transformed, mean-centered and divided by the standard deviation of each variable before performing statistical analysis. All the statistical analyses, such as ANOVA, PCA, PLS-DA, HCA, were performed by using MetaboAnalyst 3.0 [23]. The Minimum Standards of Reporting Checklist contains details of the experimental design, and statistics, and resources used in this study (Additional file 2).

Results

HPLC detection

As the only certificated quality marker by Chinese Pharmacopoeia (edition 2015) [8], cyasterone was detected in four groups by HPLC. The results showed that the content of cyasterone in each sample could meet the minimum requirement (≥0.030%) of Chinese Pharmacopoeia. However, the 4-years growth ages plants have the highest content of cyasterone (0.087%), followed by 3-years group (0.076%), 2-year group (0.065%) and 1-year group (0.039%) (details see Additional file 3). These results were also partial proved by previous studies [15]. Therefore, considered the content of marker compound, herbs with 1–4 growth years ages were all qualified and the 4th year was the best harvest year.

GC–MS data extraction

To obtain an overview of annual metabolic changes in roots of C. officinalis, we carried on the GC–MS approach to all samples. The representative GC–MS chromatograms showed obvious variation in different growth ages (Fig. 1a–d). In total, 752 chromatographic peaks were detected and then numbered 1–752 in sequence of retention time. Peak 442 was contributed by ribitol as reference substance. In order to remove the systematic noise, we just extracted those peaks that were successfully discovered (peak area value >0) at least 6 times in either groups (n = 8). In result, 341 peaks (not include peak 442) were retained. Among them, 166 peaks were given identified chemical name (details see Additional files 1, 4). It should be noted that 4 chemicals were identified twice. They were 3-hydroxypropionic acid (peak 99 and 107), aspartic acid (peak 295 and 349), xylitol (peak 431 and 432), and diglycerol (peak 446 and 457). This may result from the insufficient precision of methods. To the end, the final dataset was composed of all the 166 peaks of 32 samples and their peak area values, which was used to the following ANOVA, PCA, HCA, PLS-DA etc.

One-way ANOVA

We firstly carried on univariate analysis method, ANOVA, to have an overview of all 166 metabolites data, attempted to simply find potentially important metabolites. In result, 63 metabolites showed potentially significant difference about their content between 4 groups using the standard $P < 0.05$ (detail see Additional file 5). Compared with the 1st growth year (group A), 15 metabolites changed significantly when herbs grew for two years (group B), while 40 metabolites changed in 3rd year (group C) and 32 metabolites in 4th year (group D). This trend was as well illustrated in Fig. 2a, which clearly showed us most metabolic variations happened in 3rd year after sawing. Similar trend was also revealed in

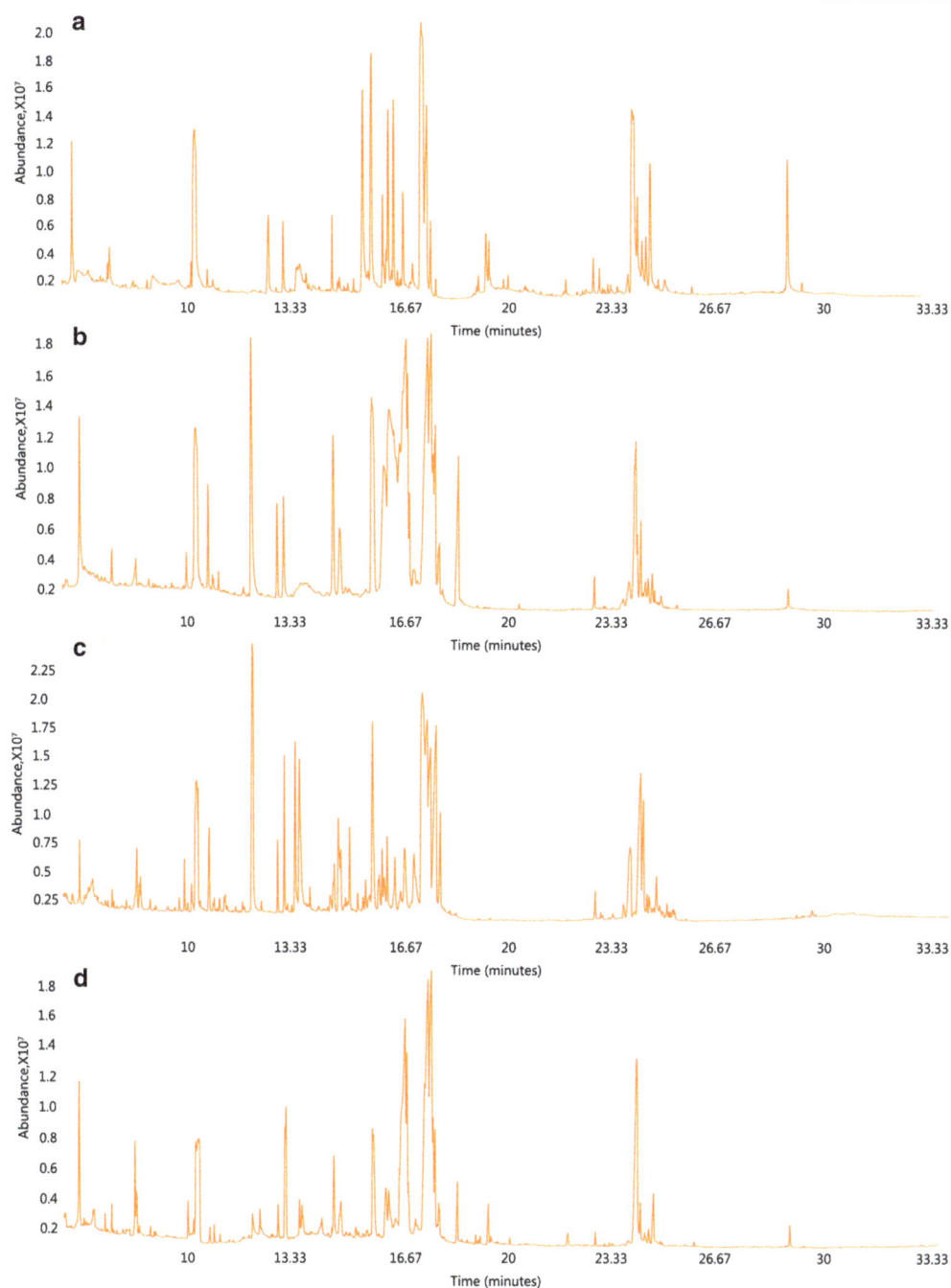

Fig. 1 Representative GC–MS chromatogram of each group. **a** Sample with 1 growth age. **b** Sample with 2 growth ages. **c** Sample with 3 growth ages. **d** Sample with 4 growth ages

Fig. 2b by comparing the number of metabolites changed significantly between previous year and following year. Therefore, we speculated that the 3rd year, when the most large-scale of metabolites changed, more likely a turning point for *C. officinalis* metabolism.

Top 10 typical metabolites were listed Additional file 5, using the standard of $P < 0.0001$. In Fig. 3 their changes in different growth years were illustrated by box plots, which showed that those metabolites more or less prone to accumulate in some certain years. For instance, xylitol

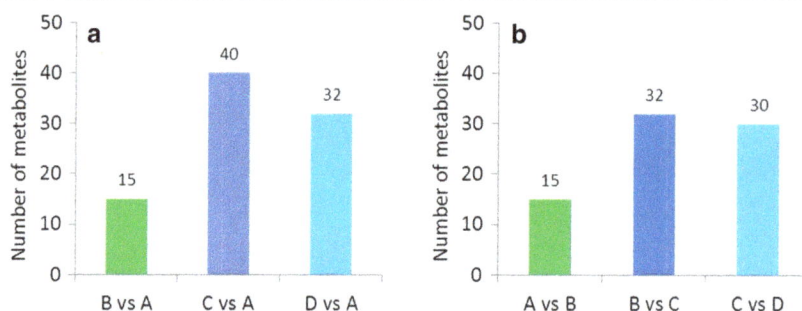

Fig. 2 Number of metabolites that changed significantly. **a** *Each column* shows the number of significantly changed metabolites (*P* < 0.05, ANOVA) with respect to the first growth year for the next 3 groups. **b** *Each column* shows the number of significantly changed metabolites (*P* < 0.05, ANOVA) with respect to the previous growth year for group B, group C and group D

and citramalic acid were hardly detected in the first 3 growth years until grew for 4 years. While mannose and oxalic acid accumulated rich in fist year but decreased during the 2–4 years. Gluconic acid, 3-hydroxybutyric acid, glutaric acid and cellobiose were easily detected in 3–4 years while little existed in 1–2 years. However, this trend was inverted for pipecolinic acid and ribonic acid.

Cluster analysis

To have a further visually insight on every metabolite content change in different growth years. We performed a heat-map combined with HCA, using extracted dataset composed by 63 metabolites filtered by ANOVA (*P* < 0.05). As illustrated in Fig. 4, 32 samples trended to separate into 3 classes. Samples with same growth age had trend to cluster in same class. For instance, samples of group C all clustered in class III and group D all clustered in class II. Seven samples from group A and 6 samples from group B were together clumped in class I and further separated into two subclasses. Unusually, the rest 3 samples of group A or B, A2, B1, B5, were together put into class III. This means that those 3 samples were more similar to group C. The fact that only group D was clustered in an independent class, class II, indicated that its metabolic profile was stabilized when herbs of 4 growth age. Therefore, compared with the traditional cultivation, more proper harvest time for *C. officinalis* may be the 4th year after sowing because of the micro-change in metabolic profile between samples.

Showed in Fig. 4, 4 metabolite classes were found in the heat-map, each of which revealed the content distribution in different sample classes or growth years. Metabolites in Class (1), like glycine (peak 217), 2-hydroxy-3-isopropylbutanedioic acid (peak 379), valine (peak 157), were least abundant in 3 growth years than any other growth ages. However, metabolites in class (4), like 2-deoxyerythritol (peak 199), acetol (peak 430), citramalic acid (peak 322), were most abundant in

4 growth years. Most of metabolites in Class (2), like ribonic acid (peak 424), pipecolinic acid (peak 253), *N*-carbamylglutamate (peak 537), had high content in the 1–2 growth years compared with the next 3 or 4 growth years, while metabolites in class (3), like gluconic acid (peak 618), 3-hydroxypropionic (peak 99), glutaric acid (peak 277), cellobiose (peak 674), lactic acid (peak 47), trended to accumulate in 3–4 growth years when compared with 1–2 growth years.

PCA

As one of common used unsupervised methods of multivariate analysis, we performed PCA on the 166 metabolites dataset. Considering only the first two principal components, PC1 and PC2, explained 27.8% variance. An obvious separation between the earliest (group A and group B) and latest (group C and group D) growth years in Fig. 5a was discovered, which exhibited the notable metabolic difference between them. The considerable overlap between the group A and group B indicated their metabolic profiles were similar. This fact as well had been told by Fig. 4, where group A and group B were clustered in two subclasses although belonged to a same upper class. Compared with earliest growth years, the latest groups, group C or group D, were better separated due to samples of group D gathered more closely in this PCA score plot. This result proved again that group D had less internal difference relatively.

PLS-DA

Principal component analysis analysis demonstrated the presence of discriminating factors which allowed the separation between earliest growth years and latest years. However, this kind of unsupervised method did not allow observing well separation of every two groups, such as group A/group B or group C/group D. To verify whether our current metabolites dataset provided enough information could detail the significant

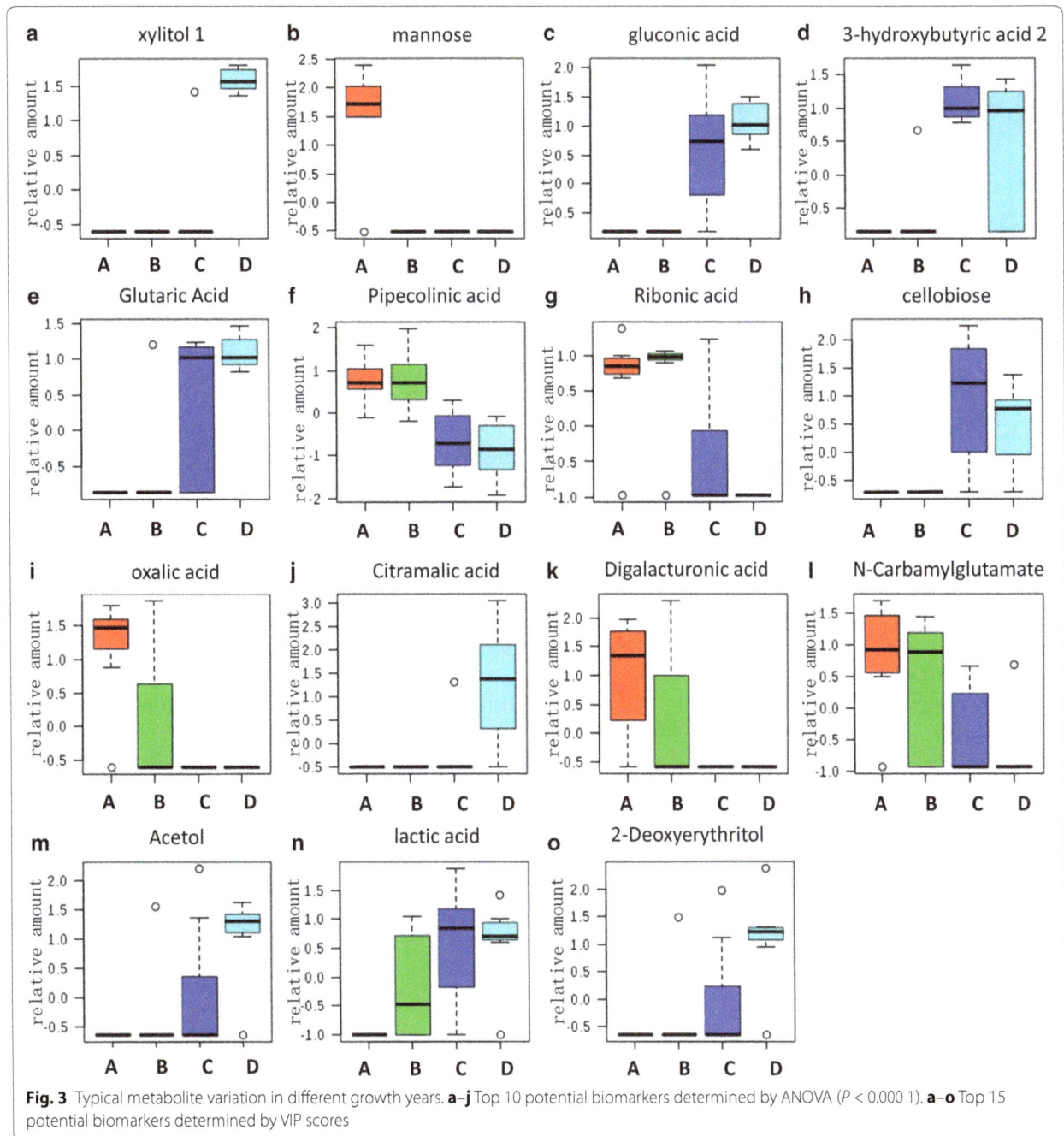

Fig. 3 Typical metabolite variation in different growth years. **a–j** Top 10 potential biomarkers determined by ANOVA ($P < 0.000\ 1$). **a–o** Top 15 potential biomarkers determined by VIP scores

difference of any two groups, we decided to use a supervised method as PLS-DA. In result, this method dose exhibited the ability to discriminate each group in three dimensional score plot with three principle components (Fig. 5b), accounting for 32.1% variance. As showed in Fig. 5a, b, the main factor that drived the separation between each group was PC1. In order to summarize the importance of metabolites for constructing PC1, we listed the top 15 metabolites with high variable influence on projection (VIP) score (Fig. 6a). They were gluconic acid, xylitol, glutaric acid, pipecolinic acid, ribonic acid, mannose, oxalic acid, digalacturonic acid, lactic acid, 2-deoxyerythritol, acetol, 3-hydroxybutyric acid, citramalic acid, *N*-carbamylglutamate, and cellobiose. These results were correlated with main loadings of PLS regression (Fig. 6b). In order to verify whether those 15 metabolites have ability to discriminate different growth years as potential chemical markers, we re-performed

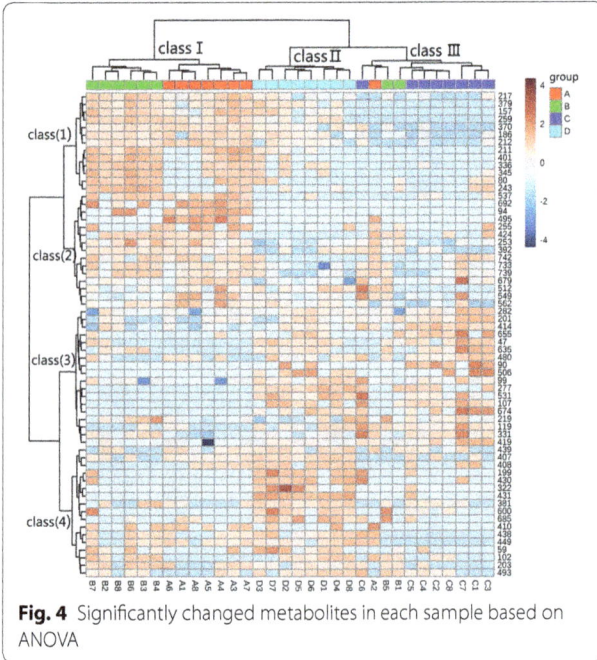

Fig. 4 Significantly changed metabolites in each sample based on ANOVA

PLS-DA based on 15 metabolites. Luckily, the new score plot (Fig. 7) who produced by this simple dataset was very similar with the score plot produced by 166 metabolites (Fig. 5b). That means, using the 15 metabolites to evaluate the quality of herbs is feasible.

Discussion

Unlike LC–MS or NMR, GC–MS we used in the present study prefers to offer information about primary metabolites, such as sugar, protein, lipid and organic acids et al. Generally, primary metabolites could be the precursors for the secondary metabolites, like various terpenoids including cyasterone. In the present study, a wild range of variation of primary metabolites that related sugar metabolism showed regular change in different growth years, like mannose, acetol and D-glyceric acid (detail see Additional file 3). Those metabolites related sugar metabolism pathway could further offer some important metabolic intermediates, like pyruvic acid and phosphoglyceraldehyde, which were used in the biosynthesis pathways of terpenoids [24].

In the current Chinese Pharmacopoeia, one of the most important methods for herb quality control is to evaluate the content of one or more chemical compounds. However, this method ignores the synergistic effect of multiple compounds, which is much emphasized in clinical application of traditional Chinese medicine [25]. Therefore, a better method to evaluate the herbal quality is to characterize the metabolic profile with a wide range of chemical compositions, other than just simply assessing one or several chemical compounds. Generally, herbs with a similar metabolic characterization would have similar properties. In the present study, 166 metabolites were synergistically used to investigate the herbal quality

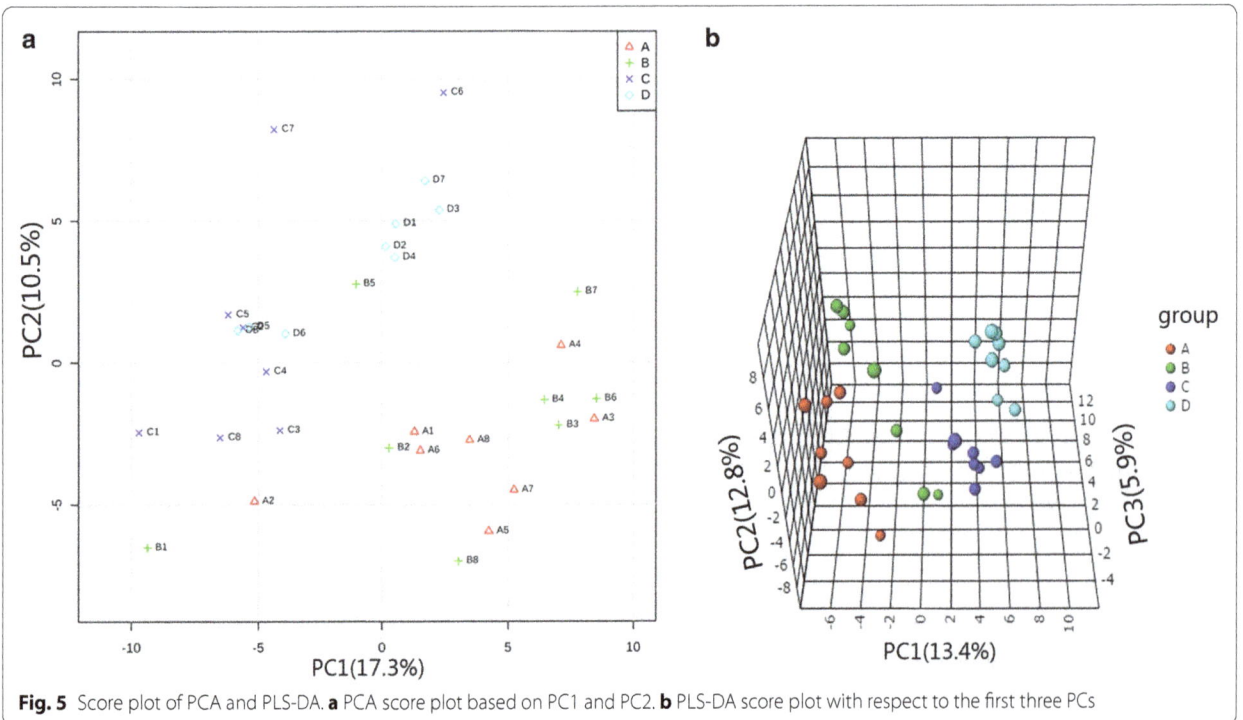

Fig. 5 Score plot of PCA and PLS-DA. **a** PCA score plot based on PC1 and PC2. **b** PLS-DA score plot with respect to the first three PCs

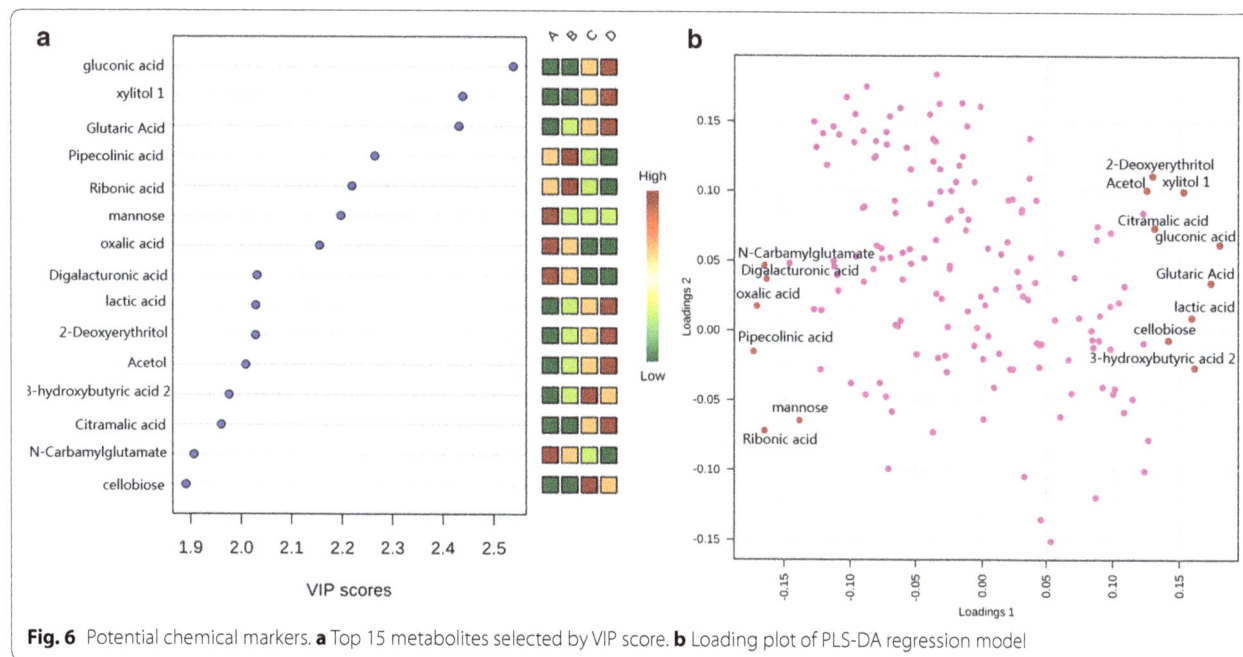

Fig. 6 Potential chemical markers. **a** Top 15 metabolites selected by VIP score. **b** Loading plot of PLS-DA regression model

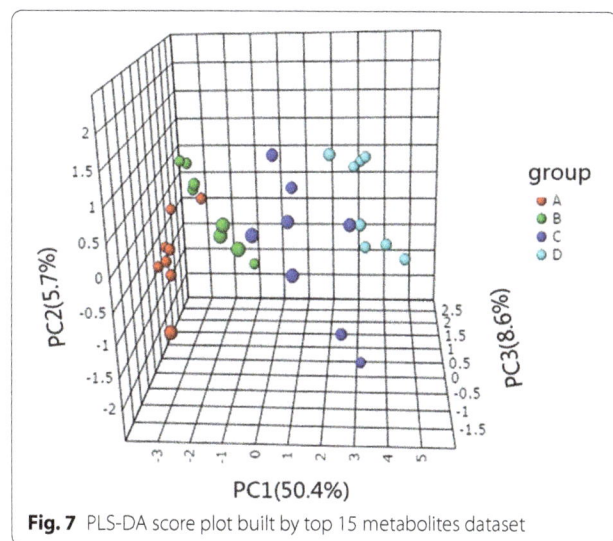

Fig. 7 PLS-DA score plot built by top 15 metabolites dataset

and successfully revealed the unique chemical patterns of samples with different growth ages. Compared with the single chemical marker assessing, this method provided more chemical information of plants in an overall perspective.

Based on current analytical techniques, it is impossible to obtain the truly whole compositions of medicinal plants. Ideally, the represented metabolites are unique components that contribute to the therapeutic effects of herbal medicines. However, for many plants, the accurate pharmacological compounds are still unclear. Therefore,

other chemical components that is of interest for quality control purposes are also used to as markers. As the different role on quality control, those markers could further be classified into eight categories regardless whether they are active compounds [26]. In the present study, we selected 15 metabolites as potential chemical markers for quality control mainly because of their ability to evaluate the herbal consistency and discriminate the different growth ages.

Quality control of herbal medicines aims to ensure their authentication, consistency, safety and efficacy. As the variation on quality control purpose, various chemical markers or analysis techniques should be used at different conditions. In this study, we established a GC–MS approach to reveal the variation on *C. officinalis* with different growth ages and found out several marker compounds to discriminate them. However, it should be noted that herbal quality is affected by climate factors, like precipitation, sunlight, temperature et al., which were not actually measured in this study. Therefore, in order to test the discrimination efficacy of these markers, followed multi-plot demonstration for several years is recommended.

Conclusions

The results mentioned above showed that the chemical profile of *C. officinalis* could be quite different when collected in different growth years. Gluconic acid, xylitol, glutaric acid, pipecolinic acid, ribonic acid, mannose, oxalic acid, digalacturonic acid, lactic acid,

2-deoxyerythritol, acetol, 3-hydroxybutyric acid, citra-malic acid, *N*-carbamylglutamate, and cellobiose are the main 15 discrimination metabolites between different growth years. With the aim to boost the consistency of herbal quality, *C. officinalis* is recommended to harvest in 4th growth year based on the information provided by GC–MS. The method of GC–MS combined with multivariate analysis is a powerful tool to discriminate the different herbal growth age.

Abbreviations
GC–MS: gas chromatography–mass spectrum; GAP: good agriculture practice; LC–MS: liquid chromatography–mass spectrum; HPLC: high performance liquid chromatography; NMR: nuclear magnetic resonance; ANOVA: analysis of variance; PCA: principal component analysis; PLS-DA: partial least squares discriminant analysis; HCA: hierarchical cluster analysis; PC: principal component; VIP: variable influence on projection.

Authors' contributions
MT conceived the research project and offered main research materials. ZL, XS, SY, MJ and MD, performed the experiment and collected the data. KT analyzed the data and wrote the manuscript. JC and JL revised the manuscript. All authors read and approved the final manuscript.

Author details
[1] College of Agronomy, Sichuan Agricultural University, Chengdu 611130, People's Republic of China. [2] Maize Institute, Sichuan Agricultural University, Chengdu 611130, People's Republic of China. [3] Institute for New Rural Development, Sichuan Agricultural University, 608 Room, No. 1 building, 211 Huiming Road, Wenjiang District, Chengdu City 611130, Sichuan Province, People's Republic of China.

Acknowledgements
The field management and herbal collection were supported by Wen-guang Li and QiXiang farmer professional cooperative. The GC–MS detection was supported by Biotree company in Shanghai, China.

Competing interests
The authors declare that they have no competing interests.

Funding
This study was supported by the grant from the National Key Technology Support Program (2011BAI13B02-7). This program aimed to boost herbal quality of *Cyathula officinalis* by optimizing its cultivation techniques.

References
1. Li YH, Chen F, Wang JF, Wang Y, Zhang JQ, Guo T. Analysis of nine compounds from *Alpinia oxyphylla* fruit at different harvest time using UFLC-MS/MS and an extraction method optimized by orthogonal design. Chem Cent J. 2013;7:134.
2. Douglas JA, Follett JM, Parmenter GA, Sansom CE, Perry NB, Littler RA. Seasonal variation of biomass and bioactive alkaloid content of goldenseal, *Hydrastis canadensis*. Fitoterapia. 2010;7:925.
3. He CE, Wei J, Jin Y, Chen S. Bioactive components of the roots of *Salvia miltiorrhizae*: changes related to harvest time and germplasm line. Ind Crop Prod. 2010;3:313.
4. Gao CY, Lu YH, Tian CR, Xu JG, Guo XP, Zhou R, Hao G. Main nutrients, phenolics, antioxidant activity, DNA damage protective effect and microstructure of *Sphallerocarpus gracilis* root at different harvest time. Food Chem. 2011;2:615.
5. Xin-Yue SO, Ying-Dong LI, Yan-Ping SH, Ling JI, Juan CH. Quality control of traditional Chinese medicines: a review. Chin J Nat Med. 2013;6:596.
6. Goodarzi M, Russell PJ, Vander Heyden Y. Similarity analyses of chromatographic herbal fingerprints: a review. Anal Chim Acta. 2013;804:16.
7. Zhang B, Peng Y, Zhang Z, Liu H, Qi Y, Liu S, Xiao P. GAP production of TCM herbs in China. Planta Med. 2010;76(17):1948.
8. Commission Chinese Pharmacopoeia. Pharmacopoeia of People's Republic of China. Beijing: China Medical Science Press; 2015. p. 38–9.
9. Park HY, Lim H, Kim HP, Kwon YS. Downregulation of matrix metalloproteinase-13 by the root extract of *Cyathula officinalis* Kuan and its constituents in IL-1beta-treated chondrocytes. Planta Med. 2011;13:1528.
10. Han X, Shen S, Liu T, Du X, Cao X, Feng H, Zeng X. Characterization and antioxidant activities of the polysaccharides from *Radix Cyathulae officinalis* Kuan. Int J Biol Macromol. 2015;72:544.
11. Feng H, Du X, Tang J, Cao X, Han X, Chen Z, Chen Y, Zeng X. Enhancement of the immune responses to foot-and-mouth disease vaccination in mice by oral administration of a Novel polysaccharide from the roots of *Radix Cyathulae officinalis* Kuan (RC). Cell Immunol. 2013;2:111.
12. Lai JN, Chen HJ, Chen CC, Lin JH, Hwang JS, Wang JD. Duhuo Jisheng Tang for treating osteoarthritis of the knee: a prospective clinical observation. Chin Med. 2007;2(1):4.
13. Ni LJ, Xu XL, Zhang LG, Shi WZ. Quantitative evaluation of the in vitro effect and interactions of active fractions in Yaotongning-based formulae on prostaglandin E 2 production. J Ethnopharmacol. 2014;154:807.
14. Wu J, Yuan Q, Zhang D, Zhang X, Zhao L, Zhang X, Ruan J. Evaluation of Chinese medicine Qian-Yu for chronic bacterial prostatitis in rats. Indian J Pharmacol. 2011;5:532.
15. Zhou R. Phytochemical investigation on two plants, *Cyathula officinalis* Kuan and Combretum griffithii. Chengdu: Chengdu Institute of Organic Chemistry, Chinese Academy of Science; 2004.
16. Zhang XJ, Qiu JF, Guo LP, Wang Y, Li P, Yang FQ, Su H, Wan JB. Discrimination of multi-origin chinese herbal medicines using gas chromatography–mass spectrometry-based fatty acid profiling. Molecules. 2013;18(12):15329.
17. Hu C, Xu G. Metabolomics and traditional Chinese medicine. TrAC, Trends Anal Chem. 2014;61:207.
18. Buriani A, Garcia-Bermejo ML, Bosisio E, Xu Q, Li H, Dong X, Simmonds MS, Carrara M, Tejedor N, Lucio-Cazana J, Hylands PJ. Omic techniques in systems biology approaches to traditional Chinese medicine research: present and future. J Ethnopharmacol. 2012;3:535.
19. Xiang Z, Wang XQ, Cai XJ, Zeng S. Metabolomics study on quality control and discrimination of three Curcuma species based on gas chromatograph–mass spectrometry. Phytochem Anal. 2011;5:411.
20. Liu F, Bai X, Yang FQ, Zhang XJ, Hu Y, Li P, Wan JB. Discriminating from species of *Curcumae Radix* (Yujin) by a UHPLC/Q-TOFMS-based metabolomics approach. Chinese medicine. 2016;11:21.
21. Fan QJ, Liu JL, Sun L, Zheng SL, Yuan JC, Tian ML, Kong FL. Development of fingerprinting for quality evaluation of *Cyathula officinalis* Kuan by LC-DAD-ESI-Q-TOF MS/MS coupled with multivariate statistical analysis. Anal Methods. 2015;7(8):3395.

22. Kind T, Wohlgemuth G, Lee DY, Lu Y, Palazoglu M, Shahbaz S, Fiehn O. FiehnLib: mass spectral and retention index libraries for metabolomics based on quadrupole and time-of-flight gas chromatography/mass spectrometry. Anal Chem. 2009;24:10038.

23. Xia J, Sinelnikov IV, Han B, Wishart DS. MetaboAnalyst 3.0–making metabolomics more meaningful. Nucleic Acids Res. 2015;W1:251.

24. Zhan AY, You XL, Zhan YG. Biosynthetic pathway and applications of plant terpenoid isoprenoid. Lett Biotechnol. 2010;1:131.

25. Wang L, Zhou GB, Liu P, Sun JH, Liang Y, Yan XJ, et al. Dissection of mechanisms of Chinese medicinal formula Realgar-Indigo naturalis as an effective treatment for promyelocytic leukemia. Proc Natl Acad Sci. 2008;12:4826.

26. Li S, Han Q, Qiao C, Song J, Cheng CL, Xu H. Chemical markers for the quality control of herbal medicines: an overview. Chin Med. 2008;3:7.

17

Advances in bio-active constituents, pharmacology and clinical applications of rhubarb

Yu-Jie Cao[1], Zong-Jin Pu[1], Yu-Ping Tang[1,2]* ⓘ, Juan Shen[1], Yan-Yan Chen[2], An Kang[1], Gui-Sheng Zhou[1] and Jin-Ao Duan[1]

Abstract

Rhubarb is one of the most ancient, commonly used and important herbs in Chinese medicine. The modern researches of rhubarb clarified the efficacies, ingredients and mechanisms in a more scientific and rigorous way. The main chemical compositions of rhubarb include anthraquinones, anthrones, stilbenes, tannins, polysaccharides etc. These compositions show extensive pharmacological activities including regulating gastrointestinal, anticancer, antimicrobial, hepatoprotective, anti-inflammatory, protecting cardiovascular, cerebrovascular and so on. This paper reviews the recent studies on the active ingredients, pharmacological effects, clinical application and functional mechanism.

Keywords: Rhubarb, Ingredients, Pharmacological activities, Clinical application, Functional mechanism

Background

Rhubarb is a collective name of various perennial plants of the genus *Rheum* L. from Polygonaceae family. This plant has important economic value, not only referred to a few edible rhubarbs [1], but also used as purgative drug in China since the third millennium BC [2], firstly recorded in *Shen Nong's Herbal Classic*. Rhubarb has been suggested to exert eliminating heat, purging fire, cooling blood, dispersing blood stasis, dredging collateral antidotal and purgative effects, used to treat constipation, diabetic nephropathy, chronic renal failure, acute pancreatitis, gastrointestinal bleeding and other diseases [3].

There are articles summarizing the research progresses of rhubarb on treating acute organophosphorus pesticide poisoning [4], acute ischemic stroke [5], acute pancreatitis [6], chronic kidney disease [7] in recent years. Zheng [8] summarized the researches of rhubarb containing the isolation, pharmacological activities, and phytochemical analysis. But there is no article to associate the different components of rhubarb with diseases. In this article, we not only introduce the active ingredients, pharmacology, applications and mechanism of rhubarb, but also summarize the relationship between ingredients and pharmacologic action.

Chemical components

Back in the early years of the nineteenth century, the chemical compositions of officinal rhubarb had been researched [3]. In recent years, unofficial rhubarbs with rich resources are also studied. Although they are different species, the main composition of these rhubarb species is similar. Scientists and medics isolated various types of compounds from rhubarb, containing anthraquinones and their glycosides, anthrones and their glycosides, stilbenes, butyrophenones and chromones, tannins, saccharides and so on [9].

Anthraquinones

Anthraquinones are the main characteristic as well as pharmacodynamic ingredients of rhubarb [10, 11]. The proportion of anthraquinones ranges from 3 to 5% in different species [3]. More than 30 anthraquinones have

*Correspondence: yupingtang@njucm.edu.cn
[2] College of Pharmacy and Shaanxi Collaborative Innovation Center of Chinese Medicinal Resources Industrialization, Shaanxi University of Chinese Medicine, Xianyang 712046, China
Full list of author information is available at the end of the article

been isolated and identified from rhubarb [12]. They are divided into free type and combination type. Free anthraquinones mainly contain rhein, emodin, aloe-emodin, chrysophanol, physcion, isoemodin, chrysaron, isoemodin, laccaic acid D. Combination anthraquinones are the glycosides combined by free anthraquinones and glycosyl. There are many kinds of anthraquinone glycosides, containing aloe-emodin-8-glucoside, emodin-8-glucoside, rhein-8-glucoside, physcion diglucoside, emodin-6-glucoside etc. [3, 9]. Main structures of anthraquinones (1–11) are as follows (Fig. 1) [3, 8, 12].

Rhein has the ability of protecting kidney [13], inhibiting the formation of renal fibrosis [14], improving diabetic nephropathy [15] and lipid disorders [16]. Rhein also has a strong inhibitory effect on common clinical anaerobes [17].

Emodin has a wide range of pharmacological effects, including anti-tumor [18], anti-microbial [19], antioxidant [20], anti-inflammatory [21]. It also can bring high blood pressure down, decrease blood lipids and improve microcirculation, protect liver and kidney [17].

Chrysophanol has a protective effect on the nervous system, improving the activity of antioxidant enzyme, reducing the damage of oxygen free radicals to cells [22].

Physcion also has neuroprotective effect, inhibiting the inflammatory response after cerebral ischemia and reducing the nerve damage caused by reperfusion [23]. Besides, physcion has anti-tumor effects on a variety of carcinoma cells, mainly through inhibiting cell proliferation, inducting apoptosis and blocking cell cycle [24].

Aloe-emodin, another important active compound of rhubarb, has attracted much attention, due to its various effects such as cardiovascular protection, hepatoprotective activities, anti-tumor, antibacterial, antifungal, antiviral, anti-inflammatory, immune regulation, laxative [17, 25].

Anthraquinone glycosides process the characteristic of antioxidant, anticancer, anti-inflammatory, laxative and many others biological properties [26], laxative activity strongest among them.

Anthrones and dianthrone

Anthrones and dianthrone, also characteristic components of rhubarb, are related to purgative activity. Mainly these include rheinosides A–D, palmidin A, B, C, rheidin A, B, C, and sennosidin A–F, etc. [9]. 26 anthrones have been isolated from the species of this genus [8]. Sennosides have a strong cathartic effects though translating to anthraquinones in vivo. The main structures of anthrones and dianthrone (12–25) are as follows (Fig. 2) [3, 8, 12].

Stilbenes

Stilbenes are important components of rhubarb, concerning antihyperlipidemic, antioxidant and hepatoprotective effect [3, 27]. So far, there are 31 compounds found in rhubarb belonging to stilbenes [12], such as rhapontigenin, isorhapontigenin and rhaponticin. Some representative

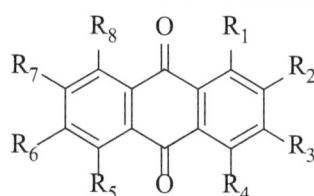

		R_1	R_2	R_3	R_4	R_5	R_6	R_7	R_8
1	Rhein	H	COOH	H	OH	OH	H	H	H
2	Emodin	H	CH_3	H	OH	OH	H	OH	H
3	Chrysophanol	H	CH_3	H	OH	OH	H	H	H
4	Aloe emodin	H	CH_2OH	H	OH	OH	H	H	H
5	Physcion	H	CH_3	H	OH	OH	H	OCH_3	H
6	Isoemodin	H	CH_3	OH	H	OH	H	H	OH
7	Laccaic acid D	H	OH	COOH	CH_3	OH	H	OH	OH
8	Aloe-emodin-8-oglucoside	OH	H	H	H	H	CH_2OH	H	OGlu
9	Chrysophanol-8-glucoside	OH	H	CH_3	H	H	H	H	OGlu
10	Physcion-8-glucoside	OH	H	CH_3	H	H	CH_3	H	OGlu
11	Physcion diglucoside	OH	H	CH_3	H	H	CH_3	H	$OGlu^6{\rightarrow}^1Glu$

Fig. 1 Main structures of rhubarb anthraquinones

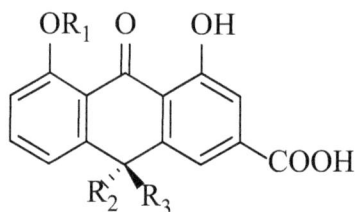

		R_1	R_2	R_3
12	Rheinoside A	Glu	Glu	OH
13	Rheinoside B	Glu	OH	Glu
14	Rheinoside C	Glu	Glu	H
15	Rheinoside D	Glu	H	Glu

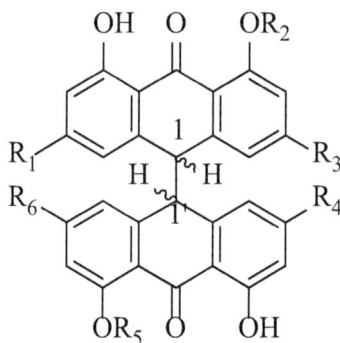

		R_1	R_2	R_3	R_4	R_5	R_6
16	Palmidin A	CH_2OH	H	H	OH	H	CH_3
17	Palmidin B	CH_2OH	H	H	CH_3	H	H
18	Palmidin C	CH_3	H	H	OH	H	CH_3
19	Rheidin A	OH	H	CH_3	COOH	H	H
20	Rheidin B	H	H	CH_3	COOH	H	H
21	Rheidin C	H	H	CH_3	COOH	H	OCH_3
22	Sennosidin A	COOH	H	H	COOH	H	H
23	Sennosidin C	COOH	H	H	CH_2OH	H	H
24	Sennoside A	COOH	Glu 1-1'trans	H	COOH	Glu 1-1'trans	H
25	Sennoside C	COOH	Glu 1-1'meso	H	COOH	Glu 1-1'meso	H

Fig. 2 Main structures of rhubarb anthrones and dianthrones

structures of stilbenes (26–28) are showed at Fig. 3 [3, 8, 12].

Tannins

Since the 1880s, the discovery that rhubarb tannins reduced the content of BUN, sparked great interest and attention of scholars both at home and abroad. Tannins in rhubarb generally account for 10–30% [28]. It can be divided into hydrolytic type and condensation type. Gallic acid and d-cate-chin are the monomers of these tannins. Studies have discovered that tannins are the active elements owing to the stypticity and constipate activity of rhubarb [29]. It has been proved that tannins can adjust genotoxicity, oxidative stress, inflammation and apoptosis [30]. Total

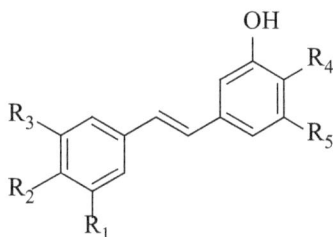

		R₁	R₂	R₃	R₄	R₅
26	Rhaponticin	OH	H	OH	OCH₃	H
27	Piceatannol 3'-O-glucopyranoside	H	OH	OGlu	H	OH
28	Resveratroloside	H	OGlu	H	H	OH

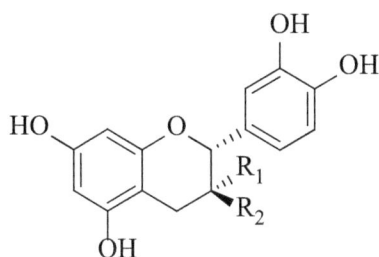

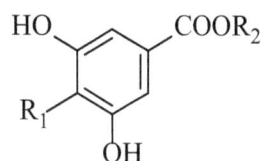

		R₁	R₂
29	(+)-Catechin	H	OH
30	(-)-Epicatechin	OH	H

		R₁	R₂
31	Gallic acid	OH	H
32	4-O-methyl gallic acid	OCH₃	H
33	Glucogallin	OH	Glu

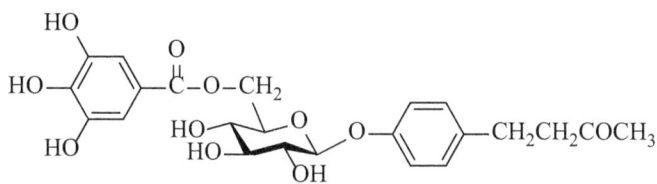

Lindleyin
34

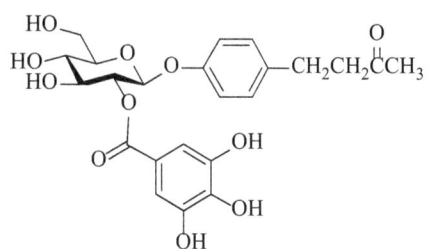

Isolindleyin
35

Fig. 3 Main structures of rhubarb stilbenes, tannins, butyrophenones and chromones

tannins extract can protect the kidney of K₂Cr₂O₇-injured rats by treating CrNT as a free radical scavenger [31]. The basic structures of tannins (29–33) recorded at Fig. 3.

Butyrophenones and chromones

6 butyrophenones and 14 chromones have been isolated from rhubarb already. Lindleyin and Isolindleyin whose structures are showed at Fig. 3, have been confirmed possessing anti-inflammatory and analgesic activity [32]. Chromones are of expanding coronary vessels, decreasing blood pressure, removing cholesterol, antibacterial and other activities [3].

Polysaccharides

Polysaccharides play multiple roles and have extensive bioactivities in life process, with an immense potential in healthcare, food and cosmetic industries, due to their therapeutic effects and relatively low toxicity [33]. It has been proved that rhubarb polysaccharides have the following pharmacological activity, lowering the blood sugar, protecting liver, promoting the proliferation of intestinal epithelial cell, antineoplastic, anti-senescence and etc. [34].

We list the main active ingredient groups, representative component and mainly pharmacological activity, showing the relationship between these components and effects. Rhubarb contains several different active ingredients. Each active ingredient often has different pharmacological activities, acting on multiple targets. One pharmacological activity may also be caused by a variety of ingredients. There is a synergistic effect among these components. The relationship is summarized in Fig. 4.

Pharmacology

Digestive system

Purgative

Rhubarb has been used as a first-choice herb for constipation in clinic for thousands of years in China. Its purgative activity is definite. Processing can change the potency and efficacy of Chinese herb. The purgative activity is different in raw rhubarb and its processed products [35].

Active ingredients and mechanism of purgation: Combination anthraquinones, including sennosides, rheinosides and anthraquinone aglyconesa, are considered as the main bioactive constituents of the laxative effect [26, 36], playing the most important role in stimulating the intestine and leading to diarrhea [37]. Combined anthraquinone is metabolized into free metabolise in intestinal canal to exerting laxative effect [38]. Sennoside A, the strongest purgative composition, is rarely absorbed in the intestine, most of them reached the colon, metabolized into rhein anthrone and rhein in the intestine [39]. After giving chloramphenicol, the active of *Escherichia coli* restrained, the purging effect of sennoside A and C weaken, anthrone in the colon is also greatly reduced [40]. When the free anthraquinone derivatives were injected to the colon of rat, the re-absorption of water and electrolyte would be inhibited, resulted in diarrhea [41]. Most of free anthraquinones are absorbed before arriving colon. Therefore, combined anthraquinones play drastic effect by means of metabolizing into free anthraquinones. It is thought that anthraquinones can stimulate the nerve plexus within the mucosa and intestinal smooth muscles, promoting peristalsis [9]. The rhubarb extractives and the anthraquinone derivatives can antagonize the adrenaline effectively, which can inhibit the contraction of the smooth muscle in vitro system of isolated intestine [37]. It also regulates the colon cholinergic neuron of constipating rats [42]. Besides, Rhubarb effectively down-regulates the expression of AQ4P in rat's proximal colon, and rhein/emodin can suppress the AQ4P expression of LoVo cells in vitro [43]. Sennoside A may decrease AQP3 expression in the colon to inhibit water transport from the luminal to the vascular side, leading to laxation [39]. The mechanism of its purgative activity is summarized as Fig. 5 [3, 9, 38, 44, 45].

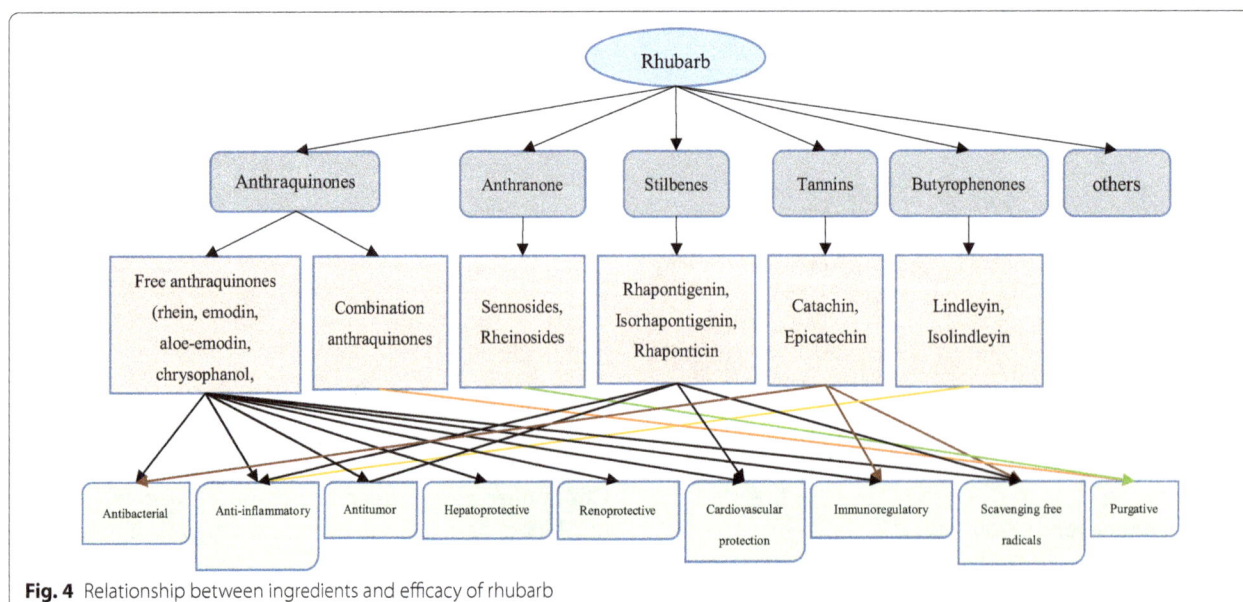

Fig. 4 Relationship between ingredients and efficacy of rhubarb

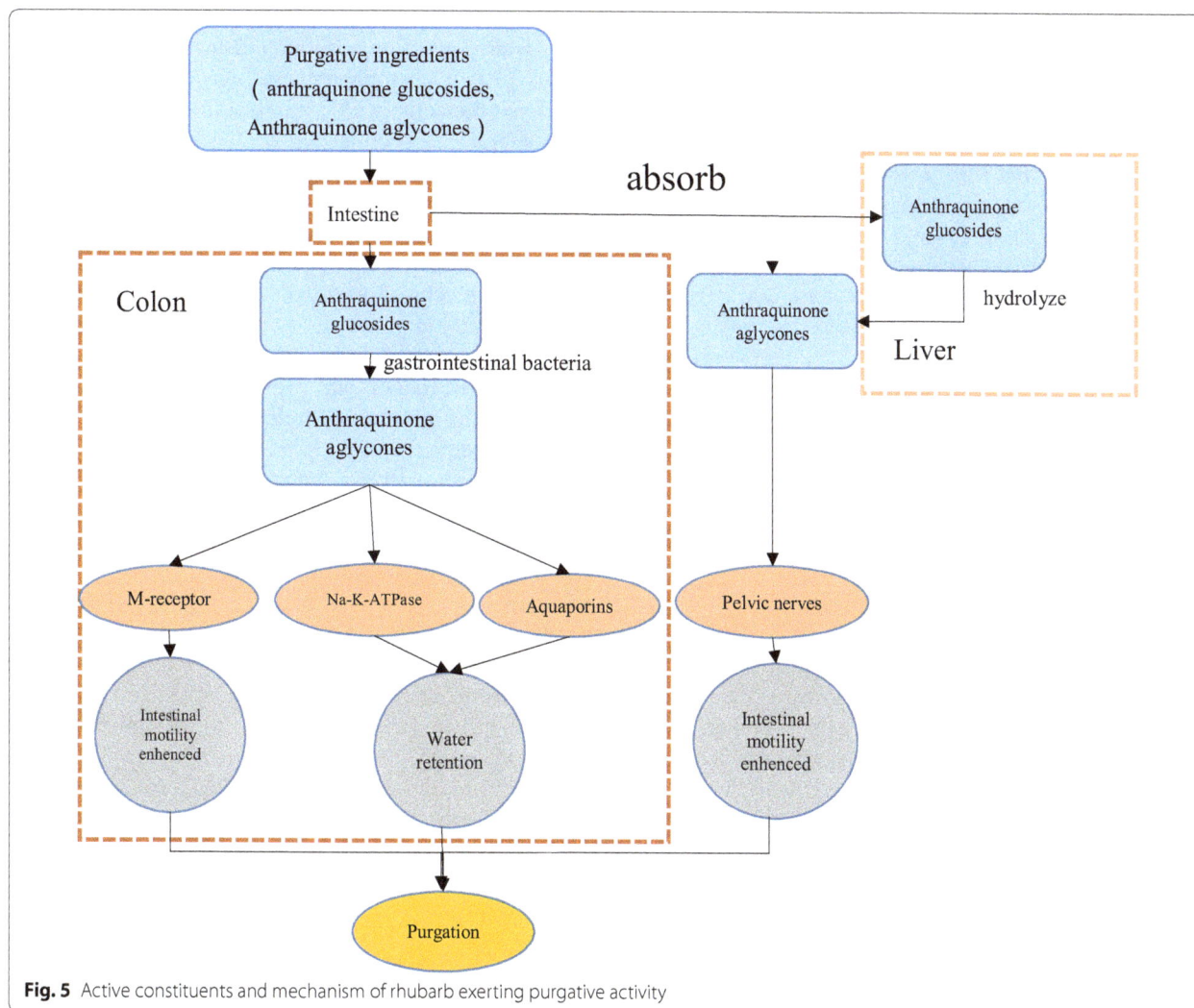

Fig. 5 Active constituents and mechanism of rhubarb exerting purgative activity

Hepatoprotective

Liver-protective function is an important part of studies on rhubarb in recent years. Rhubarb anthraquinones and tannins have a biphasic effect on liver, protection and damage. Anthraquinones showed stronger improvement on liver fibrosis and liver cell injury than tannins, and high dose tannins may injury liver in some extent [46]. Rhubarb and its free anthraquinones are also investigated in hepatic encephalopathy [47], liver fibrosis [48, 49], intrahepatic cholestasis [50] and so on.

Cardiovascular system

Promoting blood circulation and hemostasis

Rhubarb not only processes the effect of hemostasis but also improves hemorheology, stopping bleeding without leaving congestion. Charred rhubarb significantly improved the plasma viscosity, hematocrit, FIB, PT,

APTT and TT in the acute blood stasis rats [51], owning the best effect.

Mechanism of promoting blood circulation and Hemostasis: It is confirmed that chrysophanol and tannin are associated with the hemostasis effect. Chrysophanol can short the time of clotting, increase the number of platelets, promote blood coagulation in mice and tannin has a convergence effect, to promote local vasoconstriction [52]. Zhang found the main hemostasis mechanism of micron rhubarb charcoal was to produce prothrombin and thrombin by activating both endogenous and exogenous blood coagulation factor [53]. It is also believed that the pharmacological basis of promoting blood circulation is inhibiting the activity of Na^+-K^+-ATPase, to increase the plasma osmotic pressure, leading the water in the organization transferring into the blood vessels, increasing blood volume, helping with relieving microcirculation disturbance [54].

Hypolipidemic

Rhubarb has the effect of preventing and treating high blood lipids, reducing the TC, LDL, TG levels caused by high fat diet [55]. Rhubarb polysaccharide can reduce the blood lipid of diabetic atherosclerosis rats [56]. It has been confirmed that rhein and rheum emodin can regulate blood lipids, inhibit the formation of hyperlipidemia, prevent atherosclerosis [56, 57].

Mechanism of hypolipidemic: It promotes the excretion of cholesterol, improves blood rheology characteristics, decreases the release of inflammatory factors to maintain the balance of fat metabolism, inhibits the synthesis of cholesterol and triglyceride to achieve the purpose of regulating blood lipids [58]. Chen [59] found chrysophanol can reduce the blood lipid levels of zebrafish after high-fat diet, the mechanism may reduce the absorption of lipids in intestinal tract.

Urinary system
Kidney protection

Kidney protecting effect of rhubarb is owing to the combination of various pharmacological activities itself. Rhubarb, with anti-bacterial, anti-inflammatory, enhancing immunization, diuretic, regulating metabolism and other effects, protects the damaged kidney tissue, promotes protein synthesis, speeds up the excretion of waste and so on [3]. Rhubarb is commonly used in clinical practice to treat kidney disease such as chronic functional failure and diabetic nephropathy.

Mechanism of kidney protection: In recent years, the renal protective effect of rhubarb [60] and its active components, especially emodin [61] and rhein [62, 63], have raised widespread concern. But generally accepted views on the therapeutical mechanism have not been attained [64]. Rhein has the effect of improving the metabolism of glycolipid, reducing the excretion of urinary protein and anti-oxidative stress, which may be one of the mechanisms to prevent and treat diabetic nephropathy [65]. Emodin mainly involves cells and cytokines, such as TGF-β, CTGF, MCP-1, and TSP-1 to achieve the purpose of treating kidney diseases [66].

Nervous system

Rhubarb exerts an antipyretic effect by acting on the central nervous system. The mechanism of rhubarb antipyretic effect may be related to deduct the production of PGE_2 and cAMP in hypothalamus and down-regulate central body temperature [67]. Chrysophanol improved the learning and memory function of cerebral ischemia–reperfusion injured mice, increasing its anoxia tolerance capability, repairing the damage of brain tissue pathomorphism, so as to protect brain [68]. Besides the central nervous system, rhubarb also acts on the peripheral

nervous system. It can improve the cholinergic nerve decreasing caused by constipation in colonic myenteric plexus [42]. Chrysophanol and physcion significantly improved the activity of hypoxia-injured cells, enhanced cell survival rate, protected and improved the ultrastructure of hypoxia-induced neurons [69].

Respiratory system

Rhubarb is also used to treat acute respiratory distress syndrome in clinic. Rhubarb, combining with Shenfu injection, can improve the condition of patients with acute respiratory distress syndrome, such as improving organ dysfunction and respiratory mechanics index, increasing the oxygenation index, shortening mechanical ventilation time [70]. Rhubarb also has a good therapeutic effect on respiratory failure caused by other diseases.

Others
Anti-inflammatory

Rhubarb has the effect of heat-clearing and detoxifying for its anti-inflammatory effects, used to treat inflammations caused by a variety of reasons. Rhubarb remitted the degree of auricular swelling and foot swelling in mice and rats, reduced total protein and LTB4 in airbag synovitis exudates [71].

Mechanism of anti-inflammatory: Currently, studies of rhubarb anti-inflammatory mechanism are focused on its monomer components such as emodin, rhein and aloe-emodin. Eodin can reduce the level of IL-6 in periodontal tissue of periodontitis rats [72]. Due to intervention effect of emodin lipid nano-microbubble, the protein expressions of p-P38, p-ERK, p-JNK and the release levels of inflammation cytokine, such as TNF-α, IL-1β, IL-6, were significantly decreased [73]. Rhein reduced the level of inflammatory factors caused by type II diabetes mellitus [74]. Hu [75] found aloe-emodin was also the bioactive component of rhubarb related to anti-inflammatory effect. Aloe-emodin could decrease the production of proinflammatory cytokine in LPS-induced RAW264.7 macrophages by inhibiting NF-κB, MAPK, and PI3K pathways.

Antitumor

A number of studies have shown that the anthraquinones of rhubarb could inhibit the growth and proliferation of various cancer cells [8]. Its extract and active monomers including aloe-emodin, emodin and rhein, are researched on multiple cancer models [76–78].

Mechanism of antitumor: to determine and identify the possible molecular mechanisms of anti-cancer effect of rhubarb, medical practitioners focused on the free anthraquinones of rhubarb and emodin is the most frequently studied element among the active constituents.

Firstly, emodin inhibited the proliferation of tumor cell and induced apoptosis. Liu [79] found emodin inhibit the growth of human pancreatic cancer cell line Panc-1, and this inhibition effect was obvious connected with concentration and time. Secondly, it could inhibit the growth of tumor blood vessels. He [80] investigated the 95% ethanol extract and four subsequent fractions of rhubarb root and five anthraquinones extract on zebrafish model by quantitative endogenous alkaline phosphatase assay and staining assay, finding the anthraquinones with acidic or polar, hydrophilic substitution at C-6 or C-3 positions, played a substantial role in inhibiting angiogenesis. Then, rhubarb inhibited carcinoma cell metastasis. Tsai found rhubarb extract inhibit HA22T cell migration in wound healing in a dose-dependent manner [81].

Anti-bacterial

It has been confirmed that anthraquinone derivatives of rhubarb have remarkable antibacterial activity on several experimental bacterial strains in vitro [82, 83]. *Staphylococcus aureus* are often used on experiment because it is sensitive to rhubarb. Zhou [84] proposed rhubarb exerted antibacterial activity by changing the membrane permeability, inhibiting the synthesis of proteins and respiratory metabolism. Liu investigated on Emodin's effect and mechanisms on anti-MRSA in vitro and vivo, discovering that Emodin can destroy the cytoderm and cytomembrane structure of methicillin-resistant *Staphylococcus aureus* [85].

Anti-fibrosis

Many studies showed that rhubarb and its active components principally refer to emodin and rhein, could ameliorate organ fibrosis including renal, liver, lung, pancreas, cardiovascular system and so on [86, 87].

Mechanism of anti-fibrosis: Xu [88] summarized the mechanism for rhein ameliorating renal fibrosis as follows: inhibiting the infiltration of inflammatory cell, the transdifferentiating of renal tubular epithelial cells, the expression of profibrotic cytokines and blocking the activation of interstitial fibroblast. Wang [49] investigated the inhibitory effect and possible mechanism of emodin on hepatic fibrosis caused by CCl_4, finding that emodin exerted anti-hepatic fibrosis effect for inhibiting the activation of hepatic stellate cell though up-regulation the expression of Smad7 and down-regulation the expression of α-SMA in liver tissue. Liu [87] observed the influence of emodin on bleomycin-induced pulmonary fibrosis in rats, explored its protective mechanisms, proposing emodin may protect against rats with pulmonary fibrosis by enhancing antioxidation and anti-inflammatory ability.

Application

With the deep research on rhubarb, a traditional diarrhea drugs, its clinical application is widened, not only used to treat the constipation, but also other diseases.

Constipation

Rhubarb has a significant diarrhea effect, used to treat constipation caused by various reasons on clinic [89–91]. Yu found that umbilicus compressing of Rhubarb and Mirabilite achieved satisfactory and safe efficacy on constipation patients with orthopedic surgery by observing their bristol stool scale, defecation frequency and total effective rate [92]. Clinically, rhubarb often plays a curative effect through acupoint application rather than oral administration.

Diabetic nephropathy and chronic renal failure

Rhubarb is one of the most popular traditional Chinese herbs used in treating diabetic nephropathy (DN) and chronic renal failure (CRF) [93].

A large number of related literatures reported that rhubarb was often used in conjunction with other drugs in the treatment of diabetic nephropathy. Liu [94] found the SCr, BUN, Alb and FBG significantly improved after the patients treated with rhubarb compound. Rhubarb could improve the condition of diabetic nephropathy patients by reducing the excretion of urinary protein, lowering blood lipid, improving renal function, regulating the abnormal expression of TGF-β1, MMP-2, MMP-9 and MCP-1 in the blood of diabetic nephropathy patients, inhibiting renal inflammation and fibrosis process [95].

Rhubarb soda tablets combined with Jinshuibao Capsule significantly reduced Scr and BUN levels in patients with chronic renal failure [96]. Xiao [97] summarized the clinical and laboratory study on the rhubarb in the treatment of CRF. He found rhubarb and its prescriptions had a definite curative effect on CRF by ameliorating azotemia, preventing nephritic compensatory hypertrophy and high metabolism situation, and so on.

Acute pancreatitis

Rhubarb can promote the secretion and discharge of pancreatic juice, increase pancreatic juice flow. It is used to treat acute edema and hemorrhagic necrotizing pancreatitis [6].

Rhubarb and mirabilite external application reduced the risk of abdominal distension and stomachache, reducing the probability of complications in patients with acute pancreatitis. The relevant laboratory indicators were closer to normal and the average hospital stay was significantly shorter [98].

Rhubarb inhibited the inflammatory response, improved intestinal microcirculation and restored normal intestinal absorption, to exert the function of treating AP [99]. The free anthraquinone of rhubarb and the rhubarb decoction could attenuate kidney injury induced by acute pancreatitis [100].

Gastrointestinal bleeding

Rhubarb has hemostatic effect, used to treat gastrointestinal bleeding clinically. Conventional treatment combined with rhubarb powder exerting better therapeutic effect on the upper gastrointestinal bleeding by comparing control group and observation group [101]. Tan found rhubarb reduced curative time and increased the recovery rate of gastrointestinal bleeding caused by severe brain injury [102].

Others

In addition to the above diseases, rhubarb is also used to treat a variety of liver and kidney diseases, gastrointestinal dysfunction, cancers, hemorrhoid, periodontitis and so on [3].

Toxicity

It has been confirmed that rhubarb has varying degrees of toxicity on liver, kidney, gastrointestinal tract, reproductive system and blood systems, may possess teratogenicity and reproductive toxicity [103]. It is thought that gastrointestinal tract, liver, kidney are potential target organs of its toxicity.

Gastrointestinal toxicity of rhubarb characterized by diarrhea, constipation and melanosis [104]. Anthraquinones in rhubarb have purgative effect, while tannic acid and other components causing diarrhea. Small doses of rhubarb did not cause diarrhea, on the contrary inducing secondary constipation after discontinuation [26].

Yan [105] administrated total rhubarb anthraquinones on S.D. rats for 13 weeks to induce nephrotoxicity, finding the renal tubule epithelial cells swelled and denatured in tissue slice. Da [106] compared the toxicity of rhein and emodin in human renal tubular epithelial cells (HK-2), discovering that both emodin and rhein induced the apoptosis of HK-2 cells, having significant cytotoxic effect and the cytotoxicity of emodin on HK-2 cells was stronger than Rhein.

Animal experiments and clinical application confirmed rhubarb has hepatoprotective and choleretic effect. However, under certain conditions, rhubarb may damage liver [47]. Wang [107] investigated the effect of total extracts from prepared rhubarb on normal and pathological animals within a high dose range, finding prepared rhubarb showed bidirectional effects in hepatoprotection and hepatotoxicity, which could protect liver in CCl_4 injured chronic hepatic injury, but had a certain hepatotoxic effect to normal animals.

Besides, rhubarb is of reproduction toxicity. Wang [108] explored the abortion effect and mechanism induced by rhubarb extract. The result showed that rhubarb extract not only interfered the stability of pregnancy state in pregnant mice for its purgative activity, but also directly affected endometrial environment in early embryonic mice, resulting in abortion. Administrating rhubarb for 30 days induced a significant toxic effect on testis in adult rats by promoting interstitial cell apoptosis, affecting the synthesis of testosterone, reducing spermic formation, and the injury degree was dose-dependent [109].

Conclusion and perspectives

Rhubarb is one of the oldest and most frequently used herbal medicines in China, Korea, Japan, and other Asian countries. In this article, we summarize the active ingredients, pharmacological effects, functional mechanisms of rhubarb, as well as its clinical applications. There are about 200 compounds isolated from rhubarb, including anthraquinones, anthrones, stilbenes, flavonoids, acylglucosides, and pyrones. Most of the studies focused on exploring the bioactivities of anthraquinones. These constituents have shown extensive pharmacological activities, including cathartic, anticancer, hepatoprotective, anti-inflammatory, anti-microbial, analgesic effects and so on.

Pharmacological effects of rhubarb are extensive. In clinic, it is used to treat various diseases, such as constipation, acute pancreatitis, gastrointestinal bleeding, DN, CRF and so on. But rhubarb is not suitable for long-term using to avoid producing toxic and side effects. It is an important direction for the development of rhubarb that reducing its toxicity, through compatibility, processing, changing the dosage or administration route et al., to play a better therapeutic role.

Main active ingredients of rhubarb, rhein, emodin, chrysophanol and so on, have extensive pharmacological activities with low toxic and side effects, possessing good application prospects. At present, rhein is studied as a drug candidate to treat cancer. The potential anti-tumor mechanisms may block cell cycle, induce apoptosis and control metastasis. Some scholars are also committed to develop rhein as a new drug for diabetic nephropathy. Lindleyin whose pharmacological action is similar to aspirin, is expected to be developed as a new anti-inflammatory and analgesic drug. Developing and applying monomer compounds divided from rhubarb is another development direction of rhubarb.

Abbreviations

TCM: Traditional Chinese Medicine; ALT: alanine aminotransferase; AST: aspartate transaminase; LPS: lipopolysaccharide; MAO: monoamine oxidase;

GSH-ST: glutathione *S*-transferase; α-SMA: alpha smooth muscle actin; P-gp: *P*-glycoprotein; AP: acute pancreatitis; TNF-α: tumor necrosis factor-α; IL-1β: interleukin 1β; IL-6: interleukin 6; TC: total cholesterol; LDL: low density lipoprotein; TG: triglyceride; CRF: chronic renal failure; TGF-β: transforming growth factor-β; MMP: mitochondrial membrane potential; MCP: monocalcium phosphate; Cr: creatinine; UN: urea nitrogen; LTB4: leukotrienes B4; NF-κB: nuclear transcription factor-kappa B; MAPK: mitogen-activated protein kinase; PI3K: phosphatidylinositol 3 kinase.

Authors' contributions

Y-PT proposed the framework of this paper. AK and J-AD implemented the thought of this paper. Y-JC wrote this paper. Z-JP, JS Collated the references. All authors read and approved the final manuscript.

Author details

¹ Jiangsu Collaborative Innovation Center of Chinese Medicinal Resources Industrialization, and Jiangsu Key Laboratory for High Technology Research of TCM Formulae, and National and Local Collaborative Engineering Center of Chinese Medicinal Resources Industrialization and Formulae Innovative Medicine, Nanjing University of Chinese Medicine, Nanjing 210023, Jiangsu, China. ² College of Pharmacy and Shaanxi Collaborative Innovation Center of Chinese Medicinal Resources Industrialization, Shaanxi University of Chinese Medicine, Xianyang 712046, China.

Acknowledgements

Not applicable.

Competing interests

The authors declare that they have no competing interests.

Consent for publication

Not applicable.

Funding

National Basic Research Program of China (973 Program) (2011CB505300, 2011CB505303), National Natural Science Foundation of China (81603258), 333 High-level Talents Training Project Funded by Jiangsu Province (BRA2016387), and the Priority Academic Program Development of Jiangsu Higher Education Institutions (PAPD).

References

1. Hu YP, Wang L, Li Y. Application of molecular techniques in the research of germplasm resources of Rheum. Biotech Bull. 2010;12:64–8.
2. Barceloux DG. Rhubarb and oxalosis (Rheum species). Dis Mon. 2009;55:403–11.
3. Jiao D, Du SJ. Study on rhubarb. Shanghai: Shanghai Science and Technology Press; 2000. p. 273–307.
4. Wang L, Pan S. Adjuvant treatment with crude rhubarb for patients with acute organophosphorus pesticide poisoning: a meta-analysis of randomized controlled trials. Complement Ther Med. 2015;23:794–801.
5. Lu L, Li HQ, Fu DL, Zheng GQ, Fan JP. Rhubarb root and rhizome-based Chinese herbal prescriptions for acute ischemic stroke: a systematic review and meta-analysis. Complement Ther Med. 2014;22:1060–70.
6. Zhou Y, Wang L, Huang X, Li H, Xiong Y. Add-on effect of crude rhubarb to somatostatin for acute pancreatitis: a meta-analysis of randomized controlled trials. J Ethnopharmacol. 2016;194:495–505.
7. Wang H, Song H, Yue J, Li J, Hou YB, Deng JL. *Rheum officinale* (a Traditional Chinese Medicine) for chronic kidney disease. Cochrane Database Syst Rev. 2012;7:CD008000.
8. Zheng QX, Wu HF, Guo J, Nan HJ, Chen SL, Yang JS, Xu XD. Review of rhubarbs: chemistry and pharmacology. Chin Herbal Med. 2013;5:9–32.
9. Fu XS, Chen F, Liu XH, Xu H, Zhou YZ. Progress in research of chemical constituents and pharmacological actions of Rhubarb. Chin J New Drugs. 2011;20:1534–8.
10. Guan Q, Liang S, Wang Z, Yang Y, Wang S. 1H NMR-based metabonomic analysis of the effect of optimized rhubarb aglycone on the plasma and urine metabolic fingerprints of focal cerebral ischemia-reperfusion rats. J Ethnopharmacol. 2014;154:65–75.
11. Ma LP, Zhao L, Hu HH, Qin YH, Bian YC, Jiang HD, Zhou H, Yu LS, Zeng S. Interaction of five anthraquinones from rhubarb with human organic anion transporter 1 (SLC22A6) and 3 (SLC22A8) and drug–drug interaction in rats. J Ethnopharmacol. 2014;153:864–71.
12. Gao LL. Studies on the chemical constituents and biological activity of *Rheum tanguticum* Maxim.et Balf., *Rhenm officinale* Bail. and *Rheum palmatum* L. Doctor, Graduate School of Peking Union Medical College, Beijing, China; 2012.
13. Tan ZH, Shen YJ, Zhao JN, Li YH, Zhang J. Effects of rhein on the function of human mesangial cells in high glucose environment. Acta Pharm Sin. 2004;39:881–6.
14. Su J, Yin LP, Zhang X, Li BB, Liu L, Li H. Influence of rhein intervention on the expression of HGF and BMP7 in renal tissue of rats with chronical allograft nephropathy. Chin J Clin Pharmacol. 2011;16:1114–20.
15. Wang WY, Zhao Y, Liu XD, Feng YJ, Suo W, Hang G. Preparation of rhein solid dispersion and its effects on experimental diabetic nephropathy in rats. West Chin J Pharm Sci. 2012;27:32–5.
16. Liu QY, Yu SJ. Effects of Rhein on resistin m RNA expression of adipose tissue and plasma free fatty acid in diabetic obese rats. Chin J Tradit Chin Med Pharm. 2009;19:1061–3.
17. Ji YS. Pharmacology and application of active ingredients of Traditional Chinese Medicine. Beijing: People's Medical Publishing House; 2011. p. 95–117.
18. Cui Y, Lu P, Song G, Liu Q, Zhu D, Liu X. Involvement of PI3K/Akt, ERK and p38 signaling pathways in emodin-mediated extrinsic and intrinsic human hepatoblastoma cell apoptosis. Food Chem Toxicol. 2016;92:26–37.
19. Li L, Song X, Yin Z, Jia R, Li Z, Zhou X, Zou YF, Li LX, Yin LZ, Yue GZ, Ye G, Lv C, Shi WJ, Fu YP. The antibacterial activity and action mechanism of emodin from *Polygonum cuspidatum* against *Haemophilus parasuis* in vitro. Microbiol Res. 2016;186–187:139–45.
20. Brkanac SR, Geric M, Gajski G, Vujcic V, Garaj-Vrhovac V, Kremer D, Domijan AM. Toxicity and antioxidant capacity of *Frangula alnus* Mill. bark and its active component emodin. Regul Toxicol Pharmacol. 2015;73:923–9.
21. Chen YK, Xu YK, Zhang H, Yin JT, Fan X, Liu DD, Fu HY, Wan B. Emodin alleviates jejunum injury in rats with sepsis by inhibiting inflammation response. Biomed Pharmacother. 2016;84:1001–7.
22. Zhao YM, Fang YL, Li JC, Duan YX, Zhao HH, Gao L, Luo YM. Neuroprotective effects of Chrysophanol against inflammation in middle cerebral artery occlusion mice. Neurosci Lett. 2016;630:16–22.
23. Tong Y, Jin Z. Research progress of pharmacological effect of physcion. Chin Arch Tradit Chin Med. 2015;33:938–40.
24. Chen X, Gao H, Han Y, Ye J, Xie J, Wang C. Physcion induces mitochondria-driven apoptosis in colorectal cancer cells via downregulating EMMPRIN. Eur J Pharmacol. 2015;764:124–33.
25. Tabolacci C, Cordella M, Turcano L, Rossi S, Lentini A, Mariotti S, Nisini R, Sette G, Eramo A, Piredda L, Maria RD, Facchiano F, Beninati S. Aloe-emodin exerts a potent anticancer and immunomodulatory activity on BRAF-mutated human melanoma cells. Eur J Pharmacol. 2015;762:283–92.
26. Duval J, Pecher V, Poujol M, Lesellier E. Research advances for the extraction, analysis and uses of anthraquinones: a review. Ind Crops Prod. 2016;94:812–33.
27. Li HL, Wang AB, Huang Y, Liu DP, Wei C, Williams GM, Zhang CN, Liu G, Liu YQ, Hao DL, Hui RT, Lin M, Liang CC. Isorhapontigenin, a new res-

veratrol analog, attenuates cardiac hypertrophy via blocking signaling transduction pathways. Free Radic Biol Med. 2005;38:243–57.

28. Dai WS, Zhao RH, Chen HB. Content determination of tannins in *Rheum officinale* by Casein method. Lishizhen Med Mater Med Res. 2003;14:324–6.

29. Zhong HY, Zhang M, Dai Y, Zhang HF. Effect of tannin contained in Radix et Rhizoma Rhei and Radix Polygoni Multiflori on small intestinal propulsion. Lishizhen Med Mater Med Res. 2006;17:2478–9.

30. Shahid A, Ali R, Ali N, Hasan SK, Bernwal P, Afzal SM, Vafa A, Sultana S. Modulatory effects of catechin hydrate against genotoxicity, oxidative stress, inflammation and apoptosis induced by benzo(a) pyrene in mice. Food Chem Toxicol. 2016;92:64–74.

31. Zeng LN, Ma ZJ, Zhao YL, Zhang LD, Li RS, Wang JB, Zhang P, Yan D, Li Q, Jiang BQ, Pu SB, Lu Y, Xiao XH. The protective and toxic effects of rhubarb tannins and anthraquinones in treating hexavalent chromium-injured rats: the Yin/Yang actions of rhubarb. J Hazard Mater. 2013;246–247:1–9.

32. Nan HJ, Xu XD, Chen SL, Bai ZC. Research progress in *Rheum* plants. Nat Prod Res Dev. 2009;21:690–701.

33. Lei S. Bioactivities, isolation and purification methods of polysaccharides from natural products: a review. Int J Biol Macromol. 2016;92:37–48.

34. Xie Y, Li GW, Ma YM. Research progress in rhubarb polysaccharides. Chin J New Drugs. 2010;19:755–8.

35. Li H, Wang J, Qu Y, Xiao X. Analysis on changes of purgative biopotency in different processed products of rhubarb. Chin J Chin Mater Med. 2012;37:302–4.

36. Takayama K, Tsutsumi H, Ishizu T, Okamura N. The influence of rhein 8-*O*-β-D-glucopyranoside on the purgative action of sennoside A from rhubarb in mice. Biol Pharm Bull. 2012;35:2204–8.

37. Feng TS, Yuan ZY, Yang RQ, Zhao S, Lei F, Xiao XY, Xing DM, Wang WH, Ding Y, Du LJ. Purgative components in rhubarbs: adrenergic receptor inhibitors linked with glucose carriers. Fitoterapia. 2013;91:236–46.

38. Qu Y, Wang JB, Li HF, Wang Q, Xiao XH, He YZ. Study on relationship of laxative potency and anthraquinones content traditional Chinese drugs containing. Chin J Chin Mater Med. 2008;33:806–8.

39. Kon R, Ikarashi N, Nagoya C, Takayama T, Kusunoki Y, Ishii M, Ueda H, Ochiai W, Machida Y, Sugita K, Sugiyama K. Rheinanthrone, a metabolite of sennoside A, triggers macrophage activation to decrease aquaporin-3 expression in the colon, causing the laxative effect of rhubarb extract. J Ethnopharmacol. 2014;152:190–200.

40. Nie K. Research and thinking on pharmacological action of rhubarb. J ShanDong Univ Trad Chin Med. 2009;33:239–62.

41. Lemmens L, Borja E. The influence of dihydroxyanthracene derivatives on water and electrolyte movement in rat colon. J Pharm Pharm. 1976;28:498–501.

42. Wang XW, Liu HF, Xu M. Effect of rhubarb on changes of cholinergic nerves in colonic myenteric plexus for chronic slow transit constipation rat. Chongqing Med. 2008;37:1685–7.

43. Zhang WS, Li F, Bao JQ, Wang SC, Shang GW, Li JC, Wang CH. Regulatory effect of anthraquinone derivatives from rhubarb on Aquaporin 4 expression in colon of rats and in LoVo cell line. Chin J Integr Trad West Med. 2008;28:818–23.

44. Li GF. Analysis on pharmacological effects and clinical application of rhubarb. Guide Chin Med. 2013;16:317–8.

45. Li F, Wang SC, Wang X, Ren QY, Wang W, Shang GW, Zhang L, Zhang SH. Novel exploration of cathartic pharmacology induced by rhubarb. Chin J chin mater med. 2006;4:481–4.

46. Qin LS, Zhao HP, Zhao YL, Ma ZJ. Protection and bidirectional effect of rhubarb anthraquinone and tannins for rats liver. Chin J Integr Trad West Med. 2014;34:698–703.

47. Qiu H, Mao DW, Wei AL. Preventive and therapeutic effects of rhubarb extract on hepatic encephalopathy in rats with acute hepatic failure. Chin Med Mat. 2002;25:573–5.

48. Zhang LL, Zhang HY, Wang LM, Li XJ, Jia JT, Lv ML, Fan YM, Zhang CY, Liu MS, Zhao ZF, Han DW, Cheng J. Protective effect of emodin on lung injury induced by hepatic fibrosis in rats. Chin J Pathophys. 2014;30:291–6.

49. Wang XL, Zhang YB, Li XY, Niu YC, Qi YQ, Zhu LQ, Dong MX. Effects of emodin on hepatic fibrosis in rats and underlying mechanisms. Chin

Med Pharmaco Clinic. 2013;4:56–8.

50. Xiong XL, Yan SQ, Qin H, Zhou LS, Zhang LL, Jiang ZX, Ding Y. Protective effect of emodin pretreatment in young rats with intrahepatic cholestasis. Chin J Contemp Pediatr. 2016;18:165–71.

51. Sui F, Yan MJ, Li Y. L N, Xiao YQ, Li L. Comparison of the actions on blood stasis of rhubarb with different prepared methods. Chin Med Pharmaco Clinic. 2012;6:90–3.

52. Wang RQ. Clinical observation of the treatment of micron rhubarb charcoal in peptic ulcer bleeding and the mechanism of platelet system. Master, Hubei College of Traditional Chinese Medicine, Hubei, China; 2007.

53. Zhang S, Shi ZH, Hao JJ, Wang RQ. Hemostatic mechanism of micron rhubarb charcoal. J Chengdu University Trad Chin Med. 2007;30:54–5.

54. Wang GD, Yan T. Clinical application and research of rhubarb. Sichuan: Sichuan Science and Technology Press; 2013.

55. Wang ZW, Guo M, Ma D, Wang RJ. Effects of rhubarbs from different regions on blood lipid and antioxidation of hyperlipidemia rats. Chin J Appl Physiol. 2015;31:278–81.

56. Wang YM, Tian LH, Zhang J. Effects of rhubarb polysaccharide on blood glucose, blood lipids, hepatic lipase activity in rats with diabetic atherosclerosis. Mod Med J Chin. 2008;10:6–9.

57. Zhou SP, Zhou LL, Han W, Wu HP, Li H. Regulating effect of emodin on lipid metabolism and plasma fibrinogen in hyperlipidemic model. Chin J Trad Med Sci Tech. 2007;14:349–50.

58. Du L, Yuan B, Zhang BX, Zhang YL, Gao XY, Wang Y. Study on mechanism for anti-hyperlipidemia efficacy of rhubarb through assistant analysis systems for acting mechanisms of Traditional Chinese medicine. Chin J Chin Mater Med. 2015;40:3703–8.

59. Chen K, Wang CQ, Fan YQ, Han ZH, Wang Y, Gao L, Zeng HS. Lipid-lowering effect of seven traditional Chinese medicine monomers in zebrafish system. Sheng Li Xue Bao. 2017;69:55–60.

60. Wu YX. Clinical application of Dahuang in the treatment of diabetic nephropathy. Clin J Chin Med. 2013;5:29–30.

61. Bi LM. The Research about the effects of fluvastatin and emodin on the expression of MCP-1 on diabetic kidney rats. Master, Nanjing University of Chinese Medicine, Jiangsu, China; 2007.

62. Peng LL. Integrin-linked kinase regulates the ratio of MMP-9/TIMP-1 in tubular epithelial Myofibroblast transdifferentiation of diabetic nephropathy and the role of rhein. Doctor, Central South University, Hunan, China; 2012.

63. Ai ZH, Cai HW, Zhong ZH. Therapeutic effects of rhein on experimental diabetic nephropathy in rats. Acta Acad Med Mil Tert. 2004;26:304–6.

64. Gu LB, Wan YG, Wang M. Advances in molecular mechanism of rhubarb in the treatment of diabetic nephropathy. Chin J Chin Mater Med. 2003;28:703–5.

65. Wang M. Protective effect of rhein on kidney in obese diabetic rats and its mechanism. Doctor, Liaoning University of TCM, Liaoning, China; 2008.

66. Qi ZQ, Hu HZ, Wang XS, Li W. Review on molecular and cellular mechanism researches of emodin for treating kidney disease. Global Chin Med. 2015;9:1145–8.

67. Li Y, Yan MJ, Sui F, Lin N, Liu LL, Xiao YQ, Li L, Ma CY. Study on antipyretic effect and mechanism of alcohol extracts from different processed rhubarb. J Chin Med Mater. 2012;35:1224–7.

68. Yan J. Study on neuroprotective effects and mechanism of chrysophanol liposomes on cerebral ischemia–reperfusion injured mice. Doctor, Hebei Med University, Hebei, China; 2014.

69. Zhang M. The laboratory investigation of the effects on emodin and chrysophanol to hypoxic damaged neural cell. Master, Lanzhou University, Gansu, China; 2010.

70. Lin MX, Wu J, Zhuang R, Wang BJ, Jin SW. Influence of rhubarb combined shenfu injection on respiratory functions of acute respiratory distress syndrome patients. Chin Arch Tradit Chin Med. 2013;6:1465–7.

71. Wang ZW, Guo M, Ma D, Tuo HY, Wang RQ. Analysis of anti-inflammatory effect and mechanism of *Rheum tanguticum* cultivated in South of Gansu. Chin J Exp Tradit Med Form. 2016;22:158–61.

72. Du JD, Yu ZH, He FD. Effect of emodin on the expression of osteocalcin and interleukin-6 in periodontal tissues of periodontitis rats. Clin Med. 2009;29:92–5.

73. Jang YN, Mo HY, Ren H. Effect of emodin lipid nano-microbubble on MAPK signal pathway and inflammation cytokine in AT-II cells by mechanical stretch. Chin Med Mat. 2013;36:967–71.

74. Huang M, Ma J, Yang CH, Lu B, Guo P, Shao JQ, Du H, Wang J. Effects of rheinic acid on markers of insulin secretion, inflammation and oxidative injury in db/db mice. Chin Remed Clin. 2013;13:976–9.

75. Hu B, Zhang H, Meng X, Wang F, Wang P. Aloe-emodin from rhubarb (*Rheum rhabarbarum*) inhibits lipopolysaccharide-induced inflammatory responses in RAW264.7 macrophages. J Ethnopharmacol. 2014;153:846–53.

76. Lin SZ. Study on the effects of emodin on pancreatic cancer and its mechanisms. Doctor, Zhejiang University, Zhejiang, China; 2011.

77. Wang RT, Yin H, Dong SB, Yuan W, Liu YP, Liu C. Research progress of emodin anti-gallbladder carcinoma. Chin J Chin Mater Med. 2014;39:1976–8.

78. Li RF, Yang FJ, Zhao J, Ye YT, Xu WQ. Effects of dihydroxy anthraquinones compound on radiosensitivity of cervical carcinoma HeLa cells. Chin Pharm. 2011;15:1353–6.

79. Liu A, Deng ZF, Hu JX, Han SW, Huang LL, Ke PY, Lin SZ. Effect of emodin on cell proliferation and apoptosis of human pancreatic cancer cell line Panc-1. Chin Tradit Herbal Drugs. 2011;42:756–9.

80. He ZH, He MF, Ma SC, But PP. Anti-angiogenic effects of rhubarb and its anthraquinone derivatives. J Ethnopharmacol. 2009;121:313–7.

81. Tsai KH, Hsien HH, Chen LM, Ting WJ, Yang YS, Kuo CH, Tsai CH, Tsai FJ, Tsai HJ, Huang CY. Rhubarb inhibits hepatocellular carcinoma cell metastasis via GSK-3-beta activation to enhance protein degradation and attenuate nuclear translocation of beta-catenin. Food Chem. 2013;138:278–85.

82. Li CL, Ye YW, Sun JY. Study on antimicrobial activity of emodin and aloe-emodin. Chin J Pharmacol Toxicity. 1989;5:381–1234.

83. Tian B, Hua YJ, Ma XQ, Wang GL. Relationship between antibacterial activity of aloe and its anthaquinone compounds. Chin J Chin Mater Med. 2003;28:1034–7.

84. Zhou L, Yun BY, Wang YJ, Xie MJ. Antibacterial mechanism of emodin on *Staphylococcus aureus*. Chin J Biochem Mol Biol. 2011;27:1156–60.

85. Liu M. Investigation on its Anti-MRSA effects of emodin in vitro and in vivo, and its mechanism. Doctor, Third Military Medical University, Chongqing, China; 2015.

86. Li J, Yin LB, Zhang X, Li BB, Liu L, Li H. Influence of rhein intervention on the expression of HGF and BMP7 in renal tissue of rats with chronical allograft nephropathy. Chin J Clin Pharm Therap. 2011;16:1114–20.

87. Liu LJ, Qian H, Zhang P. Protective effect of emodin on rats with pulmonary fibrosis and its partial mechanisms. Chin Pharmacol Bull. 2015;31:266–72.

88. Xu K, Zhang L. Research progress of rhein acid on renal fibrosis. J New Chin Med. 2012;44:119–21.

89. Gu QP, Liu JJ, Xie JF. Clinical observation on 100 cases of chronic constipation treated by rhubarb combined with *Lactobacillus* in Elderly. Strait Pharm J. 2015;27:118–9.

90. Luo HQ, Lin XJ, Liu XM. Clinical effect and nursing of hot compress with fructus evodiae and coarse salt combined with acupoint sticking of rhubarb in prevention of constipation after stroke. Zhong Xi Yi Jie He Hu Li. 2015;1:4–8.

91. Liu SX, Zhao CZ, Yang DD. Clinical study on umbilical area applying rhubarb and borneol to prevent constipation for acute myocardial infarction patients. Hu Li Yan Jiu. 2010;24:881–2.

92. Yu XF. Observation of clinical efficacy on constipation after orthopedic surgery treated with umbilicus compress of rhubarb and mirabilite in the patients. Shi Jie Zhong Xi Yi Jie He Za Zhi. 2014;6:614–6.

93. Zhu W, Wang XM. Progress in study on mechanisms of rhubarb in treating chronic renal failure. Chin J Integr Trad West Med. 2005;25:471–5.

94. Liu HF, Zhang CY. Comprehensive nursing rhubarb compound enema decoction high colon dialysis treatment for diabetic nephropathy phase IV and V clinical observation. Hu Li Tian Di. 2016;1:184–6.

95. Xiong ZH. The study of intervention effect and molecular mechanism of rhubarb used in diabetic nephropathy. Doctor, Guangzhou University of Chinese Medicine. Guangzhou, China; 2012.

96. Wang JN. Clinical observation of the combined treatment of rhubarb soda and jinshuibao capsule on chronic renal failure. Chin J Clin Rational Drug Use. 2013;6:67–8.

97. Xiao W, Deng HZ, Ma Y. Summarization of the clinical and laboratory study on the rhubarb in treating chronic renal failure. Chin J Chin Mater Med. 2002;27:241–4.

98. Sun BQ, Zhu GB. Clinical observation on treatment of rhubarb and mirabilite on severe acute pancreatitis. J Emerg Tradit Chin Med. 2017;23:1155–6.

99. Zhang Y, Wang P, Yang YM, Zang Y, Yu YP, Meng XL, Chen XR. Protective effect of rhubarb free Anthraquinone on intestinal barrier injury in beagle dogs induced by severe acute pancreatitis. Chin J Exp Tradit Med Form. 2013;19:172–6.

100. Wang LL, Liu YQ, Cheng L, Fan L, Xiong YX. The influence of free anthraquinone of rhubarb in sever acute pancreatitis induced kidney injury. Chin Med Pharmaco Clin. 2015;31:31–4.

101. Wang SZ. Forty cases with UPPer gastrointestinal hemorrhage treated with oral administration of raw dahuang powder. Henan Trad Chin Med. 2015;35:2798–9.

102. Liao SF, Chen HM, Zhang YQ, Wang YC. Clinical study on controlling upper gastrointestinal bleeding by early nasogastric feeding rhubarb powder after severe brain injuries. Mod Med J China. 2004;14:105–7.

103. Guo P, Zhang TJ, Zhu XY, He YZ. Study on toxicity of Radix et Rhizoma Rhei and countermeasure for its attenuation. Chin Tradit Herbal Drugs. 2009;40:1671–4.

104. Du C, Wang CL, Fan BL. Advances in research on target organ of rhubarb and its specific toxicity. J Toxicol. 2015;29:461–4.

105. Yan M, Zhang LY, Sun LX, Jiang ZZ, Xiao XH. Nephrotoxicity study of total rhubarb anthraquinones on Sprague Dawley rats using DNA microarrays. J Ethnopharmacol. 2006;107:08–11.

106. Wang QX. Study on the toxicity and its mechanism of rhubarb and its major constituents. Doctor, Academy of Military Medical Sciences, Beijing, China; 2007.

107. Wang YH, Zhao HP, Wang JB, Zhao YL, Xiao XH. Study on dosage-toxicity/efficacy relationship of prepared rhubarb on basis of symptom-based prescription theory. Chin J Chin Mater Med. 2014;39:918–23.

108. Wang HF, Guo B, Ma XP, Xue RC. Reproductive toxicity study of rhubarb extract on early pregnancy mice and its preliminary mechanism. Chin J Immun. 2016;32:184–8.

109. Hu XC. Study on the reproductive toxicity of rhubarb in male rats. Master, Chengde Medical College, Hebei, China, 2012.

18

Seeing the unseen of Chinese herbal medicine processing (*Paozhi*)

Xu Wu[1], Shengpeng Wang[2*], Junrong Lu[3,4], Yong Jing[3], Mingxing Li[1], Jiliang Cao[2], Baolin Bian[5] and Changjiang Hu[3*]

Abstract

Processing (*Paozhi*) represents a unique Chinese pharmaceutic technique to facilitate the use of Chinese herbal medicines (CHMs) for a specific clinical need in the guidance of Traditional Chinese Medicine (TCM) theory. Traditionally, most CHMs require a proper processing to meet the needs of specific clinical syndromes before being prescribed by TCM practitioners. During processing, significant changes in chemical profiles occur, which inevitably influence the associated pharmacological properties of a CHM. However, although processing is formed in a long-term practice, the underlying mechanisms remain unclear for most CHMs. The deepening understanding of the mechanism of processing would provide scientific basis for standardization of processing. This review introduced the role of processing in TCM and several typical methods of processing. We also summarized the up-to-date efforts on the mechanistic study of CHM processing. The processing mechanisms mainly include the following aspects: (i) directly reducing contents of toxic constituents; (ii) structural transformation of constituents; (iii) improving solubility of constituents; (iv) physically changing the existing form of constituents; (v) and influence by excipients. These progress may give new insights into future researches.

Keywords: Processing, Chinese herbal medicines, Decoction pieces, Standardization, Mechanism

Background

Processing, *Paozhi* in Chinese, is an ancient Chinese pharmaceutic technique to facilitate the use of Chinese herbal medicines (CHMs) for a specific clinical need in the guidance of Traditional Chinese Medicine (TCM) theory [1]. Processing of CHMs develops along with the history of TCM and promotes the formation of TCM theory in long-term practice, even wine serves as part of the ancient Chinese character 'medicine' for all its important role. Most CHMs need to be elaborately processed to become decoction pieces prior to their final consumption in the clinic or manufacture of proprietary drugs [2]. Processing represents a unique Chinese pharmaceutic

approach that differentiates CHMs from other medicinal herbs in the world. In Chinese Pharmacopoeia (CP, 2015 edition), decoction piece(s) and related processing method(s) are clearly listed as a specific item of a CHM, and some decoction pieces like Astragali Radix Preparata Cum Melle are recorded as a separate CHM with independent quality control standards and indications [3]. In contrast, only few processed medicinal herbs and processing methods are recorded in the pharmacopoeias of other countries [4].

Processing encompasses a series of techniques such as cutting, crushing, roasting, baking, and stir-frying with or without liquid/solid excipient, by which decoction pieces with different therapeutic potency can be derived from the same herb [1]. For instance, Pinelliae Rhizoma (PR) is a commonly used CHM for the treatment of phlegm-induced cough, vomit and headache [5]. Four processed PR are recorded in the latest CP, namely raw PR, PR Praeparatum (PRP, processed with

*Correspondence: sxwsp@163.com; hhccjj204@126.com
[2] State Key Laboratory of Quality Research in Chinese Medicine, Institute of Chinese Medical Sciences, University of Macau, Macao, China
[3] College of Pharmacy, Chengdu University of Traditional Chinese Medicine, Liutai Avenue, Wenjiang District, Chengdu, Sichuan, China
Full list of author information is available at the end of the article

15% Glycyrrhizae Radix et Rhizoma and 10% lime), PR Praeparatum cum Zingibere et Alumine (PRZA, processed with 25% Zingiberis Rhizoma Recens and 12.5% alume) and PR Praeparatum cum Alumine (PRPA, processed with 20% alume) [3]. These decoction pieces produced by different processing methods are developed to reduce the toxicity of PR [6] and to guide and concentrate its therapeutic effects. Raw PR is often externally used for treatment of carbuncle and furuncle, PRP is inclined to relieve phlegm-caused cough, dizziness and headache, while PRZA and PRPA are respectively prescribed for phlegm-caused vomit and cough (Fig. 1).

Generally, processing can reduce toxicity, reinforce efficacy, alter energetic nature and therapeutic direction, as well as improve flavor of CHMs, thereby increase the therapeutic effectiveness and applicability of CHMs in individualized treatment. However, despite the extensive use of processed CHM, the underlying mechanisms of processing remain unclear for most CHMs to date. During the processing, particularly under heating and/or moist conditions, complicated changes in herbal components of CHMs may occur: the contents be increased or decreased; structures be changed; and/or novel compounds be formed. In many cases, the contents and structures of

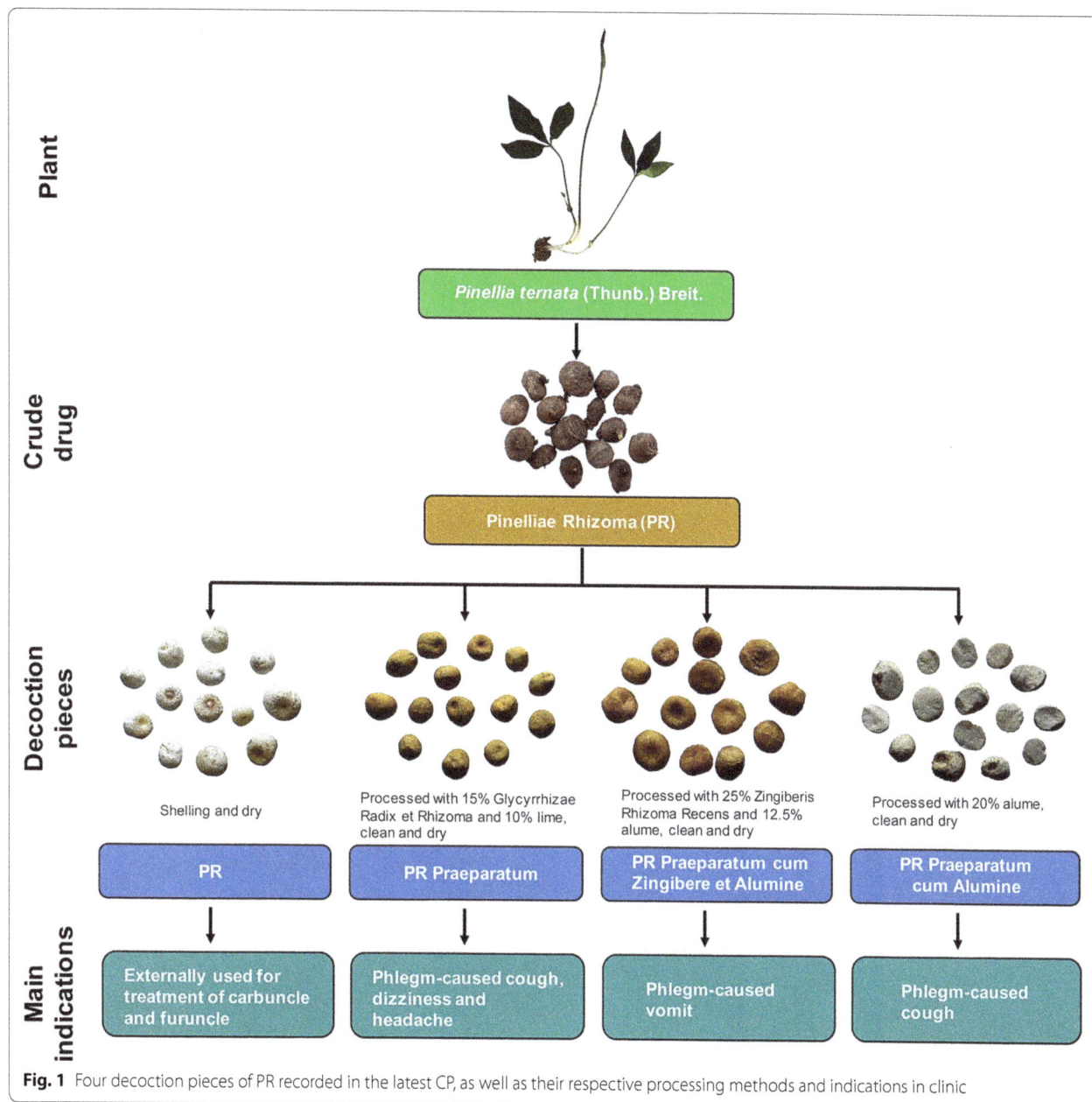

Fig. 1 Four decoction pieces of PR recorded in the latest CP, as well as their respective processing methods and indications in clinic

constituents may be altered simultaneously. Along with these changes mediated by processing, the pharmacological activity of a certain CHM may be changed accordingly. Therefore, investigation of the chemical and pharmacological changes of CHM before and after processing is key for understanding of underlying mechanisms. In the past few decades, emerging studies have been carried out to elucidate the mechanisms of processing. Herein, this review summarizes the up-to-date knowledge on these aspects, aiming to provide new insights to future researches.

Methods of processing

The first recordation of processing can be dated back to 200 BC in Recipes for 52 Ailments (*Wushi'er Bingfang*), in which some classical methods like burning, calcining, stewing, and soaking were listed [7]. In the Northern and Southern dynasties, Master Lei's discourse on processing (*Leigong Paozhi Lun*) appeared as the earliest book that systemically described the principles and methods of processing [8]. Afterwards, there are a series of monographs of processing that record and summarize the experiences of TCM practitioners. In broad terms, processing describes every procedure involved in preparing raw plants (or animal or mineral) into decoction pieces. In this review we mainly discuss these specific methods applied when the CHMs are cleaned, cut, and dried. Some commonly used processing methods are described below and listed in Table 1.

Stir-frying

Cleaned and cut crude CHMs are fried in a pot, with or without the aid of excipients, while being constantly stirred until a certain degree of frying is obtained.

Stir-frying without excipients

Usually there are three degrees of stir-frying evaluated by the color in appearance and/or odor of a specific herb: stir-frying till yellow, till charred, and till carbonized (black outside and charred inside). Crataegi Fructus is a typical CHM that can be stir-fried until different degrees for distinct therapeutic purpose [9]. Un-processed Crataegi Fructus can promote digestion and invigorate blood circulation while stir-fried Crataegi Fructus is mainly used for indigestion. In contrast, charred Crataegi Fructus and carbonized Crataegi Fructus are used for the treatment of indigestion-caused diarrhea and gastrointestinal hemorrhage, respectively.

Stir-frying with liquid excipients

In order to reinforce and/or guide the efficiency of the herbs, many liquid excipients like yellow rice wine, vinegar and honey are often added to the crude herbs prior to stir-frying. For instance, processing with wine can enhance the effect of Angelicae Sinensis Radix in invigorating blood circulation [10], and wine-fried Angelicae Sinensis Radix is widely prescribed in many famous

Table 1 Typical processing methods and representative processed CHMs listed in CP (2015 edition)

Processing method	Excipient	Representative processed CHM
Stir-frying (清炒)	–	Stir-fried Ziziphi Spinosae Semen (炒酸棗仁)
		Charred Crataegi Fructus (焦山楂)
		Carbonized Rhei Radix Et Rhizoma (大黃炭)
Stir-frying with liquid excipients (炙)	Yellow rice wine (酒)	Wine-fried Rhei Radix Et Rhizoma (酒大黃)
	Vinegar (醋)	Vinegar-fried Curcumae Rhizoma (醋莪術)
	Salt water (鹽)	Salt-fried Alpiniae Oxyphyllae Fructus (鹽益智仁)
	Fresh ginger juice (薑)	Ginger-fried Magnoliae Officinalis Cortex (薑厚樸)
	Refined honey (蜜)	Honey-fried Astragali Radix (炙黃芪)
Stir-frying with solid excipients (炒)	Wheat bran (麥麩)	Bran-fried Dioscoreae Rhizoma (麩炒山藥)
	Rice (米)	Rice-fried Mylabris (米斑蝥)
	River sand (砂)	Zingiberis Rhizoma Praeparatum (sand-fried Zingiberis Rhizoma 炮薑)
Steaming (蒸)	–	Ginseng Radix Et Rhizoma Rubra (Steamed Ginseng 紅參)
	Yellow rice wine (酒)	Wine-steamed Corni Fructus (酒萸肉)
	Vinegar (醋)	Vinegar-steamed Schisandrae Chinensis Fructus (醋五味子)
Boiling (煮)	Zingiberis Rhizoma Recens and alume	Arisaematis Rhizoma Preparatum (制天南星)
	Glycyrrhizae Radix et Rhizoma and lime	Pinelliae Rhizoma Praeparatum (法半夏)
Stewing (煨)	Straw paper (草紙)	Straw paper-stewed Aucklandiae Radix (煨木香)
	Wheat bran (麥麩)	Wheat bran-stewed Myristicae Semen (麩煨肉豆蔻)
Water trituration (水飛)	–	Water-triturated Cinnabaris (朱砂粉)
Calcining (煅)	–	Calcined Haematitum (煅赭石)

TCM formulae including Danggui Buxue decection, Siwu Decoction and Longdan Xiegan Pills.

Stir-frying with solid excipients

Similar to liquid excipient-assisted stir-frying, stir-frying with solid excipients also helps to extend the utility of CHMs. Stir-frying with rice represents an important approach of TCM practitioners to reduce the toxicity of some poisonous CHMs such as Mylabris [11] and reinforce the effect of many spleen-tonifying CHMs including Codonopsis Radix [12].

Steaming

Steaming is a commonly used processing method to alter the properties of various CHMs by steaming the crude herbs with or without additional excipients. For example, steaming raw Polygoni Multiflori Radix with black bean juice can turn the anti-malarial and defecating effects to tonifying effects like liver and kidney replenishing, hair blackening, and bone strengthening [13, 14].

Boiling

Boiling CHMs in water or in a herbal decoction can also (i) minimize the side effect of CHMs, such as Glycyrrhizae Radix decoction boiled Polygalae Radix to reduce the irritation on throat [15]; or (ii) enhance the therapeutic effect, such as vinegar boiled Curcumae Rhizoma to reinforce the effect in removing blood stasis.

Stewing

Wrapping CHMs in moistened papers, bran or mud, and heating until the envelop becomes cracked or charred is another approach to reduce the undesired constituents and reinforce the astringent effect of CHMs. Wheat bran-stewed Myristicae Semen is the major form of Myristicae Semen in clinical application due to reduced irritant oils [16]. Stewing using moistened straw paper endows Aucklandiae Radix with stronger astringent property and enhance the anti-diarrhea effect [17].

Other processing methods

Many other methods are widely applied to guarantee the safety and effectiveness of CHMs. For instance, water trituration is a repetitious and complicated process by grounding mineral CHMs with water to obtain extremely fine powder. Many mineral and crustaceous CHMs can be calcined directly or indirectly in the flames to render these hard CHMs crisp and thus easy to crush.

Advances in understanding the mechanism of processing

Processing is an important feature of CHM, which is formed early in the history of TCM and has developed along with its clinical practice. The methods and purposes of processing are usually different for different herbs, while processing might have multiple influences on a certain herb. In TCM theory, disease is often a result of imbalance between Yin and Yang in human body. It is believed that processing can adjust the nature (heat, warm, cold and cool) of a certain CHM to facilitate the symptomatic and accurate prescription by TCM practitioners and help equilibrate the balance between Yin and Yang in human body. In this regard, traditionally, most CHMs require proper processing before being prescribed. Processing may directly reduce the contents of toxic constituents, transform the structure of constituents, or increase the solubility of active constituents (Fig. 2). Efforts have been made in recent years to understand the traditional aspect of processing. Some representative evidences in elucidating the mechanisms of CHM processing are displayed in Table 2.

Directly reducing contents of toxic constituents

The primary concept of detoxification is to reduce the contents of toxic constituents in CHM. Processing has been proved as a useful means to reduce the toxicity of certain CHMs. Toxic compounds usually possess unique physical characteristics. Based on this, specific processing methods may efficiently reduce their contents in the corresponding CHMs.

Mylabris (Banmao), is derived from the blister beetles *Mylabris phalerata* Pallas or *M. cichorii* Linnaeus, and is a famous poisonous CHM using for treating cancers [59, 60]. The internal use of Banmao often leads to serious nephrotoxicity which is lethal [61]. Traditionally, Mylabris is stir-frying processed with or without the presence of rice. In recent years, Mylabris is also processed with sodium hydroxide solutions. Both methods have been proved to reduce its toxicity [62]. It has been demonstrated that cantharidin, a terpenoid defensive toxin, is responsible for the therapeutic action as well as toxicity of Mylabris [63–65]. Therefore, control of the contents of cantharidin is key for safe and effective use of Mylabris. A number of studies show that cantharidin can be readily sublimated when the processing temperature reaches 120 °C, and thus its contents in raw materials are significantly reduced [66]. Furthermore, in alkaline condition of sodium hydroxide solution, cantharidin becomes the form of cantharidinate sodium, which is less nephrotoxic than the original form [67, 68]. Based on

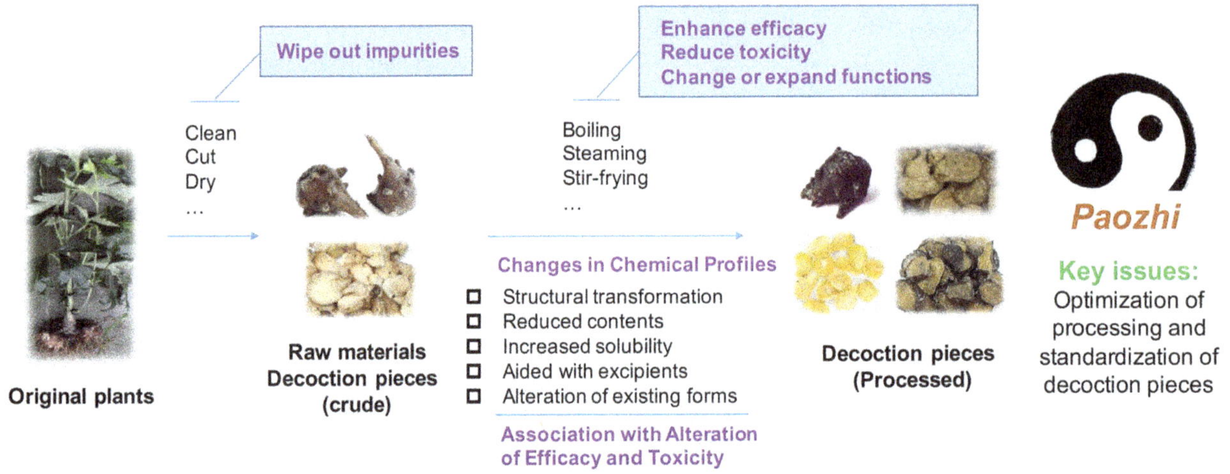

Fig. 2 Understanding of traditional aspects of CHM processing (*Paozhi*) via advanced chemical and pharmacological evaluations. *Paozi* results in complex changes in chemical profiles of CHMs via structural transformation, reduced contents, increased solubility, alteration of existing form of constituents and influence by excipients. Inevitably, these chemical changes lead to alteration of efficacy and/or toxicity of CHMs. *Paozi* can adjust the nature (heat, warm, cold and cool) of a certain CHM to facilitate the symptomatic and accurate prescription by TCM practitioners and help equilibrate the balance between Yin and Yang in human body. As a traditional technique, the key issues in modernization of *Paozi* are the optimization of processing method and the standardization of decoction pieces. The processing of Aconitum root is illustrated as a representative

these findings, different processing methods result in the decreased contents of highly-toxic cantharidin and thus reduce the toxicity of Mylabris.

Crotonis Semen (Badou, in Chinese) is the dried fruit of *Croton tiglium* L., and is used in TCM for treatment of ascites, constipation, diphtheritis, acute laryngitis and laryngeal obstruction [69]. Raw Crotonis Semen is highly toxic and can cause hemolysis and severe diarrhea. It is demonstrated that the toxic components mainly exist in the Croton oil [70, 71]. Traditional processing method to remove oil from Crotonis Semen can remarkably reduce the contents of toxic constituents, resulting in reduced toxicity.

Structural transformation of constituents

Many methods of processing, such as stir-frying, steaming and boiling, necessitate the heating and/or moist conditions, which inevitably leads to complex chemical changes in processed CHMs. Structural transformation of herbal components is one of the most common consequences due to processing. Herbal components may undergo oxidation, decomposition, isomerization, hydrolysis and/or reaction with other constituents, eventually, to form novel compounds [72]. This often results in alteration of pharmacological or toxicological properties of processed CHMs compared to the raw ones. Some of CHMs, including the Aconitum root, Ginseng Radix et Rhizome and Rhei Radix et Rhizoma, have been demonstrated to possess distinct chemical profiles after processing and show reduced toxicity or altered therapeutic activities.

Aconitum root: decomposing of highly toxic components during processing leads to detoxification

Chuanwu (*Aconiti* Radix, the mother root of *A. carmichaeli*), Fuzi (*A. Lateralis* Radix, the daughter root of *A. carmichaeli*) and Caowu (*A. kusnezoffii* Radix, the root of *A. kusnezoffii*) are three most popular Aconitum herbs used in TCM and are documented in the latest CP [73, 74]. Raw Aconitum plants are extremely dangerous, and can only applied in external use. They are used in decoction, proprietary medicines and other formulations only after being properly processed (repeated boiling or steaming). Aconitum root induces remarkable cardiotoxicity and neurotoxicity. The toxidrome of acute aconite poisoning is a combination of cardiovascular, neurological, gastrointestinal and other symptoms [75]. Despite their toxicity and narrow therapeutic window, Aconitum root has been widely used in TCM due to their anti-inflammatory, analgesic and cardiotonic properties [76]. Till now, there are six different types of processed Aconitum medicinals, including Zhichuanwu, Yanfuzi, Danfupian, Heishunpian, Baifupian and Zhicaowu, which are documented in the latest CP. Regardless of the distinct processing methods, many researches have demonstrated that properly processed Aconitum root showed reduced toxicity [77, 78].

The toxicity of Aconitum herbs is mainly due to the presence of Aconitum alkaloids at high concentrations [79, 80]. These alkaloids have been found to target voltage-sensitive sodium channels in myocardium, nerves and muscles, and cause cardiotoxicity and

Table 2 Mechanisms of processing of representative CHMs

Decoction pieces		Purpose and major mechanisms of processing	References
Crude CHM	**Processed CHM (processing method)**		
Aconiti Radix, Chuanwu 川乌 Aconiti Lateralis Radix, Nifuzi 泥附子	Aconiti Radix Cocta, Zhichuanwu 制川乌 (soaking, boiling or steaming) Aconiti Lateralis Radix Praeparata, Yanfuzi 盐附子 (soaking) Aconiti Lateralis Radix Praeparata, Danfupian 淡附片 (soaking in salt water, boiling with Glycyrrhizae Radix and black bean) Aconiti Lateralis Radix Praeparata, Heishunpian 黑顺片 (soaking in salt water, staining and steaming) Aconiti Lateralis Radix Praeparata, Baifupian 白附片 (soaking in salt water, peeling and steaming) Paofupian炮附片 (sand-scorch of Heishunpian or Baifupian)	*Purpose* Reducing toxicity *Mechanisms* Structural transformation of toxic constituents: (1) highly toxic diester diterpene alkaloids hydrolyze or decompose into monoester diterpene alkaloids of low toxicity or non-toxic non-esterfied diterpene alkaloids. (2) Diester diterpene alkaloids react with components in Glycyrrhizae Radix to generate lipo-alkaloids of low-toxicity. On the other hand, the resultant alkaloids have considerable anti-inflammatory and analgesic effects	[18–20]
Aconiti Kusnezoffii Radix, Caowu 草乌	Aconiti Kusnezoffii Radix Cocta, Zhicaowu 制草乌 (soaking in water and boiling)		
Pinelliae Rhizoma, Banxia 半夏	Pinelliae Rhizoma Praeparatum, Fabanxia 法半夏 (soaking with water and then with Glycyrrhizae Radix juice) Pinelliae Rhizoma Praeparatum Cum Zingibere et Alumine, Jiangbanxia 姜半夏 (soaking with water, boiling with ginger and alum) Pinelliae Rhizoma Praeparatum Cum Alumine, Qingbanxia 清半夏 (soaking with alum solution)	*Purpose* Reducing toxicity *Mechanisms* (1) Physically changed crystal structure: alum solution changes the structure of needle-like calcium oxalate crystals and dissolves the lectin in the crystals, which decreases the side effect. (2) Detoxifying components from excipients: a compound gingerol from ginger juice can effectively inhibit Banxia-induced inflammation	[21–25]
Typhonii Rhizoma, Baifuzi 白附子	Zhibaifuzi 制白附子 (soaking with alum solution)		
Rhei Radix et Rhizoma, Dahuang 大黄	Jiudahuang 酒大黄 (stir-frying with alcohol) Shudahuang 熟大黄 (steaming or steaming with alcohol) Dahuangtan 大黄炭 (charring)	*Purpose* Changing functions and reducing toxicity *Mechanisms* (1) Decomposing of conjugated anthraquinones into the corresponding free anthraquinones; (2) reduced contents of tannins; (3) after processing, Dahuangtan has no effect on blood circulation	[26–28]
Angelicae Sinensis Radix, Danggui 当归	Jiudanggui 酒当归 (stir-frying with alcohol)	*Purpose* Enhancing efficacy *Mechanisms* (1) Increasing the solubility of ferulic acid; (2) decreasing the content of Z-ligustilide. Both ferulic acid and Z-ligustilide are biological constituents, but high concentration of Z-ligustilide is irritant	[10, 29–31]
Ginseng Radix et Rhizoma, Renshen 人参	Ginseng Radix et Rhizoma Rubra, Hongshen 红参 (steaming)	*Purpose* Enhancing efficacy and reduced side effect *Mechanisms* (1) Structural transformation of ginsenosides via hydrolysis of sugar moieties and/or epimerization of 20(S)-type into 20(R)-type; (2) Maillard reaction on reducing sugars and amino acids to form phenol compounds; (3) degradation of denichine which has neurotoxicity. These changes contribute to enhanced anti-oxidant, anti-cancer and immue-modulating effects, and reduced side effect	[32–37]
Strychni Semen, Maqianzi 马钱子	Zhimaqianzi 制马钱子 (stir-frying with sand)	*Purpose* Reducing toxicity *Mechanisms* Decomposition and oxidation of highly-toxic strychnine and brucine to generate isostrychnine, isobrucine, brucine N-oxide and strychnine N-oxide	[38–41]

Table 2 continued

Decoction pieces		Purpose and major mechanisms of processing	References
Crude CHM	**Processed CHM (processing method)**		
Mylabris, Banmao 斑蝥	Mibanmao 米斑蝥 (stir-frying with rice)	*Purpose* Reducing toxicity *Mechanisms* Reducing contents of toxic constituents: stir-frying of Banmao facilitates sublimation of cantharidin when the processing temperature reaches 120 °C, and the content of cantharidin is significantly reduced	[42]
Crotonis Fructus, Badou 巴豆	Crotonis Semen Pulveratum, Badoushuang 巴豆霜 (partially removal of croton oil)	*Purpose* Reducing toxicity *Mechanisms* Reduced contents of toxic constituents: processing via removal of Crotonis oil which contains toxic constituents reduces toxicity of Badou	[43]
Atractylodis Macrocephalae Rhizoma, Baizhu 白術	Fuchaobaizhu 麸炒白術 (stir-frying with bran)	*Purpose* Enhancing efficacy *Mechanisms* Structural transformation via decomposing atractylone into Atractylenolide I and II during processing	[44, 45]
Genkwa Flos, Yuanhua 芫花	Cuyuanhua 醋芫花 (stir-frying with vinegar)	*Purpose* Reducing toxicity and enhancing efficacy *Mechanisms* (1) The contents of Yuanhuacine and genkwadaphnin which are highly toxic are decreased; (2) the contents of bioactive flavonoids, including genkwanin, 3'-hydroxy-genkwanin and apigenin, are increased, likely due to the transformation of flavonoid glycosides into the respective glycones	[46]
Glycyrrhizae Radix et Rhizoma, Gancao 甘草	Glycyrrhizae Radix et Rhizoma Praeparata Cum Melle, Zhigancao 炙甘草 (stir-frying with honey)	*Purpose* Enhancing efficacy *Mechanisms* Hydrolysis of glycosides such as glycyrrhizin, liquiritin apioside and isoliquiritin apioside into glycyrrhetinic acid, liquiritigenin and isoliquiritigenin, respectively, with enhanced anti-inflammatory effect	[47]
Calamina, Luganshi 爐甘石	Duanluganshi 煆爐甘石 (calcining)	*Purpose* Enhancing efficacy *Mechanisms* Decomposing ZnCO3 into ZnO which has better antimicrobial activity	[48, 49]
Leaves of *Baphicacanthus cusia* (Nees) Bremek., *Polygonum tinctorium* Ait. or *Isatis indigotica* Fort.	Indigo Naturalis, Qingdai 青黛	*Purpose* Enhancing efficacy *Mechanisms* Decomposing isatan B or indole glycoside and further condensed to form indigos and indirubin, the active constituents	[50]
Kansui Radix, Gansui 甘遂	Cugansui 醋甘遂 (stir-frying with vinegar)	*Purpose* Reducing toxicity *Mechanisms* (1) Conversion of the highly-toxic 3-Acyl ester components into the non-toxic 20-acyl ester components; (2) reaction of diterpenes with acetic acid to form acetylated diterpenes with poor solubility which decreases toxicity	[51, 52]
Sinapis Semen, Jiezi 芥子	Chaojiezi 炒芥子 (Stir-frying)	*Purpose* Reducing side effect *Mechanisms* Inactivation of myrosase via heating to retain the glucosinolates, including sinalbrin	[53]
Xanthii Fructus, Cang'erzi 蒼耳子	Chaocang'erzi 炒蒼耳子 (stir-frying)	*Purpose* Reducing toxicity *Mechanisms* Decomposing β-D-Fructofuranosyl-α-D-glucopyranoside and other glycosides	[54]
Epimedii Folium, Yinyanghuo 淫羊藿	Zhiyinyanghuo 炙淫羊藿 (stir-frying with mutton fat)	*Purpose* Enhancing efficacy *Mechanisms* Decomposing flavonoid glycosides to form secondary glycosides or aglycones, which results in enhanced gonadal function	[55, 56]
Coptidis Rhizoma, Huanglian 黄連	Jiuhuanglian 酒黄連 (stir-frying with alcohol)	*Purpose* Enhancing efficacy *Mechanisms* (1) Increased solubility of the contents of berberine, palmatine, coptisine and jatrorrhizine; (2) decomposing of berberine to form a novel compound berberubine which has anticancer activity	[57, 58]

neurotoxicity [81, 82]. C_{19}-diterpenoid-type alkaloids are found to be the main constituents of aconitum [73]. These alkaloids are further classified into four types: diester diterpenoid alkaloids (DDA), such as aconitine, mesaconitine, and hypaconitine; monoester diterpenoid alkaloids (MDA), such as benzoylaconine, benzoylhypaconine, and benzoylmesaconine; non-ester diterpenoid alkaloids (NDA), such as aconine, mesaconine, and hypaconine; and lipoalkaloids. A series of studies have demonstrated that the DDA can be decomposed into MDA by losing an acetic acid at C-8 position during processing, which further undergo elimination of a benzoylic acid at C-14 position to generate NDA, or substitution with a fatty acid acyl group at C-8 position to form lipoalkaloids [18–20]. For instance, at the heating and moist condition (boiling or steaming), aconitine, mesaconitine and hypaconitine could be firstly converted into benzoylaconine, benzoylmesaconine and benzoylhypaconine, respectively, and further transformed into aconine, mesaconine, and hypaconine, respectively [83, 84]. After processing, the contents of the DDA (aconitine, mesaconitine and hypaconitine) were significantly reduced in Fuzi [84]. Since DDA are much toxic (100- to 400-fold) than MDA and lipoalkaloids, decomposing of DDA has been identified as the main mechanism for detoxification of aconitum processing [73]. Notably, MDA and lipoalkaloids also display remarkable anti-inflammatory and analgesic effects.

Traditionally, the processing of Aconitum root is monitored by tasting the spicy flavor which should gradually fade to certain extent. With the understanding of the underlying mechanisms, processing of aconitum is now controlled by determination of the marker alkaloids. For instance, as recorded in the latest CP, the total contents of DDA-type constituents should not be higher than 0.02% (g/g), while the contents of NDA-type constituents should be no less than 0.01% (g/g).

Ginseng: structural transformation of ginsenosides during processing results in enhanced efficacy

Ginseng Radix et Rhizome (Renshen, in Chinese) has been traditionally used in TCM for thousands of years, and is also one of the most popular functional food in Asian countries [85, 86]. Ginsenosides, the triterpene saponins, have been found to be the main bioactive constituents in ginseng, which are responsible for anti-oxidant, antidiabetic, immune modulatory, anti-inflammatory and anti-cancer properties [87–89]. Their structures are mainly grouped into dammarane type with 20(S)-protopanaxadiol and 20(S)-protopanaxatriol as the aglycone and oleanane type [90].

White ginseng (the fresh ginseng air-dried) and the processed one, Hongshen (the fresh ginseng steamed for 2–3 h and dried), are two types of ginseng products available in the market. Traditionally, Hongshen is considered to be more powerful in "boosting yang" than the White ginseng [91, 92]. Several reports have suggested that certain activities of Hongshen are better than the White ginseng [93]. During processing (steaming), complex chemical changes occur in terms of ginsenosides. The malonyl-ginsenosides, which are only found in the white ginseng, are de-malonylated and converted into the corresponding ginsenosides [94, 95]. The sugar chains at C-20 and/or C-3 are further hydrolyzed [95]. Furthermore, the 20(S)-type ginsenosides can be transformed into 20(R)-type [90, 94, 95]. As a result, the chemical profile of White ginseng and Hongshen are considerably different. The polar ginsenosides in White ginseng becomes the less polar ones. The characteristic ginsenosides in Hongshen include 20(S)-, 20(R)-Rg_3, Rk_3, Rh_4, Rk_1, Rg_5, etc., which have been demonstrated to exhibit more potent anti-cancer, anti-diabetic, and anti-inflammatory effects [96, 97]. Therefore, structural transformation of ginsenosides during processing results in enhanced efficacy of the steamed ginseng.

Improved solubility of active constituents

Emerging evidences indicate that processing improves the solubility of herbal constituents in certain CHMs. Under heating condition, excipients used in processing such as wine and vinegar often help active constituents more easily to dissolve from a complex texture. Eventually, the processed CHMs show enhanced efficacy.

Coptidis Rhizoma (Huanglian, in Chinese) is derived from the dried rhizome of *Coptis chinensis* Franch., *C. deltoidea* C. Y. Cheng et Hsiao or *C. teeta* Wall, and is traditionally used for toothache, dysentery, hypertension, inflammation and liver diseases [98, 99]. Alkaloids, such as berberine, palmatine, epiberberine and coptisine, are found to be one of the main types of active constituents [100]. It is reported that the dissolution rate of total alkaloids in wine-processed Coptidis Rhizoma reaches 90%, while that in raw medicinals is only 58%. After processing, the contents of berberine, palmatine, coptisine and jatrorrhizine that were detected in the processed Coptidis Rhizoma were significantly increased [57]. This observation is also seen on Angelicae Sinensis Radix (Danggui, in Chinese). Danggui, the dried root of *Angelica sinensis* (Oliv.) Diels., is a famous CHM and has been used for more than 2000 years in China as a dietary supplement for women's health [10]. A recent study showed that yellow wine-processed Danggui displays a significant increase in solubility of ferulic acid, one of the major biological components [10].

Physically changing the existing form of constituents

Processing can also change the existing form of constituents in CHMs, which may influence their actions. One example is the PR, the dried tuber of *P. ternata* (unb.) Breit. It is first recorded in Shen-Nong-Ben-Cao-Jing (Shen Nong's Herbal Classic, B.C. 100–200), and is widely used in TCM to treat cough, phlegm, vomiting and cancer [25, 101]. Similar to the Aconitum, raw PR is very toxic and can be only applied for external use. In order to reduce its toxicity, alum solution is always used in the processing of PR. Recent studies showed that aluminium ions in the alum solution were capable of complexing with oxalic acid in calcium oxalate of raphides, which helped to dissolve calcium oxalate and thus altered the unique rigid crystal structure [24]. This further led to the dissolve and degradation of the lectin inside the raphides [24]. As a result, the pro-inflammatory effect of raphides was significantly decreased. Therefore, physically structural alteration of needle-like calcium oxalate crystals contributes to the reduction of toxicity of PR during processing.

Influences of excipients

Excipients, including wine, vinegar, ginger juice, honey, rice, Glycyrrhizae Radix et Rhizoma, Euodiae Fructus and mutton fat, are frequently used in processing of CHMs to meet different purposes, and sometimes play an important role. Wine, vinegar and honey are commonly used as solvents to promote the solubility of several types of naturally-occurring compounds. As discussed above, wine can help the dissolve of active constituents of Danggui and Huanglian [10, 57]. Meanwhile, some excipients can react with the constituents in specific CHMs. For instance, during vinegar-assisted processing the toxic diterpenes in Kansui Radix (Gansui) can react with acetic acid to form acetylated diterpenes with poor solubility, which results in reduced toxicity [51, 52].

Notably, some excipients themselves, such as Glycyrrhizae Radix et Rhizoma, Euodiae Fructus and honey, are derived from CHMs and have their own therapeutic effects. Several studies show that constituents from these excipients are important for reducing toxicity and/or enhancing efficacy. As above described, 25% juice of Zingiberis Rhizoma Recens is used in the processing of PR Praeparatum cum Zingibere et Alumine (Jiangbanxia). It is demonstrated that gingerol derived from the ginger juice can remarkably inhibit Banxia-induced inflammation, which contributes to the detoxification effect [102]. Euodiae Fructus (Wuzhuyu) is the dried fruit of *E. rutaecarpa* (Juss.) Benth., *E. rutaecarpa* (Juss.) Benth. *var. officinalis* (Dode) Huang, or *E. rutaecarpa* (Juss.) Benth. *var. bodinieri* (Dode) Huang, and its processed products are produced by boiling raw materials with

Glycyrrhizae Radix [103, 104]. Studies have shown that Glycyrrhizae Radix can enhance the analgesic effects of Wuzhuyu. After processing, the content of hydroxyevodiamine is reduced significantly, while that of evocarpine is increased [105].

Conclusion and future perspectives

Processing is formed in long-term practice with a systematic theory, and represents one of the therapeutic wisdoms of TCM. Since most crude materials of CHMs require proper processing before being used, standardization of processing is a prerequisite for standardization of CHM. However, it is of much difficulty in terms of this aspect. Firstly, the methods of processing vary significantly in different regions of China [7]. For certain CHMs, there is no unified processing practice for all areas of China. Although there are a total of 618 decoction pieces that have been adopted in the latest CP, a large number of processed CHMs are not covered. Most CHMs recorded in the local standards of different provinces have used different methods [106]. The use of excipients also sometimes varies [106]. Secondly, even in the latest CP, the processing practice is not accurately described. It is reported that the bioactive or toxic constituents can be changed over time and processing temperature [107–109]. The use of excipients is also important. For instance, different types and concentration of wine have distinct impact on the main compositions and contents of the alkaloids of *Coptis chinensis* [110]. Notably, there is no standards for most excipients used. Based on these facts, it is difficult to control the procedure of processing in practice. Traditionally, pharmaceutical workers process CHMs mainly according to their experiences to judge the color, flavor or appearance of CHMs. In a recent study, Fei et al. analyzed the color values of the peel and flesh of Crataegi Fructus and constructed related mathematical functions to effectively evaluate the processing degree of Crataegi Fructus [9]. Some researchers have also suggested to use novel techniques such as microwaves, which can be easily controlled [111, 112]. However, whether these new evaluation systems or techniques are able to produce qualified products still needs more assessment before applying to industry. Till now, the efforts for optimization and standardization of processing are still largely needed.

Another challenge is the standardization of decoction pieces, especially the processed CHMs. At current stage, there are no quality control standards for most processed CHMs. As described in this review, there are complex chemical changes in processing which are usually associated with alterations in pharmacological effects. Therefore, the deepening understanding of the underlying mechanisms of processing is of great significance for the standardization of CHMs including the selection of markers.

Investigation of the mechanisms of processing has been ongoing for several decades. With the development of novel concepts, techniques and models, great advances have been achieved, although most parts of processing remain unclear. In this review, we have summarized current progress with regards of processing mechanisms into the following aspects: (i) directly reducing contents of toxic constituents; (ii) structural transformation of constituents; (iii) improving solubility of constituents; (iv) physically changing the existing form of constituents; (v) influence by excipients. Most studies have focused on changes in chemical profiles of processed CHMs. The application of new technologies such as NMR, GC–MS and LC–MS has greatly facilitated the qualitative and quantitative analysis of herbal constituents, even at trace concentrations [41, 113–115]. Due to the changed chemical profiles, the finding of chemical markers that are pharmacologically relevant is essential for evaluating the processing practice. Several studies have demonstrated that "omics" studies are efficient and may at least partially represent holistic perspectives [116–119]. In a recent report, targeted glycomics and untargeted metabolomics were used to investigate the overall chemical characterization of Rehmanniae Radix [116]. The obtained data were further processed by multivariate statistical analysis. Finally, the processing-induced chemical transformation was summarized to evoke the mechanism behind processing. In another study, metabolomics study revealed seven chemical markers of raw and processed Atractylodis Macrocephalae Rhizoma [118]. However, despite these advances, most studies do not investigate the association of chemical and pharmacological changes. It is always valuable to assess the contribution of alteration of chemical compositions and formation of novel compounds to changed bioactivities of a CHM.

As mentioned above, decoction pieces are the only form directly applied in clinical practices. However, many studies have used the raw herb, instead of the decoction pieces, for chemical and pharmacological evaluations, which do not take into consideration of the chemical changes during processing of CHMs. This would possibly or sometimes inevitably lead to bias in understanding the traditional use of CHMs. Therefore, it is essential to use decoction pieces, especially the processed ones, for modern CHM researches.

Taken together, standardization of processing methods of CHM is a prerequisite to maintain the quality and guarantee the safety of CHM. To set up unified and scientific processing practices of CHM, further efforts should be paid to elucidate the mechanism of processing using advanced and comprehensive technologies.

Abbreviations
CHM: Chinese herbal medicine; CP: Chinese Pharmacopoeia; PR: Pinelliae Rhizoma; PRP: PR Praeparatum; PRZA: PR Praeparatum cum Zingibere et Alumine; PRPA: PR Praeparatum cum Alumine; TCM: Traditional Chinese Medicine.

Authors' contributions
SW and CH designed the study. JL and JC conducted the literature search. XW and SW drafted the manuscript and prepared tables and figures. YJ, ML and BB contributed to revisions of the manuscript. All authors read and approved the final manuscript.

Author details
[1] Laboratory of Molecular Pharmacology, Department of Pharmacology, School of Pharmacy, Southwest Medical University, Luzhou, Sichuan, China. [2] State Key Laboratory of Quality Research in Chinese Medicine, Institute of Chinese Medical Sciences, University of Macau, Macao, China. [3] College of Pharmacy, Chengdu University of Traditional Chinese Medicine, Liutai Avenue, Wenjiang District, Chengdu, Sichuan, China. [4] West China School of Pharmacy, Sichuan University, Chengdu, Sichuan, China. [5] Institute of Chinese Materia Medica, China Academy of Chinese Medical Sciences, Beijing, China.

Acknowledgements
Not applicable.

Competing interests
The authors declare that they have no competing interests.

Consent for publication
Not applicable.

Funding
This review was supported by the Research Fund of the University of Macau (MYRG2016-00143-ICMS-QRCM) and Macau Science and Technology Development Fund (071/2017/A2).

References
1. Sheridan H, Kopp B, Krenn L, Guo D, Sendker J. Traditional Chinese herbal medicinal preparation: invoking the butterfly effect. Science. 2015;350:S64–6.
2. Wang S, Wu X, Tan M, Gong J, Tan W, Bian B, Chen M, Wang Y. Fighting fire with fire: poisonous Chinese herbal medicine for cancer therapy. J Ethnopharmacol. 2012;140:33–45.
3. Commission. Chinese Pharmacopoeia. 2015 edition. Beijing: China Medical Science Press; 2015.
4. Guo P, Brand E, Zhao Z. Chinese medicinal processing: a characteristic aspect of the ethnopharmacology of Traditional Chinese Medicine. In: Heinrich M, Jäger AK, editors. Ethnopharmacology, ch26. Hoboken: Wiley; 2015. p. 303–16.
5. Zhang ZH, Zhao YY, Cheng XL, Dai Z, Zhou C, Bai X, Lin RC. General toxicity of Pinellia ternata (Thunb.) Berit. in rat: a metabonomic method for profiling of serum metabolic changes. J Ethnopharmacol. 2013;149:303–10.
6. Yu H, Pan Y, Wu H, Ge X, Zhang Q, Zhu F, Cai B. The alum-processing mechanism attenuating toxicity of Araceae Pinellia ternata and Pinellia pedatisecta. Arch Pharm Res. 2015;38:1810–21.

7. Zhao Z, Liang Z, Chan K, Lu G, Lee EL, Chen H, Li L. A unique issue in the standardization of Chinese materia medica: processing. Planta Med. 2010;76:1975–86.

8. Sionneau P. Pao Zhi: an introduction to the use of processed Chinese medicinals. Boulder: Blue Poppy Enterprises Inc.; 1995.

9. Fei C, Dai H, Wu X, Li L, Lu T, Li W, Cai B, Yin W, Yin F. Quality evaluation of raw and processed Crataegi Fructus by color measurement and fingerprint analysis. J Sep Sci. 2017. https://doi.org/10.1002/jssc.201700575.

10. Zhan JY, Zheng KY, Zhu KY, Bi CW, Zhang WL, Du CY, Fu Q, Dong TT, Choi RC, Tsim KW, Lau DT. Chemical and biological assessment of Angelicae Sinensis Radix after processing with wine: an orthogonal array design to reveal the optimized conditions. J Agric Food Chem. 2011;59:6091–8.

11. Zhang Z, Wang Z, Sun S, Li J, Zhang G, Miao M. Pharmacological action of various processed *Mylabris phalerata* Pallas. China J Chin Meteria Med. 1990;15:214–7.

12. Zhou Y, Lei H, Li F, He F, Bai D, Zhou C. Discussion of processing principle of Dangshen. World Chin Med. 2009;4:161–3.

13. Zhang L, Ma WF, Li J, He J, Zhang P, Zheng F, Zhang BL, Gao XM, Chang YX. Influence of processing on pharmacokinetic of typical constituents in radix polygoni multiflori after oral administration by LC-ESI-MS/MS. J Ethnopharmacol. 2013;148:246–53.

14. Liang Z, Chen H, Yu Z, Zhao Z. Comparison of raw and processed Radix Polygoni Multiflori (Heshouwu) by high performance liquid chromatography and mass spectrometry. Chin Med. 2010;5:29.

15. Feng XD, Gao GW, Huang HX. Research on the quality changes in pre-and-post-processed pieces of radix polygalae. J Chin Med Mater. 2008;31:818–20.

16. Yuan Z, Liu H, Wang J, Jia T, Chen J. Optimization of bran-roasted processing technology of sliced myristicae semen by orthogonal test. Chin J Inf TCM. 2016;23:74–6.

17. Wen JX, Zhao D, Deng J. Influence of processing methods on the chemical composition of the essential oil from *Aucklandia lappa*. J Chin Med Mater. 2012;35:1397–401.

18. Hao Y, Zifeng P, Yufeng Z, Fengrui S, Zhiqiang L, Shuying L. Analysis of norditerpenoid alkalods in processing radix aconiti lateralis preparata with radix glycyrrhizae preparata by electrospray ionization tandem mass spectrometry. Chin J Anal Chem. 2007;35:959–63.

19. Wu W, Liang Z, Zhao Z, Cai Z. Direct analysis of alkaloid profiling in plant tissue by using matrix-assisted laser desorption/ionization mass spectrometry. J Mass Spectrom. 2007;42:58–69.

20. Wang J, van der Heijden R, Spijksma G, Reijmers T, Wang M, Xu G, Hankemeier T, van der Greef J. Alkaloid profiling of the Chinese herbal medicine Fuzi by combination of matrix-assisted laser desorption ionization mass spectrometry with liquid chromatography-mass spectrometry. J Chromatogr A. 2009;1216:2169–78.

21. Mao ZC, Peng ZS. Progress on research of rapid propagation system of *Pinellia ternata*. China J Chin Materia Med. 2003;28:193–5.

22. Zhong LY, Wu H, Zhang KW, Wang QR. Study on irritation of calcium oxalate crystal in raw *Pinellia ternata*. China J Chin Materia Med. 2006;31:1706–10.

23. Wu H, Ge X, Yu H, Chen L. Comparisons of crystal form of raphides to toxicity raphides in four poisonous herbs of Araceae family. China J Chin Materia Med. 2010;35:1152–5.

24. Yu H, Pan Y, Wu H, Ge X, Zhang Q, Zhu F, Cai B. The alum-processing mechanism attenuating toxicity of Araceae *Pinellia ternata* and Pinellia pedatisecta. Arch Pharmacal Res. 2015;38:1810–21.

25. Tao S, Yong T, Tsui MS, Hua Y, Fu XQ, Li T, Chi LC, Hui G, Li YX, Zhu PL. Metabolomics reveals the mechanisms for the cardiotoxicity of Pinelliae Rhizoma and the toxicity-reducing effect of processing. Sci Rep. 2016;6:34692.

26. Liu Y, Li L, Xiao YQ, Yao JQ, Li PY, Yu DR, Ma YL. Global metabolite profiling and diagnostic ion filtering strategy by LC-QTOF MS for rapid identification of raw and processed pieces of *Rheum palmatum* L. Food Chem. 2016;192:531–40.

27. Feng S, Meijuan Y, Yan L, Yongqing X, Li L. Comparision of the actions on blood stasis of rhubarb with different prepared methods. Pharmacol Clin Chin Mater Med. 2012;6:90–3.

28. Wang JB, Ma YG, Zhang P, Jin C, Sun YQ, Xiao XH, Zhao YL, Zhou CP. Effect of processing on the chemical contents and hepatic and renal toxicity of rhubarb studied by canonical correlation analysis. Acta Pharmaceutica Sinica. 2009;44:885–90.

29. Zheng YZ, Choi RJ, Xie HQ, Cheung AW, Duan R, Guo AJ, Zhu JT, Chen VP, Bi CW, Zhu Y. Ligustilide suppresses the biological properties of Danggui Buxue Tang: a Chinese herbal decoction composed of Radix Astragali and Radix Angelica sinensis. Planta Med. 2010;76:439–43.

30. Du J, Bai B, Kuang X, Yu Y, Wang C, Ke Y, Xu Y, Tzang AH, Qian ZM. Ligustilide inhibits spontaneous and agonists- or K+ depolarization-induced contraction of rat uterus. J Ethnopharmacol. 2006;108:54–8.

31. Suzuki A, Yamamoto M, Jokura H, Fujii A, Tokimitsu I, Hase T, Saito I. Ferulic acid restores endothelium-dependent vasodilation in aortas of spontaneously hypertensive rats. Am J Hypertens. 2007;20:508–13.

32. Kang KS, Kim HY, Baek SH, Yoo HH, Park JH, Yokozawa T. Study on the hydroxyl radical scavenging activity changes of ginseng and ginsenoside-Rb2 by heat processing. Biol Pharm Bull. 2007;30:724–8.

33. Kwon SW, Sang BH, Park IH, Kim JM, Man KP, Park JH. Liquid chromatographic determination of less polar ginsenosides in processed ginseng. J Chromatogr A. 2001;921:335–9.

34. Sun BS, Gu LJ, Fang ZM, Wang CY, Wang Z, Lee MR, Li Z, Li JJ, Sung CK. Simultaneous quantification of 19 ginsenosides in black ginseng developed from *Panax ginseng* by HPLC-ELSD. J Pharm Biomed Anal. 2009;50:15–22.

35. Sangmyung L, Hyunju S, Chungsig C, Hung TM, Min BS, Kihwan B. Ginsenosides from heat processed ginseng. Chem Pharm Bull. 2009;57:92–4.

36. Kang KS, Kim HY, Yamabe N, Yokozawa T. Stereospecificity in hydroxyl radical scavenging activities of four ginsenosides produced by heat processing. Bioorg Med Chem Lett. 2006;16:5028–31.

37. Ha YW, Lim SS, Ha IJ, Na YC, Seo JJ, Shin H, Son SH, Kim YS. Preparative isolation of four ginsenosides from Korean red ginseng (steam-treated Panax ginseng C. A. Meyer), by high-speed counter-current chromatography coupled with evaporative light scattering detection. J Chromatogr A. 2007;1151:37–44.

38. Han Q, Li S, Qiao C, Song J, Cai Z, Pui-Hay-But P, Shaw P, Xu H. A simple method to identify the unprocessed Strychnos seeds used in herbal medicinal products. Planta Med. 2008;74:458–63.

39. Haghi G, Hatami A, Safaei A. Hydrophilic-interaction chromatography with UV detection for analysis of strychnine and brucine in the crude seeds of Strychnos nux-vomica and their processed products. Chromatographia. 2010;71:327–30.

40. Choi YH, Sohn YM, Kim CY, Oh KY, Kim J. Analysis of strychnine from detoxified Strychnos nux-vomica seeds using liquid chromatographyelectrospray mass spectrometry. J Ethnopharmacol. 2004;93:109–12.

41. Wu W, Qiao C, Liang Z, Xu H, Zhao Z, Cai Z. Alkaloid profiling in crude and processed Strychnos nux-vomica seeds by matrix-assisted laser desorption/ionization-time of flight mass spectrometry. J Pharm Biomed Anal. 2007;45:430–6.

42. Zhao LN, Shi YB, Zhang ZL, Zhang BS. Comparison of total cantharidin contents in blister beetle before and after processed by HPLC. Chin J Exp Tradit Med Formul. 2010;16:39–41.

43. Fan H. Processing principle of common toxic components of toxic Traditional Chinese Medicines. China J Chin Med. 2014;29:1335–6.

44. Wang K, Chen L, LI W, Ke H, Chang C Wang. Analysis of the sesquiterpenoids in processed Atractylodis Rhizoma. Chem Pharm Bull. 2007;55:50–6.

45. Li W, Wen HM, Cui XB, Zhang KW. Process mechanism of Atractylodes macrocephala and conversion of sesquiterpenes. China J Chin Materia Med. 2006;31:1600–3.

46. Geng L, Sun H, Yuan Y, Liu Z, Cui Y, Bi K, Chen X. Discrimination of raw and vinegar-processed Genkwa Flos using metabolomics coupled with multivariate data analysis: a discrimination study with metabolomics coupled with PCA. Fitoterapia. 2013;84:286–94.

47. Sung M, Li P. Chemical analysis of raw, dry-roasted, and honey-roasted licorice by capillary electrophoresis. Electrophoresis. 2004;25:3434–40.

48. Guo YM, Yu KF, Liu YH, Zhao JZ, Wang ZC, Zhang HB. Analysis on processing mechanism of Calamine. Chin J Chin Mater Med. 2005;30:596–9.

49. Zhou L, Xu C, Zhang L, Ding A. Processing mechanism of calamine. China J Chin Materia Med. 2010;35:1556–9.

50. Yang M, Liu Z, Su Z, Zou W. Study on mechanism of precursors transforming into indigo and indirubinin blue-genera plants. China J Chin Materia Med. 2010;35:928–31.

51. Liu Y, Liu Z, Song F, Liu S. Optimization of preparing process condition of kansui roots by electrospray ionization mass spectrometry. J Chin Mass Spectrom Soc. 2010;31:72–8.

52. Bicchi C, Appendino G, Cordero C, Rubiolo P, Ortelli D, Veuthey JL. HPLC-UV and HPLC-positive-ESI-MS analysis of the diterpenoid fraction from caper spurge (Euphorbia lathyris) seed oil. Phytochem Anal. 2001;12:255–62.

53. Shen HB, Peng GP, Xie BZ. Comparison of the content of sinalbrin in Sinapis Semen before and after the process. China J Chin Materia Med. 1987;12:18–20.

54. Ruan G, Li G. The study on the chromatographic fingerprint of Fructus xanthii by microwave assisted extraction coupled with GC-MS. J Chromatogr B Anal Technol Biomed Life Sci. 2007;850:241–8.

55. Jin X, Jia X, Sun E, Wang J, Chen Y, Cai B. Research on variation regularity of five main flavonoids contents in epimedium and processed epimedium. China J Chin Materia Med. 2009;34:2738–42.

56. Rui N. Action of the drug herba epimedii on the testosterone of mouse plasma and its accessory sexual organ before and after processing. China J Chin Materia Med. 1989;14:18–20.

57. Liu F, Zhang ZQ, Lai JY, Bei HU. Determination of four kinds of alkaloids from Rhizoma Coptis and processed Rhizoma Coptis by HPLC. Chin Tradit Patent Med. 2010;32:1925–8.

58. Park KD, Lee SH, Kim JH, Kang TH, Moon JS, Kim SU. Synthesis of 13-(substituted benzyl) berberine and berberrubine derivatives as antifungal agents. Bioorg Med Chem Lett. 2006;16:3913–6.

59. Nakatani T, Konishi T, Miyahara K, Noda N. Three novel cantharidin-related compounds from the Chinese blister beetle, Mylabris phalerata Pall. Chem Pharm Bull. 2004;52:807–9.

60. Huh JE, Kang KS, Ahn KS, Saiki I, Kim DH, Kim SH. Mylabris phalerata induces apoptosis by caspase activation following cytochrome c release and Bid cleavage. Life Sci. 2003;73:2249–62.

61. Cheng KC, Lee HM, Shum SF, Yip CP. A fatality due to the use of cantharides from Mylabris phalerata as an abortifacient. Med Sci Law. 1990;30:336–40.

62. Zhang Z, Wang Z, Sun S, Li J, Zhang G. Studies on the pharmacological action of various processed Mylabris phalerata pallas. China J Chin Materia Med. 1990;15:22–5.

63. Honkanen RE. Cantharidin, another natural toxin that inhibits the activity of serine/threonine protein phosphatases types 1 and 2A. FEBS Lett. 1993;330:283–6.

64. Li W, Xie L, Zheng C, Yi Z, Sun Y, Yi M, Xu Z, Xiao H. Cantharidin, a potent and selective PP2A inhibitor, induces an oxidative stress-independent growth inhibition of pancreatic cancer cells through G2/M cell-cycle arrest and apoptosis. Cancer Sci. 2010;101:1226–33.

65. Eisner T, Smedley SR, Young DK, Eisner M, Roach B, Meinwald J. Chemical basis of courtship in a beetle (Neopyrochroa flabellata): Cantharidin as "nuptial gift". Proc Natl Acad Sci USA. 1996;93:6499–503.

66. Liu YF, Zhao LN, Zhang ZL. Determination of cantharidin in Mylabris after processing with potash by HPLC. Chin Arch Tradit Chin Med. 2010;3:487–8.

67. Dandan W. Study on a new method for processing of Mylabris. ShiZhen J Tradit Chin Med Res. 1996;1:40–1.

68. Tian JH, Lu D, Tian B, Li JY. Cantharidinate sodium injection in the treatment of bladder cancer after surgery in 23 cases. J Tradit Chin Med. 2004;45:768.

69. Wang X, Hou L, Xiaoping S, Tang F. Mechanisms of Semen Crotonis Pulveratum and Rhubarb intervening CD4+ CD25+/CD4+ Treg in rats with ulcerative colitis. Pharmacol Clin Chin Mater Med. 2013;2:127–9.

70. Kim MS, Kim HR, So HS, Lee YR, Moon HC, Ryu DG, Yang SH, Lee GS, Song JH, Kwon KB. Crotonis fructus and its constituent, croton oil, stimulate lipolysis in OP9 adipocytes. EvidenceBased Complemen Alter Med. 2014;2014:780385.

71. Belman S, Troll W. The inhibition of croton oil-promoted mouse skin tumorigenesis by steroid hormones. Can Res. 1972;32:450–4.

72. Cai B, Qin K, Hao W, Hao C, Lu T, Zhang X. Chemical mechanism during chinese medicine processing. Prog Chem. 2012;77:637–49.

73. Singhuber J, Ming Z, Prinz S, Kopp B. Aconitum in Traditional Chinese Medicine-a valuable drug or an unpredictable risk? J Ethnopharmacol. 2009;126:18–30.

74. Xie Y, Jiang ZH, Zhou H, Xu HX, Liu L. Simultaneous determination of six aconitum alkaloids in proprietary Chinese medicines by high-performance liquid chromatography. J Chromatogr A. 2005;1093:195–203.

75. Chan TY. Aconite poisoning following the percutaneous absorption of Aconitum alkaloids. Forensic Sci Int. 2012;223:25–7.

76. Shaheen F, Ahmad M, Khan MTH, Jalil S, Ejaz A, Sultankhodjaev MN, Arfan M, Choudhary MI, Atta-ur-Rahman. Alkaloids of Aconitum laeve and their anti-inflammatory, antioxidant and tyrosinase inhibition activities. Phytochemistry. 2005;66:935–40.

77. Liu M, Cao Y, Lv D, Zhang W, Zhu Z, Zhang H, Chai Y. Effect of processing on the alkaloids in aconitum tubers by HPLC-TOF/MS. J Pharm Anal. 2017;7:170–5.

78. Nyirimigabo E, Xu Y, Li Y, Wang Y, Agyemang K, Zhang Y. A review on phytochemistry, pharmacology and toxicology studies of Aconitum. J Pharm Pharmacol. 2015;67:1–19.

79. Chan TY. Aconitum alkaloid poisoning related to the culinary uses of aconite roots. Toxins. 2014;6:2605–11.

80. Chan TY. Aconitum alkaloid poisoning because of contamination of herbs by aconite roots. Phytother Res. 2015;30:3–8.

81. Borcsa B, Fodor L, Csupor D, Forgo P, Th MA, Hohmann J. Diterpene alkaloids from the roots of Aconitum moldavicum and assessment of Nav 1.2 sodium channel activity of aconitum alkaloids. Planta Med. 2014;80:231–6.

82. Borcsa B, Fodor L, Csupor D, Forgo P, Hohmann J. Assessment of the Nav1.2 sodium channel activity of Aconitum diterpene and norditerpene alkaloids. Planta Med. 2013;79:1258.

83. Liu Y, Tan P, Li F, Qiao Y. Study on the aconitine-type alkaloids of Radix Aconiti Lateralis and its processed products using HPLC-ESI-MSn. Drug Test Anal. 2013;5:480–4.

84. Qiu XH, Jie HE. Effect on the contents of ester-type alkaloids in Radix Aconiti Laterlis Preparata by different decocting time and compatibility dosage of Radix Glycyrrhizae. Lishizhen Med Mater Med Res. 2007;12:3015–7.

85. Wong AS, Che CM, Leung KW. Recent advances in ginseng as cancer therapeutics: a functional and mechanistic overview. Nat Prod Rep. 2015;32:256–72.

86. Wang CZ, Cai Y, Anderson S, Yuan CS. Ginseng metabolites on cancer chemoprevention: an angiogenesis link? Diseases. 2015;3:193–204.

87. Xie CL, Li JH, Wang WW, Zheng GQ, Wang LX. Neuroprotective effect of ginsenoside-Rg1 on cerebral ischemia/reperfusion injury in rats by downregulating protease-activated receptor-1 expression. Life Sci. 2015;121:145–51.

88. Zhang XH. Xian-Xiang Xu. Ginsenoside Ro suppresses interleukin-1β-induced apoptosis and inflammation in rat chondrocytes by inhibiting NF-κB. Chin J Nat Med. 2015;13:283–9.

89. Siraj FM, Sathishkumar N, Kim YJ, Kim SY, Yang DC. Ginsenoside F2 possesses anti-obesity activity via binding with PPAR and inhibiting adipocyte differentiation in the 3T3-L1 cell line. J Enzyme Inhib Med Chem. 2015;30:9–14.

90. Wei W, Le S, Zhe Z, Guo Y, Liu S. Profiling and multivariate statistical analysis of Panax ginseng based on ultra-high-performance liquid chromatography coupled with quadrupole-time-of-flight mass spectrometry. J Pharm Biomed Anal. 2015;107:141–50.

91. Chu C, Xu S, Li X, Yan J, Liu L. Profiling the ginsenosides of three ginseng products by LC-Q-TOF/MS. J Food Sci. 2013;78:C653–9.

92. Zhang HM, Li SL, Zhang H, Wang Y, Zhao ZL, Chen SL, Xu HX. Holistic quality evaluation of commercial white and red ginseng using a UPLC-QTOF-MS/MS-based metabolomics approach. J Pharm Biomed Anal. 2012;62:258–73.

93. Lee JI, Ha YW, Choi TW, Kim HJ, Kim SM, Jang HJ, Choi JH, Choi MH, Chung BC, Sethi G. Cellular uptake of ginsenosides in Korean white ginseng and red ginseng and their apoptotic activities in human breast cancer cells. Planta Med. 2011;77:133–40.

94. Xie Y, Luo D, Cheng Y, Ma J, Wang Y, Liang Q, Luo G. Steaming-Induced chemical transformations and holistic quality assessment of red ginseng derived from panax ginseng by means of HPLC-ESI-MS/MSn-based multicomponent quantification fingerprint. J Agric Food Chem. 2012;60:8213–24.

95. Xiao SY, Luo GA. Chemical reactions of ginsenosides in red ginseng processing by HPLC/MS/MS. Chin Tradit Herbal Drugs. 2005;1:40–3.

96. Lee ES, Choi JS, Kim MS, You HJ, Ji GE, Kang YH. Ginsenoside metabolite compound K differentially antagonizing tumor necrosis factor-α-induced monocyte-endothelial trafficking. Chem Biol Interact. 2011;194:13–22.

97. Wang CZ, Aung HH, Zhang B, Sun S, Li XL, He H, Xie JT, He TC, Du W, Yuan CS. Chemopreventive effects of heat-processed Panax quinquefolius root on human breast cancer cells. Anticancer Res. 2008;28:2545–51.

98. Qian XC, Zhang L, Tao Y, Huang P, Li JS, Chai C, Li W, Di LQ, Cai BC. Simultaneous determination of ten alkaloids of crude and wine-processed Rhizoma Coptidis aqueous extracts in rat plasma by UHPLC-ESI-MS/MS and its application to a comparative pharmacokinetic study. J Pharm Biomed Anal. 2015;105:64–73.

99. Tan HL, Chan KG, Priyia P, Acharaporn D, Surasak S, Tahir MK, Learn-Han L, Bey-Hing G. Rhizoma Coptidis: a potential cardiovascular protective agent. Front Pharmacol. 2016;7:362.

100. Hyunah J, Min BS, Yokozawa T, Jehyun L, Yeongshik K, Jaesue C. Anti-Alzheimer and antioxidant activities of coptidis rhizoma alkaloids. Biol Pharm Bull. 2009;32:1433–8.

101. Lee JY, Park NH, Lee W, Kim EH, Jin YH, Seo EK, Hong J. Comprehensive chemical profiling of Pinellia species tuber and processed Pinellia tuber by gas chromatography-mass spectrometry and liquid chromatography-atmospheric pressure chemical ionization-tandem mass spectrometry. J Chromatogr A. 2016;1471:164–77.

102. Yu HL, Mao SH, Zhao TF, Wu H, Pan YZ, Shu CY. Antagonistic effect of gingerols against TNF-α release, ROS overproduction and RIP3 expression increase induced by lectin from *Pinellia ternata*. China J Chin Materia Med. 2015;40:3630–5.

103. Pan X, Bligh SW, Smith E. Quinolone alkaloids from Fructus Euodiae show activity against methicillin-resistant *Staphylococcus aureus*. Phytother Res. 2014;28:305–7.

104. Yin YY, Liu SS, Han LW, Qiu-Xia HE, Zhang QW, Liu KC, Yan LH, Wang ZM. Chemical components of alkaloids from euodiae fructus and their antiangiogenic activities. Chin J Exp Tradit Med Formul. 2016;22:45–53.

105. Kano Y, Qine Z, Komatsu K. On the evaluation of the preparation of Chinese medicinal prescriptions. VI. The changes of the alkaloid contents by processing of Evodia fruit, Yakugaku Zasshi. J Pharm Soc Japan. 1991;111:32–5.

106. Guo P, Brand E, Zhao Z. Chinese medicinal processing: a characteristic aspect of the ethnopharmacology of Traditional Chinese Medicine. Hoboken, New Jersey, United States: Wiley; 2000. p. 132–40.

107. Zhang L, Shu X, Tang Y, Ding A, Duan J. Study on preparation processing technique of Radix Kansui stir baked with vinegar. China J Chin Mater Med. 2009;34:681–4.

108. Mubai S, Zhu J. Processing technology and quality of red ginseng. J Changchun Univ Chin Med. 2014;30:611–3.

109. Zhangchi N, Zhiqian S, Chun W, Yuanyan L, Honglian Z, Jiahe G, Xinling M, Zhenli L. Effects of processed temperature and time on color and contents of six types of Boswellic acids in Frankinense. Mod Tradit Chin Med Mater MedicaWorld Sci Technol. 2017;19:508–15.

110. Chen K, Yuan J. The effects of processing the Coptis chinensis using different types of wine on the main components of alkaloids. Adv Anal Chem. 2016;6:14–9.

111. Zhu X, Wang C, Wang X, Cai M, Deng S. Effects of different processing methods on the determination of trigonelline in Fructus Cannabis decoction pieces. J Pharm Res. 2016;35:19–21.

112. Liu LH. Optimization of microwave extraction process of total alkaloid from *Aconitum flavum*. Med Plant. 2010;1:93–5.

113. Wu X, Zhu L, Ma J, Ye Y, Lin G. Adduct ion-targeted qualitative and quantitative analysis of polyoxypregnanes by ultra-high pressure liquid chromatography coupled with triple quadrupole mass spectrometry. J Pharm Biomed Anal. 2017;145:127–36.

114. Guo S, Duan JA, Qian D, Wang H, Tang Y, Qian Y, Wu D, Su S, Shang E. Hydrophilic interaction ultra-high performance liquid chromatography coupled with triple quadrupole mass spectrometry for determination of nucleotides, nucleosides and nucleobases in Ziziphus plants. J Chromatogr A. 2013;1301:147–55.

115. Hankemeier T. Traditional processing strongly affects metabolite composition by hydrolysis in *Rehmannia glutinosa* roots. Chem Pharm Bull. 2011;59:546–52.

116. Li Z, Xu JD, Zhou SS, Qian M, Ming K, Hong S, Li XY, Duan SM, Xu J, Li SL. Integrating targeted glycomics and untargeted metabolomics to investigate the processing chemistry of herbal medicines, a case study on Rehmanniae Radix. J Chromatogr A. 2016;1472:74–87.

117. Zhang CE, Niu M, Li Q, Zhao YL, Ma ZJ, Xiong Y, Dong XP, Li RY, Feng WW, Dong Q. Urine metabolomics study on the liver injury in rats induced by raw and processed Polygonum multiflorum integrated with pattern recognition and pathways analysis. J Ethnopharmacol. 2016;194:299–306.

118. Shan GS, Zhang LX, Zhao QM, Xiao HB, Zhuo RJ, Xu G, Jiang H, You XM, Jia TZ. Metabolomic study of raw and processed Atractylodes macrocephala Koidz by LC–MS. J Pharm Biomed Anal. 2014;98:74–84.

119. Sun H, Ni B, Zhang A, Wang M, Dong H, Wang X. Metabolomics study on Fuzi and its processed products using ultra-performance liquid-chromatography/electrospray-ionization synapt high-definition mass spectrometry coupled with pattern recognition analysis. Analyst. 2012;137:170–85.

iTRAQ-based proteomic analysis to identify the molecular mechanism of Zhibai Dihuang Granule in the Yin-deficiency-heat syndrome rats

Chang-Ming Liu[1], Jing Chen[1], Su Yang[1], Ting-Ting Jiang[2], Zhong-Liang Chen[1], Hui-Hui Tu[1], Lian-Gen Mao[1], Yu-Ting Hu[2], Lin Gan[2], Zhong-Jie Li[1] and Ji-Cheng Li[1,2]*

Abstract

Background: Zhibai Dihuang Granule (ZDG) is a traditional Chinese medicine which has been used to treat Yin-deficiency-heat (YDH) syndrome for thousands of years in China. However, little work has been conducted to explore the molecular mechanism of ZDG in YDH syndrome, and the processes of YDH syndrome prevention and treatment have been developed slowly. The present study was aimed to explore the therapeutic mechanism of ZDG on YDH syndrome.

Methods: The YDH syndrome rats were induced by hot Chinese herbs, then treated by ZDG orally for 1 week. Body weight was measured every 2 days. After sacrifice, blood samples were collected and the thymus, adrenal glands, spleen, and liver were immediately removed and weighed. iTRAQ-based proteomics approach was applied to explore the serum protein alterations with the treatment of ZDG, and to investigate the underlying mechanism of ZDG in treating YDH syndrome.

Results: The body weights of YDH syndrome rats were significantly decreased compared with control group, and increased in ZDG treated rats. The relative weights of thymus in YDH syndrome rats were increased compared with the control rats, and significantly decreased in after ZDG treatment. In the proteomic analyses, seventy-one proteins were differentially expressed in the YDH syndrome group and the ZDG treated group, including 10 up-regulated and 61 down-regulated proteins. Gene ontology analysis revealed that the differentially expressed proteins were mostly related to immune response, and pathway enrichment analysis showed that these proteins were enriched in coagulation and complement cascades. Enzyme-linked immunosorbent assay was performed to detect the protein levels in coagulation and complement cascades, and the results showed that complement component 5 levels were significantly increased, while fibrinogen gamma chain levels were significantly decreased in the ZDG treated group.

Conclusions: We found that ZDG treatment could lead to proteins alteration in immune response, especially in coagulation and complement cascades. ZDG can up-regulate the proteins in the complement cascade to eliminate pathogens, and down-regulate the proteins in the coagulation cascade to suppress inflammation. Our study provides experimental basis to understand the therapeutic mechanism of ZDG and revealed that ZDG can regulate coagulation and complement cascades in treating YDH syndrome.

Keywords: Herbal medicine, Zhibai Dihuang Granule, TCM, Proteomic analysis, Coagulation, Complement

*Correspondence: lijichen@zju.edu.cn
[1] Institute of Cell Biology, Zhejiang University, Hangzhou, People's Republic of China
Full list of author information is available at the end of the article

Background

Yin-deficiency-heat (YDH) syndrome is a common sub-health status in traditional Chinese medicine (TCM) characterized by fatigue, emaciation, five center (the palms, soles, and chest) heat, dry mouth, and tidal fever. If left untreated, YDH syndrome may develop into disease states, such as recurrent oral-ulcer, swollen gums and throat. YDH syndrome frequently occurs in individuals with yin-deficiency constitution, one of the most common pathological constitution in general population [1]. It is usually caused by long-term psychological stress, so it prevails especially among white collar workers and college students [2]. It has been reported that the incidence of YDH syndrome is significantly higher in individuals aged 15–34 than that in other age groups [1]. With the quickening pace of modern life and the increasing occupational stress, YDH syndrome is presenting a great challenge in China.

However, as a sub-health status, the appropriate conventional medicine to treat YDH syndrome is lacking. In TCM theory, the mechanism of YDH syndrome is considered as the deficiency of body fluid, especially in the mucous epithelium. It leads to the deterioration of moistening function, which finally result in the hyperactivity of internal heat in the body. Zhibai Dihuang Granule (ZDG), a classic traditional herbal medicine characterized by the function of nourishing Yin and suppressing internal heat, is commonly used to treat YDH syndrome clinically. ZDG is made from *Cornus officinalis, Rehmannia glutinosa, Dioscorea oppositifolia, Phellodendron amurense, Anemarrhena asphodeloides, Paeonia suffruticosa, Alisma plantago-aquatica* and *Poria cocos* [3]. *Anemarrhena asphodeloides* possesses the function of clearing away heat, nourishing Yin and moistening dryness. *Phellodendron amurense* is commonly used for purging pathogenic fire and expelling dampness. *Rehmannia glutinosa* possesses the effects of kidney-nourishing and essence-enriching. *Cornus officinalis* tonifies the liver and kidney, and *Dioscorea oppositifolia* invigorate spleen. *Paeonia suffruticosa* and *Alisma plantago-aquatica* display the activities of eliminating the internal heat [4]. The combination of these herbs may enhance the therapeutic effect on YDH syndrome. Currently, ZDG has been used not only in YDH syndrome management, but also to treat the concomitant symptoms of other diseases such as, diabetic nephropathy [5] and apoptosis of renal tubular cells [3]. However, owning to the diversity of the ingredients, and the complexity of the interaction between ZDG and the human body, the molecular mechanisms of therapeutic effects of ZDG are poorly understood. Furthermore, herbal medicine differs from the modern Western medicine in substance, methodology and philosophy [6], which impede Western countries from recognizing and accepting the therapeutic effects of the herbal medicine. Thus, there is an urgent need to reveal the therapeutic mechanism of ZDG on YDH syndrome.

Unlike the conventional medicine, herbal medicine usually treats patients in a holistic manner. As systems biology explores the complicated interactions among biological system components [7], it offers significant advantages to study the specific symptoms in TCM and the herbal medicine's mechanism of action. Proteomics, one of the important part of systems biology, has developed to be a powerful tool to study protein changes in physiological conditions, illness, and the response to outside stimuli [8]. Proteomics provides systematic quantitative and qualitative mapping of the whole proteome in tissue, cultured cells and blood, and identify altered proteins as potential drug targets or biomarkers. Accordingly, by analyzing protein alterations before and after TCM treatment, the mechanism of action of TCM remedies can be explained and fully understood. In this study, iTRAQ-coupled 2D LC–MS/MS was used to explore alterations in serum protein levels after ZDG treatment. Furthermore, a series of bioinformatics approaches were applied to explore the therapeutic mechanism of ZDG.

Methods

The minimum standards of reporting checklist (Additional file 1) contains details of the experimental design, statistics, and resources used in this study.

Herbal medicine and animal experiments

The Chinese herbs such as, Fuzi (*Aconitum carmichaeli*, harvested in Sichuan province), Ganjiang (*Zingiber officinale Roscoe*, harvested in Guangdong province), and Rougui (*Cinnamomum cassia Presl*, harvested in Sichuan province), which are characterized by pungent and hot nature, were used to induce YDH syndrome in animal models [9–11]. Briefly, dried Fuzi, Ganjiang and Rougui (600 g each) were immersed in 4.5 L distilled water for 0.5 h. Then, the herbs were boiled with high heat, followed by simmering with gentle heat three times (25 min for the first time, 30 min for the second time, and 40 min for the third time). Finally, the extracts were merged together, then filtered, and concentrated to 2 g/mL. ZDG (batch no. 161204, each bottle containing 200 granules, 1.7 g for 10 granules), purchased from Zhongjing Wanxi Pharmaceuticals Ltd. Co. (Nanyang, China), was ground to a fine powder with a mortar and pestle and then dissolved in distilled water at a concentration of 0.57 g/mL. Female Sprague–Dawley rats (180–220 g) were purchased from the Experimental Animal Center of Zhejiang Province. The rats were raised at a temperature-controlled (21–23 °C) and 12 h light/dark cycle room with free access to standard rat diet and water. All rats were acclimatized to the environment for 1 week before the experiments. The rats were randomly divided into the control group (N = 24), the YDH syndrome group (N = 20) and the ZDG treated group (N = 20). The rats in the control group were given sterile saline solution (2 mL/100 g) via gavage, and the rats in the YDH syndrome group and the ZDG treated group were given equal amount of Chinese herbal decoction via gavage for 2 weeks. On day 14, rats in the ZDG treated group (N = 20) were given ZDG (8.64 g/kg/day, via gavage) for 7 days, and rats in the YDH syndrome group and the control group were given equal amount of sterile saline solution for 7 days. The body weight of rats in each group was weighed every 5 days throughout the experiment. All rats were sacrificed at the end of the third week, and the blood samples were collected in the vacutainer tubes, and then clotted at room temperature for 1 h, followed by the centrifugation at $1500 \times g$ for 10 min at 4 °C to separate serum. The serum was aliquoted immediately in sterile centrifuge tubes and stored at − 80 °C. The thymus, adrenal glands, spleen, and liver were immediately removed and weighed. The experimental procedures were approved by the Zhejiang University Institutional Animal Care and Use Committee (China) and performed in compliance with the Guide for the Care and Use of Laboratory Animals, National Research Council (US) Institute for Laboratory Animal Research, 1996.

iTRAQ-2D LC–MS/MS based proteomic analysis
Protein extraction
Serum samples from three group (18 rats per group) were subjected to protein extraction. In each sample, high abundant proteins albumin and IgG were removed using Pierce™ Albumin/IgG Removal Kit. Protein concentration was determined with 2-D Quant kit (GE Healthcare, Chicago, USA) according to the manufacturer's instructions.

Trypsin digestion
The protein sample (100 µg) was reduced with 10 mM DTT (Sigma, St. Louis, MO, USA) for 1 h at 37 °C and alkylated at room temperature with 20 mM IAA (Sigma, St. Louis, MO, USA) for 45 min. Finally, trypsin was added with the ratio of protein:trypsin = 50:1 for the first digestion overnight and with the ratio of protein:trypsin = 100:1 for the second digestion for 4 h.

iTRAQ labeling
After digestion with trypsin, the peptides were desalted by using Strata X C18 SPE column and vacuum-dried. Then, the peptides were reconstituted in 0.5 M TEAB

and processed for iTRAQ labeling according to the manufacturer's protocol. Briefly, nine samples (three biological replicates per group) were labeled with the iTRAQ tags as control group (113 tags), YDH syndrome group (114 tags), and ZDG treated group (116 tags), and incubated at room temperature for 2 h. The labeled samples were then pooled and dried by vacuum centrifuging.

Strong cation exchange (SCX) fractionation
The pooled samples were subjected to Agilent 300 Extend C18 column (5 µm particles, 4.6 mm ID, 250 mm length, Phenomenex, CA, USA) for fractionation. Briefly, the samples were re-suspended with buffer A (25 mM NaH_2PO_4 in 25% ACN, pH 2.6) and loaded onto the SCX column. The samples were then eluted with a gradient of buffer A at the flow rate of 1 mL/min for 10 min, 5–65% buffer B (25 mM NaH_2PO_4, 1 M KCl in 25% ACN, pH 2.6) for 11 min, and 65–100% buffer B for 1 min. The eluted peptides were combined into 18 fractions and dried by vacuum centrifuging.

LC–MS/MS analysis
The fractions were then subjected to a reversed-phase pre-column (Acclaim PepMap 100, Thermo Fisher Scientific, CA, USA) on an EASY-nLC 1000 UPLC system. Briefly, the fractions were re-suspended in buffer A (0.1% FA in 2% ACN) and loaded onto the column at 6 µL/min for 5 min. Then, the fractions were then eluted with 6–22% buffer B (0.1% FA in 98% ACN) for 26 min, 22–35% buffer B for 8 min, followed by a 3-min linear gradient to 80%, then holding at 80% for 3 min at a constant flow rate of 400 nL/min.

The eluted peptides were then subjected to NSI source followed by tandem mass spectrometry (MS/MS) in Q Exactive™ plus (ThermoFisher Scientific, CA, USA). The intact peptides were detected at a resolution of 70,000 in the Orbitrap. The peptides with normalized collision energy (NCE) setting of 30 were selected for MS/MS, and ion fragments were detected at a resolution of 17,500 in the Orbitrap. A data-dependent procedure that alternated between one MS scan followed by 20 MS/MS scans was applied for the top 20 precursor ions above a threshold ion count of 10,000 in the MS survey scan with 30.0 s dynamic exclusion. The electrospray voltage was set as 2.0 kV. Automatic gain control (AGC) was applied to prevent overfilling of the Orbitrap, and $5e^4$ ions were accumulated for generation of MS/MS spectra. For MS scans, the m/z scan range was 350–1800. Fixed first mass was set as 100 m/z. Each SCX fraction was analyzed twice.

Database search
The MS/MS data were searched against *Uniprot Rattus norvegicus* database by using Mascot search engine

(v.2.3.0). Trypsin was set as cleavage enzyme allowing on more than 2 missing cleavages. For precursor ions, the mass error was set to 10 ppm, and for fragment ions, the mass error was set to 0.02 Da. Oxidation on Met was considered as variable modification, and carbamidomethylation on Cys was considered as fixed modification. Proteins with the false discovery rate (FDR) $\leq$ 1% were considered for further analysis. Protein ratios with the fold changes $\geq$ 1.20 or $\leq$ 0.83, and a p value less than 0.05 were considered significant.

Bioinformatics analysis

The interaction gene networks of the identified proteins were analyzed by GeneMANIA (http://www.genemania.org/). The interaction networks of the identified proteins were analyzed by STRING (Search Tool for the Retrieval of Interacting Genes/Proteins) database (http://string-db.org/). The biological process, molecular function and cellular component were analyzed by searching gene ontology (GO) database (http://geneontology.org/). The pathway analysis was performed by Kyoto Encyclopedia of Genes and Genomes (KEGG) pathway database (http://www.genome.jp/kegg/mapper.html).

Enzyme-linked immunosorbent assay (ELISA)

Based on the bioinformatics analysis and fold changes of differentially expressed proteins, we selected serum proteins involved in coagulation and complement cascades for ELISA validation. Rat C4b-binding protein alpha chain (C4bpa) ELISA kit (Cusabio, detection limit 39 ng/mL), rat complement fragment 5 (C5) ELISA kit (Cusabio, detection limit 2.34 ng/mL), and rat complement component 9 (C9) ELISA kit (Cusabio, detection limit 1.56 ng/mL) were proteins in the complement cascade. Rat coagulation factor VII (F7) ELISA kit (Cusabio, detection limit 0.195 ng/mL), rat fibrinogen alpha chain (Fga) ELISA kit (Cusabio, detection limit 0.025 µg/mL), rat fibrinogen beta chain (Fgb/Ab1-181/Ab1-216/Ac1-581) ELISA kit (Cusabio, detection limit 0.156 µg/mL), and rat von Willebrand Factor (vWF) ELISA kit (Cusabio, detection limit 0.078 ng/mL) were proteins in the coagulation cascade. ELISA was performed according to the manufacturer's instructions.

Statistical analysis

The experimental data was analyzed using the GraphPad Prism 5 (GraphPad Software Inc., USA). Comparison between two groups were performed using Mann–Whitney test, and multiple comparisons were performed using one-way ANOVA. The data were expressed as mean ± standard deviation (SD). p value less than 0.05 was considered statistically significant.

Results

ZDG increased the body weight in YDH syndrome rats

Throughout the 14-day construction period of YDH syndrome animal model, rats in the YDH syndrome group and ZDG treated group had lower body weight than that in the control group (Fig. 1). At the end of the second week, the body weight in the YDH syndrome group and ZDG treated group were significantly decreased than the control group ($p < 0.001$, Table 1). During the 7-day ZDG treated period, the body weight of rats (256.50 ± 11.53, day 21) increased in the ZDG treated group, compared to the rats in the YDH syndrome group (250.45 ± 8.96, day 21, Table 1).

Effect of ZDG on the relative organ weight in YDH syndrome rats

At the end of animal experiments, the liver, spleen, thymus, and adrenal glands were immediately removed and relative weights of the organs in each group were calculated. The results indicated that the relative weights of liver, spleen and adrenal glands showed no significant differences in the three groups, while the relative weights of thymus in YDH syndrome rats were increased compared with the control rats, and significantly decreased ($p = 0.017$) compared with the ZDG treated rats (Fig. 2).

Effect of ZDG on the serum protein expression in YDH syndrome rats

In the iTRAQ-2D LC–MS/MS analyses, a total of 1049 proteins were identified with three biological replicates, among which 997 proteins were quantified (see

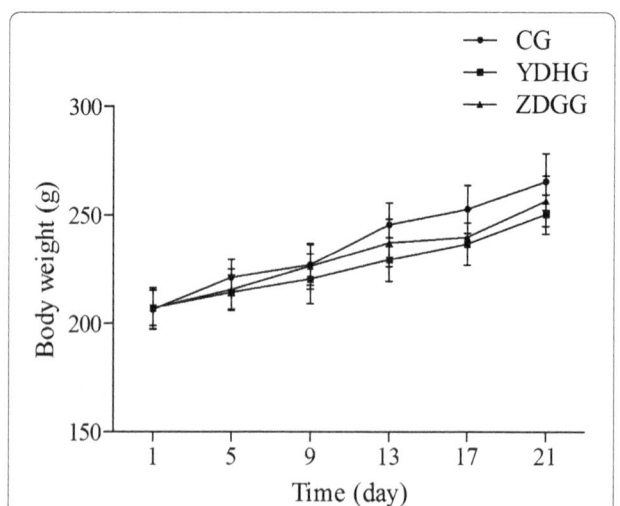

Fig. 1 Effects of ZDG on body weight in YDH syndrome rats. Body weight was measured every 5 days. *YDHG* YDH syndrome group, *ZDGG* ZDG treated group, *CG* control group. The values are presented as the mean ± SD

Table 1 Effect of ZDG on body weight in YDH syndrome rats

	CG		YDHG		ZDGG	
	Mean	SD	Mean	SD	Mean	SD
Day 1	206.50	9.16	207.26	8.21	207.15	9.48
Day 5	221.36	8.38	214.48**	7.83	215.68*	9.49
Day 9	227.00	9.47	220.62*	11.45	226.38	10.60
Day 13	245.60	9.99	229.45***	10.07	237.19**	10.97
Day 17	252.64	10.98	236.65***	9.83	239.82**	12.93
Day 21	265.40	13.10	250.45***	8.96	256.50*	11.53

SD standard deviation, *CG* control group, *YDHG* YDH syndrome group, *ZDGG* ZDG treated group

* Significant difference from the control group on the same day (Mann–Whitney U-test. * $p < 0.05$, ** $p < 0.01$, *** $p < 0.001$)

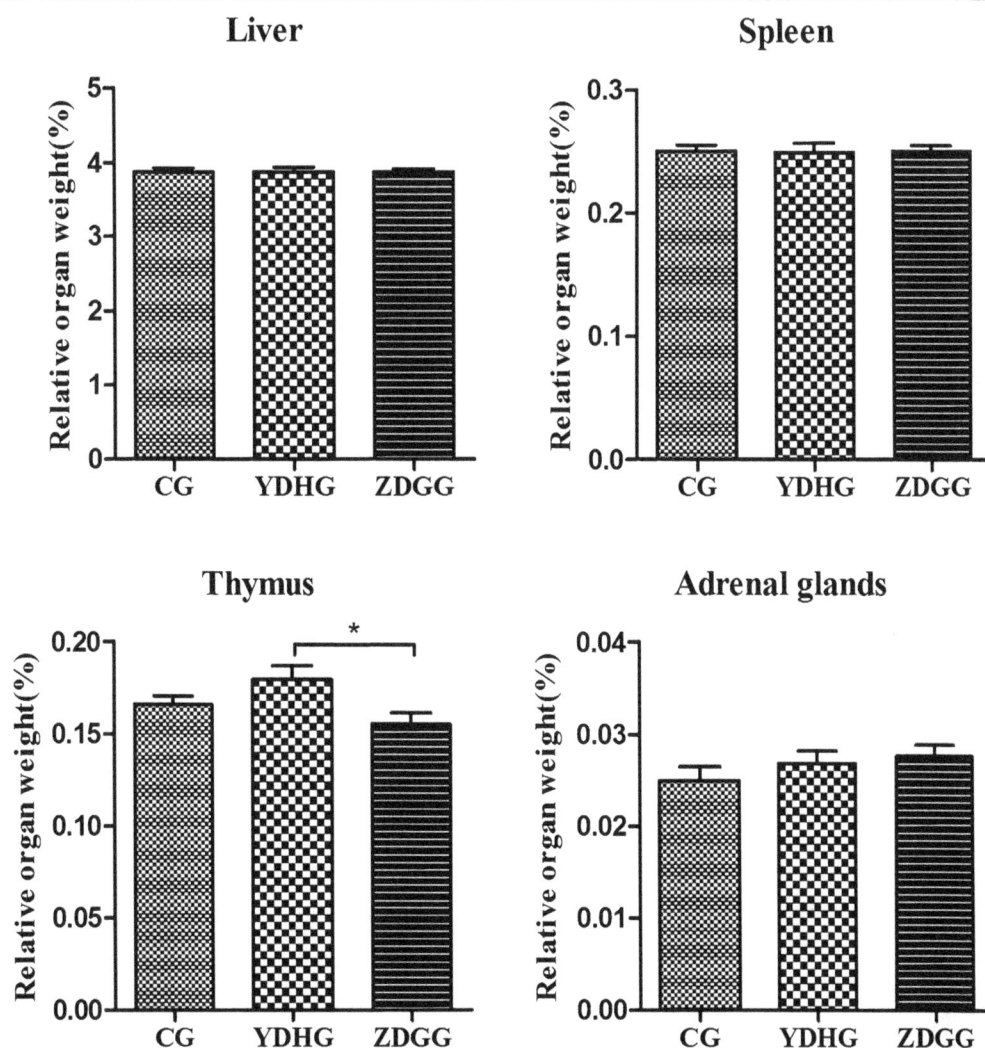

Fig. 2 Comparison of relative organs weight in YDHG, ZDGG and CG. The values are presented as mean ± SD. Differences in each group were determined by using the Mann–Whitney U-test, and $p < 0.05$ indicates statistical significance. *Significant difference ($p < 0.05$). *CG* control group, *YDHG* YDH syndrome group, *ZDGG* ZDG treated group

Additional file 2). Among the quantified proteins, 71 proteins (10 up-regulated and 61 down-regulated proteins) showed statistically significant changes (at least a 1.20-fold change and $p < 0.05$) in the YDH syndrome group and ZDG treated group (Fig. 3). According to the expression profiles of proteins in the YDH syndrome group, ZDG treated group and control group, we classified the differentially expressed proteins into 6 clusters (Fig. 4). The fold change and regulated type of the differentially expressed proteins were presented in Additional file 3.

Among 10 up-regulated proteins in the ZDG treated group, the GO analysis indicated that most proteins were involved in humoral immune response (5 proteins), complement activation (5 proteins), activation of immune response (5 proteins), immune effector process (5 proteins), innate immune response (5 proteins),

immunoglobulin mediated immune response (4 proteins), B cell mediated immunity (4 proteins), complement activation (classical pathway, 4 proteins), humoral immune response mediated by circulating immunoglobulin, lymphocyte mediated immunity (4 proteins), positive regulation of immune response (5 proteins), and adaptive immune response based on somatic recombination of immune receptors built from immunoglobulin superfamily domains (4 proteins), indicating that the up-regulated proteins mainly participated in immune response (Fig. 5a). Among the 61 down-regulated proteins, the GO analysis revealed that most proteins were associated with proteolysis (13 proteins), blood coagulation (6 proteins), coagulation (6 proteins), hemostasis (6 proteins), and platelet activation (5 proteins), revealing a great abundance in coagulation in down-regulated proteins (Fig. 5b). The interacted gene network analyzed by GenMANIA (http://genemania.org/) indicated that most genes encoding the differential proteins were co-expressed (Fig. 6).

KEGG pathway and STRING analyses showed that most differentially expressed proteins in the ZDG treated group were enriched in coagulation and complement cascades (Fig. 7). Besides, the proteins in coagulation cascades displayed down-regulation, while those in complement cascades displayed up-regulation (Fig. 8, Additional file 4).

Validation of proteins expression in coagulation and complement cascades

ELISA was performed to detect the serum expression of the proteins in coagulation and complement cascades. The results showed that serum expression of C4bpa and C5 levels were significantly increased in the ZDG treated group compared with the YDH syndrome group ($p = 0.028$, $p = 0.018$, respectively). C5 and C9 showed the trend of returning to normal after ZDG treatment. Serum expression of F7 and Fgg were significantly decreased in the ZDG treated group compared with the YDH syndrome group ($p = 0.007$, $p = 0.033$, respectively), and Fgg returned to normal. The levels of Fga, and vWF were lower in the ZDG treated group than the YDH syndrome group, and Fga was showed the trend of returning to normal after ZDG treatment, but no significant difference was observed (Fig. 9). In conclusion, serum expression of C5, C9, Fga, and Fgg were observed the trend of returning to normal condition in the ZDG treated group. The results revealed increased levels of proteins in complement cascade and decreased levels of proteins in coagulation cascade after ZDG treatment.

Quality control validation of MS data

The MS data validation is shown in supplementary figures. The mass error of all the identified peptides was

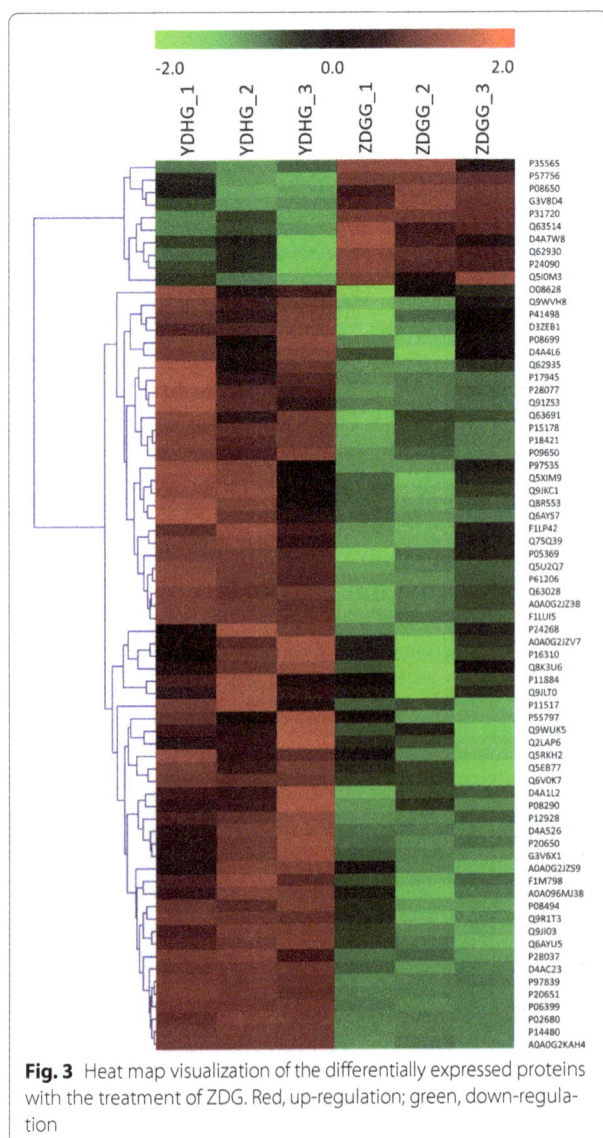

Fig. 3 Heat map visualization of the differentially expressed proteins with the treatment of ZDG. Red, up-regulation; green, down-regulation

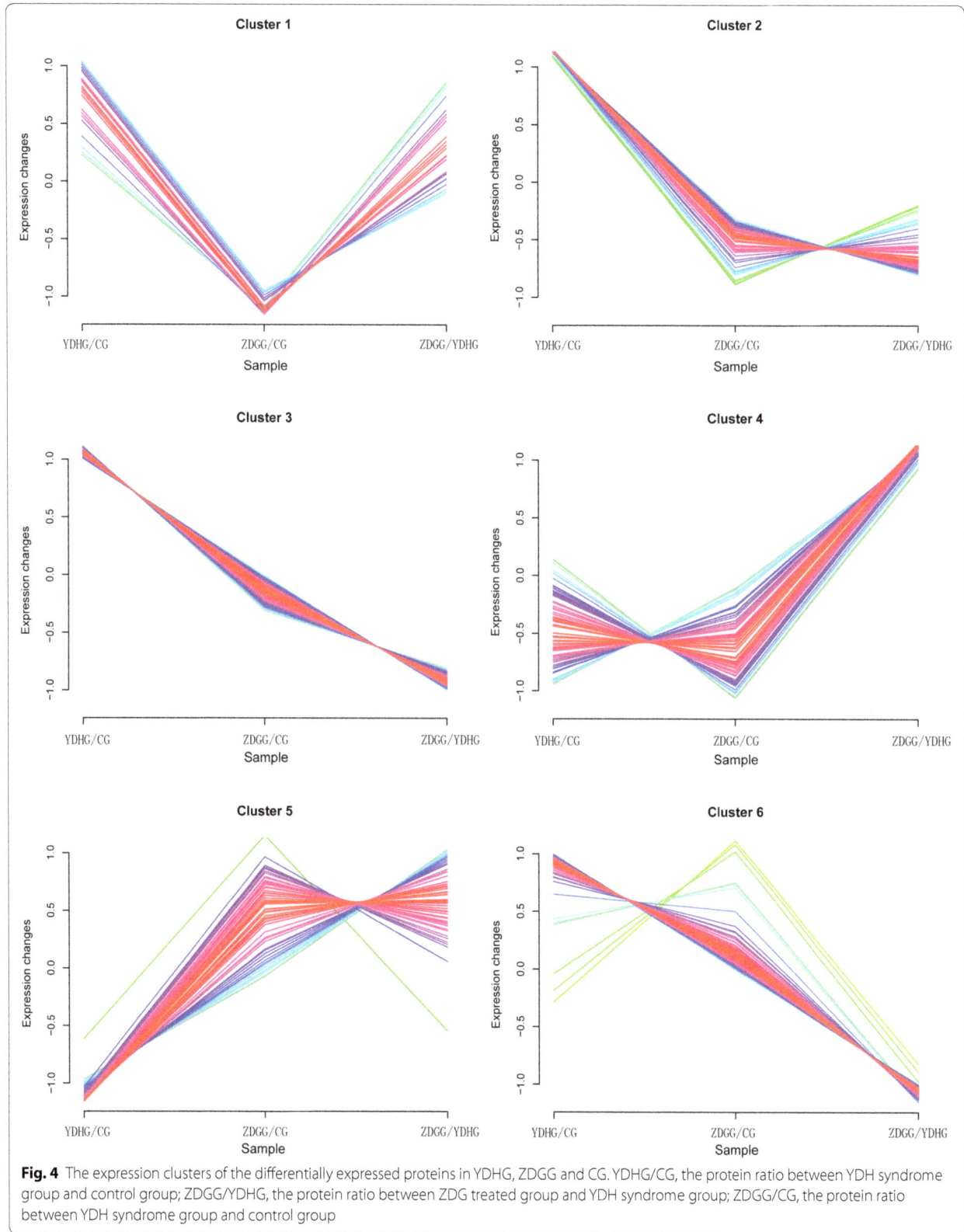

Fig. 4 The expression clusters of the differentially expressed proteins in YDHG, ZDGG and CG. YDHG/CG, the protein ratio between YDH syndrome group and control group; ZDGG/YDHG, the protein ratio between ZDG treated group and YDH syndrome group; ZDGG/CG, the protein ratio between YDH syndrome group and control group

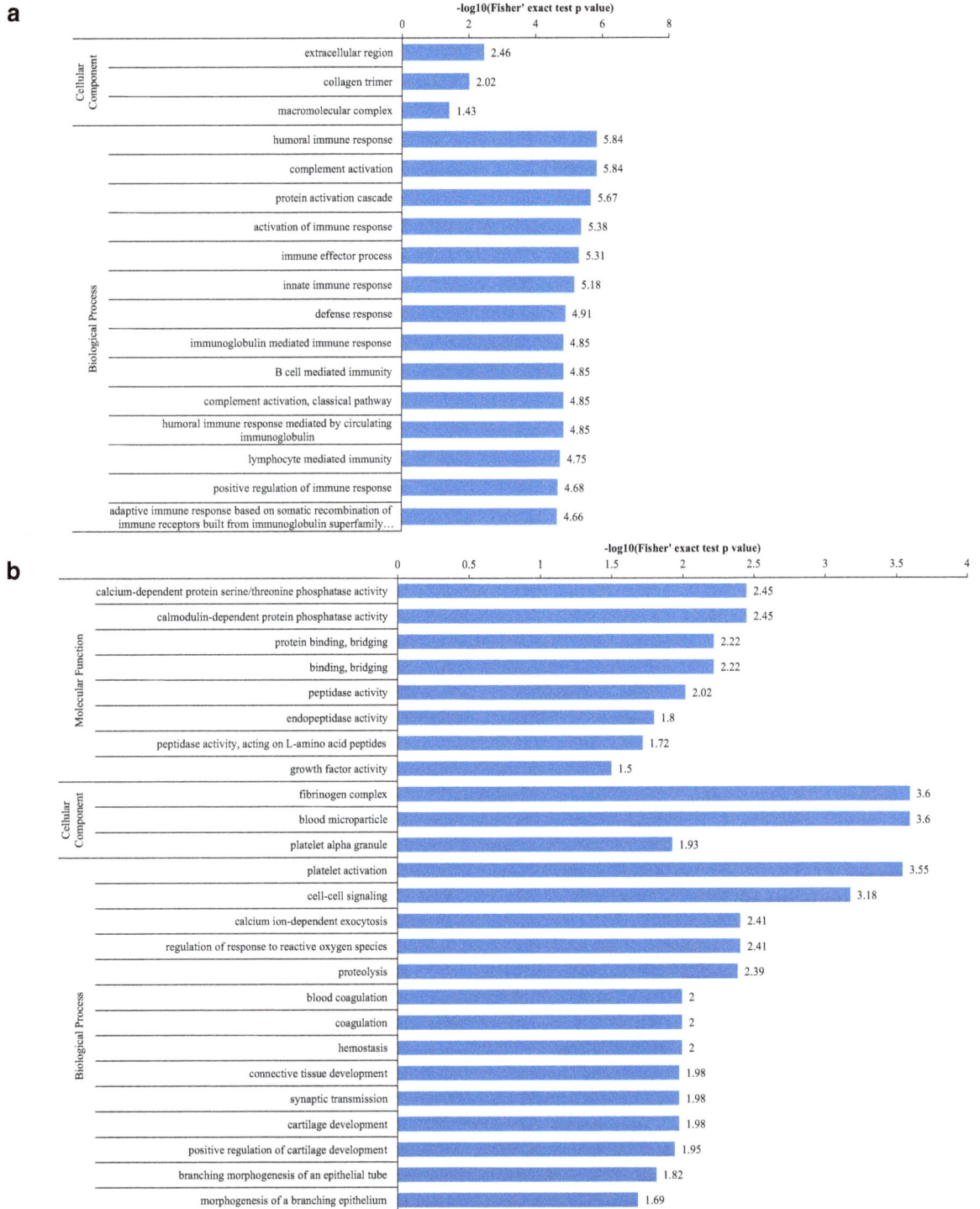

Fig. 5 Bioinformatics data mining of the set of differentially expressed proteins with the treatment of ZDG. The GO terms are sorted by −log10 of the Fisher's exact test p value, which indicates the enrichment significance of GO terms. **a** GO enrichment analysis of up-regulated proteins. **b** GO enrichment analysis of down-regulated proteins

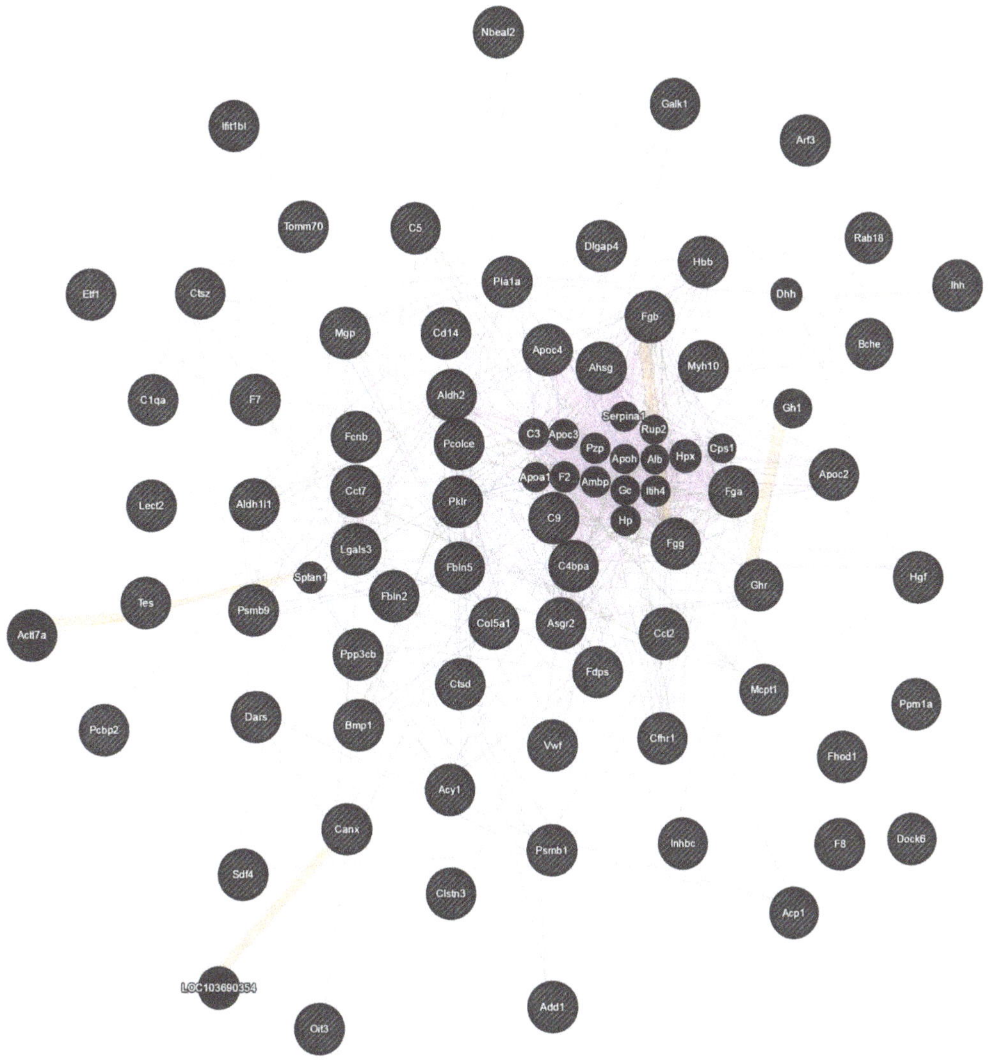

Fig. 6 The interacted gene network of the differentially proteins analyzed by GenMANIA. Purple line, co-expression; orange line, predicted; blue line, co-localization; yellow line, shared protein domains

checked, and the distribution of mass error was near zero and most of them were < 0.02 Da, indicating that the mass accuracy of the MS data fits the requirement. The length of most peptides was distributed between 8 and 16, which agree with the property of tryptic peptides. Pearson correlation analysis was used to estimate repeatability in three repeats of the MS data (see Additional file 5).

Discussion

YDH syndrome is common in TCM practice. Although the mechanisms of YDH syndrome are still unclear, it is widely believed that the excessive consumption of Yin results in the pathological condition called "internal heat" in TCM theory. YDH syndrome has been demonstrated

to be associated with depressed immunity and enhanced inflammation. Previous study revealed the decreased immunological substances [12] and increased inflammatory cytokines [13] in YDH constitution. Individuals with YDH syndrome present with five center (the palms, soles, and chest) heat, tidal fever, recurrent oral-ulcer, swollen gums and throat, which is closely related to the inflammatory reaction. Inflammation is an immune response characterized by the release of chemokines and cytokines [14]. Interestingly, TNF-α, IL-1β, and IL-6 levels have been shown to be up-regulated in YDH syndrome individuals [15], indicating that the inflammatory response could be enhanced in YDH syndrome. Thus, we hypothesized that YDH syndrome shares common biological basis with immune response and inflammation.

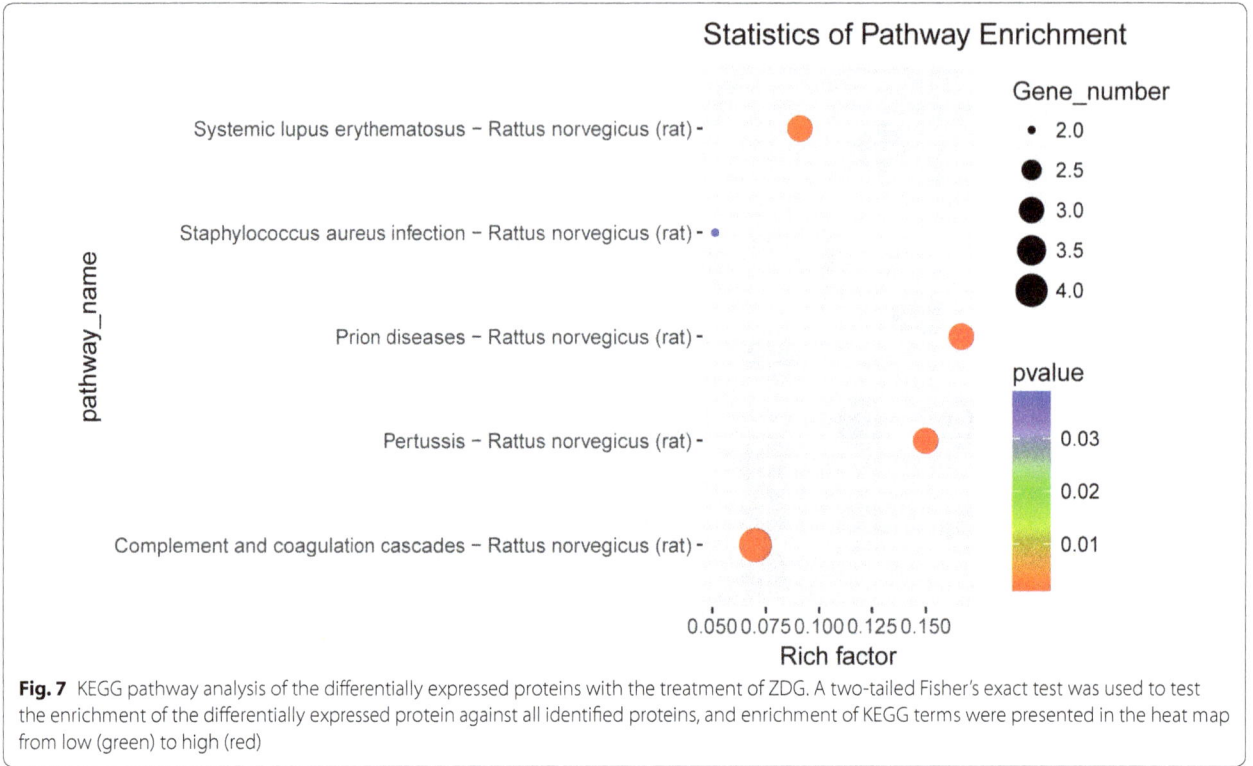

Fig. 7 KEGG pathway analysis of the differentially expressed proteins with the treatment of ZDG. A two-tailed Fisher's exact test was used to test the enrichment of the differentially expressed protein against all identified proteins, and enrichment of KEGG terms were presented in the heat map from low (green) to high (red)

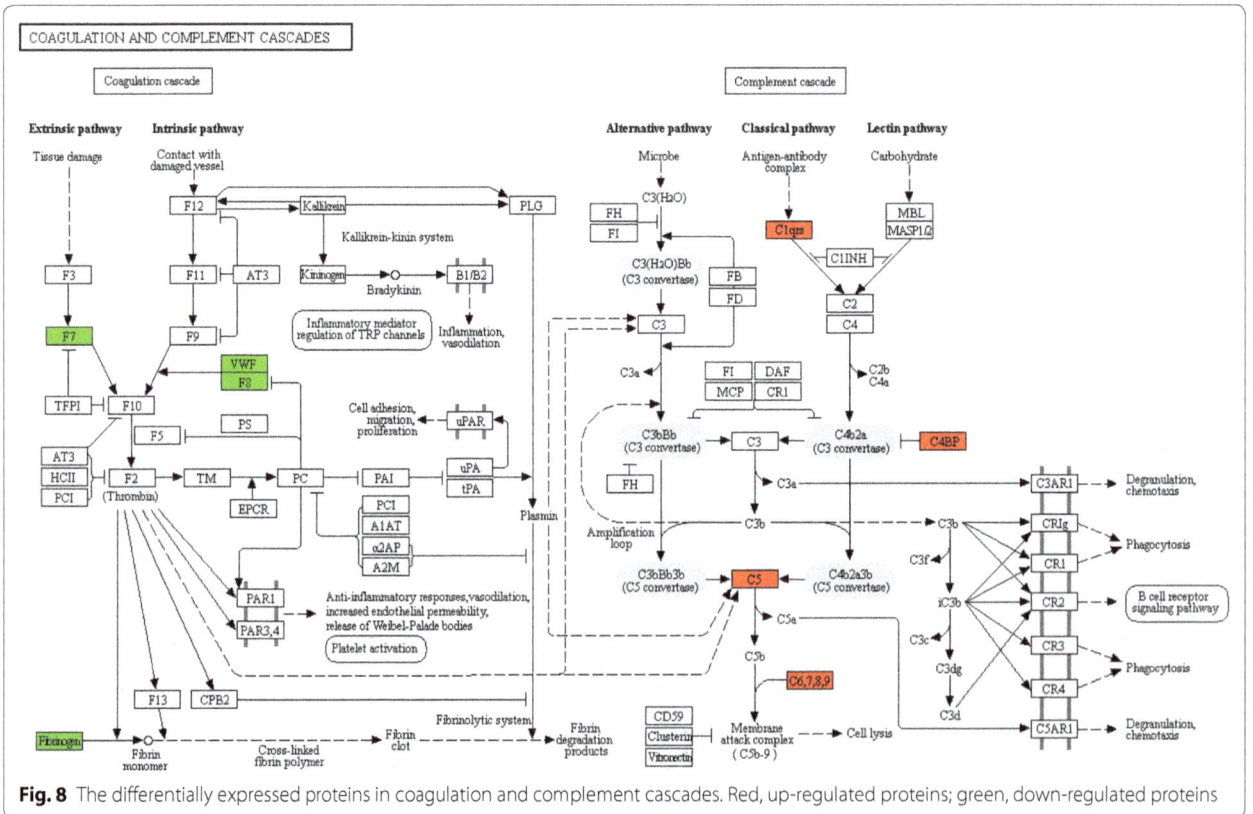

Fig. 8 The differentially expressed proteins in coagulation and complement cascades. Red, up-regulated proteins; green, down-regulated proteins

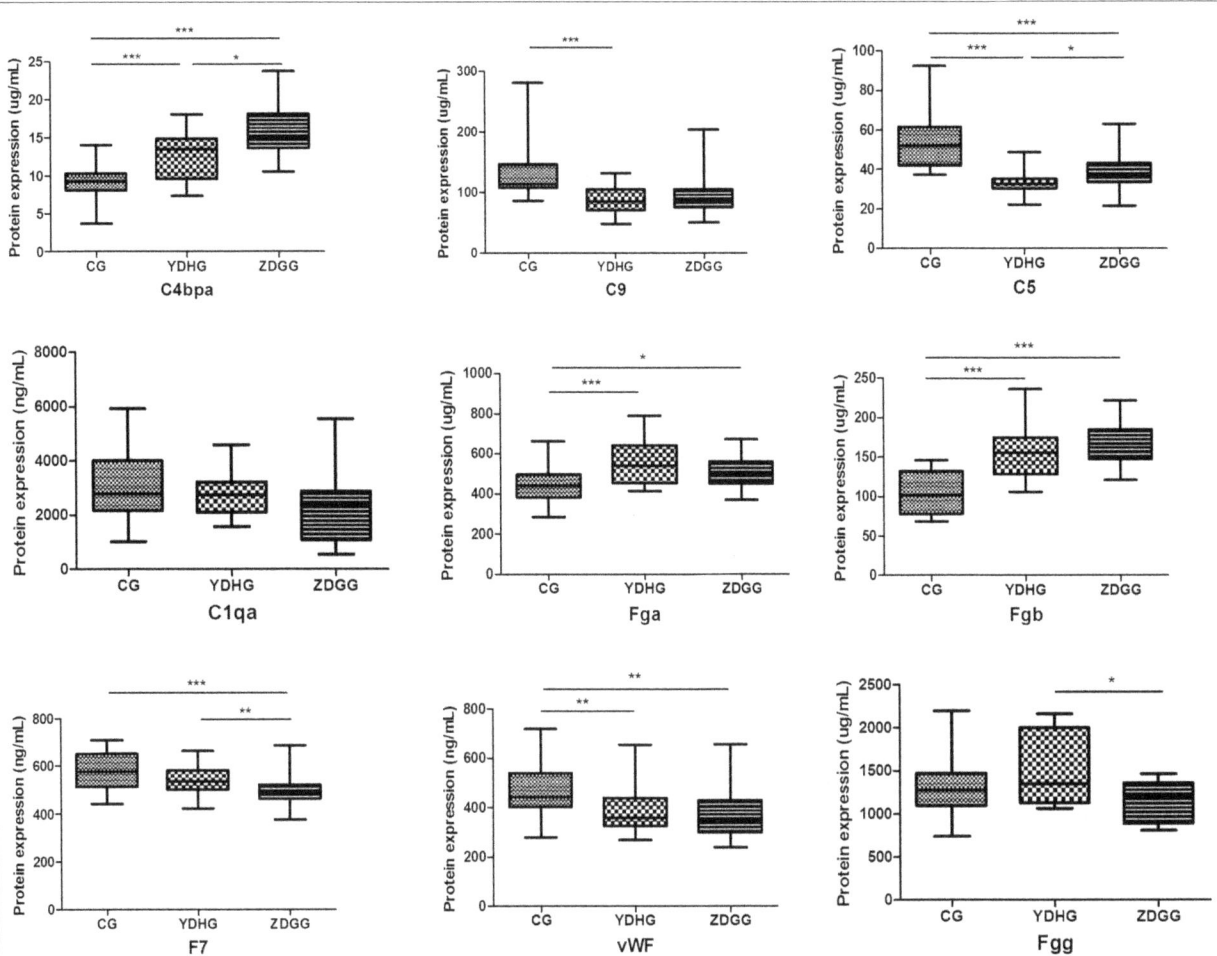

Fig. 9 Verification of the differentially expressed proteins in coagulation and complement cascades by ELISA. Proteins expression were measured in the control group (n = 24), the YDH syndrome group (n = 20) and the ZDG treated group (n = 20). p values were calculated with the Mann–Whitney U-test, *p < 0.05, **p < 0.01, ***p < 0.001. *CG* control group, *YDHG* YDH syndrome group, *ZDGG* ZDG treated group

Herbal medicines have been widely used to manage and prevent diseases. ZDG is a well-known classic traditional herbal medicine to treat YDH syndrome. ZDG shares the similar ingredients with the Liuwei Dihuang Granule (LDG) herbal medicine, which has been reported to decrease the inflammatory cells in autoimmune encephalomyelitis [16]. However, few articles have reported the therapeutic mechanism of ZDG in treating YDH syndrome. In the present study, we found that 71 serum proteins were differentially expressed with ZDG treatment. GO analysis of these proteins revealed the enrichment of immune response in up-regulated proteins, and the enrichment of coagulation in down-regulated proteins. Both KEGG and STRING analyses indicated that the differentially expressed proteins after ZDG treatment were mainly involved in the coagulation and complement cascades pathway. Therefore, we hypothesized that ZDG can treat YDH syndrome by regulating proteins in the coagulation and complement cascades pathway.

The coagulation and complement cascades pathway is highly associated with immunity and enhanced inflammation. The complement system is a key sentinel of innate immunity, while the coagulation system serves as main actor in hemostasis. Both (coagulation and complement systems) belong to the "first line of defense" against injurious stimuli and invaders [17]. There is extensive cross-talk between inflammation and coagulation [18]. Inflammation induces activation of coagulation, and coagulation proteases modulate inflammation [17]. The extrinsic coagulation cascade is initiated by the combination of factor VII (F7) and the tissue factor (TF). The activated factor VII (F7a) activates both factor X (F10) and factor IX (F9), and the activated factor X (F10a) has pro-inflammatory properties [19]. However, in the intrinsic coagulation cascade, vWF prevents factor VIII (F8) from being activated, consequently inhibiting the activation of F9 and F10 [20]. F10a catalyzes prothrombin into thrombin, the key hydrolytic enzyme in the coagulation cascade, which induces up-regulation of various pro-inflammatory cytokines, including monocyte chemotacticprotein-1, IL-6, IL-8, and macrophage migration [20–22]. In our proteomics study, F7 and vWF were decreased after the ZDG treatment, indicating that ZDG can inhibit the enzymes in both extrinsic and intrinsic coagulation cascades. Fibrinogen, assembled by α-chain (Fga), β-chain (Fgb), and γ-chain (Fgg) participate in inflammatory response. Fibrin, the production of fibrinogen, regulates the generation of inflammatory cytokine in vivo [22, 23]. Fibrinogen was found to be down-regulated with the treatment of ZDG in the proteomics experiments, and the serum levels of Fga and Fgg were confirmed to be decreased by ELISA. Therefore, the repressed fibrinogen level by ZDG treatment could result in the suppression of inflammatory response.

Complement was initially thought to be the heat-sensitive fraction in human plasma which improves the antibodies in their capacity to eliminate pathogens. Activation of the complement cascade enhances the immune function. In classical pathway (CP), the recognition of pathogens occurs directly via contacting the pathogen-associated molecular patterns (PAMPs) by C1q, followed by activation of C1r and C1s [24]. C4 and C2 are subsequently cleaved by the activated C1s to form C4b2a [25]. As a C3 convertase, C4b2a cleaves C3 into the fragments C3a and C3b, the latter can be covalently bound to the pathogens via its exposed thioester [26]. When C3b reaches a certain amount on the surface of pathogens, the terminal pathway (TP) of complement is initiated. In TP, the C3 convertase C3bBb and C4b2a can interact with C3 to form C3bBb3b and C4b2a3b, both of which are C5 convertases. C5 is cleaved by these convertases to generate C5a and C5b, and the latter in combination with C6, C7, C8, and C9 form the membrane attack complex (MAC) [27]. Previous studies have demonstrated that the sublytic MAC can drive inflammation by activating NLRP3 inflammasome and triggering the release of cytokines IL-1β and IL-18 [28, 29]. Our results revealed the increased serum levels of C4bp, C5, and C9 after ZDG treatment, indicating that ZDG can enhance the activation of the complement cascade, and improve the ability to eliminate pathogens.

Conclusions
In summary, treatment with ZDG significantly increased the protein expression in the complement cascade to promote the complement activation, and enhanced the ability to eliminate pathogens in immune process. Besides,

ZDG also decreased the protein expression in the coagulation cascade to alleviate the inflammation. The results suggested that ZDG could treat YDH syndrome by regulating complement and coagulation cascades pathway.

Abbreviations
ZDG: Zhibai Dihuang Granule; YDH: Yin-deficiency-heat; GO: gene ontology; ELISA: enzyme-linked immunosorbent assay; KEGG: Kyoto Encyclopedia of Genes and Genomes; C4bpa: complement component 4 binding protein alpha; C5: complement component 5; C9: complement component 9; F7: coagulation factor VII; Fga: fibrinogen alpha chain; Fgg: fibrinogen gamma chain; vWF: von Willebrand Factor; TCM: traditional Chinese medicine; DTT: dithiothreitol; IAA: 3-indoleacrylic acid; iTRAQ: isobaric tags for relative and absolute quantification; SPE: solid phase extraction; SCX: strong cation exchange; ACN: acetonitrile; FA: formic acid; UPLC: ultra performance liquid chromatography; NCE: normalized collision energy; AGC: automatic gain control; LDG: Liuwei Dihuang Granule; TF: tissue factor; PAMPs: pathogen-associated molecular patterns; CP: classical pathway; TP: terminal pathway; MAC: membrane attack complex; NLRP3: NACHT, LRR and PYD domains-containing protein 3; SD: standard deviation.

Authors' contributions
JCL conceived the study. CML, SY, TTJ, HHT, ZLC and LGM performed the animal experiments. CML, JC and SY performed the proteomics experiment and ELISA. ZJL, YTH and LG performed statistical analyses. JCL and CML coordinated the research and drafted the manuscript. All authors read and approved the final manuscript.

Author details
Institute of Cell Biology, Zhejiang University, Hangzhou, People's Republic of China. ² South China University of Technology School of Medicine, Guangzhou, People's Republic of China.

Acknowledgements
Not applicable.

Competing interests
The authors declare that they have no competing interests.

Funding
This work was supported by grants from the National Natural Science Foundation of China (No. 81573709), the National Basic Research Program of China (No. 2014CB543002).

References
1. Wang Q, Zhu YB. Epidemiological investigation of constitutional types of Chinese medicine in general population: base on 21,948 epidemiological investigation data of nine provinces in China. China J Tradit Chin Med Pharm. 2009;24:7–12.
2. Yu HJ, Wang Y, Yang LP. Epidemiological investigation of Yin deficiency and Yang deficiency constitutions in TCM of Henan University. Liaoning J Tradit Chin Med. 2013;40:619–21.
3. Hsu YH, Chen TH, Wu MY, Lin YF, Chen WL, Cheng TH, Chen CH. Protective effects of Zhibai Dihuang Wan on renal tubular cells affected with gentamicin-induced apoptosis. J Ethnopharmacol. 2014;151:635–42.

4. Liu H, Tang H, Guo ZC. Clinical Study on Zhibai Dihuang decoction combined with endocrine therapy in treating Kidney-yin deficiency type of advanced prostate cancer. Chin J Inform TCM. 2016;23:24–7.

5. Kanwar YS, Wada J, Sun L, Xie P, Wallner EI, Chen S, Chugh S, Danesh FR. Diabetic nephropathy: mechanisms of renal disease progression. Exp Biol Med (Maywood). 2008;233:4–11.

6. Cheung F. TCM made in China. Nature. 2011;480:S82–3.

7. Oberg AL, Kennedy RB, Li P, Ovsyannikova IG, Poland GA. Systems biology approaches to new vaccine development. Curr Opin Immunol. 2011;23:436–43.

8. Hussain MA, Huygens F. Proteomic and bioinformatics tools to understand virulence mechanisms in *Staphylococcus aureus*. Curr Proteomics. 2012;9:2–8.

9. Zhou YS, Fan YL, Zhang YP, Jiang XL, Zou SJ, Wang LF. Development of animal model of heat syndrome due to insufficiency of yin fluids. Chin J Basic Med TCM. 2001;7:23–5.

10. Han B, Wang S, Li L, Wang Y, Zhao H. Gene expression profiling of rat livers with yin-deficiency-heat syndrome. J Tradit Chin Med. 2013;33:378–83.

11. Yang CP, Xue CM. The establisment and the influence on the antioxidant effect of yin-deficiency mice model induced by pungent Chinese herbs. J Sichuan Tradit Chin Med. 2004;22:14–5.

12. Wang JM. The application of doctrine of Yin and Yang in the immune response. J Zhejiang Coll Tradit Chin Med. 1979;5:4–5.

13. Wang Q, Ren XJ, Yao SL, Wu HD. Clinical observation on the endocrinal and immune functions in subjects with yin-deficiency constitution. Chin J Integr Med. 2010;16:28–32.

14. Medzhitov R. Inflammation 2010: new adventures of an old flame. Cell. 2010;140:771–6.

15. Yan HF, Ma JL, Zhu HH, Qu K, Qu F, Fan XH, Bai J, Zeng XR. Yin deficiency syndrome vexing heat in chest, palms and soles was related to TNF-α IL-1β IL-6 clinical observation. Chin Arch Tradit Chin Med. 2008;26:293–5.

16. Liu Y, Zhao H, Zhang J, Zhang P, Li M, Qi F, Wang Y, Kou S, Zheng Q, Wang L. The regulatory effect of liuwei dihuang pills on cytokines in mice with experimental autoimmune encephalomyelitis. Am J Chin Med. 2012;40:295–308.

17. Choi G, Schultz MJ, Levi M, van der Poll T. The relationship between inflammation and the coagulation system. Swiss Med Wkly. 2006;136:139–44.

18. Esmon CT. The interactions between inflammation and coagulation. Br J Haematol. 2005;131:417–30.

19. Cirino G, Cicala C, Bucci M, Sorrentino L, Ambrosini G, DeDominicis G, Altieri DC. Factor Xa as an interface between coagulation and inflammation—molecular mimicry of factor Xa association with effector cell protease receptor-1 induces acute inflammation in vivo. J Clin Invest. 1997;99:2446–51.

20. Saenko EL, Shima M, Sarafanov AG. Role of activation of the coagulation factor VIII in interaction with vWf, phospholipid, and functioning within the factor Xase complex. Trends Cardiovasc Med. 1999;9:185–92.

21. Asokananthan N, Graham PT, Fink J, Knight DA, Bakker AJ, McWilliam AS, Thompson PJ, Stewart GA. Activation of protease-activated receptor (PAR)-1, PAR-2, and PAR-4 stimulates IL-6, IL-8, and prostaglandin E2 release from human respiratory epithelial cells. J Immunol. 2002;168:3577–85.

22. Szaba FM, Smiley ST. Roles for thrombin and fibrin(ogen) in cytokine/chemokine production and macrophage adhesion in vivo. Blood. 2002;99:1053–9.

23. Ljungman P, Bellander T, Schneider A, Breitner S, Forastiere F, Hampel R, Illig T, Jacquemin B, Katsouyanni K, von Klot S, et al. Modification of the interleukin-6 response to air pollution by interleukin-6 and fibrinogen polymorphisms. Environ Health Perspect. 2009;117:1373–9.

24. Arlaud GJ, Gaboriaud C, Thielens NM, Rossi V, Bersch B, Hernandez JF, Fontecilla-Camps JC. Structural biology of C1: dissection of a complex molecular machinery. Immunol Rev. 2001;180:136–45.

25. Muller-Eberhard HJ, Polley MJ, Calcott MA. Formation and functional significance of a molecular complex derived from the second and the fourth component of human complement. J Exp Med. 1967;125:359–80.

26. Law SK, Dodds AW. The internal thioester and the covalent binding properties of the complement proteins C3 and C4. Protein Sci. 1997;6:263–74.

27. Berends ET, Kuipers A, Ravesloot MM, Urbanus RT, Rooijakkers SH. Bacteria under stress by complement and coagulation. FEMS Microbiol Rev. 2014;38:1146–71.

28. Laudisi F, Spreafico R, Evrard M, Hughes TR, Mandriani B, Kandasamy M, Morgan BP, Sivasankar B, Mortellaro A. Cutting edge: the NLRP3 inflammasome links complement-mediated inflammation and IL-1beta release. J Immunol. 2013;191:1006–10.

29. Triantafilou K, Hughes TR, Triantafilou M, Morgan BP. The complement membrane attack complex triggers intracellular Ca2+ fluxes leading to NLRP3 inflammasome activation. J Cell Sci. 2013;126:2903–13.

PERMISSIONS

All chapters in this book were first published in CM, by BioMed Central; hereby published with permission under the Creative Commons Attribution License or equivalent. Every chapter published in this book has been scrutinized by our experts. Their significance has been extensively debated. The topics covered herein carry significant findings which will fuel the growth of the discipline. They may even be implemented as practical applications or may be referred to as a beginning point for another development.

The contributors of this book come from diverse backgrounds, making this book a truly international effort. This book will bring forth new frontiers with its revolutionizing research information and detailed analysis of the nascent developments around the world.

We would like to thank all the contributing authors for lending their expertise to make the book truly unique. They have played a crucial role in the development of this book. Without their invaluable contributions this book wouldn't have been possible. They have made vital efforts to compile up to date information on the varied aspects of this subject to make this book a valuable addition to the collection of many professionals and students.

This book was conceptualized with the vision of imparting up-to-date information and advanced data in this field. To ensure the same, a matchless editorial board was set up. Every individual on the board went through rigorous rounds of assessment to prove their worth. After which they invested a large part of their time researching and compiling the most relevant data for our readers.

The editorial board has been involved in producing this book since its inception. They have spent rigorous hours researching and exploring the diverse topics which have resulted in the successful publishing of this book. They have passed on their knowledge of decades through this book. To expedite this challenging task, the publisher supported the team at every step. A small team of assistant editors was also appointed to further simplify the editing procedure and attain best results for the readers.

Apart from the editorial board, the designing team has also invested a significant amount of their time in understanding the subject and creating the most relevant covers. They scrutinized every image to scout for the most suitable representation of the subject and create an appropriate cover for the book.

The publishing team has been an ardent support to the editorial, designing and production team. Their endless efforts to recruit the best for this project, has resulted in the accomplishment of this book. They are a veteran in the field of academics and their pool of knowledge is as vast as their experience in printing. Their expertise and guidance has proved useful at every step. Their uncompromising quality standards have made this book an exceptional effort. Their encouragement from time to time has been an inspiration for everyone.

The publisher and the editorial board hope that this book will prove to be a valuable piece of knowledge for researchers, students, practitioners and scholars across the globe.

LIST OF CONTRIBUTORS

Run-sheng Zheng, Wen-li Wang, Jing Tan, Hui Xu, Ruo-ting Zhan and Wei-wen Chen
Research Centre of Chinese Herbal Resource Science and Engineering, Guangzhou University of Chinese Medicine, Guangzhou, China
Key Laboratory of Chinese Medicinal Resource from Lingnan, Ministry of Education, Guangzhou University of Chinese Medicine, Guangzhou, China

So-Youn Jung, Kyoung-Min Kim and Young Kyun Kim
College of Korean Medicine, Dong-Eui University, Yangjeong-ro, Busanjin-gu, Busan 47227, Republic of Korea

Suin Cho
School of Korean Medicine, Pusan National University, Yangsan, Gyeongnam 50612, Republic of Korea

Sehyun Lim
School of Public Health, Far East University, Chungbuk 27601, Republic of Korea

Chiyeon Lim
College of Medicine, Dongguk University, Ilsandong-gu, Gyeonggi-do 10326, Republic of Korea

He-Ting Zhang, Hai-Yan Duan, Xiao-Mei Xie and Ling Zhang
School of Pharmacy, Anhui University of Chinese Medicine, Hefei 230031, China

Hua-Sheng Peng
School of Pharmacy, Anhui University of Chinese Medicine, Hefei 230031, China
State Key Laboratory Breeding Base of Dao-di Herbs, China Academy of Chinese Medical Sciences, Beijing 100700, China

Jun Wang
School of Pharmacy, Anhui University of Chinese Medicine, Hefei 230031, China
School of Pharmacy, Bozhou Vocational and Technical College, Bozhou 236800, China

Ming-En Cheng and Dai-yin Peng
School of Pharmacy, Anhui University of Chinese Medicine, Hefei 230031, China

Institute of TCM Resources Protection and Development, Anhui Academy of Chinese Medicine, Hefei 230031, People's Republic of China

Yanqiong Zhang, Xia Mao, Jing Su, Shihuan Tang, Haiyu Xu and Hongjun Yang
Institute of Chinese Materia Medica, China Academy of Chinese Medical Sciences, No. 16, Nanxiaojie, Dongzhimennei, Beijing 100700, China

Ya Geng
School of Basic Medicine, Shandong University of Traditional Chinese Medicine, Jinan 250300, China

Rui Guo, Junfang Li and Xuefeng Xiao
College of Pharmacy, Tianjin University of Traditional Chinese Medicine, Tianjin 300193, China

Qian Chen
School of Pharmaceutical Sciences, Wenzhou Medical University, Wenzhou 325035, China

Ni Ai, Jie Liao, Xin Shao, Yufeng Liu and Xiaohui Fan
Pharmaceutical Informatics Institute, College of Pharmaceutical Sciences, Zhejiang University, Hangzhou 310058, China

Jer-Yiing Houng, Hsia-Fen Hsu and Li-Wen Fang
Department of Nutrition, I-Shou University, No.8, Yida Rd., Yanchao District, Kaohsiung City 82445, Taiwan

Tzong-Shyuan Tai
Department of Medical Research, E-Da Hospital, Kaohsiung City 82445, Taiwan
School of Medicine for International Students, I-Shou University, Kaohsiung City 82445, Taiwan

Shu-Ching Hsu
National Institute of Infectious Diseases and Vaccinology, NHRI, Miaoli County 35053, Taiwan
Department of Medical Research, Show-Chwan Memorial Hospital, Changhua County 50008, Taiwan

Tzann-Shun Hwang
Graduate Institute of Biotechnology, Chinese Culture University, Taipei City 11114, Taiwan

Chih-Jiun Lin
Department of Leisure and Recreation Management, Da-Yeh University, Changhua County 51591, Taiwan

Jin-Fa Tang, Wei-Xia Li, Fan Zhang, Yu-Hui Li, Ying-Jie Cao, Ya Zhao and Xue-Lin Li
The First Affiliated Hospital of Henan University of Chinese Medicine, No. 19, Renmin Road, Jinshui District, Zhengzhou 450000, People's Republic of China

Zhi-Jie Ma
Beijing Friendship Hospital Affiliated to Capital Medical University, No. 95, Yongan Road, Xuanwu District, Beijing 100050, China

Wenbo Peng, Romy Lauche, Jane Frawley and Jon Adams
Australian Research Centre in Complementary and Integrative Medicine (ARCCIM), University of Technology Sydney, Ultimo, NSW, Australia

David Sibbritt
Australian Research Centre in Complementary and Integrative Medicine (ARCCIM), University of Technology Sydney, Ultimo, NSW, Australia
Australian Research Centre in Complementary and Integrative Medicine (ARCCIM), Faculty of Health, University of Technology Sydney, Level 8, Building 10, 235-253 Jones St, Ultimo, NSW 2007, Australia

Caleb Ferguson
Centre for Cardiovascular and Chronic Care, University of Technology Sydney, Ultimo, NSW, Australia

Jiu Chun
Department of Clinical Korean Medicine, Graduate School, Kyung Hee University, Seoul 02447, Republic of Korea

Sun Haeng Lee and Jin Yong Lee
Department of Clinical Korean Medicine, Graduate School, Kyung Hee University, Seoul 02447, Republic of Korea
Department of Pediatrics of Korean Medicine, Kyung Hee University Korean Medicine Hospital, Kyung Hee University Medical Center, Seoul 02447, Republic of Korea

Gyu Tae Chang
Department of Clinical Korean Medicine, Graduate School, Kyung Hee University, Seoul 02447, Republic of Korea
Department of Pediatrics of Korean Medicine, Kyung Hee University Hospital at Gangdong, Dongnam-ro 892, Gangdong-gu, Seoul 05278, Republic of Korea

Hyun Jeong Lee, Young-Sik Kim, Donghun Lee and Hocheol Kim
Department of Herbal Pharmacology, College of Korean Medicine, Kyung Hee University, Seoul 02447, Republic of Korea

Sung Hyun Lee
Korea Institute of Science and Technology for Eastern Medicine (KISTEM), NeuMed Inc., Seoul 02440, Republic of Korea

Yulin Zhang, Yeer Liang and Chengwei He
State Key Laboratory of Quality Research in Chinese Medicine, Institute of Chinese Medical Sciences, University of Macau, N22-7038, Avenida da Universidade, Taipa, Macao 999078, China

Chi-Ren Liao and Kun-Chang Wu
Department of Chinese Pharmaceutical Sciences and Chinese Medicine Resources, College of Biopharmaceutical and Food Sciences, China Medical University, Taichung 40402, Taiwan

Yang Zhao
Department of Chinese Pharmaceutical Sciences and Chinese Medicine Resources, College of Biopharmaceutical and Food Sciences, China Medical University, Taichung 40402, Taiwan
Key Laboratory for Information System of Mountainous Areas and Protection of Ecological Environment, Guizhou Normal University, Guiyang 550001, China

Yuan-Shiun Chang
Department of Chinese Pharmaceutical Sciences and Chinese Medicine Resources, College of Biopharmaceutical and Food Sciences, China Medical University, Taichung 40402, Taiwan
Chinese Crude Drug Pharmacy, China Medical University Hospital, Taichung 40402, Taiwan

Xin Zhou
Key Laboratory for Information System of Mountainous Areas and Protection of Ecological Environment, Guizhou Normal University, Guiyang 550001, China

Chun-Pin Kao
Department of Nursing, Hsin Sheng College of Medical Care and Management, Taoyuan 32544, Taiwan

Yu-Ling Ho
Department of Nursing, Hungkuang University, Taichung 43302, Taiwan

Yiqun Li, Huiting Cao, Mengzhu Liu, Benyong Zhang, Liwei Guo, Jinao Duan, Xueping Zhou and Huaxu Zhu
Jiangsu Collaborative Innovation Center of Chinese Medicinal Resources Industrialization, Nanjing University of Chinese Medicine, Nanjing 210023, China

Qichun Zhang
Jiangsu Collaborative Innovation Center of Chinese Medicinal Resources Industrialization, Nanjing University of Chinese Medicine, Nanjing 210023, China
Department of Pharmacology, School of Pharmacy, Nanjing University of Chinese Medicine, Nanjing 210023, China

Xinlong Zhang and Donglei Shi
Jiangsu Key Laboratory for High Technology Research of TCM Formulae, Nanjing University of Chinese Medicine, Nanjing 210023, China

Huai Y. Wang
HKUST Shenzhen Research Institute, Hi-Tech Park, Nanshan, Shenzhen 518000, China

Amy G. W. Gong, Tina T. X. Dong and Karl W. K. Tsim
HKUST Shenzhen Research Institute, Hi-Tech Park, Nanshan, Shenzhen 518000, China
Division of Life Science and Center for Chinese Medicine, The Hong Kong University of Science and Technology, Clear Water Bay, Hong Kong, China

Y. Z. Zheng
Department of Biology, Hanshan Normal University, Chaozhou 521041, Guangdong, China

Xiaofeng Xu and Xuanyi Chen
Department of Gynecology, Suzhou Hospital Affiliated to Nanjing University of Chinese Medicine, No. 18 Yangsu Road, Gusu District, Suzhou 215009, Jiangsu Province, China

Yong Tan
Department of Gynecology, The No.1 Clinical Medical College, Nanjing University of Chinese Medicine, No. 138 Xianlin Avenue, Xianlin University City, Nanjing 210046, Jiangsu Province, China

Guorong Jiang, Lurong Zhang and Guoqiang Liang
Institute of Traditional Chinese Medicine, Suzhou Hospital Affiliated to Nanjing University of Chinese Medicine, No. 18 Yangsu Road, Gusu District, Suzhou 215009, Jiangsu Province, China

Rensheng Lai
Department of Pathology, Jiangsu Hospital of Traditional Chinese Medicine, No.155 Hanzhong Road, Qinhuai District, Nanjing 210002, Jiangsu Province, China

Chiyeon Lim
College of Medicine, Dongguk University, Ilsandong-gu, Gyeonggi-Do 10326, Republic of Korea

Sehyun Lim
School of Public Health, Far East University, Chungbuk 27601, Republic of Korea

Byoungho Lee
Kyunghee Naseul Korean Medicine Clinic, Bucheon-si, Gyeonggi-do 14548, Republic of Korea

Buyeo Kim
Department of Medical Research, Korea Institute of Oriental Medicine, Daejeon 34054, Republic of Korea

Suin Cho
School of Korean Medicine, Yangsan Campus of Pusan National University, Yangsan-si 50612, Republic of Korea

Kai Tong, Xu Sun, Shen Yan, Mei-jie Jiang, Meng-sheng Deng and Ji Chen
College of Agronomy, Sichuan Agricultural University, Chengdu 611130, People's Republic of China

Meng-liang Tian
College of Agronomy, Sichuan Agricultural University, Chengdu 611130, People's Republic of China
Institute for New Rural Development, Sichuan Agricultural University, 608 Room, No. 1 building, 211 Huiming Road, Wenjiang District, Chengdu City 611130, Sichuan Province, People's Republic of China

Zhao-ling Li
Maize Institute, Sichuan Agricultural University, Chengdu 611130, People's Republic of China

Jing-wei Li
Institute for New Rural Development, Sichuan Agricultural University, 608 Room, No. 1 building, 211 Huiming Road, Wenjiang District, Chengdu City 611130, Sichuan Province, People's Republic of China

Yu-Jie Cao, Zong-Jin Pu, Juan Shen, An Kang, Gui-Sheng Zhou and Jin-Ao Duan
Jiangsu Collaborative Innovation Center of Chinese Medicinal Resources Industrialization, and Jiangsu Key Laboratory for High Technology Research of TCM Formulae, and National and Local Collaborative Engineering Center of Chinese Medicinal Resources Industrialization and Formulae Innovative

Yu-Ping Tang
Jiangsu Collaborative Innovation Center of Chinese Medicinal Resources Industrialization, and Jiangsu Key Laboratory for High Technology Research of TCM Formulae, and National and Local Collaborative Engineering Center of Chinese Medicinal Resources Industrialization and Formulae InnovativeMedicine, Nanjing University of Chinese Medicine, Nanjing 210023, Jiangsu, China
College of Pharmacy and Shaanxi Collaborative Innovation Center of Chinese Medicinal Resources Industrialization, Shaanxi University of Chinese Medicine, Xianyang 712046, China

Yan-Yan Chen
College of Pharmacy and Shaanxi Collaborative Innovation Center of Chinese Medicinal Resources Industrialization, Shaanxi University of Chinese Medicine, Xianyang 712046, China

Xu Wu and Mingxing Li
Laboratory of Molecular Pharmacology, Department of Pharmacology, School of Pharmacy, Southwest Medical University, Luzhou, Sichuan, China

Shengpeng Wang and Jiliang Cao
State Key Laboratory of Quality Research in Chinese Medicine, Institute of Chinese Medical Sciences, University of Macau, Macao, China

Yong Jing and Changjiang Hu
College of Pharmacy, Chengdu University of Traditional Chinese Medicine, Liutai Avenue, Wenjiang District, Chengdu, Sichuan, China

Junrong Lu
College of Pharmacy, Chengdu University of Traditional Chinese Medicine, Liutai Avenue, Wenjiang District, Chengdu, Sichuan, China
West China School of Pharmacy, Sichuan University, Chengdu, Sichuan, China

Baolin Bian
Institute of Chinese Materia Medica, China Academy of Chinese Medical Sciences, Beijing, China

Chang-Ming Liu, Jing Chen, Su Yang, Zhong-Liang Chen, Hui-Hui Tu, Lian-Gen Mao and Zhong-Jie Li
Institute of Cell Biology, Zhejiang University, Hangzhou, People's Republic of China

Ji-Cheng Li
Institute of Cell Biology, Zhejiang University, Hangzhou, People's Republic of China
South China University of Technology School of Medicine, Guangzhou, People's Republic of China

Ting-Ting Jiang, Yu-Ting Hu and Lin Gan
South China University of Technology School of Medicine, Guangzhou, People's Republic of China

Index

S
Salvia Miltiorrhiza, 30, 33, 35, 37-38, 98-99, 171
Salviae Miltiorrhizae Radix, 171-172, 176, 178-179
Scutellariae Barbatae Herba, 110, 114
Silymarin, 9, 17
Sterigmatocystin, 1, 4, 7-8

T
Tripterygium Wilfordii, 139, 149-150, 166, 170
Triptolide, 139-145, 149
Tyrosinase, 213

U
Uterine Weight, 100-101, 103, 106

V
Vascular Endothelial Growth Factor, 112, 120-121, 123, 160, 162, 169-170

Y
Yanshu Injection, 117, 122
Yin-Deficiency-Heat Syndrome, 215

Z
Zhibai Dihuang Granule, 215-216, 226

www.ingramcontent.com/pod-product-compliance
Lightning Source LLC
Chambersburg PA
CBHW061252190326
41458CB00011B/3651